# Master Tung and TCM Acupuncture

## POINTS AND TREATMENTS

**Acupuncture Study
and Clinical Handbook**

Master Visuddhi Lee

BSc (Eng), BHMS, DHMS, D.Ac., F.F. Hom, PG (NAHI)

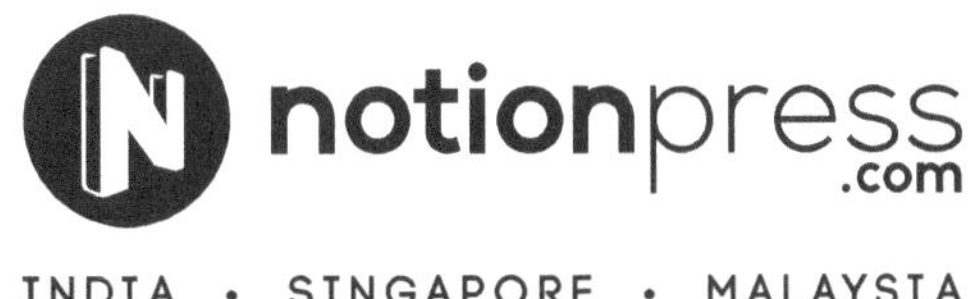

INDIA · SINGAPORE · MALAYSIA

ISBN
Paperback  979-8-89632-476-8
Hardcase  979-8-89699-987-4

# DEDICATION

To all the practitioners and seekers of healing, who strive to understand and harness the ancient wisdom of acupuncture, this book is dedicated to you. May it inspire and guide you on your journey as you explore the profound art of acupuncture.

I would like to thank my parents, who have since passed on, for instilling in me a deep respect for education and hard work. Their legacy lives on in this book.

I owe a debt of gratitude to my teachers, fellow practitioners and associates, whose guidance and mentorship have shaped me into the practitioner I am today. Without their wisdom and knowledge, this book would not have been possible.

To my students, who have challenged me to be a better teacher and healer, I am forever indebted. Your enthusiasm and dedication have inspired me to continue to pursue excellence in my work.

Last but not least, I would like to thank my patients who have entrusted me with their health and wellbeing. Your trust and support have given me the privilege of witnessing first-hand the transformative power of acupuncture.

May all be well and happy always.

Lee Chewee Hoe
Port Dickson, Malaysia
2025

# <u>CONTENTS</u>

# <u>INTRODUCTION</u>

Acupuncture is a remarkable healing art that utilizes the power of a single needle.

Acupuncture is a practice that encompasses many different schools of methodology, each utilizing the insertion of fine needles at specific points on the body. Whether it is Korean Hand Acupuncture, Scalp Acupuncture, Auricular Acupuncture, Master Tung Style Acupuncture or TCM Channel Acupuncture, the use of needles is a common thread among all schools.

While each acupuncturist may have their own preferred school, there is no inherently superior system. The patient's body is not aware of the specific system being used and will respond to the stimulus regardless. Ultimately, these different systems are merely frameworks that attempt to explain the underlying mechanisms of acupuncture.

In the heart of acupuncture, every needle insertion produces a minute injury at the site, which typically causes minimal discomfort. However, this slight stimulus to the nervous system is enough to trigger a response from the body, which involves the activation of the immune system, promotion of local blood circulation, wound healing, and modulation of pain. This basic truth transcends any particular school or system and is the key to the therapeutic benefits of acupuncture.

Master Tung Style Acupuncture is a unique style of acupuncture with its own set of points. However, its principles are still grounded in Classical Chinese Medicine.

With the increasing number of acupuncturists learning the Master Tung Acupuncture System, there is a growing need for a clinical companion that integrates the Master Tung System with the Traditional Chinese Medicine (TCM) 14 Channel System into a cohesive medical treatment plan.

In this book, we explore the synergies and unique qualities of these two systems. We aim to provide practitioners and students of acupuncture with a comprehensive resource that combines the strengths of both the Master Tung style and Traditional Chinese Medicine. Through detailed point descriptions, indications, and treatment plans, we hope to enrich your understanding and application of acupuncture.

# MASTER TUNG POINTS/ZONES DISTRIBUTION

Master Tung divided his points into 10 areas plus the dorsal trunk (DT) and ventral trunk (VT). Many of Master Tung points overlap traditional 14 channels acupuncture points and have expanded indications.

There is a numbering convention which helps to locate the area in which the point is. The sequence is related to the order in which the points were presented in Tung's original 1973 book, "Tung's Regular Meridian and Points".

Zone 1 is the fingers, zone 2 is the dorsum and palm of the hands, zone 3 is the forearms, and so on.

Traditionally, when the points numbers are setup, the zone number is "doubled". This means that zone 1 becomes 11 (one-one), zone 2 becomes 22 (two-two) and so on till zone 1010 (ten-ten). Point 22.05 is therefore the fifth point on Zone 22, on the hand. 88.03 **is** the third point on Zone 88, on the thigh.

*Credit to Alex Costa for the pics below.*

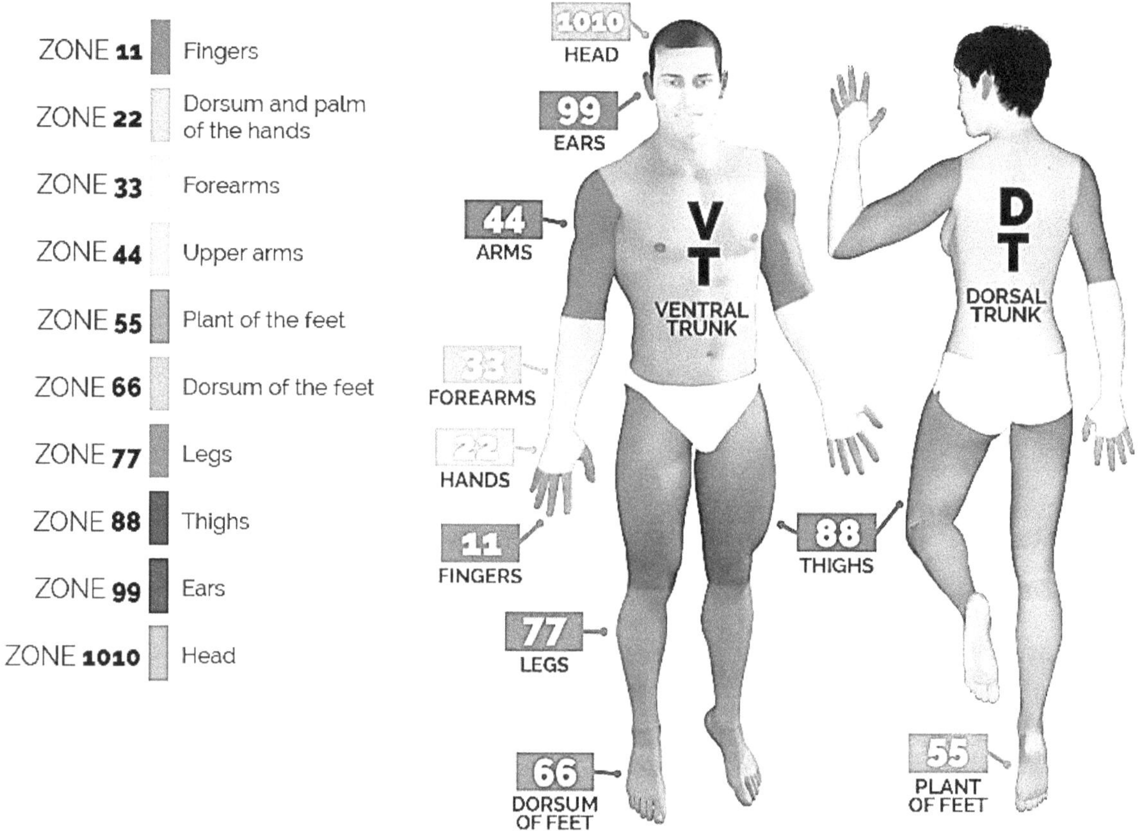

# Zone 11 – Finger (Points Location)

To help locate points on Zone 11, every finger has been drawn imaginary grid lines A-H.

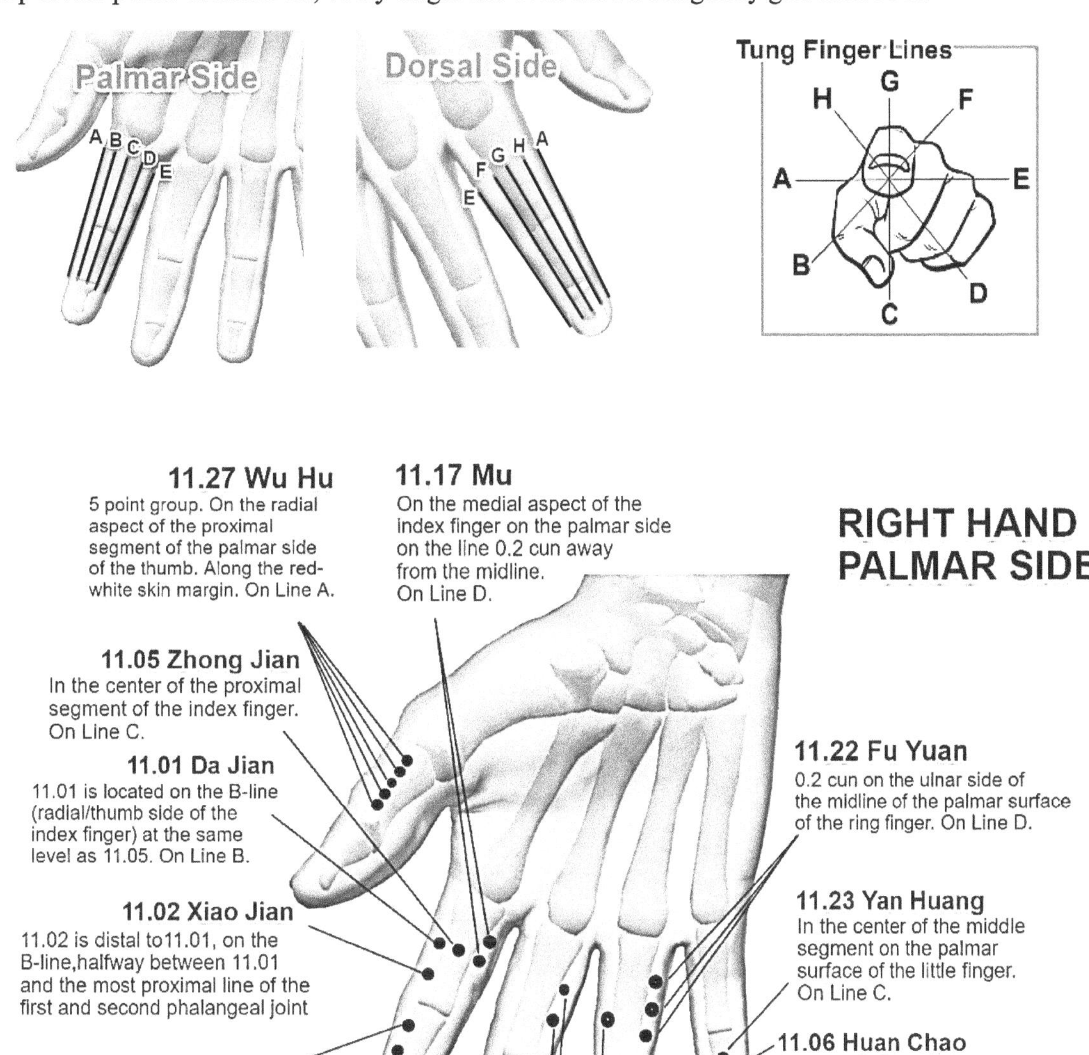



### 11.27 Wu Hu
5 point group. On the radial aspect of the proximal segment of the palmar side of the thumb. Along the red-white skin margin. On Line A.

### 11.05 Zhong Jian
In the center of the proximal segment of the index finger. On Line C.

### 11.01 Da Jian
11.01 is located on the B-line (radial/thumb side of the index finger) at the same level as 11.05. On Line B.

### 11.02 Xiao Jian
11.02 is distal to 11.01, on the B-line, halfway between 11.01 and the most proximal line of the first and second phalangeal joint

### 11.04 Wai Jian
On the second phalange, on the B-line, evenly spaced between the proximal creases of the first and second phalanx.

### 11.03 Fu Jian
On the second phalange, on the B-line, evenly spaced between the proximal creases of the first and second phalanx

### 11.18 Pi Zong
On the midline of the middle segment of the palmar middle finger on the palmar aspect. On Line C

### 11.17 Mu
On the medial aspect of the index finger on the palmar side on the line 0.2 cun away from the midline. On Line D.

### 11.21 San Yan
0.2 cun to the radial aspect of the midline of the palmar aspect of the ring finger, 0.2 cun from the second crease of the middle finger. On Line B

### 11.19 Xin Chang
0.2 cun on the ulnar side of the midline of the proximal segment on the palmar aspect of the middle finger. On Line D

**RIGHT HAND PALMAR SIDE**

### 11.22 Fu Yuan
0.2 cun on the ulnar side of the midline of the palmar surface of the ring finger. On Line D.

### 11.23 Yan Huang
In the center of the middle segment on the palmar surface of the little finger. On Line C.

### 11.06 Huan Chao
On the ulnar and palmar side of the middle segment of the ring finger, in the center between the second and third finger crease. On Line E.

### 11.20 Mu Yan
0.2 cun on the ulnar side of the midline of the middle segment on the palmar aspect of the ring finger. On Line D.

## 11.15 Zhi Shen

On the ulnar aspect of
the proximal segment
of the dorsal side of
the ring finger. On Line F.

## 11.08 Zhi Wu Jin

2 point group; evenly distributed
on the medial line of the dorsal
proximal phalanx of the index finger
along the ulnar margin of the
phalangeal bone; on the
Large Intestine channel.On Line F.

## RIGHT HAND DORSAL SIDE

## 11.14 Zhǐ Sān Zhòng

3 point group. On the
ulnar and dorsal aspect
of the proximal segment
of the ring finger.
On Line F.

## 11.13 Dan

2 point group. In the center
of the proximal segment of
the middle finger on the
dorsal side. On Line F and H.

## 11.16 Huo Xi

0.2 cun lateral to the
nail root notch of the
dorsal side of the little
finger.  Overlaps SI-1.
On Line F

## 11.07 Zhi Si Ma

3 point group; evenly distributed
on the dorsal middle phalanx of
the index finger along the ulnar
margin of the phalangeal bone;
on the Large Intestine channel.
On Line F

## 11.09 Xin Xi

2 point group. On both sides of the
middle segment of the middle finger
on the dorsal side, in the center
between the second and third
finger creases. On Line F and H.

## 11.12 Er Jiao Ming

2 point group. On the midline
of proximal segment of the
middle finger on the dorsal
side. On Line G.

## 11.11 Fei Xin

2 Point group.
On the middle segment
of the dorsal aspect
of the middle finger.
On Line G

## 11.10 Mu Huo

At the center of the distal
interphalangeal joint on the
dorsal aspect of the middle finger;
on the Pericardium channel.
On Line G

RIGHT HAND - DORSAL SIDE

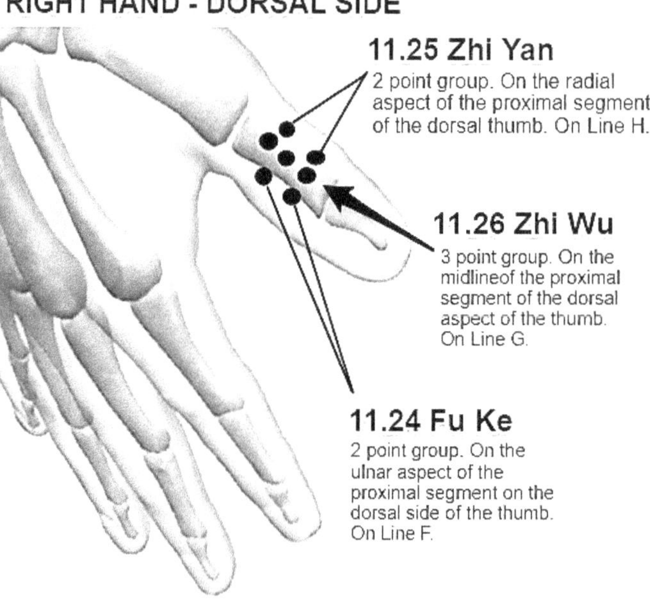

## 11.25 Zhi Yan

2 point group. On the radial
aspect of the proximal segment
of the dorsal thumb. On Line H.

## 11.26 Zhi Wu

3 point group. On the
midlineof the proximal
segment of the dorsal
aspect of the thumb.
On Line G.

## 11.24 Fu Ke

2 point group. On the
ulnar aspect of the
proximal segment on the
dorsal side of the thumb.
On Line F.

# Zone 22 – Hand (Points Location)

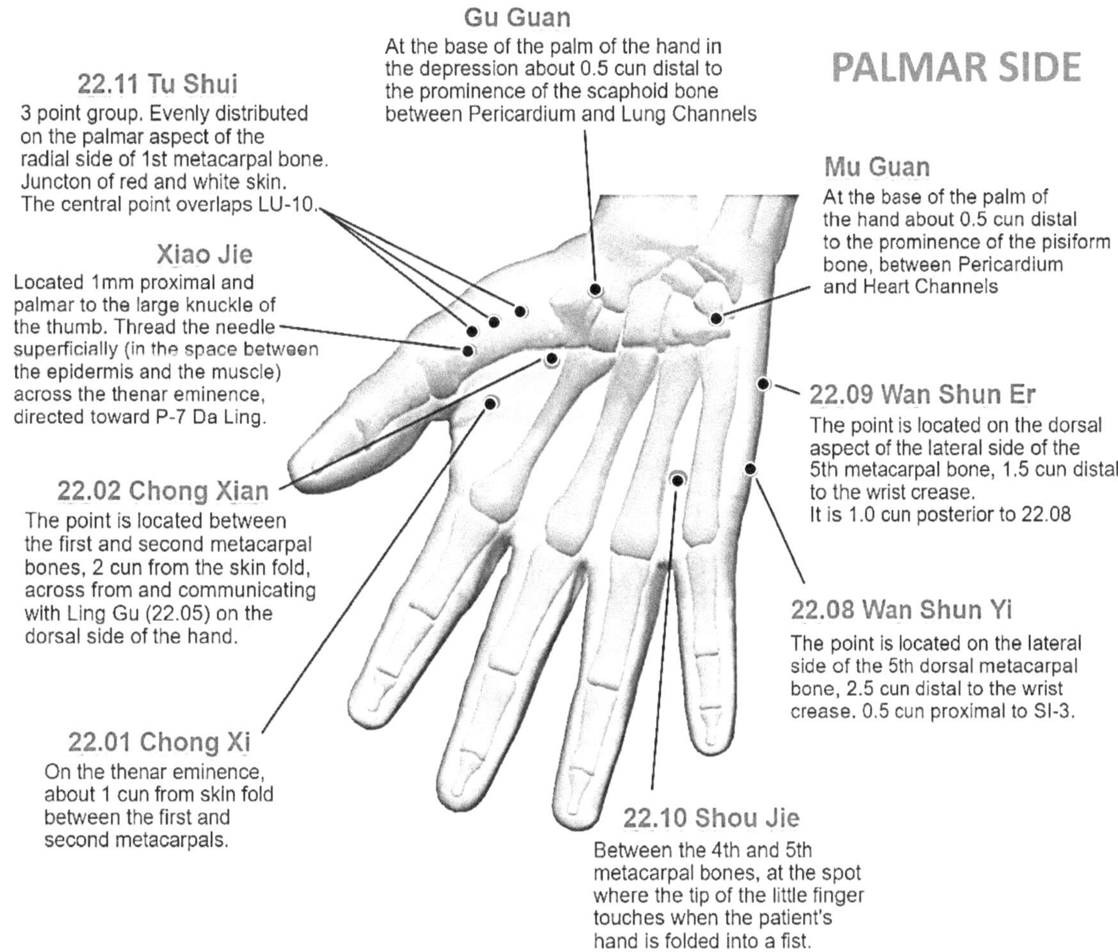

**Gu Guan**
At the base of the palm of the hand in the depression about 0.5 cun distal to the prominence of the scaphoid bone between Pericardium and Lung Channels

**PALMAR SIDE**

### 22.11 Tu Shui
3 point group. Evenly distributed on the palmar aspect of the radial side of 1st metacarpal bone. Juncton of red and white skin. The central point overlaps LU-10.

### Xiao Jie
Located 1mm proximal and palmar to the large knuckle of the thumb. Thread the needle superficially (in the space between the epidermis and the muscle) across the thenar eminence, directed toward P-7 Da Ling.

### 22.02 Chong Xian
The point is located between the first and second metacarpal bones, 2 cun from the skin fold, across from and communicating with Ling Gu (22.05) on the dorsal side of the hand.

### 22.01 Chong Xi
On the thenar eminence, about 1 cun from skin fold between the first and second metacarpals.

**Mu Guan**
At the base of the palm of the hand about 0.5 cun distal to the prominence of the pisiform bone, between Pericardium and Heart Channels

### 22.09 Wan Shun Er
The point is located on the dorsal aspect of the lateral side of the 5th metacarpal bone, 1.5 cun distal to the wrist crease. It is 1.0 cun posterior to 22.08

### 22.08 Wan Shun Yi
The point is located on the lateral side of the 5th dorsal metacarpal bone, 2.5 cun distal to the wrist crease. 0.5 cun proximal to SI-3.

### 22.10 Shou Jie
Between the 4th and 5th metacarpal bones, at the spot where the tip of the little finger touches when the patient's hand is folded into a fist. Overlaps HT-8.

## DORSAL SIDE

### 22.05 Ling Gu

The point is located in the juncture between the index finger and thumb, the 1st and 2nd dorsal metacarpal bones, 1.2 cun from 22.04, and directly opposite 22.02 .

### 22.07 Xia Bai

The point is located between the dorsal 4th and 5th metacarpal bones, 1.5 cun proximal to the metacarpophalangeal joint, 1.0 cun posterior to 22.06. Overlaps N-UE-19 Yao Tong Xue.

### Fan Hou Jie

On the dorsal aspect of the hand, 1 cun distal to 22.05 at the ulnar margin of the first metacarpal bone

### 22.04 Da Bai

On the dorsum of the hand, the point is located in the depression 0.5 cun from the joint of the index finger and thumb, or between the first and second metacarpal bones. Over laps LI-3.

### 22.06 Zhong Bai

The point is located between the dorsal metacarpal bones of the little and ring fingers, 0.5 cun proximal to the metacarpophalangeal joint. Overlaps SJ-3.

### 22.03 Shang Bai

0.5 cun proximal to the dorsal metacarpophalangeal joint of the index and middle fingers.

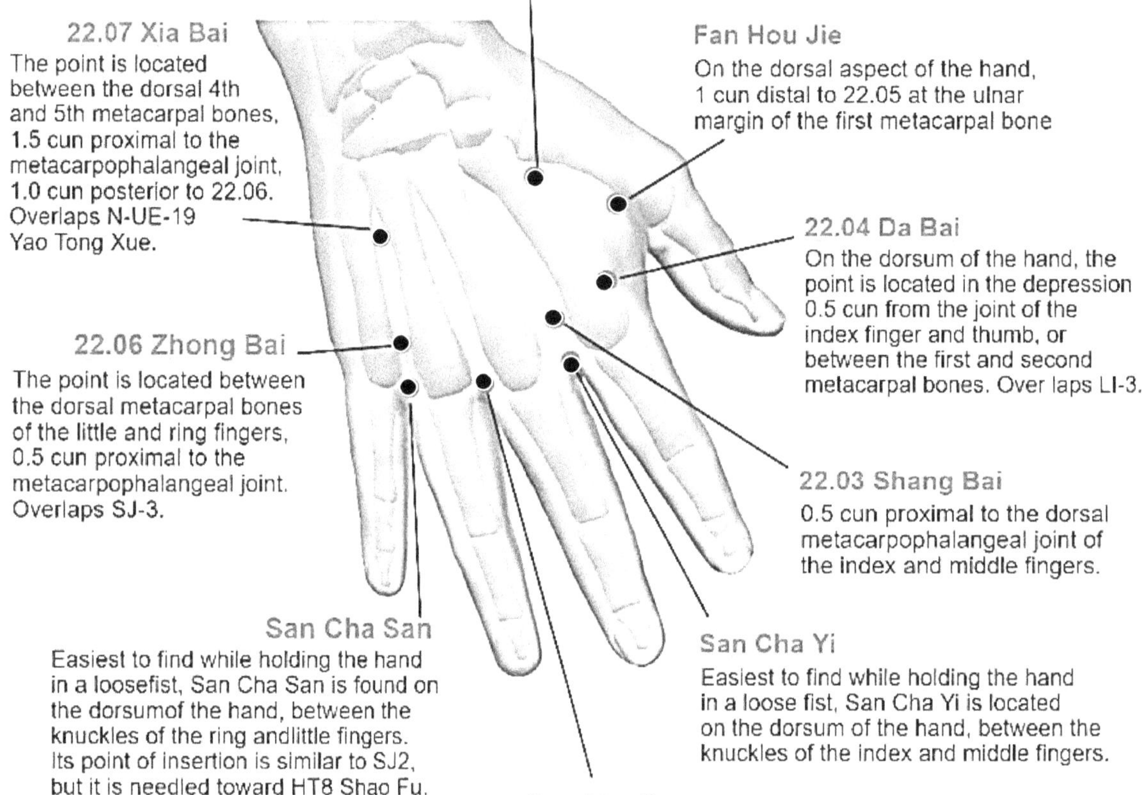

### San Cha San

Easiest to find while holding the hand in a loosefist, San Cha San is found on the dorsumof the hand, between the knuckles of the ring andlittle fingers. Its point of insertion is similar to SJ2, but it is needled toward HT8 Shao Fu.

### San Cha Yi

Easiest to find while holding the hand in a loose fist, San Cha Yi is located on the dorsum of the hand, between the knuckles of the index and middle fingers.

### San Cha Er

Easiest to find while holding the hand in a loosefist, San Cha Er is found on the dorsumof the hand, between the knuckles of the middle and ring fingers.

# Zone 33 – Forearm (Points Location)

### 33.09 Shou Qian Jin

On the lateral side of the ulna, 1.5 cun proximal to 33.08. Bet. San Jiao and Small Intestine channels.

### 33.08 Shou Wu Jin

On the lateral side of the ulna, 6.5 cun proximal to the lateral pisiform bone, 0.5 cun ulnar to 33.06.  Between San Jiao and Small Intestine channels.

### 33.06 Huo Shan

1.5 cun proximal to 33.05. On the San Jiao channel.

### 33.05 Huo Ling

2 cun proximal to 33.04. On the San Jiao channel.

### 33.04 Huo Ling

3 cun proximal to the wrist joint on the dorsal side, in the depression in the midline between the radius and ulna. Close to the border of the radius, radial side of muscle and tendon. Overlaps SJ-6. On the San Jiao channel.

### 33.07 Hua Fu Hai

2 cun proximal to Huo 33.06, on the prominence of the muscle. On the San Jiao channel. Near LI-10.

### 33.03 Qi Zheng

On the radial aspect of the forearm, halfway between LI5 and LI11, 6 cun from the wrist crease, and 2 cun posterior to 33.02. On the Large Intestine channel.

### 33.02 Qi Jiao

The point is located on the radial side of the forearm between LI5 and LI11,  4 cun proxima lto the wrist crease. On the Large Intestine channel.

### 33.01 Qi Men

The point is located on the radial side of the forearm on the line between LI5 and LI11, 2 cun proximal to the wrist crease. On the Large Intestine channel.

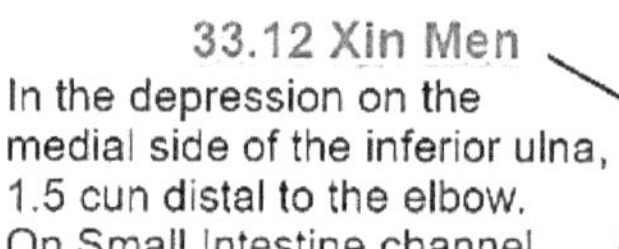

33.12 Xin Men
In the depression on the
medial side of the inferior ulna,
1.5 cun distal to the elbow.
On Small Intestine channel.

33.11 Gan Men
On the ulnar side, 6 cun
proximal to the pisiform bone.
On Small Intestine channel.

33.10 Chang Men
On the medial side of the
ulna, 3 cun proximal to
the pisiform bone.  On
Small Intestine channel.


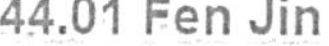

44.01 Fen Jin
On the anterior side of the humerus of the
upper arm, 1.5 cun proximal to the cubital
fossa crease (LU-5). On the Lung Channel.

33.16 Qu Ling
In the crease of the cubital fossa and on the
radial side of the tendon of m. biceps brachii.
Overlaps LU-5. On the Lung channel.

33.15 Tian Shi
On the medial aspect of the posterior radius,
3.0 cun proximal to 33.14. On the Lung
channel or Pericardium channel.

33.14 Di Shi
On the medial border of the radius
3.0 cun proximal to 33.13.  On the
Lung channelor Pericardium channel.

33.13 Ren Shi
On the medial side of the radius
of the ventral forearm, 4 cun
proximal to the wrist crease.
On the Lung channel
or Pericardium channel.

# Zone 44 – Upper Arm (Points Location)

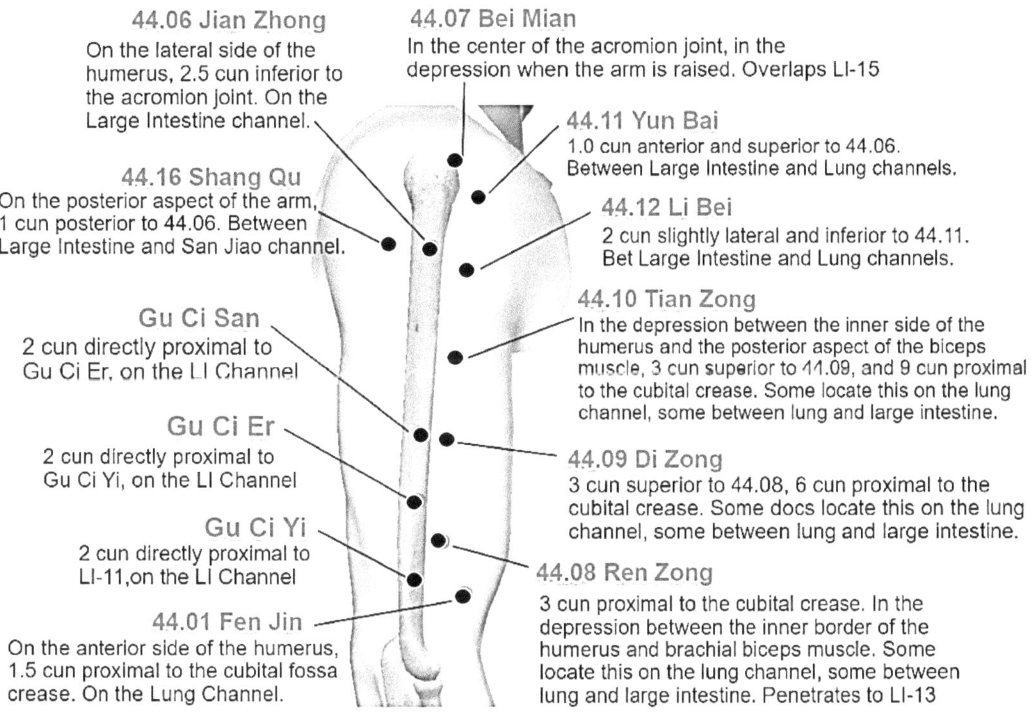

**44.06 Jian Zhong**
On the lateral side of the humerus, 2.5 cun inferior to the acromion joint. On the Large Intestine channel.

**44.16 Shang Qu**
On the posterior aspect of the arm, 1 cun posterior to 44.06. Between Large Intestine and San Jiao channel.

**Gu Ci San**
2 cun directly proximal to Gu Ci Er, on the LI Channel

**Gu Ci Er**
2 cun directly proximal to Gu Ci Yi, on the LI Channel

**Gu Ci Yi**
2 cun directly proximal to LI-11, on the LI Channel

**44.01 Fen Jin**
On the anterior side of the humerus, 1.5 cun proximal to the cubital fossa crease. On the Lung Channel.

**44.07 Bei Mian**
In the center of the acromion joint, in the depression when the arm is raised. Overlaps LI-15

**44.11 Yun Bai**
1.0 cun anterior and superior to 44.06. Between Large Intestine and Lung channels.

**44.12 Li Bei**
2 cun slightly lateral and inferior to 44.11. Bet Large Intestine and Lung channels.

**44.10 Tian Zong**
In the depression between the inner side of the humerus and the posterior aspect of the biceps muscle, 3 cun superior to 44.09, and 9 cun proximal to the cubital crease. Some locate this on the lung channel, some between lung and large intestine.

**44.09 Di Zong**
3 cun superior to 44.08, 6 cun proximal to the cubital crease. Some docs locate this on the lung channel, some between lung and large intestine.

**44.08 Ren Zong**
3 cun proximal to the cubital crease. In the depression between the inner border of the humerus and brachial biceps muscle. Some locate this on the lung channel, some between lung and large intestine. Penetrates to LI-13

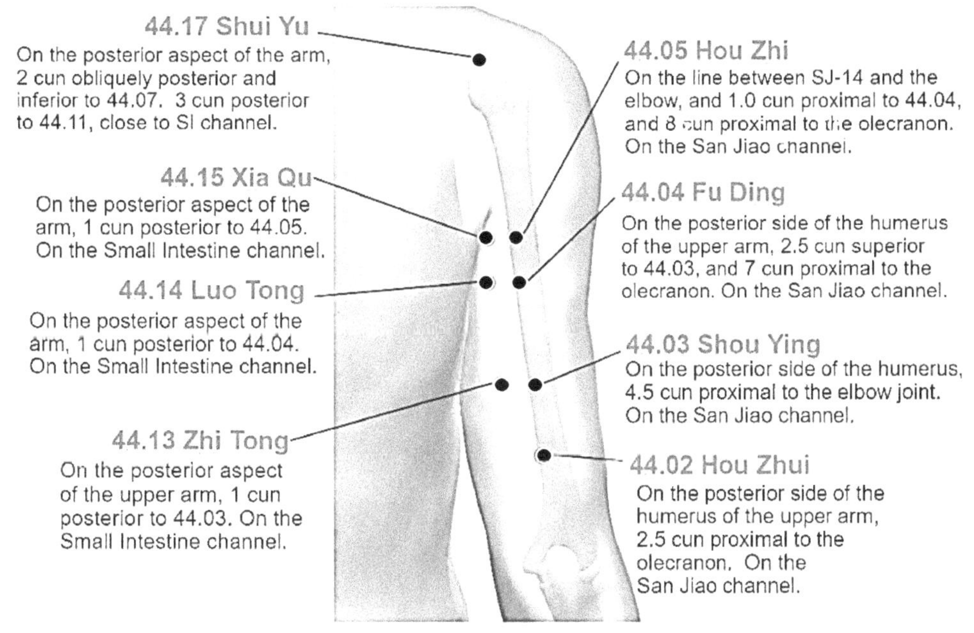

**44.17 Shui Yu**
On the posterior aspect of the arm, 2 cun obliquely posterior and inferior to 44.07. 3 cun posterior to 44.11, close to SI channel.

**44.15 Xia Qu**
On the posterior aspect of the arm, 1 cun posterior to 44.05. On the Small Intestine channel.

**44.14 Luo Tong**
On the posterior aspect of the arm, 1 cun posterior to 44.04. On the Small Intestine channel.

**44.13 Zhi Tong**
On the posterior aspect of the upper arm, 1 cun posterior to 44.03. On the Small Intestine channel.

**44.05 Hou Zhi**
On the line between SJ-14 and the elbow, and 1.0 cun proximal to 44.04, and 8 cun proximal to the olecranon. On the San Jiao channel.

**44.04 Fu Ding**
On the posterior side of the humerus of the upper arm, 2.5 cun superior to 44.03, and 7 cun proximal to the olecranon. On the San Jiao channel.

**44.03 Shou Ying**
On the posterior side of the humerus, 4.5 cun proximal to the elbow joint. On the San Jiao channel.

**44.02 Hou Zhui**
On the posterior side of the humerus of the upper arm, 2.5 cun proximal to the olecranon. On the San Jiao channel.

# Zone 55 – Plantar Surface of the Foot (Points Location)

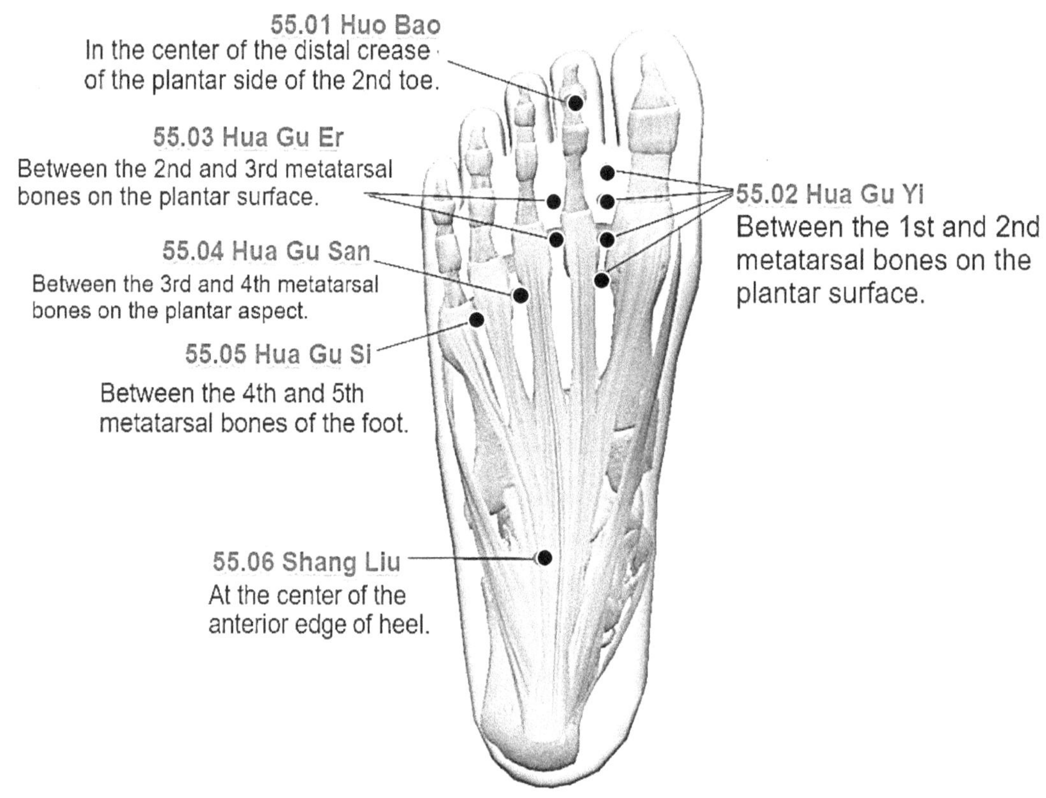

# Zone 66 – Dorsal Surface of the Foot (Points Location)

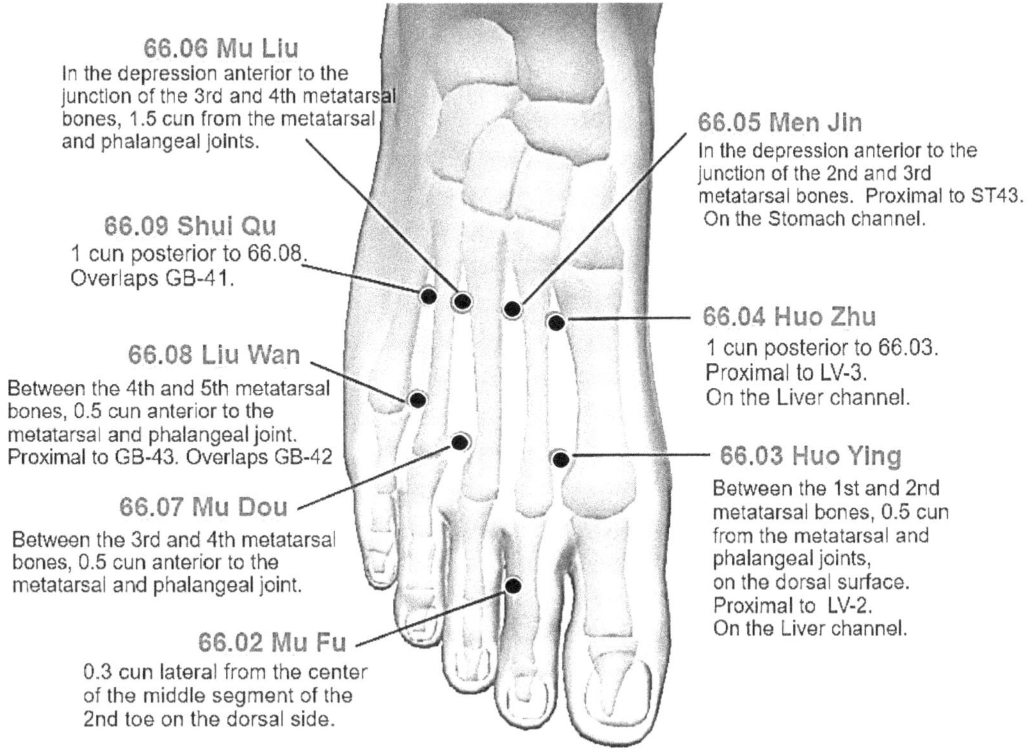



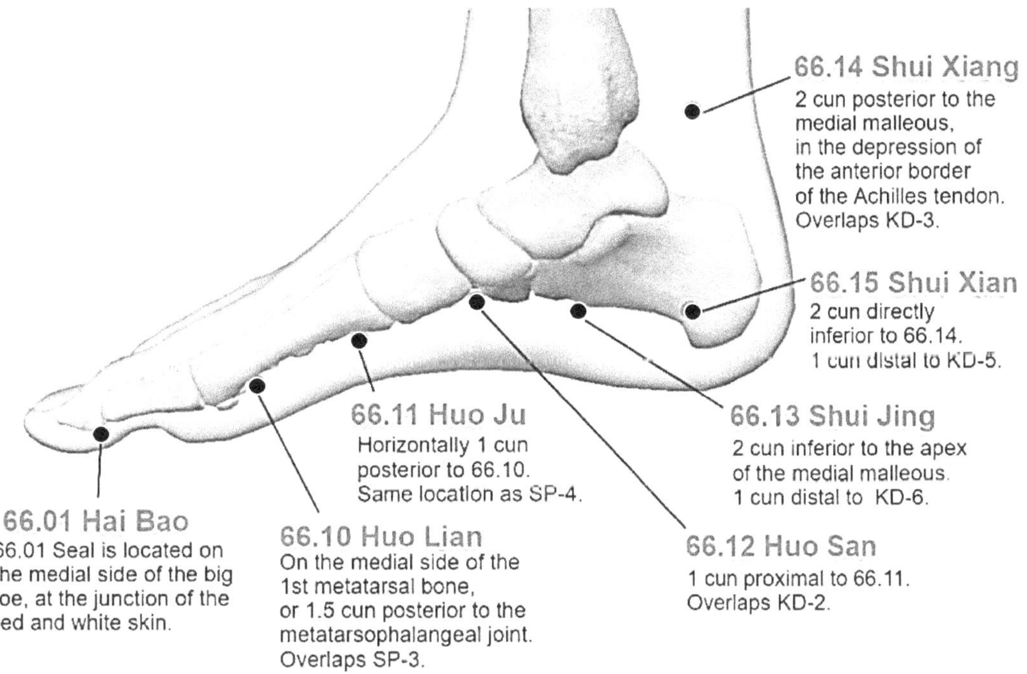

# Zone 77 – Lower Leg (Points Location)

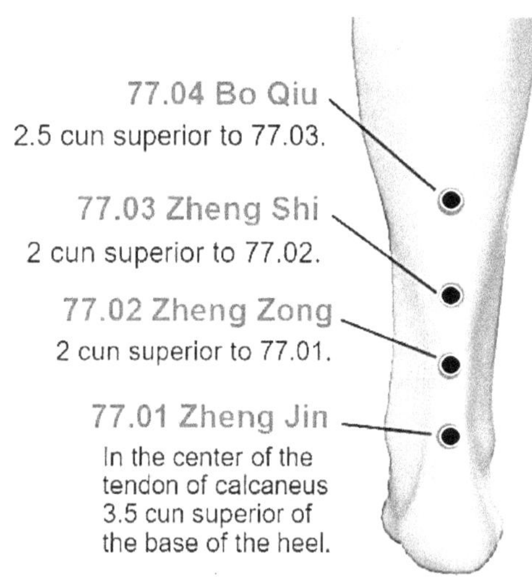



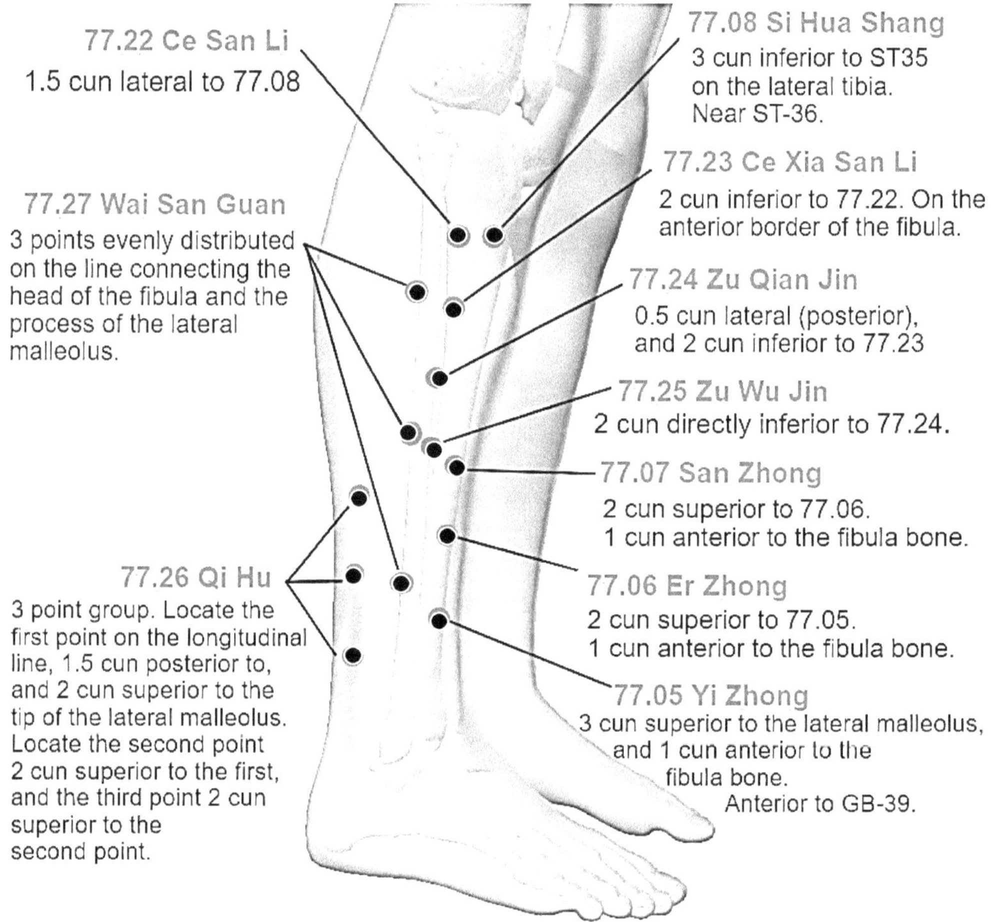

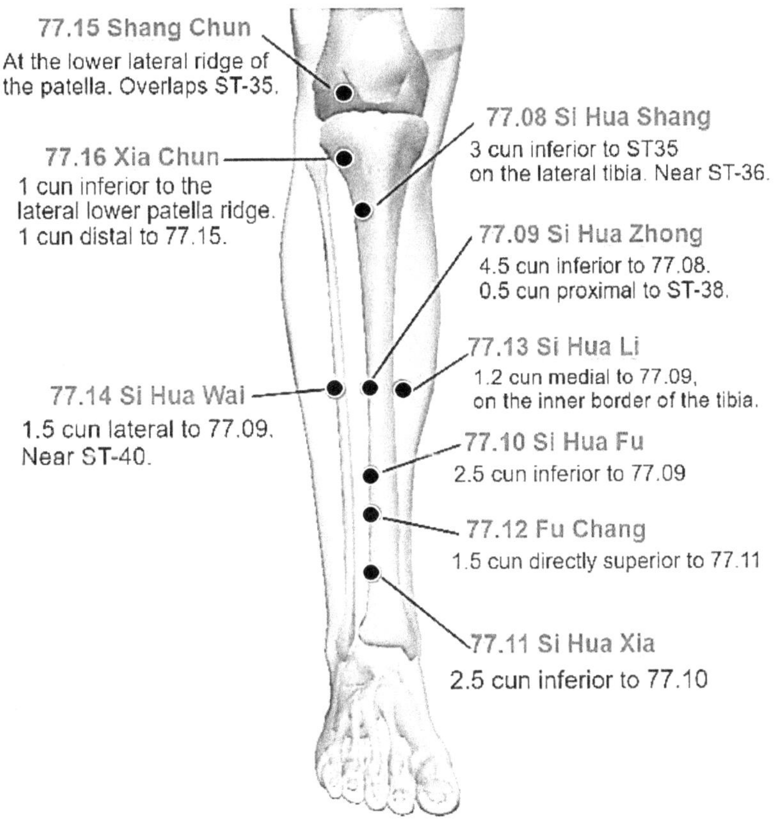


77.15 Shang Chun
At the lower lateral ridge of the patella. Overlaps ST-35.

77.16 Xia Chun
1 cun inferior to the lateral lower patella ridge. 1 cun distal to 77.15.

77.14 Si Hua Wai
1.5 cun lateral to 77.09. Near ST-40.

77.08 Si Hua Shang
3 cun inferior to ST35 on the lateral tibia. Near ST-36.

77.09 Si Hua Zhong
4.5 cun inferior to 77.08. 0.5 cun proximal to ST-38.

77.13 Si Hua Li
1.2 cun medial to 77.09, on the inner border of the tibia.

77.10 Si Hua Fu
2.5 cun inferior to 77.09

77.12 Fu Chang
1.5 cun directly superior to 77.11

77.11 Si Hua Xia
2.5 cun inferior to 77.10


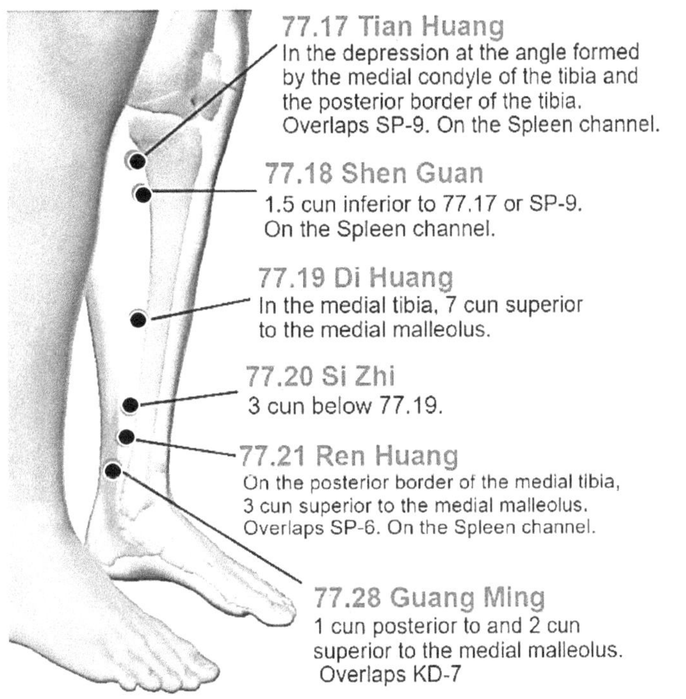


77.17 Tian Huang
In the depression at the angle formed by the medial condyle of the tibia and the posterior border of the tibia. Overlaps SP-9. On the Spleen channel.

77.18 Shen Guan
1.5 cun inferior to 77.17 or SP-9. On the Spleen channel.

77.19 Di Huang
In the medial tibia, 7 cun superior to the medial malleolus.

77.20 Si Zhi
3 cun below 77.19.

77.21 Ren Huang
On the posterior border of the medial tibia, 3 cun superior to the medial malleolus. Overlaps SP-6. On the Spleen channel.

77.28 Guang Ming
1 cun posterior to and 2 cun superior to the medial malleolus. Overlaps KD-7

# Zone 88 – Thigh (Points Location)

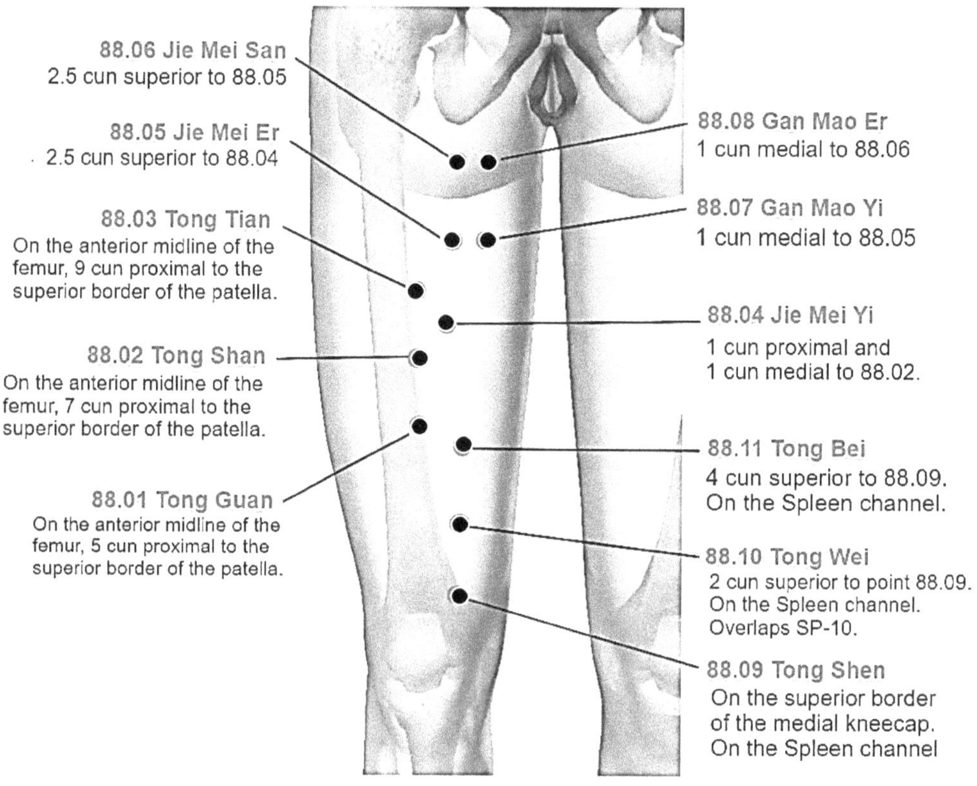


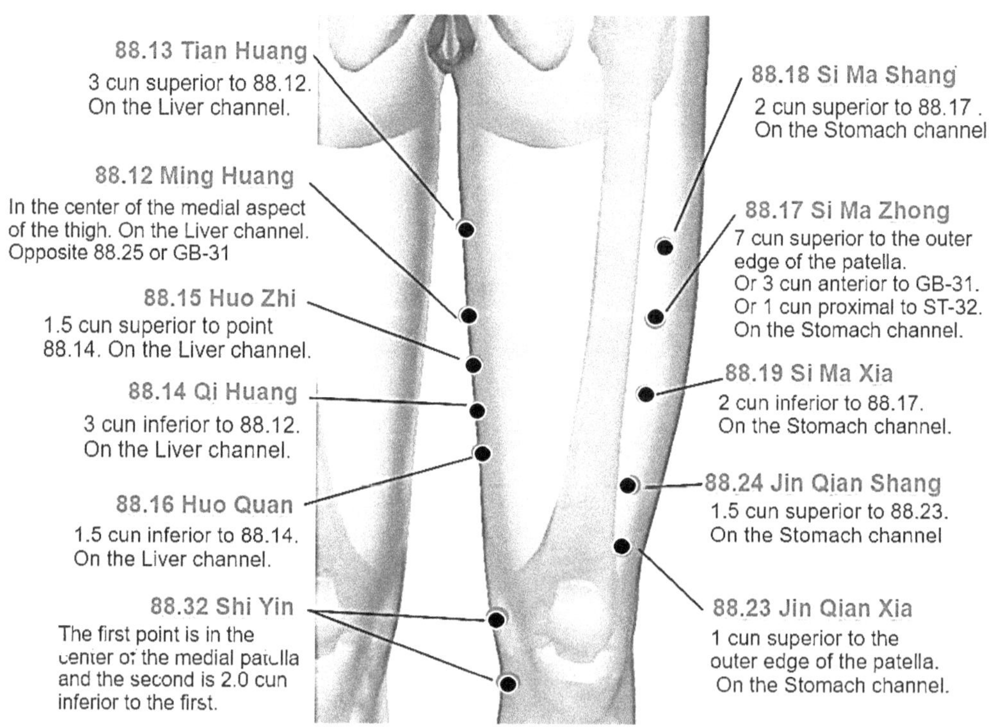

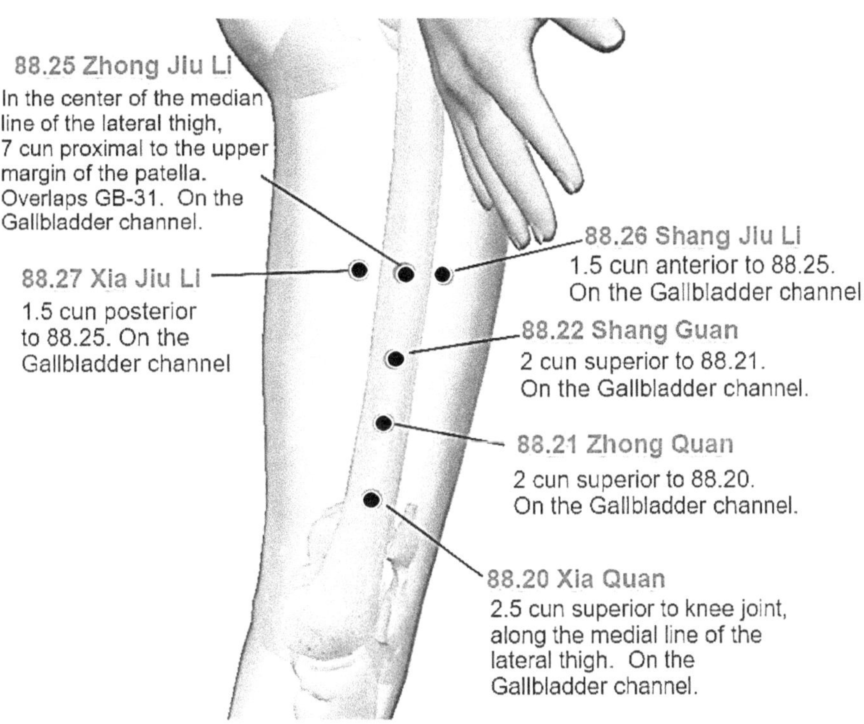
88.25 Zhong Jiu Li
In the center of the median line of the lateral thigh, 7 cun proximal to the upper margin of the patella. Overlaps GB-31. On the Gallbladder channel.
88.27 Xia Jiu Li
1.5 cun posterior to 88.25. On the Gallbladder channel
88.26 Shang Jiu Li
1.5 cun anterior to 88.25. On the Gallbladder channel.
88.22 Shang Guan
2 cun superior to 88.21. On the Gallbladder channel.
88.21 Zhong Quan
2 cun superior to 88.20. On the Gallbladder channel.
88.20 Xia Quan
2.5 cun superior to knee joint, along the medial line of the lateral thigh. On the Gallbladder channel.

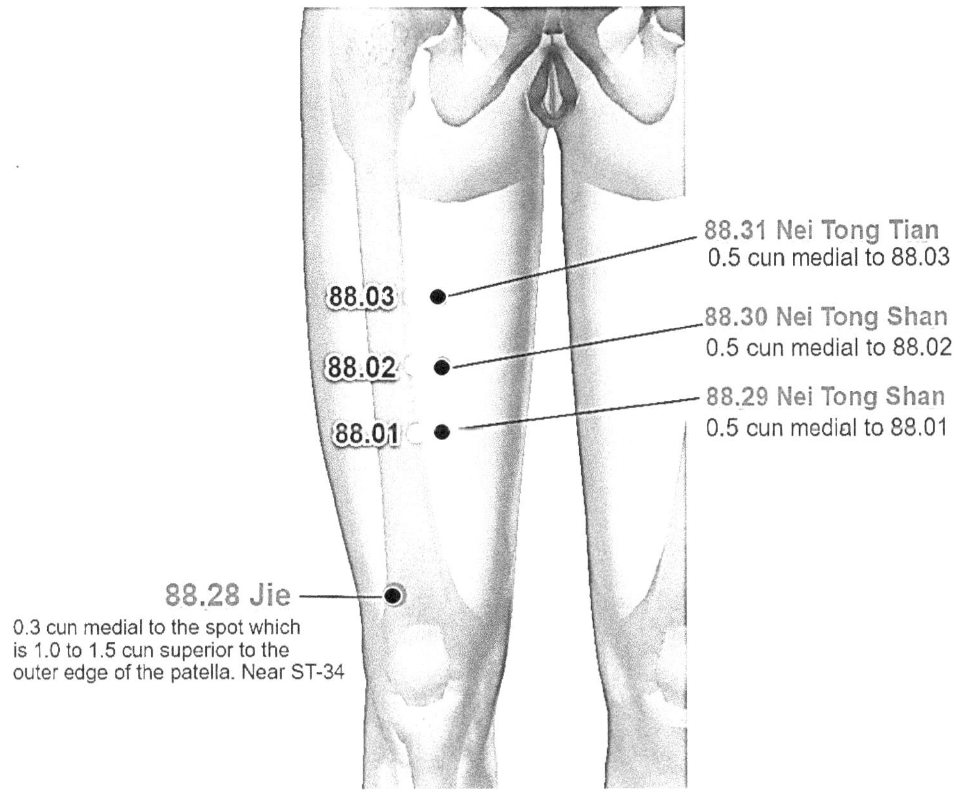
88.03
88.02
88.01
88.31 Nei Tong Tian
0.5 cun medial to 88.03
88.30 Nei Tong Shan
0.5 cun medial to 88.02
88.29 Nei Tong Shan
0.5 cun medial to 88.01
88.28 Jie
0.3 cun medial to the spot which is 1.0 to 1.5 cun superior to the outer edge of the patella. Near ST-34

# Zone 99 – Ear (Points Location)

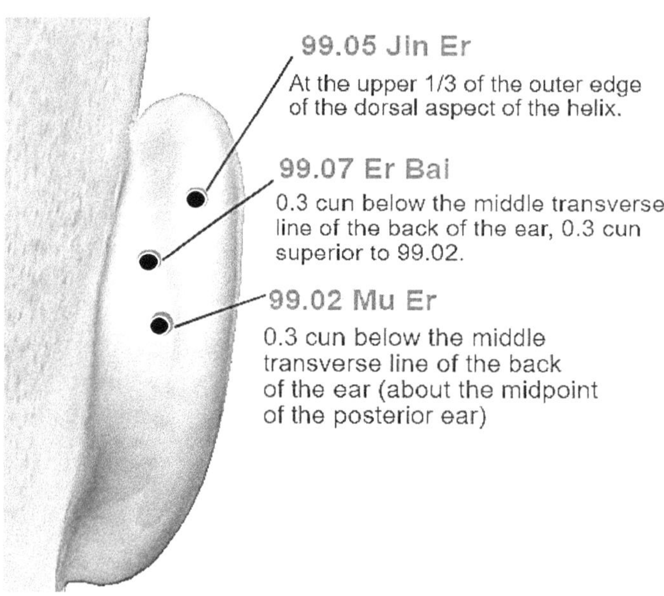



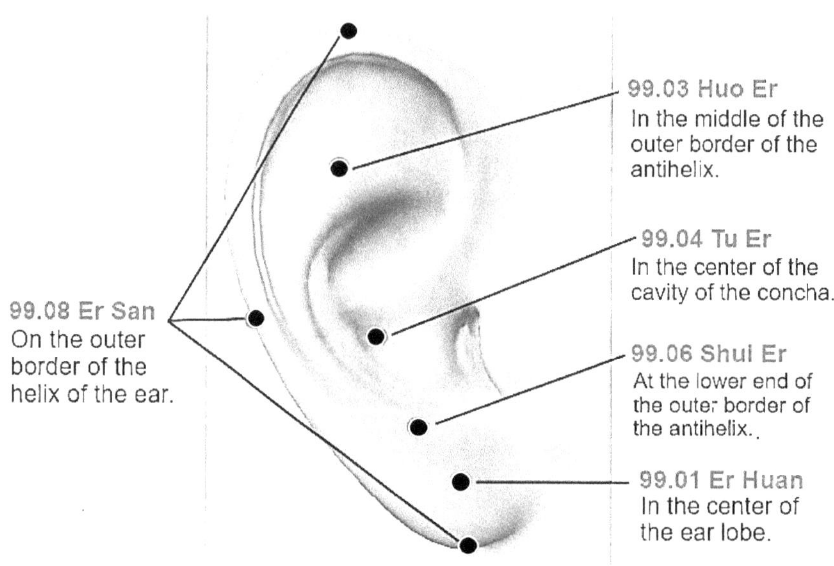

# Zone 1010 Head and Face (Points Location)

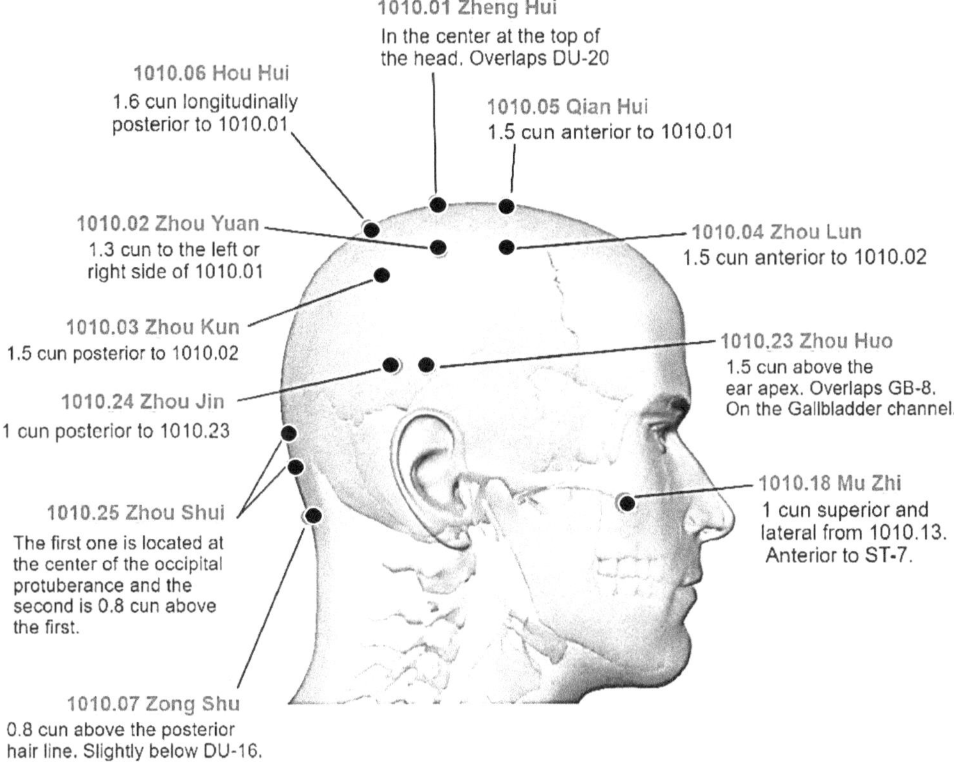


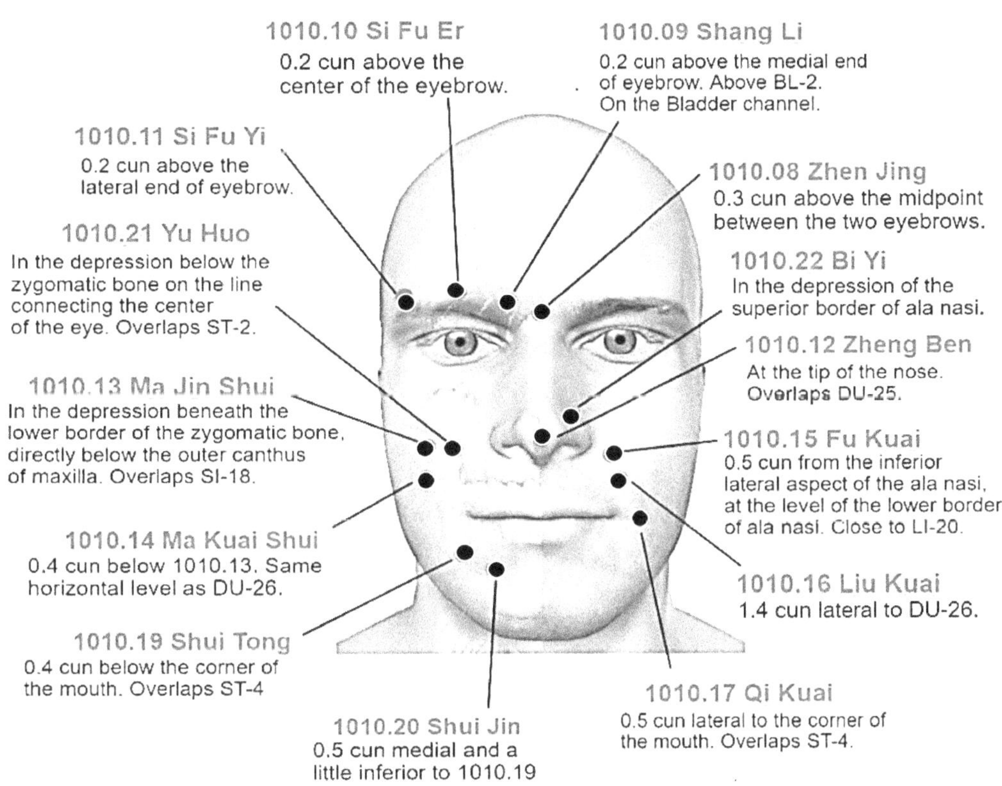

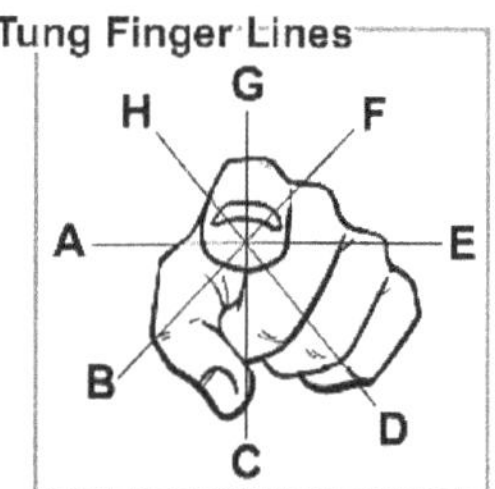

# POINTS OF THE MASTER TUNG ACUPUNCTURE SYSTEM

## ZONE 11-Finger

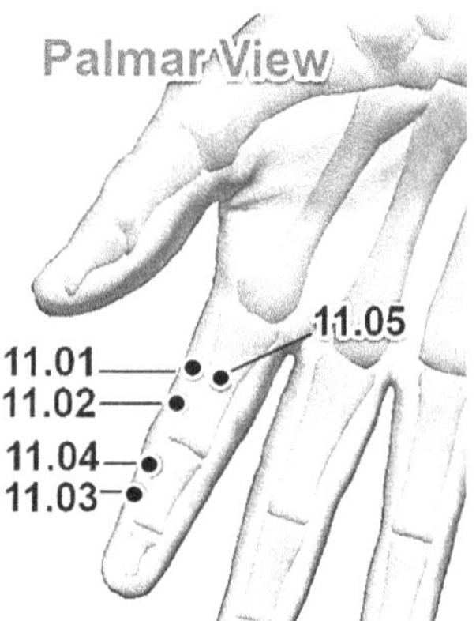

Tung Finger Lines

Palmar View

11.01
11.02
11.04
11.03
11.05

## 11.01 Dajian
### (BIG DISTANCE)

**Location:**
0.3 cun radial to the center of the proximal segment of the index finger. On Line B. (11.01 is located same level as 11.05)

**Associated Channel:** Large Intestine

**Reaction Areas:** Heart, Large Intestine, Small Intestine

**Dao Ma:** 11.01 +11.02 +11.03 +11.04+11.05 – Hernia Points

**Indications:**
- INTESTINAL OR INGUINAL HERNIA. NOT USED FOR HIATAL HERNIA. MOXA BULGING HERNIA TO ASSIST THE TREATMENT. ALSO BLEED VEINS AROUND THE MEDIAL MALLEOLUS. USE LIV-1 AS A GUIDING POINT.
- PAIN OF THE TESTIS
- URINARY TRACT INFECTION AND URETHRA PAIN (ADD 11.04)
- HEART DISEASE, PALPITATIONS, SHORTNESS OF BREATH

- ENTERITIS, INFLAMMATION OF INTESTINES ESP. IF ACCOMPANIED WITH DIARRHEA
- PAIN OF THE CORNER OF THE EYE, TMJ PAIN, TONSILLITIS, MUMPS
- FINGER NUMBNESS
- KNEE PAIN
- VERTIGO/DIZZINESS

**Manipulation/Depth of insertion:**
- For heart issues: 0.1 to 0.2 cun
- For Hernia: insert 0.2 to 0.3 cun
- For leg: 0.3-0.4 cun
- Needle adjacent to the edge of the bone
- From certain literature, needling 11.01 on both hands is contraindicated.
- Points are usually needled on the left for men and right side for women.
- If the symptoms are one sided, treat on opposite side.

**Remarks:**
- Most effective for hernia and enteritis.
- Point is effective if blue veins appear around this point or if the point is tender to palpation.

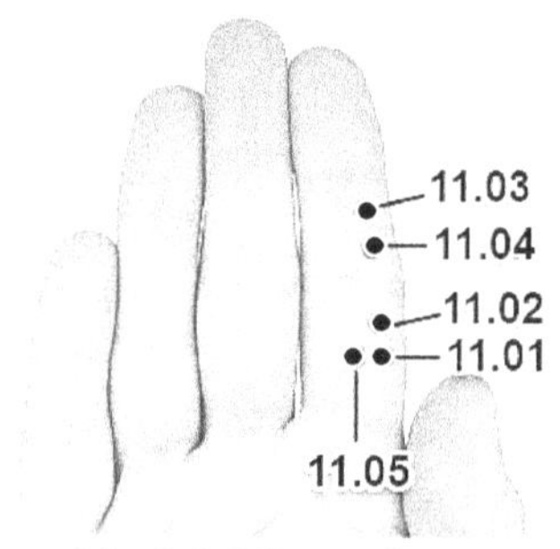

11.03
11.04
11.02
11.01
11.05

## 11.02 Xiao Jian
### (SMALL DISTANCE)

**Location:**
Upper part of the proximal segment of the index finger, 0.2 cun distal to 11.01. On Line B.

**Associated Channel:** Large Intestine

**Reaction Areas:** Lung, Heart, 6 Fu bowels*

**Indications:**
- INTESTINAL HERNIA (POINTS 11.01 TO 11.05, CHOOSE A FEW)
- BRONCHITIS, EXPECTORATION OF YELLOW SPUTUM, STUFFINESS IN THE CHEST
- IRREGULAR HEART BEAT
- KNEE PAIN
- PAIN OF THE CORNER OF THE EYE

- ENTERITIS
- LEUKORRHEA (RED AND WHITE) SWELLING OF EXTERNAL GENITALS (FEMALE).
- VERTIGO/DIZZINESS

**Manipulation**
- For heart and lung issues: shallow needling
- For Hernia and knee pain: deeper insertion
- Treat the side opposite the location of symptoms
- From certain literature, needling 11.02 on both hands are contraindicated.
- Needle adjacent to the edge of the bone

*Note: The six fu-organs refer to the gallbladder, the stomach, the small intestine, the large intestine, the bladder and the triple energizer.

## 11.03 Fu Jian
### (FLOATING DISTANCE)

**Location:**
Locate the point 0.2 cun radial from the midline of the middle segment of the index finger, 0.33 cun from the distal crease. On Line B.

**Associated Channel:** Large Intestine

**Reaction Areas:** Heart and Six bowels.

**Indications:**
- HERNIA
- URETHRITIS
- TOOTHACHE
- STOMACHACHE
- ANGINA
- PALPITATION
- IRREGULAR HEARTBEAT
- VERTIGO/DIZZINESS

**Manipulation:**
Use 0.5 cun needle; insert 0.2- 0.25 cun adjacent to the edge of the bone. Bilateral needling contraindicated.

## 11.04 Wai Jian
### (OUTER DISTANCE)

**Location:**
Locate the point 0.2 cun radial to the midline of the middle segment of the index finger, 0.66 cun away from the distal crease. On Line B.

**Associated Channel:** Large Intestine

**Reaction Areas:** Heart and Six

**Indications:** As in 11.03

**Manipulations:**
Insert 0.2 to 0.25 cun. Needle adjacent to the edge of the bone.

**Remarks:** Needle insertion to both sides simultaneously is forbidden.

# 11.05
# Zhong Jian
### (CENTER DISTANCE)

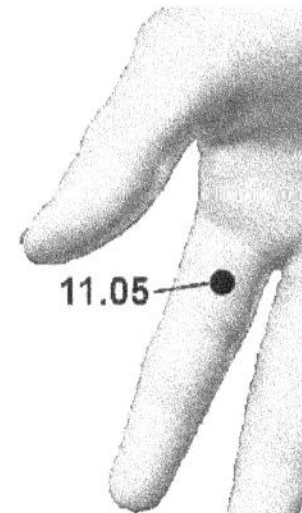

**Location:**
In the center of the proximal segment of the index finger. On Line C.

**Associated Channel:**
Large Intestine

**Reaction Areas:**
Lung, Heart and Six bowels.

**Indications:**
- ANGINA/HEART ATTACK (EMERGENCY POINT)
- PALPITATION/IRREGULAR HEARTBEAT
- SUFFOCATING SENSATION IN THE CHEST
- VERTIGO/DIZZINESS
- BLURRED VISION
- KNEE PAIN
- HERNIA
- PAIN AT THE CORNER OF THE EYE
- URETHRITIS
- TOOTHACHE

**Manipulation:**
Use 0.5 cun acupuncture needle; insert 0.1 to 0.2 cun for heart, chest, head and eye problems, insert 0.25 cun for hernia and knee pain. Pinch up the skin prior to needle insertion to avoid injury to periosteum.

Bilateral needling is contraindicated.

**Remarks:** Useful emergency point to relieve chest pain due to angina.

# 11.06 Huan Chao
### (RETURN TO THE NEST)

**Location:**
On the ulnar and palmar side of the middle segment of the ring finger, in the center between the second and third finger crease. On Line E (and/or Line A in certain text)

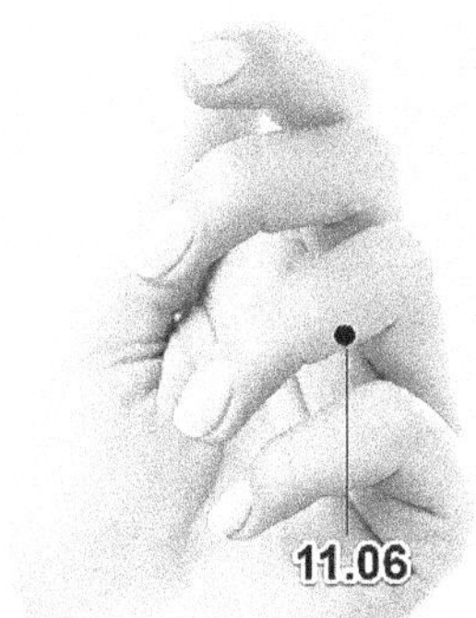

**Associated Channel:** Sanjiao

**Reaction Areas:** Liver and Kidney

**Dao Ma:** 11.06+11.24 for gynaecological issues.

**Indications:**
- INFERTILITY
- UTERINE PAIN/TUMOR, UTERITIS
- IRREGULAR MENSTRUATION
- LEUKORRHEA WITH REDDISH OR WHITE DISCHARGE
- RETROVERSION OF UTERUS
- FREQUENT URINATION
- VAGINAL SWELLING
- FREQUENT MISCARRIAGE
- GOOD FOR OVARIES
- HOLDS AND CALMS THE FETUS
- PREMENSTRUAL SYNDROME (PMS)
- MENOPAUSAL HOT FLASHES, NIGHT SWEATS,
- GYNECOLOGICAL ISSUES
- MENSTRUAL CRAMPING (DYSMENORRHEA)
- EXCESSIVE OR SCANTY MENSTRUAL BLEEDING
- BLOCKED FALLOPIAN TUBE
- HABITUAL MISCARRIAGE
- OVARIAN DISEASE
- IRREGULAR MENSES
- POLYCYSTIC OVARIAN SYNDROME (PCOS)

**Manipulation:**
Use 0.5 cun acupuncture needle; insert 0.2 to 0.3 cun. Direction of needle is perpendicular or from dorsal to palmar surface of phalange. Avoid blood vessels.

Certain text recommends 45 mins to one hour needle retention.

**Remarks:** Needle unilaterally. When using 11.06 and 11.24, needle on opposite sides to one another and vice versa (alternate between treatments).

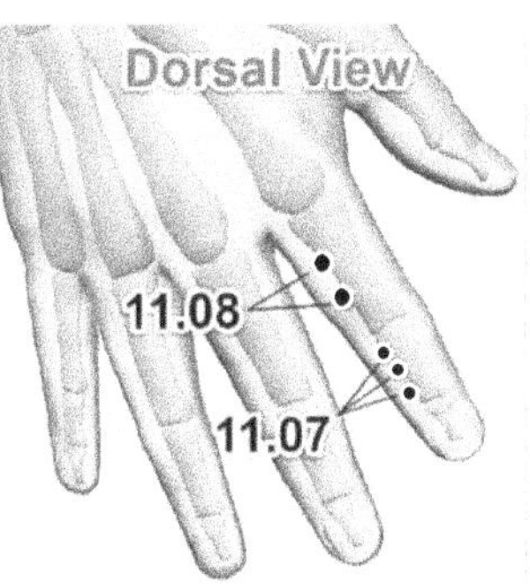


# 11.07 Zhi Si Ma
### (FINGER RAPID HORSES)

**Location:**
3 point group; evenly distributed on the dorsal middle phalanx of the index finger along the ulnar margin of the phalangeal bone; on the Large Intestine channel. On Line F.

**Associated Channel:** Large Intestine

**Reaction Areas:** Lung

**Indications:**
- PLEURISY
- PAIN OF PLEURA
- DERMATITIS
- DARK SPOTS ON THE FACE/ACNE
- RHINITIS
- TINNITUS AND OTITIS MEDIA
- SHOULDER PAIN
- STOPS LACTATION
- SKIN DISEASES
- BREAST/HYPOCHONDRIAC PAIN
- DISEASES OF THE BREAST

**Manipulation:**
Insert a needle closely along the edge of the phalanx to a depth of 0.2 to 0.3cun.

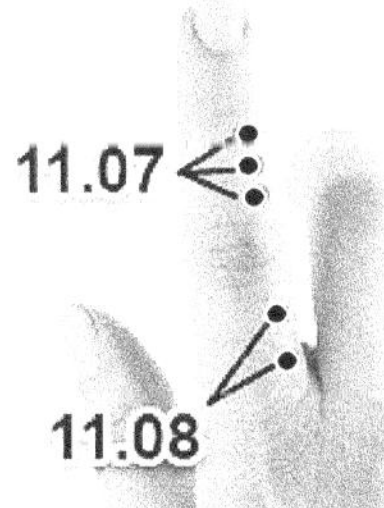


# 11.08 Zhi Wu Jin
### (FINGER 5 THOUSAND)

**Location:**
2 point group; evenly distributed on the medial line of the dorsal proximal phalanx of the index finger along the ulnar margin of the phalangeal bone.

**Associated Channel:** Large Intestine

**Reaction Areas:** Lung

**Indications:**

- ENTERITIS (INTESTINAL INFLAMMATION)
- ABDOMINAL PAIN (GASTRIC PAIN)
- FISH BONE STUCK IN THE THROAT.

**Manipulation:**
Needle closely along the edge of the phalanx to a depth of 0.2 to 0.3 cun

**Remarks:** These two points are only effective to relieve abdominal pain associated with qi stagnation. They do not serve to treat stomach and duodenal disorders such as ulcers.

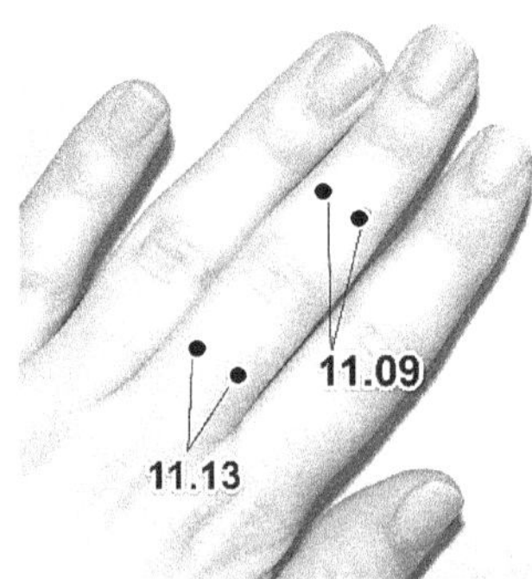

# 11.09 Xin Xi
(HEART KNEE)

**Location:**
2 point group. On both sides of the middle segment of the middle finger on the dorsal side, in the center between the second and third finger creases. On Line F and H.

**Associated Channel:** Pericardium

**Reaction Areas:** Heart

**Indications:**

- KNEE PAIN, DEGENERATIVE ESPECIALLY WITH THE ELDERLY (NOT DUE TO INJURY)
- SHOULDER AND SCAPULAR PAIN
- SPINAL PAIN
- ARTHRITIS WITH DEFORMED JOINTS.

**Manipulation:**
Use 0.5 cun acupuncture needle; insert 0.2 to 0.3 cun. Slide the needles along both sides of the medial phalange, touching the bone. Useful to needle bilateral for OA knee pain due to its systemic degenerative process.

**Remarks:** In the Tung System, all points with Heart as a Reaction area will treat knee pain.

# 11.10 Mu Huo
(WOOD FIRE)

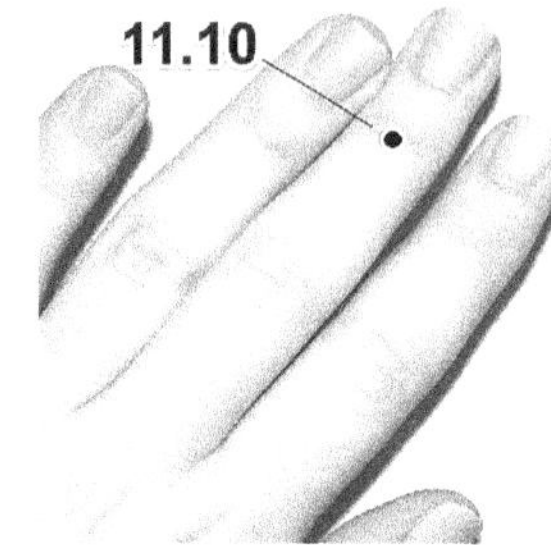

**Location:**
Palms down. Locate the point in the center of the third finger crease of the dorsal aspect of the middle finger. On line G.

**Associated Channel:** Pericardium

**Reaction Areas:** Heart and Liver

**Indications:**

- HEMIPLEGIA FROM STROKE
- STRENGTHENS THE HEART, MOVING THE BLOOD (HEART DISORDERS)
- COLD EXTREMITIES DUE TO POOR BLOOD CIRCULATION ESPECIALLY IN THE AGED
- MEDIAL KNEE PAIN

**Manipulation:**
Insert a needle superficially and horizontally towards the little finger. Can needle bilaterally. Not more than once a day.

This point can also be bled if the area appears dark or if it has surrounding dark veins.

**Caution:** Essential to follow recommended needling retention times:
1st 5 treatments for 5 minutes only,
2nd 5 treatments for 3 mins,
3rd 5 treatments for 1 minute.

Can raise blood pressure. Hence use with care for stroke patients whose conditions have not stabilized.

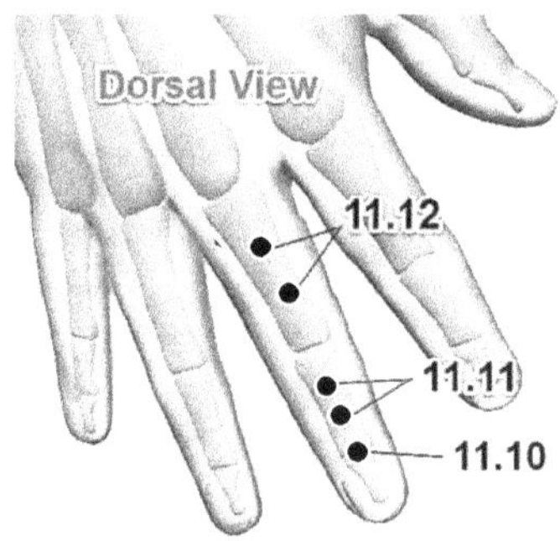


# 11.11 Fei Xin
(LUNG HEART)

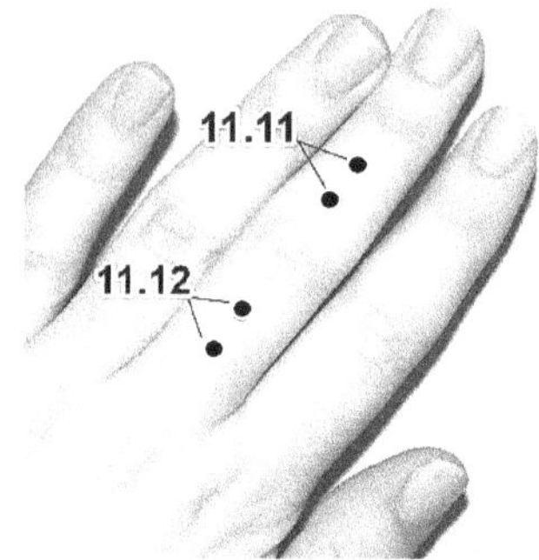

**Location:**
2 Point group. On the middle segment of the dorsal aspect of the middle finger. On Line G

**Associated Channel:** Pericardium

**Reaction Areas:** Heart and Lung

**Dao Ma:** 11.11+11.12

**Indications:**

- SPINAL DISORDERS
- VARICOSE VEINS
- SPINAL PAIN DUE TO ANKYLOSING SPONDYLITIS OR INJURY
- UPPER BACK AND NECK PAIN
- LUMBAR OR SACRAL PAIN
- COCCYX PAIN
- KNEE PAIN
- LOWER LEG/CALF MUSCLE PAIN
- HEEL PAIN
- PAIN OF ALL JOINTS

**Manipulation:**
Horizontally and superficially insert a needle towards the little finger. Pinch the skin away from the bone to access for skin. Needle bilaterally. Long needle retention may be required (up to 2 hours).

**Remarks:** Effective for spine (DU channel) related acute back pain ex. whiplash. More to treat upper spine but useful for entire spine pain.

# 11.12 Er Jiao Ming
(2 CORNER BRIGHT)

**Location:**
2 point group. On the midline of proximal segment of the middle finger on the dorsal side. On Line G

**Associated Channel:** Pericardium

**Reaction Areas:** Kidney

**Dao Ma:** 11.11+11.12

**Indications:**
- SUDDEN TWISTED BACK PAIN
- LOWER BACK PAIN
- FRONT OF FACE PAIN
- NASAL BONE PAIN
- TREATS HIGH INTRAOCULAR PRESSURE
- EYES PAIN AND PROBLEMS

**Manipulation:**
Oblique insertion towards the little finger, 0.2 cun in depth. Pulling the skin will assist needling.

Remarks: Use with 11.11 to treat pain on the spine esp. lower back pain.

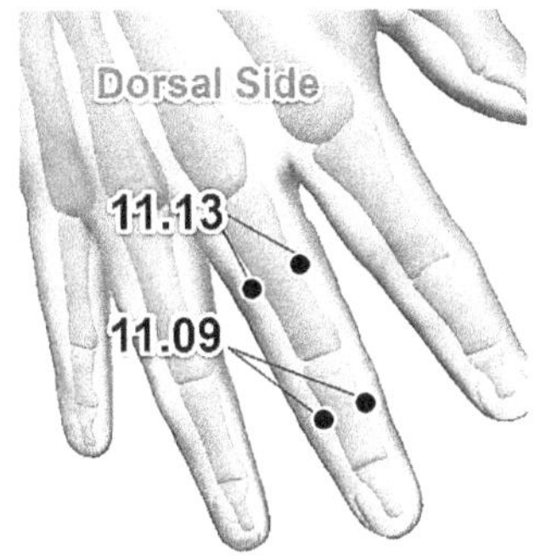


# 11.13 Dan
(GALLBLADDER)

**Location:**
2 point group. In the center of the proximal segment of the middle finger on the dorsal side. On line F, H.

**Associated Channel:** Pericardium

**Reaction Areas:** Gallbladder

**Indications:**
- HEART PALPITATION
- MORBID NIGHT CRYING OF BABIES
- KNEE PAIN.
- GALLBLADDER DISEASE
- EASILY STARTLED
- ADULT HYSTERIA
- SLEEP DISTURBANCE

**Manipulation:**
Insert 0.2 to 0.3 cun. Bleed if blood vessels visible.

**Remarks:** Usually used with 11.09 to treat arthritic knee pain (hurts more in the morning, feels better after movement due to increased blood circulation).

Useful for knee pain if there are also gallbladder indications.

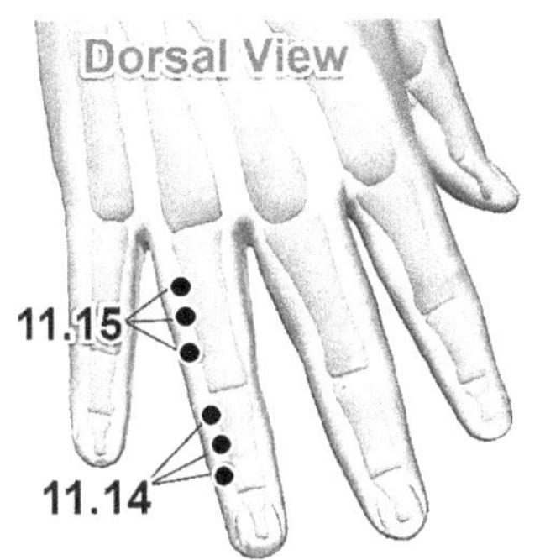


# 11.14 Zhi San Zhong
(FINGER 3 LAYER)

**Location:**
3 point group. On the ulnar and dorsal aspect of the proximal segment of the ring finger. On Line F.

**Associated Channel:** Sanjiao

**Reaction Areas:** Liver and Kidney

**Indications:**
- FACIAL PARALYSIS/BELL'S PALSY
- SWOLLEN BREAST/MASTITIS
- MUSCLE ATROPHY
- MIGRAINE/OCCIPITAL HEADACHE
- SIMILAR TO 77.05-77.07

**Manipulation:** Insert 0.2 to 0.3 cun, perpendicularly adjacent to the bone. Needle bilaterally.

**Remarks:** Useful in acute cases and to support the Dao Ma 77.05-07.


# 11.15 Zhi Shen
(FINGER KIDNEY)

**Location:**
On the ulnar aspect of the proximal segment of the dorsal side of the ring finger. On Line F.

**Associated Channel:** Sanjiao

**Reaction Areas:** Liver and Kidney

**Indications:**
- DRY MOUTH AND THIRST
- KIDNEY YIN DEFICIENCY
- HEART WEAKNESS
- UPPER BACK PAIN
- PREMATURE EJACULATION

**Manipulation:**
Insert perpendicularly 0.2 to 0.3 cun. Adjacent to the bone.

**Remarks:** Useful if upper back pain is caused by Kidney deficiency.

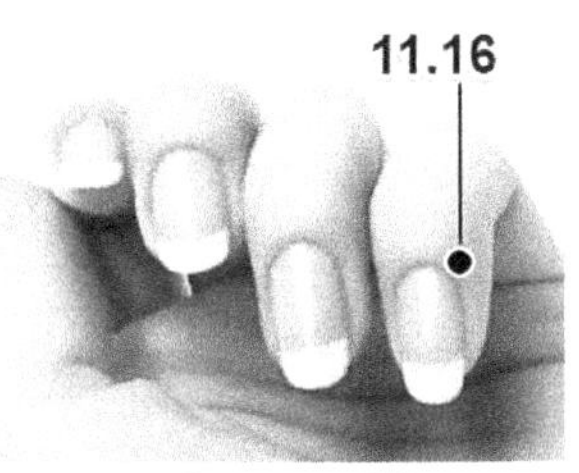


# 11.16 Huo Xi
(FIRE KNEE)

**Location:**
0.2 cun lateral to the nail root notch of the dorsal side of the little finger. On Line F.

**Overlaps:** SI-1

**Associated Channel:** Small Intestine

**Reaction Areas:** Heart

**Indications:**
- KNEE PAIN
- RHEUMATOID ARTHRITIS WITH DEFORMED JOINTS
- RHEUMATIC HEART DISEASE
- DIFFICULTY RAISING THE ARM/FROZEN SHOULDER
- PAIN DUE TO ANGER
- MENTAL DISTURBANCE/CONFUSION
- RED EYES

**Manipulation:** More effective if bled. Needle bilaterally to treat emotional and psychological conditions.

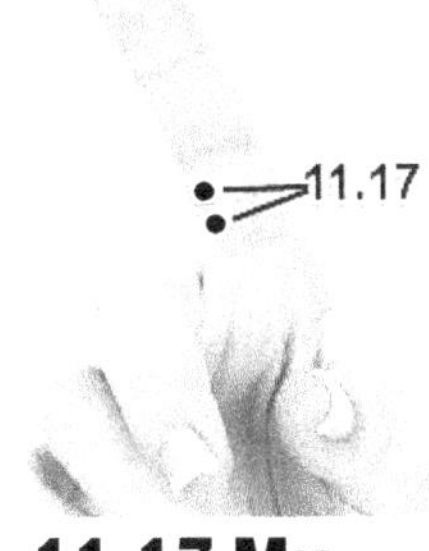


# 11.17 Mu
(WOOD POINT)

**Location:**
On the medial aspect of the index finger on the palmar side on the line 0.2 cun away from the midline. On Line D.

**Associated Channel:** Large Intestine

**Reaction Areas:** Liver

**Indications:**
- HYPERACTIVITY OF LIVER FIRE
- IRRITABILITY/ANXIETY/ANGER
- ISSUES AGGRAVATED BY ANGER

- HEADACHES
- DEPRESSION
- INSOMNIA
- DRY OR TEARING EYES.
- EXCESSIVE NASAL DISCHARGE AND CONGESTION
- PALM SWEATING
- COMMON COLD
- SKIN ITCHING/PSORIASIS

**Manipulation:** Insert 0.2-0.3 cun perpendicularly and adjacent to the bone. Usually on left side, opposite Liver position, to treat emotional issues. Bilateral needling for sinus, skin diseases, etc.

**Remarks:** 11.17 treats the "emotional" liver whereas 11.20 treats liver organ issues. Advised not to use 11.17 and 11.20 concurrently.

This point is also known as the common cold point. It can effectively stop nasal discharge upon needle insertion. The effect is quite immediate for itching as well. Usually only the proximal point is used.

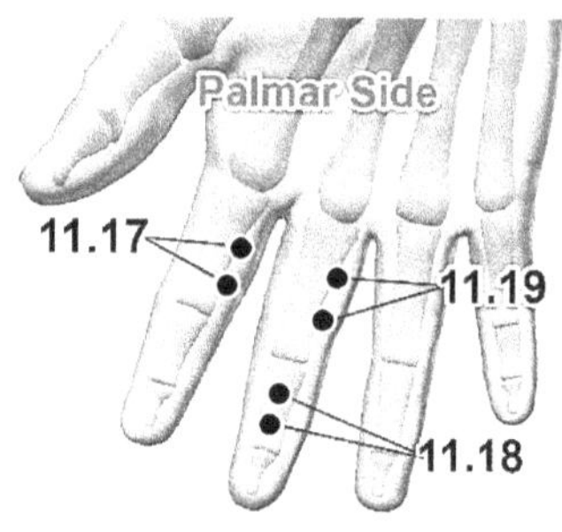


# 11.18 Pi Zhong

(SPLEEN EDEMA)

**Location:**
On the midline of the middle segment of the palmar middle finger.
On Line C

**Associated Channel:** Pericardium

**Reaction Areas:** Spleen

**Indications:**
- ENLARGEMENT OF SPLEEN
- SPLEEN DISEASE
- HICCUPS
- ABDOMINAL BLOATING IN CHILDREN

**Manipulation:** Insert 0.2 to 0.3 cun. Pinch up the skin to assist needling, insert slowly until gently contact with periosteum. Needle on right hand - opposite spleen.

# 11.19 Xin Chang

(HEART NORMAL)

**Location:**
0.2 cun on the ulnar side of the midline of the proximal segment on the palmar aspect of the middle finger. On Line D.

**Associated Channel:** Pericardium

**Reaction Areas:** Heart

**Indications:**
- HEART DISEASE
- ENLARGED HEART
- IRREGULAR HEARTBEAT
- TACHYCARDIA
- BRADYCARDIA

**Manipulation:** Insert 0.2 to 0.3 cun.

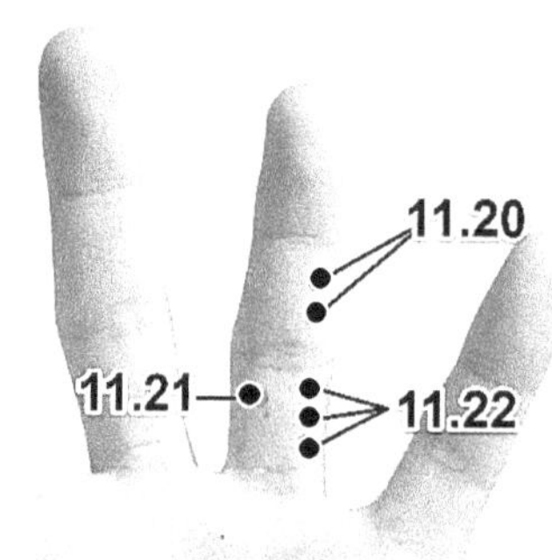


# 11.20 Mu Yan

(WOOD INFLAMMATION)

**Location:**
0.2 cun on the ulnar side of the midline of the middle segment on the palmar aspect of the ring finger. On Line D.

**Associated Channel:** Sanjiao

**Reaction Areas:** Liver

**Indications:**
- LIVER ORGAN DISEASE/PAIN
- HEPATITIS
- HEPATOMEGALY
- CIRRHOSIS (LIVER DAMAGE/FAILURE)
- HELPS RELIEVE PAIN OF LIVER CANCER
- HYPOCHONDRIAC PAIN
- INSOMNIA (DUE TO LIVER FAILURE)

**Manipulation:** Insert 0.2 to 0.3 cun perpendicularly and adjacent to the bone. On left side opposite the liver.

**Remarks:** 11.17 Mu is needled for emotional issues whereas 11.20 Mu Yan is selected for liver organ disease and liver pain. Advised not to use 11.17 and 11.20 concurrently.

# 11.21 San Yan

(THREE EYES)

**Location:**
0.2 cun to the radial aspect of the midline of the palmar aspect of the ring finger, 0.2 cun from the second crease of the middle finger, one-third of the distance between the distal crease and the proximal crease of the first phalange. On Line B

**Associated Channel:** Between Pericardium and Sanjiao

**Reaction Areas:** Heart and Lung

**Indications:**
- FATIGUE (TONIFYING POINT)
- PERSPIRATION
- INDICATIONS ARE SIMILAR TO ST-36

**Manipulation:** Insert 0.2 to 0.3 cun.

**Remarks:** Similar functions to ST-36 but not as effective, hence not a frequently used point.

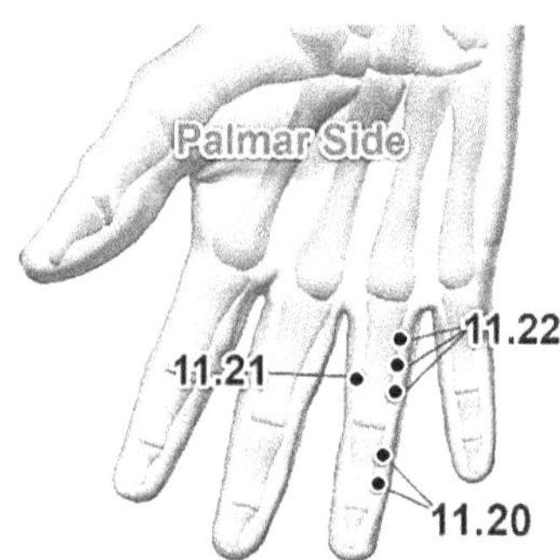


# 11.22 Fu Yuan

(RECOVER)

**Location:**
0.2 cun on the ulnar side of the midline of the palmar surface of the ring finger. On Line D.

**Associated Channel:** Sanjiao

**Reaction Areas:** Liver

**Indications:**
- RHEUMATOID ARTHRITIS
- ENLARGEMENT OF BONES
- OSTEOARTHRITIS
- PAINFUL JOINTS
- BONE STEAMING DISORDER

**Manipulation:** Insert 0.2 to 0.3 cun. Slide along the phalange.

Needle bilaterally – for multiple joints
Needle unilaterally – for single joint.

## 11.23 Yan Huang

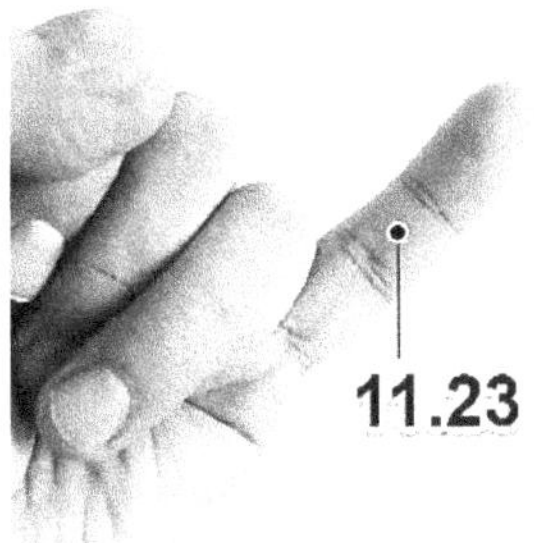

(Eye Yellow)

**Location:**
In the center of the middle segment on the palmar surface of the little finger. On Line C

**Associated Channel**: Between Heart and Small Intestine

**Reaction Areas:** Gall Bladder

**Indications:**
- Icteric sclera (hepatitis with yellow eyes)
- Jaundice

**Manipulation:** Insert 0.1 to 0.2 cun.

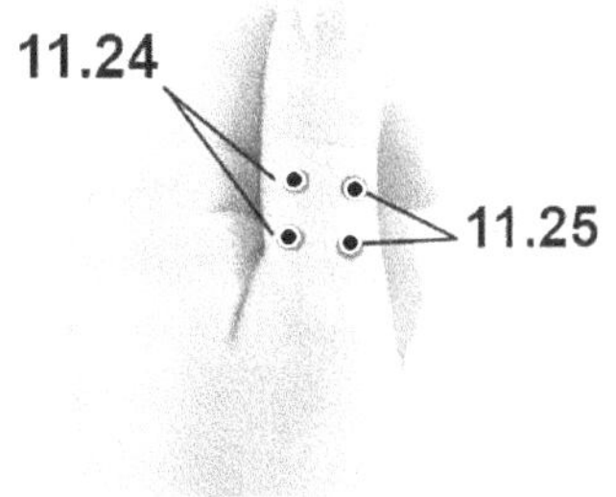

## 11.24 Fu Ke

(Gynecological)

**Location:**
2 point group. On the ulnar aspect of the proximal segment on the dorsal side of the thumb. On Line F.

**Associated Channel:** Lung

**Reaction Areas:** Uterus

**Indications:**
- Regulates hormonal activity
- Infertility
- Uteritis (pain and inflammation of uterus)
- Uterine fibroids
- Tipped uterus accompanied by low back pain and frequent urination
- Menstrual disorders: dysmenorrhea, amenorrhea, scanty/irregular menstruation

- Menopause
- Habitual miscarriage
- Distension of the lower abdomen
- Leukorrhea (Red and White)

**Manipulation:** Insert a needle closely along the edge of the phalanx to a depth of 0.2 to 0.3 cun

**Remarks:** Combines well with 11.06 and 11.17.

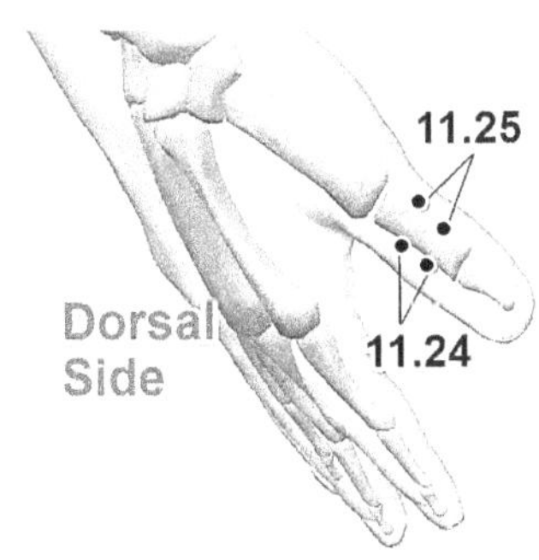

## 11.25 Zhi Xian

(Stop Drooling)

**Location:**
2 point group. On the radial aspect of the proximal segment of the dorsal thumb. On Line H.

**Associated Channel:** Lung

**Indications:**
- Drooling in adults due to brain injury
- Drooling in children.

**Manipulation:** Insert a needle closely along the edge of the phalanx to a depth of 0.2 to 0.3 cun.

## 11.26 Zhi Wu

(Control Dirt)

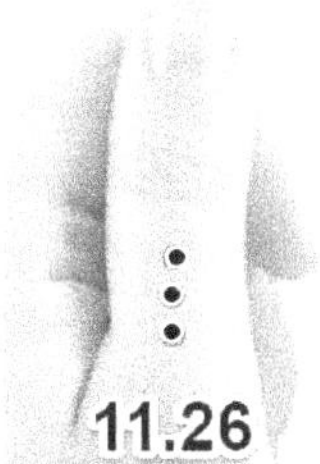

**Location:**
3 point group. On the midline of the proximal segment of the dorsal aspect of the thumb. On Line G.

**Associated Channel:** Lung

**Indications:**
- Slow healing of wounds
- Persisted carbuncles/boils
- Bedsores/frostbite/gangrene
- Blood oozing from the wound after a surgery for a tumor
- Shingles

- Surgical infection
- Malignancies

**Manipulation:** To obtain an immediate effect, bleed the points with a three-edge needle or lancet to remove dark blood. Only effective when there is a dark vessel present to bleed.

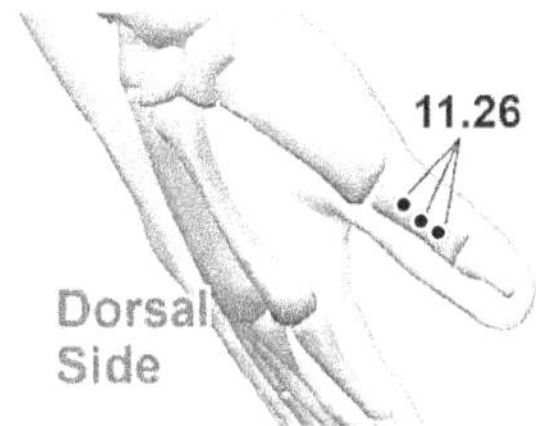

## 11.27 Wu Hu

(Five Tiger)

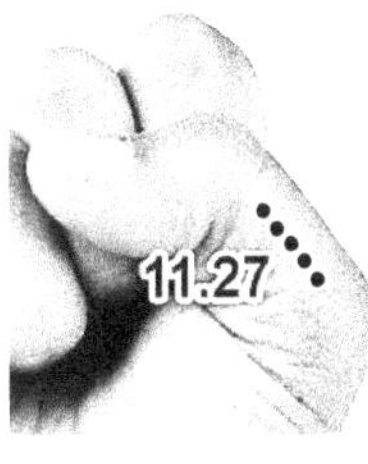

**Location:**
5 point group. On the radial aspect of the proximal segment of the palmar side of the thumb. Along the red/white skin margin. On Line A.

The points are numbered 1-5, distal to proximal:

- *11.27 #1* is located just proximal to the distal condyle of the first phalange.
- *11.27 #2* is located between Five Tigers Three and Five Tigers One.
- *11.27 #3* is located in the middle of the proximal phalange.
- *11.27 #4* is located between Five Tigers Three and Five Tigers Five.
- *11.27 #5* is located just distal to the proximal condyle of the first phalange.

**Associated Channel:** Lung

**Reaction Areas:** Spleen

**Indications:**
- Musculoskeletal joint pain
- Finger or toe pain incl. trigger finger
- General swollen joints and bones
- Rheumatoid arthritis
- Foot/ankle/heel pain
- Gout
- Hand pain
- Tendinitis, tenosynovitis
- Sore throat, pneumonia, and swollen glands.

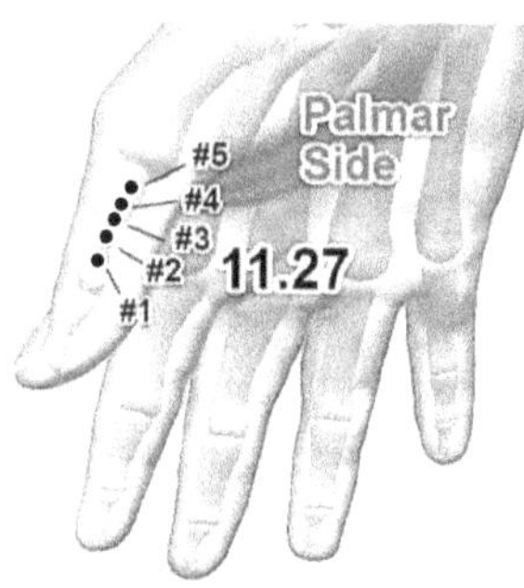



**Individual point Indications:**

• *11.27 #1 (distal):* Finger and palm pain, rheumatoid arthritis, tenosynovitis, headache

• *11.27 #2:* Deformed fingers, rheumatoid arthritis, tendinitis

• *11.27 #3 (middle):* Toe pain, gout, frontal headache

• *11.27 #4:* Instep pain, dorsum and ankle pain

• *11.27 #5 (proximal):* Heel pain

**Manipulation:**

Insert needles along the radial aspect to a depth of 0.2 to 0.4 cun, depending on the treatment of the nearby (shallow needling) or distal (deeper needling) problems. Not recommended to needle all five points in one sitting.

Needle opposite to pain but can needle on pain side when acting as Guide Points for fingers pain.

## Zhu Yuan

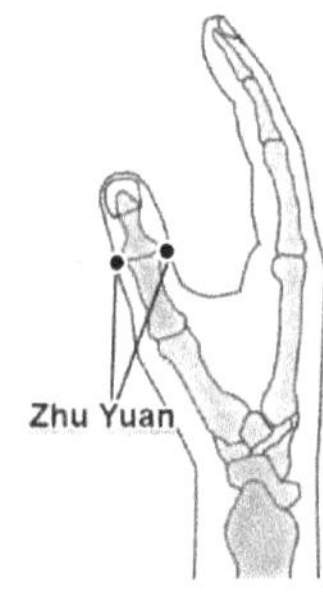



**Location:**
2 points. Locate on both sides between first and second segment of the thumb, 0.5 cun away in the ending crease. (Can acupuncture exactly on the endings of crease).

**Actions:** Rectify wind and clear heat, nourish Yin and brighten eyes.

**Indications:**
Glaucoma, cataract, Keratitis, amblyopia and any types eye or vision disorders.

**Manipulation:**
Insert 0.2 to 0.5 cun perpendicularly.

## A.07 Ye Mang

(NIGHT BLINDNESS)

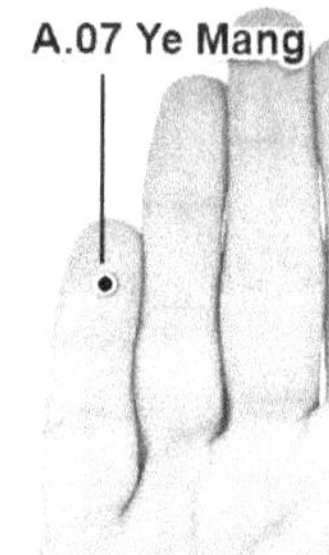



**Location:**
Located on the palmar surface of the little finger, in the center of the third phalange.

**Associated Channel:** Between Heart and Small Intestine

**Indications:**
• SEVERE NIGHT BLINDNESS

**Manipulation:**
0.2 cun bilaterally

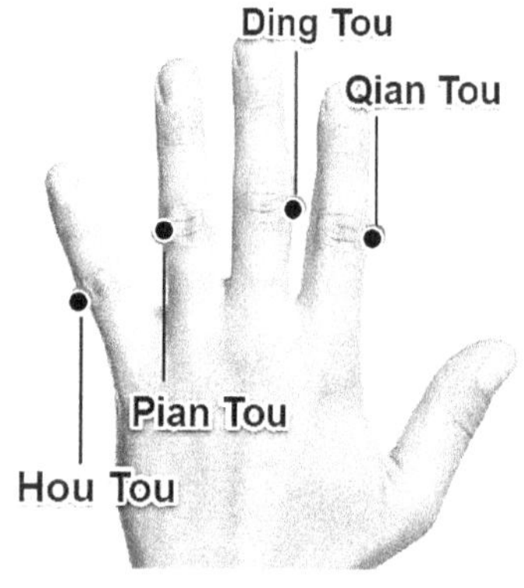



## Tou Points

**Location/manipulation:**
4 points.
**Qian Tou** and **Ding Tou** (located on Line A), needle towards the little finger.

**Pian Tou** and **Hou Tou** (located on Line E), needle towards the thumb.

Perpendicular insertion at the MIP joint where the pink and white skin meet.

**Indications:**
Headaches caused by issues in the head not other causes like hormonal changes, hypertension, etc.  Usual to needle all four points.

Qian Tou – frontal headaches

Ding Tou- vertex headaches

Pian Tou – parietal headches

Hou Tou – occipital headaches

## ZONE 22-Hand

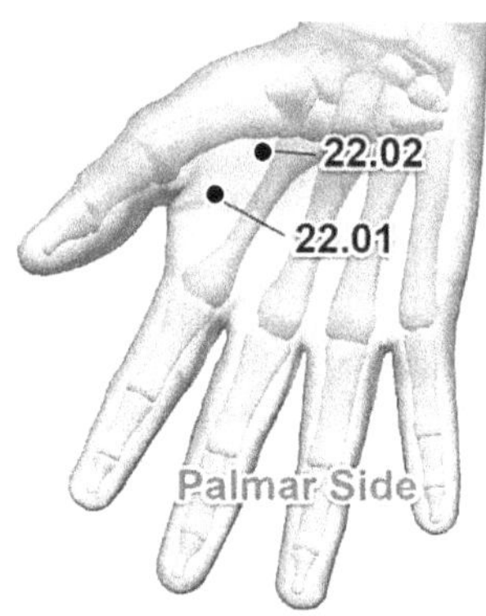



## 22.01 Chong Zi

(DOUBLE CHILD)

**Location:**
On the thenar eminence, about 1 cun from skin fold between the first and second metacarpals.

**Associated Channel:** Lung

**Reaction Areas:** Lung

**Dao Ma:** 22.01+22.02

**Indications:**
• BACK PAIN (UPPER AND SCAPULA)
• NECK AND SCAPULAR PAIN ("FALLEN PILLOW SYNDROME"
• PNEUMONIA, FEVER, BRONCHITIS
• COMMON COLD
• COUGHING
• ASTHMA, INFANTILE (MOST EFFECTIVE FOR CHILDREN)
• KNEE JOINT PAIN
• SHOULDER AND UPPER BACK
• DIFFICULTY IN OPENING AND CLOSING HANDS
• HEMIPLEGIA
• UTERINE OR OVARIAN CYSTS

**Manipulation:**
Insert 0.5 to 1.0 cun in depth.

**Remarks:** If there is pain of the neck, back and shoulder, prick any blue veins that might appear at 22.01 and 22.02 area. 22.01 is considered more for neck pain, while 22.02 more for back and shoulder pain.

## 22.02 Chong Xian

(DOUBLE FAIRY)

**Location:**
The point is located between the first and second metacarpal bones, 2 cun from the skin fold, across from and

communicating with Ling Gu (22.05) on the dorsal side of the hand.

**Associated Channel:** Lung

**Reaction Areas:** Heart, Lung

**Dao Ma:** 22.01+22.02

**Indication:**
- BACK PAIN
- PNEUMONIA
- FEVER
- HEART PALPITATION
- NECK/SHOULDER PAIN
- EFFECTIVE FOR BACK AND KNEE PAIN, ESPECIALLY AT THE BL-43 AREA
- TIP OF ACROMION
- BRONCHITIS, BRONCHIAL ASTHMA AND DIFFICULT EXPECTORATION
- HYSTEROMYOMA AND OVARIITIS
- CHEST PAIN

**Manipulation**
Insert 1.0 cun in depth. Bleed if there are blue vessels.

**Remarks:** Useful for respiratory issues.

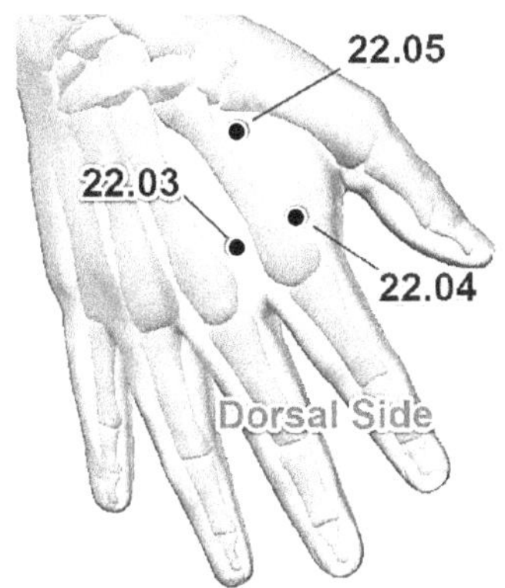


# 22.03 Shang Bai
(UPPER WHITE)

**Location:**
0.5 cun proximal to the dorsal metacarpophalangeal joint of the index and middle fingers.

**Associated Channel:** Between Pericardium and Large Intestine

**Reaction areas:** Lung, Heart, Liver

**Indications:**
- CONJUNCTIVITIS
- SORE, TIRED OR ITCHY EYES
- NECK PAIN, NEEDLE BILATERALLY
- SCIATICA
- LUMBAR AND BACK PAIN
- SHOULDER AND BACK PAIN
- STOMACH/RIB/WAIST PAIN
- LATERAL SIDE OF HEART PAIN

- SPRAIN OF THE WRIST AT RADIAL SIDE, NEEDLE DISEASED SIDE
- WEAKNESS OF FEET

**Manipulation:**
Insert 0.5 to 0.7 cun in depth.

# 22.04 Da Bai
(BIG WHITE)

**Location:**
Located on the back of the hand, just proximal and radial head of the second metacarpal bone.

**Overlaps:** LI-3

**Associated Channel:** Large Intestine

**Reaction area:** Lung.

**Dao Ma:** 22.04+22.05

**Indications:**
- ASTHMA OF CHILDREN
- HIGH FEVER OF CHILDREN (MOST EFFECTIVE)
- LOW BACK PAIN
- SCIATICA
- BRONCHITIS
- ACUTE PNEUMONIA
- COMMON COLD
- HEADACHE
- HEMIPLEGIA
- FACIAL TWITCH
- FACIAL PAIN
- TRIGEMINAL NEURALGIA
- TOOTHACHE (LOWER TEETH)
- DIARRHEA OR CONSTIPATION

**Manipulation:** Insert 0.5 to 1.0 cun deep for sciatica. Prick for child asthma, high fever and acute pneumonia.

Remarks: Treats all types of headaches

# 22.05 Ling Gu
(ADROIT BONE)

**Location:**
The point is located in the juncture between the index finger and thumb, the 1st and 2nd dorsal metacarpal bones, 1.2 cun from 22.04, and directly opposite 22.02. Fold patient's hand into a fist to locate the point.

**Associated Channel:** Large Intestine

**Reaction area:** Lung

**Dao Ma:** 22.04+22.05

**Indications**
- SCIATICA DUE TO WEAK LUNG FUNCTION, FOOT PAIN
- SP/ST THIGH SCIATICA
- LOW BACK PAIN
- ISCHIAL NERVE PAIN
- FOOT PAIN
- HEMIPARALYSIS OF NERVES
- HEMIPLEGIA
- BELL'S PALSY OR FACIAL PARALYSIS
- TRIGEMINAL NEURALGIA
- ENLARGEMENT OF BONES
- IRREGULAR MENSTRUATION
- AMENORRHEA, DYSMENORRHEA
- DIFFICULT LABOR (LABOR INDUCTION)
- BACK PAIN
- TINNITUS
- INTESTINAL PAIN
- DIZZINESS
- INSOMNIA
- HEADACHE
- CONJUNCTIVITIS
- ELBOW PAIN

**Manipulation:** Use 1.5 to 2.0 cun acupuncture needle to pierce through Zhong Xian (22.02). 0.5 to 1.5 cun deep. Alternatively, can needle under the index finger towards SI-4. Needle treatment of pregnant women is not allowed.

**Remarks:** 22.05 (Ling gu) is the main point for regulating and moving qi and blood. This point is probably the most powerful point in the Tung System.

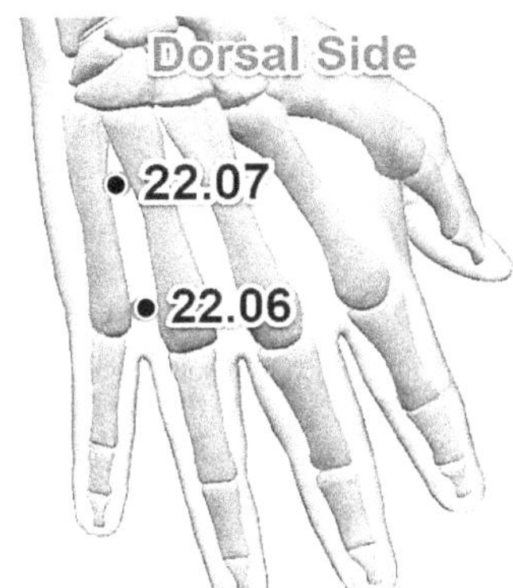


# 22.06 Zhong Bai
(CENTER WHITE)

**Location:**
The point is located between the dorsal metacarpal bones of the little and ring fingers, 0.5 cun proximal to the metacarpophalangeal joint. Fold hand into a fist to locate the point.

**Overlaps:** SJ-3

**Associated Channel:** Sanjiao

**Reaction area:** Heart, Kidney and Spleen.

**Dao Ma:** 22.06+22.07

**Indications:**
- LOW BACK DUE TO KIDNEY ISSUES
- TWISTED BACK PAIN
- SCIATICA (ESP. ALONG GB CHANNEL)
- PERIARTHRITIS OF THE SHOULDER
- PAIN OF THE SHOULDER AND BACK
- ACUTE NECK PAIN
- BONE SPURS
- NEPHRITIS
- LIMB EDEMA
- HIGH BLOOD PRESSURE
- ASTIGMATISM
- FATIGUE
- ANKLE PAIN (POSTERIOR ASPECT)
- SORENESS OF THE WAIST AND FLANK ESPECIALLY UPON STANDING-UP AND SITTING-DOWN
- VISION PROBLEMS
- TOOTHACHE
- TRIGEMINAL NEURALGIA
- TINNITUS AND SUDDEN ATTACK OF DEAFNESS
- MENIERE'S SYNDROME AND RELATED SYMPTOMS
- MIGRAINE AND VERTIGO/DIZZINESS

**Manipulation:**
Insertion of 0.3 to 0.5 cun in depth.

**Remarks:** Useful as Guide Point (needle same side as pain) for head and face issues.

# 22.07 Xia Bai
(LOWER WHITE)

**Location:**
The point is located between the dorsal 4th and 5th metacarpal bones, 1.5 cun proximal to the metacarpophalangeal joint, 1.0 cun proximal to 22.06. Fold patient's hand into a fist to locate the point

**Overlaps:** N-UE-19 Yao Tong Xue

**Associated Channel:** Sanjiao

**Reaction areas:** Heart, Kidney, Spleen

**Dao Ma:** 22.06+22.07

**Indications:**
- RENAL COLIC AND GALLBLADDER PAIN
- LOW BACK DUE TO RENAL PROBLEMS
- ACHING PAIN OF TEETH
- SLIGHT LIVER PAIN
- BACK PAIN

- DIZZINESS
- ASTIGMATISM/NEAR-SIGHTEDNESS
- FATIGUE
- SCIATICA DUE TO RENAL PROBLEMS
- ANKLE PAIN (POSTERIOR ASPECT)
- LIMB EDEMA
- AND INDICATIONS OF 22.06

**Manipulation:** Insertion of 0.3 to 0.5 cun in depth.

**Remarks:** Back pain at vertebrae T8-T12 (kidney area).

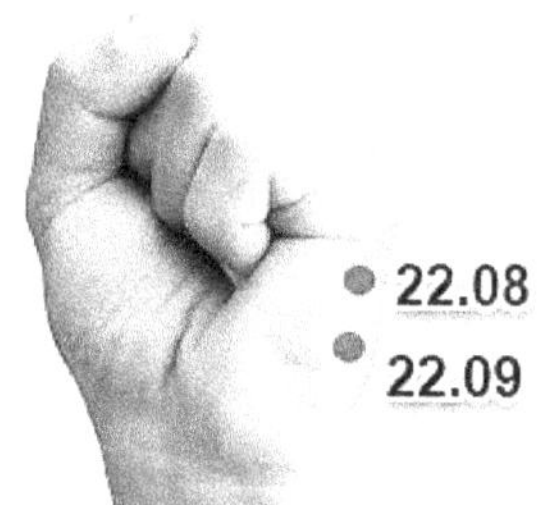


# 22.08 Wan Shun Yi
(WRIST FLOW, ONE)

**Location:**
The point is located on the lateral side of the 5th dorsal metacarpal bone, 2.5 cun distal to the wrist crease. 0.5 cun proximal to SI-3.

**Associated Channel:** Small Intestine

**Reaction area:** Kidney

**Dao Ma:** 22.08+22.09

**Indications:**
- HEADACHE
- STIFF NECK
- BLURRED VISION/EYE PAIN
- TINNITUS
- TRIGEMINAL NEURALGIA
- SCIATICA DUE TO DEFICIENCY IN THE KIDNEY
- NEPHRITIS
- EDEMA OF THE LIMBS
- HEAVINESS AND PAIN ON BOTH SIDES OF THE LOWER BACK AND WAIST
- SCIATICA/BACK PAIN (ALONG URINARY BLADDER CHANNEL)
- PAIN OF THE LUMBAR VERTEBRAE
- PAIN OF THE POPLITEAL FOSSA (BEHIND THE KNEE)
- MEDIAL ELBOW PAIN
- WRIST PAIN/CARPAL TUNNEL (ALONG SMALL INTESTINE CHANNEL)

**Manipulation:** 0.5 cun depth treats the shoulder, 1.0 cun goes to the lower back. 1.5 cun treats the leg and knee.

**Remarks:** Can replace with SI-3. Similar indications as SI-3 and SI-4. 22.08+22.09 treat kidney issues and spinal pain from neck to sacral area (along BL channel).

# 22.09 Wan Shun Er
(WRIST FLOW, TWO)

**Location:**
The point is located on the dorsal aspect of the lateral side of the 5th metacarpal bone, 1.5 cun distal to the wrist crease. It is 1.0 cun posterior to 22.08 (Wan Shun Yi).

**Associated Channel:** Small Intestine

**Reaction area:** Kidney

**Dao Ma:** 22.08+22.09

**Indications:**
- SIMILAR TO 22.08
- NOSE BLEED
- HEADACHE
- BLURRED VISION
- SCIATICA DUE TO DEFICIENCY IN THE KIDNEY
- NEPHRITIS
- EDEMA OF THE LIMBS
- HEAVINESS AND PAIN ON BOTH SIDES OF THE LOWER BACK
- BACK PAIN
- STIFFNESS AND PAIN AT THE POPLITEAL FOSSA.

**Manipulation:** 0.5 cun deep treats the shoulder, 1.0 cun goes to the lower back. 1.5 cun treats the leg and knee.

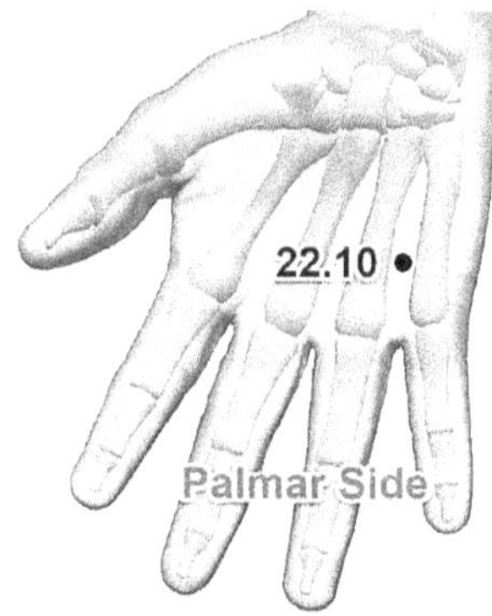


# 22.10 Shou Jie
(HAND RELEASE)

**Location:**
Between the 4th and 5th metacarpal bones, at the spot where the tip of the little finger touches when the patient's hand is folded into a fist.

**Overlaps:** HT-8

**Associated Channel:** Heart

**Reaction area:** Kidney

**Indications:**

- FAINTNESS AND NUMBNESS CAUSED BY ACUPUNCTURE NEEDLE INSERTION
- STUCK NEEDLE.
- ITCHING AND RASHES
- SWELLING AND STABBING PAIN DUE TO UNINTENDED DISTURBANCE OF QI AND BLOOD DURING NEEDLING SESSION.

**Manipulation:** Needle 0.3 to 0.5 cun for 10 to 20 minutes. Blood-letting is effective.

## 22.11 Tu Shui

(EARTH WATER)

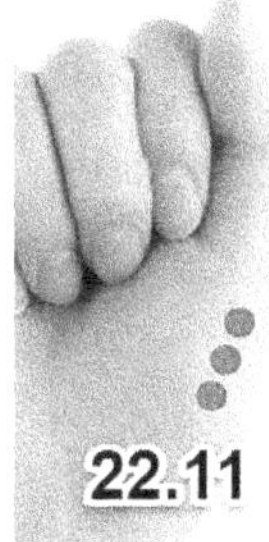

**Location:**
3 point group. Evenly distributed on the palmar aspect of the radial side of 1st metacarpal bone. Junction of red and white skin. The middle point (LU-10) is located at the mid-point of the first metacarpal bone. The second point is 0.5 cun posterior to the first one, and the third on is 0.5 cun posterior to the second one.

**Overlaps:** LU-10 (center point)

**Associated Channel:** Lung

**Reaction area:** Spleen and Kidney.

**Indications:**

- POOR DIGESTION
- GASTROENTERITIS
- DIARRHEA
- ACUTE STOMACH PAIN
- GASTRIC ULCER
- OPPOSITE SIDE PALMAR, FINGER AND HAND BONE PAIN
- SORE THROAT
- LOSS OF VOICE
- PNEUMONIA
- ASTHMA
- UTERINE FIBROIDS

**Manipulation:** Insert a needle closely along the metacarpal bone to a depth of 0.5 to 1.0 cun. Can bleed visible veins to increase effectiveness.

**Remarks:** Useful to those who have their gall bladders removed.

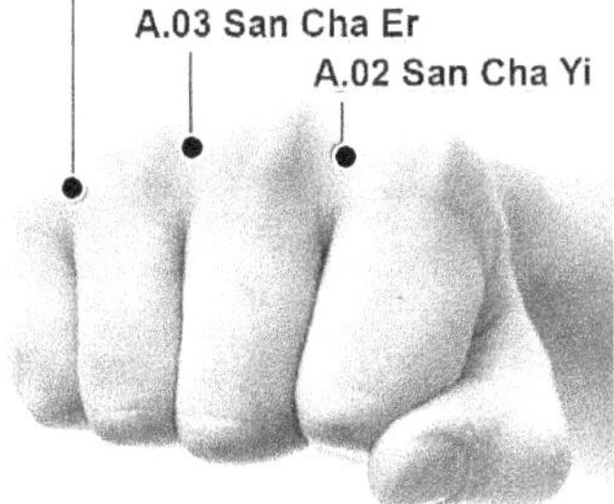


## A.02 San Cha Yi

(THREE JAM ONE)

**Location:**
Located on the dorsum of the hand, between the knuckles of the index and middle fingers.

**Associated Channel:** Between Pericardium and Large Intestine

**Indications:**

- PAIN IN THE UPPER BACK, SCAPULA, SHOULDER, UPPER EXTREMITIES, RIBS OR LOWER BACK
- LIVER AREA PAIN
- STOMACH PAIN
- EXCESSIVE UTERINE BLEEDING
- IRREGULAR MENSTRUATION

**Manipulation:** Insert needle with hand in a loose fist. Insert 1-1.5 cun deep.

## A.03 San Cha Er

(THREE JAM TWO)

**Location:**
Hold the hand in a loose fist, A.03 San Cha Er is found on the dorsum of the hand, between the knuckles of the middle and ring fingers.

**Associated Channel:** Between Pericardium and San Jiao

**Indications:**

- DISEASES OF THE FACE AND SENSORY
- ORGANS
- PALPITATIONS (SLOW PULSE)
- STOMACH PAIN
- SPINE MUSCLE PAIN
- ACUTE LUMBAR SPRAIN
- GROIN TO KNEE PAIN
- HIP JOINT/THIGH PAIN
- KNEE PAIN
- LOWER EXTREMITY PAIN

**Manipulation:** Hold the hand in a loose fist, insert 1-1.5 cun deep.

## A.04 San Cha San

(THREE JAM THREE)

**Location:**
Hold the hand in a loose fist, A.04 San Cha San is found on the dorsum of the hand, between the knuckles of the ring and little fingers

**Associated Channel:** San Jiao

**Reaction Areas:** Heart, Kidney, Spleen, Five Senses

**Indications:**

- COMMON COLD
- PROFUSE SWEATING
- HEADACHE
- SORE THROAT
- ALLERGIES, ITCHING SKIN, HIVES OR RASHES, ECZEMA, PSORIASIS, ASTHMA
- ANY DISEASE OF THE FIVE SENSES: TINNITUS, OTITIS MEDIA, EAR NERVE PAIN, DROOPING EYELIDS, FLOATERS
- FATIGUE
- AUTOIMMUNE DISORDERS
- SEVERE MUSCLE WEAKNESS
- FIBROMYALGIA/MULTIPLE SCLEROSIS
- PALPITATIONS (WITH FAST PULSE)
- CHEST AND RIB PAIN
- UPPER LEG PAIN
- LOWER BACK PAIN
- NECK AND SHOULDER PAIN
- NAUSEA AND VOMITING

**Manipulation:** 1.0 to 1.5 cun depth.

**Remarks:** San Cha San is said to be SJ-2, SJ-3, SJ-4, 22.06, 22.07, SI-3, SI-4, 22.08 and 22.09 all combined into one point. Thus, making this one of Tung's Top Point.

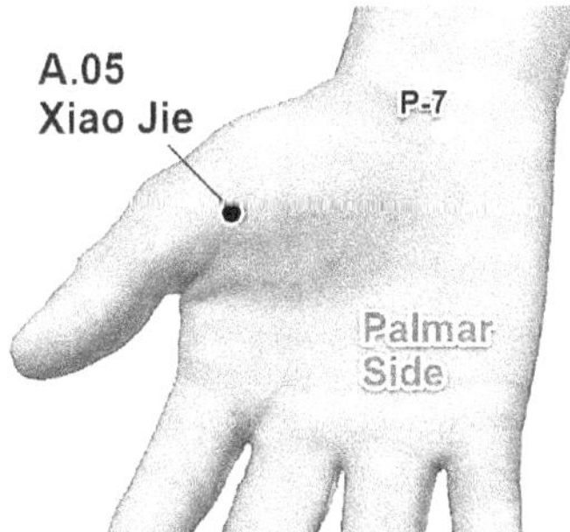


## A.05 Xiao Jie

(SMALL JOINT)

**Location:**
Xiao Jie is located 1 mm proximal and palmar to the large knuckle of the thumb.

**Associated Channel:** Lung

**Indications:**

- ACUTE OR CHRONIC ANKLE PAIN (HIGHLY EFFECTIVE)
- RHEUMATISM IN THE ANKLE
- ASTHMA
- COMMON COUGH
- DIARRHEA
- NECK PAIN
- BACK OF SHOULDER PAIN
- ELBOW, PALM AND WRIST PAIN
- CHEST PAIN
- LOWER BACK PAIN
- SCIATICA

**Manipulation:**
Thread the needle superficially (in the space between the epidermis and the muscle) across the thenar eminence, directed toward P-7.

# A.06 Ci Bai

### (NEXT WHITE)

**Location:**
Located on the dorsum of the hand, 0.5 cun proximal to the junction of the metacarpal-phalangeal joints of the middle and ring fingers.

**Associated Channel:** Between Pericardium (palmar) and San Jiao (dorsum)

**Indications:**

- LOWER LEG/CALF PAIN OR SPASM
- KNEE PAIN
- LUMBAR PAIN
- MIGRAINE
- EXCESSIVE SWEATING

**Manipulation:** Depth: 0.5 cun

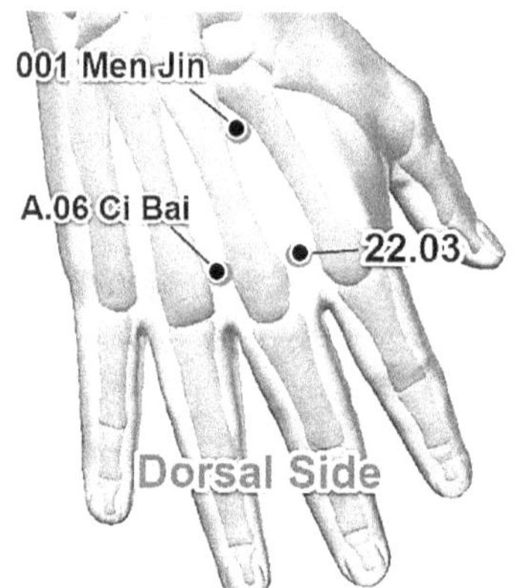


# 001 Men Jin

### (HAND GOLDEN GATE)

**Location:**
Located 1.0 cun proximal to 22.03 Shang Bai, between the second and third metacarpal bones.

**Associated Channel:** Between Pericardium and Large Intestine

**Reaction Areas:** Heart, Liver, Lung

**Indications:**

- GALLBLADDER PAIN DUE TO STONES
- KIDNEY STONE PAIN
- LOWER BACK PAIN (ACUTE)

**Manipulation:**
Insert 0.5 to 0.7 cun in depth.

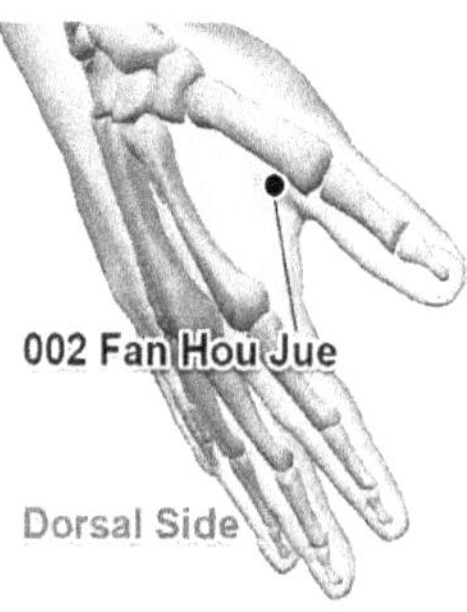


# 002 Fan Hou Jue

### (CUTTING OPPOSITE AND BEHIND)

**Location:**
Located just proximal to the distal head of the first metacarpal bone, on the ulnar side. Opposite 22.01 Double Child.

**Associated Channel:** Between Lung and Large Intestine

**Reaction Area:** Lung

**Indications:**

- UPPER BACK AND SHOULDER PAIN
- FROZEN SHOULDER

**Manipulation:** Insert 0.5 to 1.0 cun.

# Mu Guan and Gu Guan

**Location:**
**Mu Guan** is at the base of the palm of the hand about 0.5 cun distal to the pisiform bone.

**Gu Guan** is at the base of the palm of the hand in the depression about 0.5 cun distal to the scaphoid bone.

**Reaction areas:** Kidney, Lung

**Indications:**

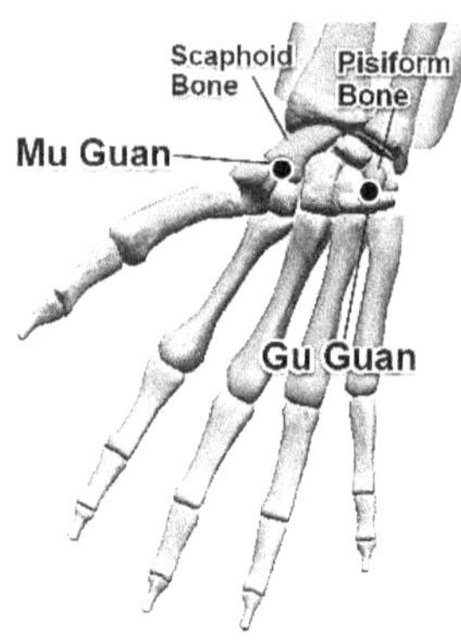


- SYSTEMIC BONE SWELLING, SYSTEMIC ARTHRITIS
- RHEUMATOID ARTHRITIS
- OSTEOARTHRITIS PAIN
- HEEL PAIN
- INSTEP PAIN
- PLANTAR FASCIITIS

**Manipulation:** Touch the bone when inserting perpendicularly. Can add P-7 to increase effectiveness when treating heel pain.

## ZONE 33-Forearm

### 33.01 Qi Men

### (THIS DOOR)

**Location:**
Located on the radial side of the forearm on the line between LI-4 and LI-11, 2 cun proximal to the wrist crease. On the Large Intestine channel.

**Associated channel:** Large Intestine

**Reaction area:** Lung.

**Dao Ma:** 33.01+33.02+33.03

**Indications:**

- HEMORRHOIDS
- CHRONIC IBS
- SPLEEN AND STOMACH DISHARMONIES
- ANAL PROLAPSE, BLEEDING
- CONSTIPATION
- IRREGULAR MENSTRUATION
- LEUCORRHEA WITH REDDISH DISCHARGE

**Manipulation:** Insertion of 0.5 to 1.0 cun in depth. Oblique insertion towards LI-11 for tonification (more common) and towards the wrist for sedation.

# 33.02 Qi Jiao
(THIS CORNER)

**Location:**
The point is located on the radial side of the forearm between LI-5 and LI-11, 4 cun proximal to the wrist crease. 2 cun posterior to 33.01. On the Large Intestine Channel.

**Associated channel:** Large Intestine

**Reaction area:** Lung.

**Dao Ma:** 33.01+33.02+33.03

**Indications:**
- HEMORRHOIDS
- ANAL PROLAPSE, BLEEDING
- CONSTIPATION
- IRREGULAR MENSTRUATION
- LEUCORRHEA WITH REDDISH DISCHARGE

**Manipulation:** Insertion of 0.5 to 1.0 cun in depth.  Oblique insertion.

# 33.03 Qi Zheng
(THIS UPRIGHTNESS)

**Location:** On the radial aspect of the forearm, halfway between LI-5 and LI-11, 6 cun from the wrist crease, and 2 cun posterior to 33.02. On the Large Intestine channel.

**Associated channel:** Large Intestine

**Reaction area:** Lung.

**Dao Ma:** 33.01+33.02+33.03

**Indications:**
- HEMORRHOIDS
- ANAL PROLAPSE, BLEEDING
- CONSTIPATION
- IRREGULAR MENSTRUATION
- LEUCORRHEA WITH REDDISH DISCHARGE

**Manipulation:** Insertion of 0.5 to 1.0 cun in depth.  Oblique insertion.

# 33.04 Huo Chuan
(FIRE THREADED)

**Location:**
3 cun proximal to the wrist joint on the dorsal side, in the depression in the midline between the radius and ulna. Close to the border of the radius, radial side of muscle and tendon. On the San Jiao channel.

**Overlaps:** SJ-6

**Associated Channel:** Sanjiao

**Reaction area:** Heart and Lung.

**Dao Ma:** 33.04+33.05+33.06

**Indications:**
- CONSTIPATION
- HEART PALPITATION (FAST HEART BEAT)
- OPPOSITE SIDE HAND/FOREARM PAIN
- CHEST PAIN AND FULLNESS
- RIB PAIN
- SPRAINED ANKLE
- STIFF NECK
- ACUTE SPRAIN IN WRIST
- ACUTE SPRAIN IN LOWER BACK.

**Manipulation:**
Insertion of 0.3 to 0.5 cun in depth.

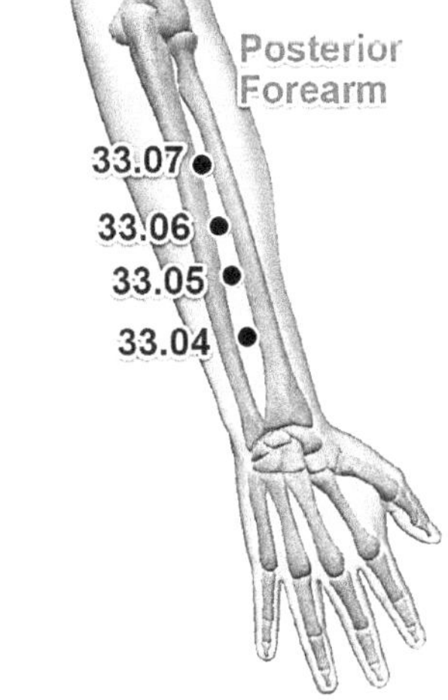


# 33.05 Huo Ling
(FIRE MOUND)

**Location:**
2 cun proximal to 33.04 (Huo Chuan - Fire Threaded).
On the San Jiao channel.

**Associated Channel:** Sanjiao

**Reaction area:** Heart

**Dao Ma:** 33.04+33.05+33.06

**Indications:**
- PAIN, STUFFINESS, AND DISTENDING FEELING IN THE CHEST
- ARM, FOREARM, HAND SPASM
- SCIATICA THAT RADIATES ALONG SHAO YANG (GB) CHANNEL.

**Manipulation:** Insertion of 0.3 to 0.5 cun in depth.

# 33.06 Huo Shan
(FIRE MOUNTAIN)

**Location:**
1.5 cun proximal to 33.05 (Huo Ling - Fire Mound). On the San Jiao channel.

**Associated Channel:** Sanjiao

**Reaction area:** Heart

**Dao Ma:** 33.04+33.05+33.06

**Indications:**
- PAIN, STUFFINESS, AND DISTENDING FEELING IN THE CHEST
- ARM, FOREARM, HAND SPASM
- SCIATICA THAT RADIATES ALONG SHAO YANG (GB) CHANNEL.

**Manipulation:** Insertion of 0.3 to 0.5 cun in depth.

# 33.07 Huo Fu Hai
(FIRE BOWELS SEA)

**Location:**
2 cun proximal to Huo 33.06, on the prominence of the muscle.
On the San Jiao channel.

**Overlaps:** LI-10

**Associated channel:** Large Intestine

**Reaction area:** Lung and Heart

**Indications:**
- ASTHMA
- COMMON COLD
- RHINITIS
- COUGH
- SHORTNESS OF BREATH (DYSPNEA)
- ANEMIA
- EXHAUSTION
- DIZZINESS
- BLURRED VISION
- RASH ON THE ARMS
- TENNIS ELBOW
- WAIST, LOWER BACK OR LEG PAIN
- SCIATICA

**Manipulation:** Insertion of 0.5 to 1.0 cun in depth.

# 33.08 Shou Wu Jin
(HAND FIVE GOLD)

**Location:**
On the lateral side of the ulna, 6.5 cun proximal from the wrist crease. 0.5 cun ulnar to 33.06.  (0.5 cun lateral to San Jiao channel).

**Associated Channel:** Between Sanjiao and Small Intestine

**Reaction area:** Liver.

**Dao Ma:** 33.08+33.09

**Indications:**
- BL OR GB SCIATICA
- ABDOMINAL PAIN
- DISTENDING FEELING OF THE LEG

- PAIN AND NUMBNESS OF THE FEET
- ADD 33.09 FOR ARM PAIN, WRIST ISSUES AND FROZEN SHOULDER.

**Manipulation:**
Insertion of 0.3 to 0.5 cun in depth.

**Remarks:** Since 33.08+33.09 improves systemic blood flow, they are useful to supplement any pain protocols.

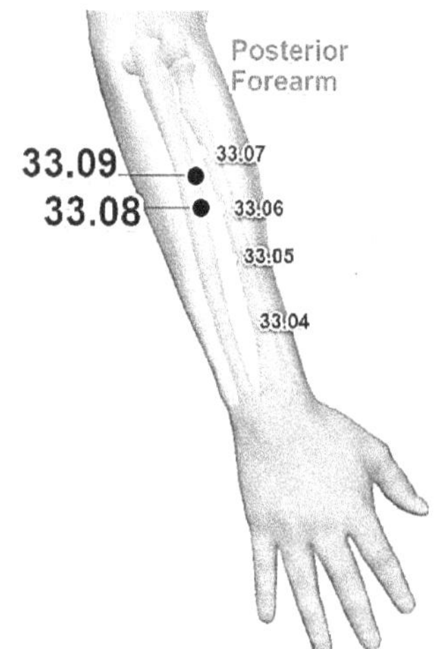


# 33.09 Shou Qian Jin

(HAND THOUSAND GOLD)

**Location:**
On the lateral side of the ulna, 1.5 cun proximal to 33.08. 8 cun proximal from the wrist crease. (0.5 cun lateral to San Jiao)

**Associated Channel:** Between Sanjiao and Small Intestine

**Reaction area:** Lung

**Dao Ma:** 33.08+33.09

**Indications:**
- BL OR GB SCIATICA
- FOREARM PAIN
- ABDOMINAL PAIN
- DISTENDING FEELING OF THE LEG
- PAIN AND NUMBNESS OF THE FEET.

**Manipulation:**
Insertion of 0.3 to 0.5 cun in depth.

# 33.10 Chang Men

(INTESTINE GATE)

**Location:** On the medial side of the ulna, 3 cun proximal to the pisiform bone. On Small Intestine channel.

**Associated Channel:** Small Intestine

**Reaction areas:** Liver and Kidney

**Dao Ma:** 33.10+33.11

**Indications:**
- ENTERITIS CAUSED BY HEPATITIS
- ACUTE ABDOMINAL PAIN
- HEPATITIS WITH INTESTINAL ISSUES
- DIARRHEA
- HEMORRHOIDS
- DIZZINESS
- BLURRED VISION

**Manipulation:** Insertion of 0.5 to 0.8 cun in depth.

**Remarks:** Treats all intestinal disorders. Useful for digestive issues caused by a gallbladder disorder.

Use acupressure on this point to control unwanted bowel movement.

# 33.11 Gan Men

(LIVER GATE)

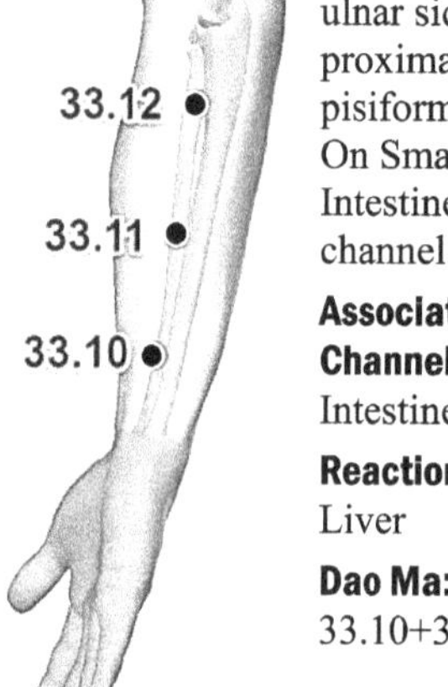


**Location:** On the ulnar side, 6 cun proximal to the pisiform bone. On Small Intestine channel.

**Associated Channel:** Small Intestine

**Reaction area:** Liver

**Dao Ma:** 33.10+33.11

**Indications:**
- ACUTE HEPATITIS (MOST EFFECTIVE)
- LOW RED BLOOD CELL COUNT
- CIRRHOSIS
- INTESTINAL PAIN
- CONSTIPATION
- JAUNDICE
- CHEST OPPRESSION
- CALF CRAMP

**Manipulation:**
Insertion of 0.3 to 0.5 cun on left side.

**Remarks:** Treats all issues caused by a congested and "sick" liver.

# 33.12 Xin Men

(HEART GATE)

**Location:**
In the depression on the medial side of the inferior ulna, 1.5 to 2.0 cun distal to the elbow. On Small Intestine channel.

**Overlaps:** SI-8

**Associated Channel:** Small Intestine

**Reaction area:** Heart

**Indications:**
- GROIN/SACRAL/COCCYX PAIN
- MEDIAL KNEE PAIN
- MEDIAL ELBOW PAIN
- CARDITIS
- HEART PALPITATIONS
- SUFFOCATING FEELING IN THE CHEST
- VOMITING
- DRY CHOLERA
- MEDIAL THIGH/GROIN PAIN
- SCIATIC PAIN ALONG THE BLADDER CHANNEL
- PAIN OF THE TAIL BONE, WHEN NEEDLING CLOSE TO THE BONE.

**Manipulation:** Insertion of 0.4 to 0.7 cun in depth.

**Remarks:** Treats heart, chest, stress, hypertension, tightness and pain in the upper chest cavity. When combined with 33.10 and 33.11, it treats those affected by poor digestion, liver congestion and weak heart (typical ailments from modern living).

# 33.13 Ren Shi

(HUMAN SCHOLAR)

**Location:**
On the medial side of the radius of the ventral forearm, 4 cun proximal to the wrist crease. On the Lung channel or Pericardium channel.

**Associated Channel:** Lung

**Reaction areas:** Heart, Lung

**Indications:**
- ASTHMA
- COUGH
- HEART DISEASE/PALPITATIONS
- PALM OR FINGER PAIN
- SHOULDER PAIN
- BACK PAIN
- CALF SPASM

**Manipulation:**
Insertion of 0.5 to 1.0 cun in depth.

**Remarks:**

0.5 insertion for asthma, finger pain, arm pain, back pain (opposite side insertion). 1 cun insertion for heart disease and heart palpitation.

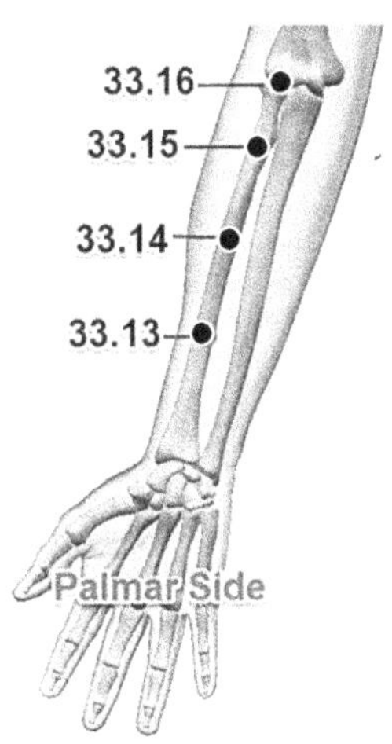


## 33.14 Di Shi
(EARTH SCHOLAR)

**Location:**
On the medial border of the radius 3.0 cun proximal to 33.13. On the Lung channel or Pericardium channel.

**Overlaps:** LU-6

**Associated Channel:** Lung

**Reaction areas:** Lung and Heart.

**Dao Ma:** 33.13+33.14+33.15

**Indications:**
- ASTHMA
- COMMON COLD
- HEADACHE
- WEAKNESS OF KIDNEY FUNCTION
- HEART DISEASE

**Manipulation:** Insert 1.0 cun for the treatment of asthma, common cold, headache, and deficiency in the kidney; insert 1.5 cun in depth to treat heart disease. An example of "deeper for further, shallower for closer".

**Remarks:** 33.14+33.15+33.16 treat all respiratory issues, allergies and heart conditions caused by a lung dysfunction.

## 33.15 Tian Shi
(HEAVEN SCHOLAR)

**Location:** On the medial aspect of the posterior radius, 3.0 cun proximal to 33.14. On the Lung channel or Pericardium channel.

**Associated Channel:** Lung

**Reaction areas:** Lung and Kidney.

**Dao Ma:** 33.13+33.14+33.15

**Indications:**

- ASTHMA (NEEDLE BOTH SIDES)
- RHINITIS
- ARM PAIN
- COMMON COLD
- CHEST FULLNESS
- UPPER ARM PAIN

**Manipulation:**
Insertion of 1.0 to 1.5 cun in depth.

## 33.16 Qu Ling
(CURVED MOUND)

**Location:**
In the crease of the cubital fossa and on the radial side of the tendon of m. biceps brachii. On the Lung channel.

**Overlaps:** LU-5

**Associated Channel:** Lung

**Reaction areas:** Heart and Lung.

**Indications:**

- BLEED FOR ASTHMA AND SHOULDER PAIN
- PNEUMONIA
- SORE THROAT
- TONSILLITIS
- SPASM
- DRY CHOLERA
- CHRONIC HEADACHE
- INFLAMMATION OF THE ELBOW JOINT
- MYOCARDIAL INFARCTION
- HEART PALPITATION
- CARDIOPLEGIA – BLEED
- STROKE WITH HEMIPLEGIA
- INFLAMMATION OF THE ELBOW
- DIARRHEA
- ACUTE GASTROENTERITIS

**Manipulation:** Insertion of 0.5 to 1.0 cun in depth. Commonly bled visible veins for any upper body issues (for spine and entire body, bleed Bl-40 area). When needling, slide by the biceps tendon.

## ZONE 44-Upper Arm

## 44.01 Fen Jin
(DIVIDING GOLD)

**Location:**
On the anterior side of the humerus of the upper arm, 1.5 cun proximal to the cubital fossa crease. On the Lung Channel. 44.01 is located on the Lung channel 3 cun distal to LU-4 and 1.5 cun proximal to LU-5

**Associated Channel:** Lung

**Reaction areas:** Lung and Heart.

**Indications:**

- COMMON COLD
- RHINITIS (NASAL INFLAMMATION)
- LARYNGITIS (THROAT INFLAMMATION)
- COUGH

**Manipulation:** Insertion of 0.5 to 1.0 cun in depth.

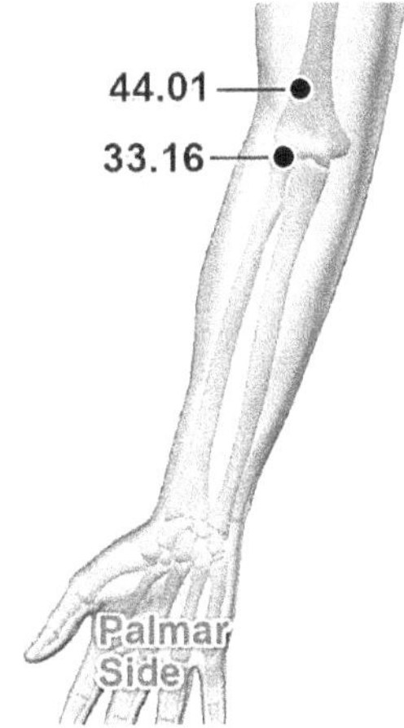


## 44.02 Hou Zhui
(BACK VERTEBRAE)

**Location:**
On the posterior side of the humerus of the upper arm, 2.5 cun proximal to the olecranon. On the San Jiao channel. 0.5 cun proximal to SJ-11

**Associated Channel:** Sanjiao

**Reaction areas:** Liver, Heart and Spine.

**Dao Ma:** 44.02+44.03

**Indications:**

- SPINE PAIN/DEGENERATION
- HERNIATED DISC OF VERTEBRAE
- NEPHRITIS
- LOWER BACK PAIN.

**Manipulation:** Insertion of 0.3 to 0.5 cun in depth. Long needle retention for one hour or more is effective.

## 44.03 Shou Ying
(HEAD WISDOM)

**Location:** On the posterior side of the humerus, 4.5 cun proximal to the elbow joint. On the San Jiao channel. 44.03 is 1.5 cun distal to SJ-12.

**Associated Channel:** Sanjiao

**Reaction areas:** Liver, Heart and Spine.

**Dao Ma:** 44.02+44.03

**Indications:**

- SPINE PAIN/DEGENERATION
- HERNIATED DISC OF VERTEBRAE
- NEPHRITIS
- LOWER BACK PAIN.

**Manipulation:** Insertion of 0.3 to 0.5 cun in depth. Long needle retention for one hour or more is effective.

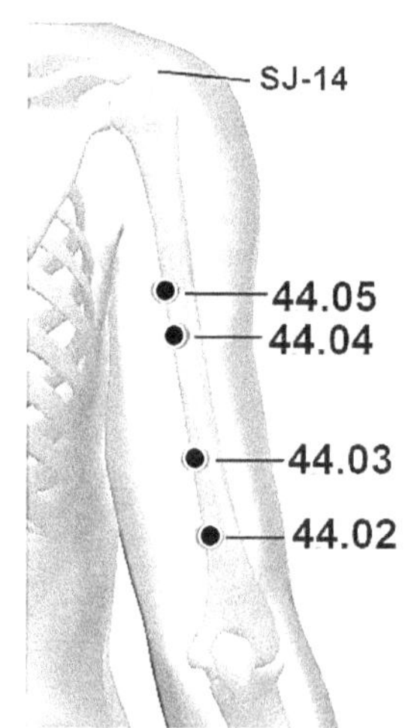


# 44.04 Fu Ding
(WEALTH APEX)

**Location:**
On the posterior side of the humerus of the upper arm, 2.5 cun superior to 44.03, and 7 cun proximal to the olecranon. On the San Jiao channel. 44.04 is 1 cun proximal to SJ-12.

**Associated Channel:** Sanjiao

**Reaction areas:** Liver and Heart.

**Dao Ma:** 44.04 +44.05

**Indications:**

- FATIGUE
- HYPOFUNCTION OF LIVER
- HYPERTENSION
- DIZZINESS
- HEADACHE
- STIFF NECK
- FACIAL PARALYSIS

**Manipulation:** Insert 0.3 cun depth for tiredness and liver weakness. 0.5 cun depth for headache, dizziness and hypertension.

# 44.05 Hou Zhi
(BACK BRANCH)

**Location:** On the line between SJ-14 and the elbow, and 1.0 cun proximal to 44.04, and 8 cun proximal to the olecranon. On the San Jiao channel. 44.05 is 2 cun proximal to SJ-12 and 1 cun distal to SJ-13.

**Associated Channel:** Sanjiao

**Reaction areas:** Heart

**Dao Ma:** 44.04 +44.05

**Indications:**

- FATIGUE
- HYPOFUNCTION OF LIVER
- HYPERTENSION
- DIZZINESS
- HEADACHE
- STIFF NECK
- FACIAL PARALYSIS
- ARTERIOSCLEROSIS
- DELAYED HEALING OF WOUNDS
- SKIN DISEASES

**Manipulation:** Insert 0.3 cun depth for tiredness and liver weakness. 0.5 cun depth for headache, dizziness and hypertension.

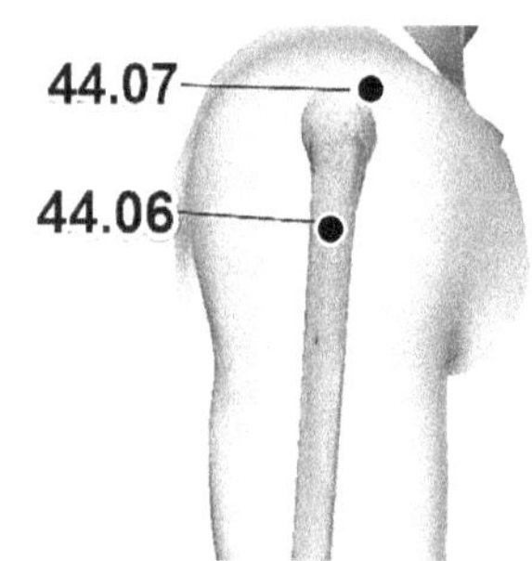


# 44.06 Jian Zhong
(SHOULDER CENTER)

**Location:**
On the lateral side of the humerus, 2.5 to 3 cun (size of deltoid varies) inferior to the acromion joint. On the Large Intestine channel.

**Associated Channel:** Large Intestine

**Reaction areas:** Heart

**Indications:**

- KNEE PAIN
- NECK RASH
- POLIO
- HEMIPLEGIA
- HEART PALPITATIONS
- ARTERIOSCLEROSIS
- NOSE BLEED
- SINUS CONGESTION

- SHOULDER PAIN (FROZEN SHOULDER)
- LEG WEAKNESS
- MUSCLE ATROPHY

**Manipulation:**
Insertion of 0.5 to 1.0 cun in depth. Palpate for tender point.

**Remarks:** Useful for nose, heart conditions, knee pain, fatigue, dampness, spleen and stomach issues, Qi and blood deficiency.

# 44.07 Bei Mian
(BACK FACE)

**Location:**
In the center of the acromion joint, in the depression when the arm is raised.

**Overlaps:** LI-15

**Associated Channel:** Large Intestine

**Reaction area:** Abdomen

**Indications:**

- FATIGUE/GENERAL WEAKNESS
- ABDOMINAL DISTENSION
- WEAK VOICE
- LEG WEAKNESS
- DEAFNESS/TINNITUS

**Manipulation:** Insertion of 0.3 to 0.5 cun in depth. Effective when bled. Bleed-cup around tender area.

# 44.08 Ren Zong
(HUMAN ANCESTOR)

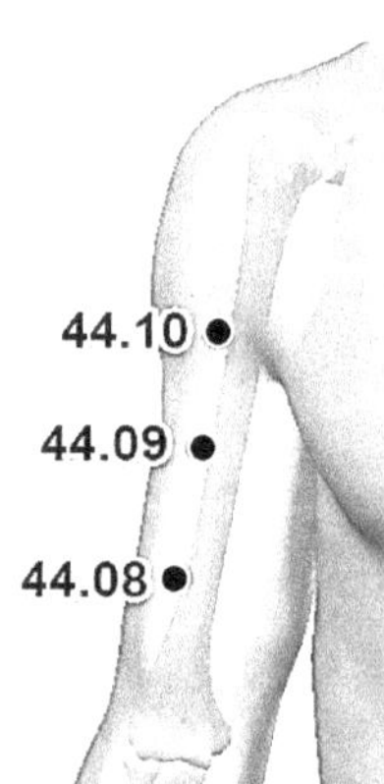


**Location:**
Flex the elbow and place the palm on the chest. Locate the point in the depression between the inner border of the humerus and the brachial biceps muscle, 3 cun superior to the cubital crease. Some locate this on the lung channel, some between lung and large intestine.

**Overlaps:** LI-13

**Associated Channel:** Lung and Large Intestine

**Reaction areas:** Lung, Heart and Liver

**Dao Ma:** 44.08+44.09+44.10

**Indications:**

- ASTHMA
- COMMON COLD
- FOOT AND HAND PAIN
- PAINFUL AND SWOLLEN ELBOW
- MOTOR IMPAIRMENT/MUSCLE ATROPHY/POLIO
- YELLOW COMPLEXION DUE TO GALLBLADDER DISEASE
- EDEMA
- SPLENOMEGALY
- LEUKEMIA

**Manipulation:** Insertion of 0.5 cun for cold and asthma; 0.8 cun for swollen arm; 1.2 cun for liver, gall bladder and spleen diseases. Precaution required because of underlying artery.

## 44.09 Di Zong
(EARTH ANCESTOR)

**Location:**
3 cun superior to 44.08, 6 cun proximal to the cubital crease. With the palm placed on the chest, locate the point in the depression between the inner border of the center of the humerus and biceps muscle, 3 cun proximal to 44.08. Some locate this on the lung channel, some between lung and large intestine. 1 cun below LI-14.

**Associated Channel:** Lung and Large Intestine

**Reaction areas:** Heart

**Dao Ma:** 44.08+44.09+44.10

**Indications:**
- RESUSCITATION POINT
- HEART DISEASE
- ARTERIOSCLEROSIS.

**Manipulation:** Insertion of 1.0 cun for mild disease; 2.0 cun for critical diseases.

## 44.10 Tian Zong
(HEAVENLY ANCESTOR)

**Location:**
With the palm placed on the chest, locate the point in the depression between the inner side of the humerus and the posterior aspect of the biceps muscle, 3 cun proximal to 44.09 and 9 cun proximal to the cubital crease. Some locate this on the lung channel, and some locate between lung and large intestine. 2 cun above LI-14.

**Associated Channel:** Lung and Large Intestine

**Reaction areas:** Legs, Six bowels

**Dao Ma:** 44.08+44.09+44.10

**Indications:**
- VAGINAL ITCHING OR PAIN
- LEUKORRHEA WITH REDDISH DISCHARGE
- CALF PAIN
- BODY ODOR
- DIABETES
- MUSCLE ATROPHY
- LOWER LEG PAIN

**Manipulation:**
Insertion of 1.0 to 1.5 cun in depth.

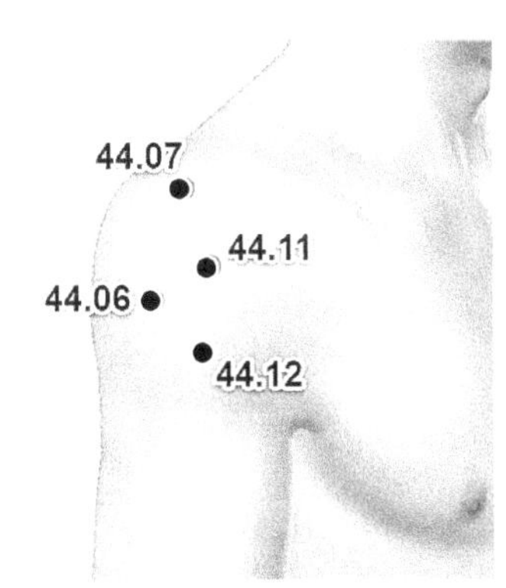


## 44.11 Yun Bai
(CLOUD WHITE)

**Location:**
1.0 cun anterior and superior to 44.06 (center of deltois muscle).  Between Large Intestine and Lung channels.

**Associated Channel:** Lung and Large Intestine

**Reaction areas:** Lung and Six bowels

**Indications:**
- VAGINITIS
- VAGINAL PAIN
- LEUKORRHEA WITH REDDISH DISCHARGE
- POLIO
- HIP AND CALF PAIN/WEAKNESS
- MUSCLE ATROPHY/HEMIPLEGIA

**Manipulation:**
Insertion of 0.3 to 0.5 cun in depth.

## 44.12 LI Bai
(PLUM WHITE)

**Location:**
2 cun slightly lateral and inferior to 44.11.  Between Large Intestine and Lung channels.

**Associated Channel:** Between Large Intestine and Lung

**Reaction areas:** Lung and Kidney

**Indications:**
- BODY ODOR
- EXCESSIVE SWEATING OF ARMPITS
- FOOT AND CALF PAIN
- POLIO

**Manipulation:**
Insertion of 0.3 to 0.5 cun in depth.

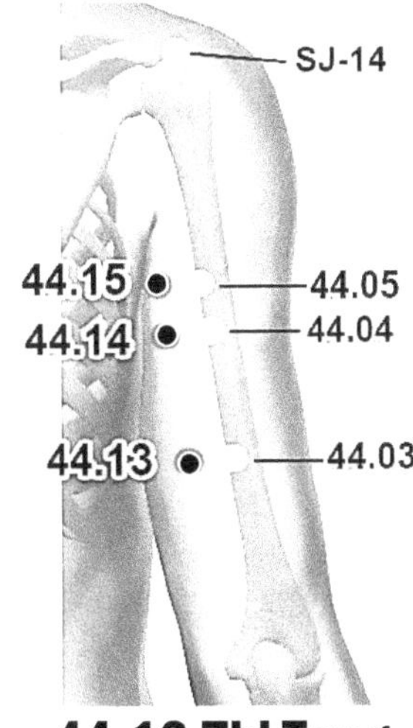


## 44.13 Zhi Tong
(BRANCH CONNECT)

**Location:**
Locate the point directly inferior to the shoulder joint, on the posterior arm, 4.5 cun superior to the cubital crease, or 1.0 cun posterior to 44.03. Insert the needle along the medial side of the humerus. On the Small Intestine channel.

**Associated Channel:** Small Intestine

**Reaction areas:** Kidney, Liver and Back

**Dao Ma:** 44.13+44.14

**Indications:**
- HYPERTENSION
- ARTERIOSCLEROSIS
- DIZZINESS
- FATIGUE
- LOWER BACK ACHING PAIN
- WEAKNESS IN UPPER/LOWER LIMBS

**Manipulation:**
Insertion of 0.6 to 1.0 cun in depth.

## 44.14 Luo Tong

(DROP CONNECT)

**Location:**
Locate the point directly inferior to the posterior acromion, on the posterior aspect of the arm, 7.0 cun above the cubital crease, or 1.0 cun posterior to 44.04. On the Small Intestine channel.

**Associated Channel:** Small Intestine

**Reaction areas:** Kidney, Liver and Back

**Dao Ma:** 44.13+44.14

**Indications:**
- HYPERTENSION DUE TO LIVER AND KIDNEY ISSUES
- ARTERIOSCLEROSIS
- DIZZINESS
- FATIGUE
- WEAKNESS OF LIMBS
- ACHING PAIN OF THE LOWER BACK

**Manipulation:**
Insertion of 0.6 to 1.0 cun in depth.

## 44.15 Xia Qu

(LOWER CURVE)

**Location:**
On the posterior aspect of the arm, directly below the posterior aspect of the acromion, 1 cun posterior to 44.05. On the Small Intestine channel.

**Associated Channel:** Small Intestine

**Reaction areas:** Liver and Lung

**Dao Ma:** 44.15+44.16

**Indications:**
- HYPERTENSION
- SCIATICA DUE TO WEAK FUNCTION OF LUNG AND LIVER
- HEMIPLEGIA
- POLIO
- NERVE DAMAGE DUE TO INJURY, STENOSIS
- DISLOCATION OF JOINTS DUE TO NERVE LOSS.
- CERVICAL INJURY.

**Manipulation:**
Insertion of 0.6 to 1.0 cun in depth.

## 44.16 Shang Qu

(UPPER CURVE)

**Location:**
On the posterior aspect of the arm, 1.0 cun posterior to 44.06.

**Associated Channel:** Between Large Intestine and Sanjiao

**Reaction areas:** Liver and Kidney

**Dao Ma:** 44.15+44.16

**Indications:**
- CIRRHOSIS
- HEPATITIS
- UPPER ARM PAIN
- LOWER LEG PAIN
- HYPERTENSION
- HEMIPLEGIA
- POLIO
- SCIATICA (LUNG AND LIVER DEFICIENT TYPE)

**Manipulation:**
Insertion of 0.6 to 1.5 cun in depth. Prick to bleed for hepatitis/cirrhosis

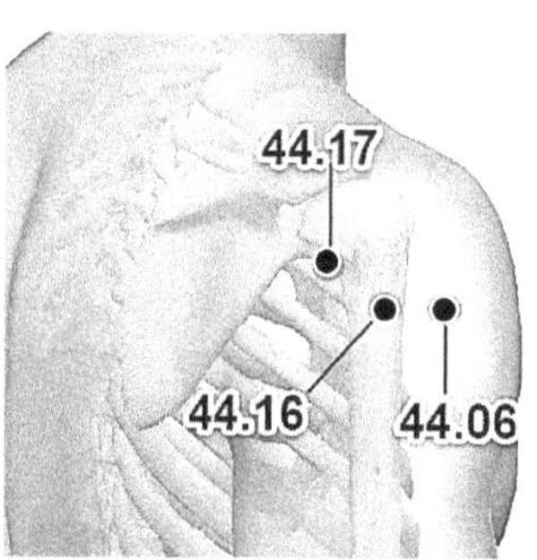


## 44.17 Shui Yu

(WATER CURVE)

**Location:**
On the posterior aspect of the arm, 2 cun obliquely posterior and inferior to 44.07. 3 cun posterior to 44.11, close to SI channel.

**Associated Channel:** Small intestine

**Reaction areas:** Kidney

**Indications:**
- NEPHRITIS
- CALCULUS OF THE KIDNEY
- LOWER BACK PAIN
- ACHING PAIN OF LEGS
- FOOT NUMBNESS AND WEAKNESS
- GENERAL DEBILITY
- PROTEINURIA
- PAIN OF THE ARM, WRIST, AND DORSUM OF HAND.

**Manipulation:**
Insertion of 0.3 to 0.5 cun in depth. Bleed to increase effectiveness.

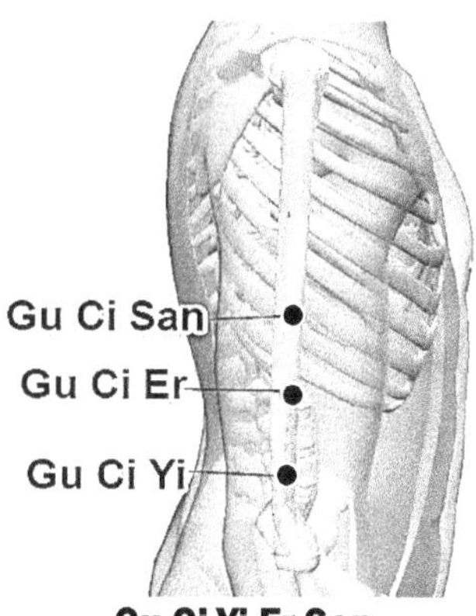


**Gu Ci Yi Er San**

(BONE SPUR ONE TWO THREE)

**Location:**
**Gu Ci Yi** is located 2 cun directly proximal to LI-11 on the LI Channel.

**Gu Ci Er** is 2 cun proximal to Gu Ci Yi on the LI Channel.

**Gu Ci San** is 2 cun proximal to Gu Ci Er on the LI Channel.

**Associated Channel:** Large Intestine

**Reaction areas:** Liver, Kidney

**Indications:**
Bone spurs, sour pain of the vertebrae, injury of the spine, back pain caused by spine issues.

**Manipulation:**
Needles should tap the humerus.

**Remarks:** While 22.05 Ling Gu treats lower back pain, Gu Ci Yi Er San treat the entire spine.

# ZONE 55-Plantar Foot

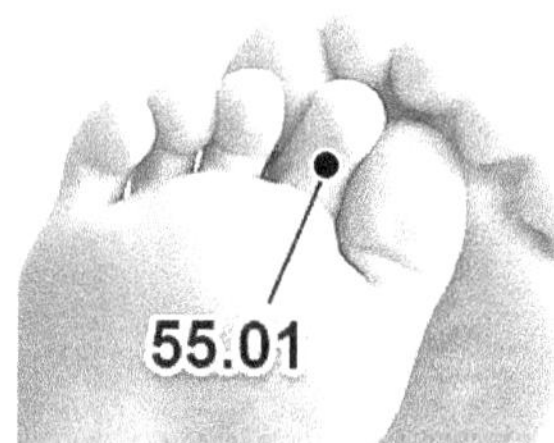


**55.01 Huo Bao**

(FIRE BAG)

**Location:**
In the center of the distal crease of the plantar side of the 2nd toe. Shared location with EX-LE-11 Du Yin.

**Associated Channel:** Stomach

**Reaction areas:** Heart and Liver

**Indications:**

- ANGINA PECTORIS/HEART ATTACK (USE PROMPT-PRICK)
- LIVER DISEASE
- DIFFICULT LABOR
- RETENTION OF PLACENTA
- EXCESSIVE BLEEDING AFTER DELIVERY
- ABNORMAL MENSTRUATION
- INTESTINAL HERNIA (ACUTE)
- NUMBNESS OF THE TOES

**Manipulation:**
Insertion of 0.3 to 0.5 cun in depth or use triangular needle. Usually bleed any veins on underside of second toe.

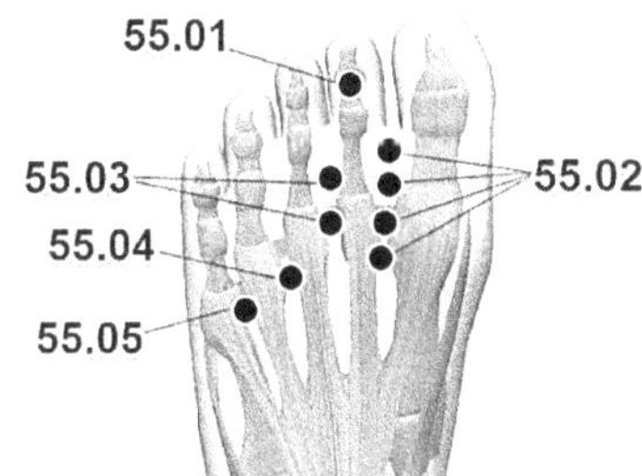


# 55.02 Hua Gu Yi
(FLOWER BONE, ONE)

**Location:**
Between the 1st and 2nd metatarsal bones on the plantar surface. The first point is located 0.5 cun posterior to the joint of the big toe and 2nd toe; the second point is 0.5 cun from the first one; the third is 0.5 cun from the second one; the fourth is 0.8 cun from the third.

**Associated Channel:** Liver

**Reaction areas:** Kidney, Lung, Spleen

**Indications:**
- CATARACTS
- GLAUCOMA
- NIGHT BLINDNESS
- NEAR/FAR SIGHTEDNESS
- OPTIC NERVE ATROPHY
- MACULAR DEGENERATION
- TRACHOMA
- CONJUNCTIVITIS
- EYE LID INFLAMMATION
- TEARS ON EXPOSURE TO WIND
- PHOTOPHOBIA
- ACHING PAIN OF THE NASAL BONE
- HEADACHE
- DEAFNESS
- TINNITUS

**Manipulation:**
Insertion of 0.5 to 1.0 cun in depth. Suitable for bilateral needling. Long needle retention required.

Can reach 55.02 from the top of the foot at LIV-2 to LIV-3 or 66.04.

**Remarks:** Commonly used for eye, head and nose issues.

# 55.03 Hua Gu Er
(FLOWER BONE, TWO)

**Location:**
Between the 2nd and 3rd metatarsal bones on the plantar surface. The first point is 1.0 cun posterior to the joint of the toes and the second point is 0.5 cun posterior to the first one.

**Associated Channel:** Stomach

**Reaction areas:** Spleen

**Indications:**
- BLOOD SUGAR ISSUES
- FINGER WEAKNESS
- ARM PAIN/WEAKNESS
- FROZEN SHOULDER

**Manipulation:**
Insertion of 0.5 to 1.0 cun in depth. 45 minutes retention.

# 55.04 Hua Gu San
(FLOWER BONE, THREE)

**Location:**
Between the 3rd and 4th metatarsal bones on the plantar aspect. 2.0 cun posterior to the joint of the two toes.

**Associated Channel:** Gallbladder

**Reaction areas:** Spleen

**Dao ma:** 55.04+55.05

**Indications:**
- LOW BACK PAIN
- SCIATICA
- SPINE PAIN
- SACRAL/COCCYX PAIN
- LEG AND FOOT NUMBNESS
- REDDENED EYE

**Manipulation:**
Insertion of 0.5 to 1.0 cun in depth.

# 55.05 Hua Gu Si
(FLOWER BONE, FOUR)

**Location:**
Patient in supine position, longitudinally 1.5 cun from the joint between the 4th and 5th metatarsal bones.

**Associated Channel:** Gallbladder

**Reaction areas:** Lung

**Dao ma:** 55.04+55.05

**Indications:**
- SACRAL/COCCYX PAIN
- SPINE PAIN
- SCIATICA
- PAIN IN THE LOWER ABDOMEN
- GASTRIC PAIN
- STOPS BLEEDING
- NUMBNESS IN THE EXTREMITIES.

**Manipulation:**
Insertion of 0.5 to 1.0 cun in depth. Bilateral.

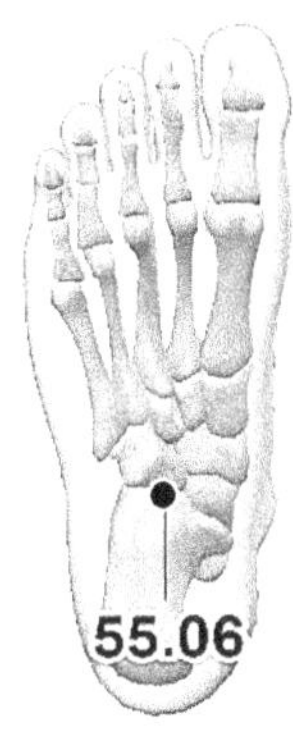


# 55.06 Shang Liu
(UPPER TUMOR)

**Location:**
Center of the anterior edge of heel.

**Variation 1:** 3 points. Add two additional points, 0.3 cun on either side of 55.06.

**Variation 2:** 2 points. Add one additional point 1.0 cun distal to 55.06.

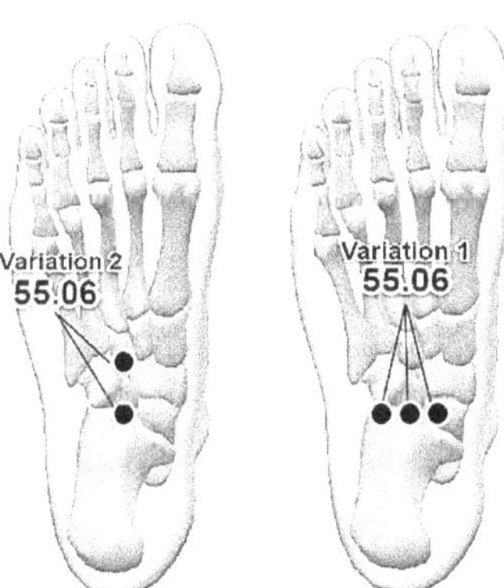


**Associated Channel:** Kidney

**Reaction area:** Cerebellum

**Indications:**
- BRAIN TUMOR
- SEVERE HEADACHE

- HYDROCEPHALUS
- CRANIAL NERVE PAIN
- CONCUSSION
- DEBILITY
- INSOMNIA
- COMA
- EPILEPSY
- HYPERTENSION

**Manipulation:**
Insertion of 0.3 to 0.5 cun in depth. Too deep may cause nausea. Upon insertion head should clear. If it does not and head feels distended, remove the needles.

**Remarks:** Treats the head and brain.

# ZONE 66-Dorsal Foot

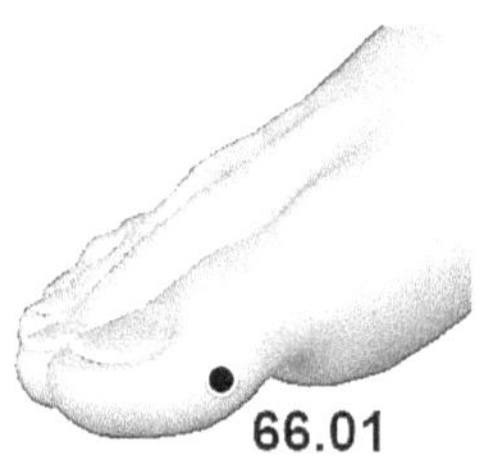

# 66.01 Hai Bao

(SEAL)

**Location:**

In the center of the posterior medial side of the big toe, anterior to SP-2.

**Associated Channel:** Spleen

**Reaction area:** Heart

**Overlaps:** Between SP-1 and SP-2

**Indications:**
- THUMB PAIN (HIGHLY EFFECTIVE)
- INDEX FINGER PAIN
- CONJUNCTIVITIS, CANTHUS PAIN
- INGUINAL HERNIA
- VAGINITIS
- EYE PAIN
- TAIL BONE PAIN
- FREQUENT URINATION

**Manipulation:**
Insertion of 0.1 to 0.3 cun in depth. Tap the distal phalanx.

**Remarks:** Great for thumb pain. Needle opposite side and combine with 11.27.

# 66.02 Mu Fu

(WOOD WIFE)

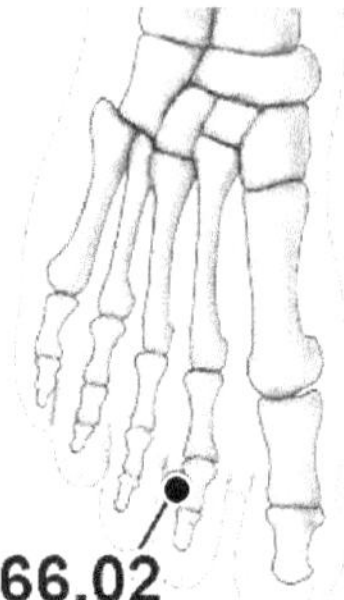

**Location:**
0.3 cun lateral from the center of the middle segment of the 2nd toe on the dorsal side.

**Associated Channel:**
Stomach

**Reaction area:** Heart

**Indications:**
- LEUKORRHEA WITH REDDISH OR WHITE DISCHARGE
- IRREGULAR MENSTRUATION
- DYSMENORRHEA, AMENORRHEA
- METRITIS, UTERINE INFLAMMATION
- BLOCKED FALLOPIAN TUBE
- INFERTILITY

**Manipulation:**
Insertion of 0.2 to 0.4 cun in depth.

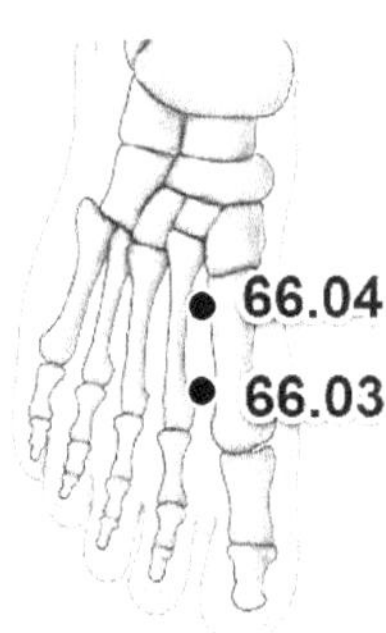

# 66.03 Huo Ying

(FIRE HARD)

**Location:**
Between the 1st and 2nd metatarsal bones, 0.5 cun from the metatarsal and phalangeal joints, on the dorsal surface. Proximal (0.5 cun posterior) to LV-2. On the Liver channel.

**Associated Channel:** Liver

**Reaction area:** Heart and Liver

**Dao ma:** 66.03+66.04

**Indications:**
- CHIN PAIN, JAW PAIN, TMJ, TINNITUS
- MYOCARDITIS
- HEART PALPITATIONS, SUDDEN REDUCTION OF BLOOD TO BRAIN, FAINTING, COMA

- HYPERTENSION
- DIZZINESS, FRIGHT
- ANXIETY AND INSOMNIA
- RETENTION OF PLACENTA
- ENLARGEMENT OF BONES
- EYE PAIN, KNEE SWELLING
- METRITIS (INFLAMMATION OF UTERINE WALL), TUMORS OF THE UTERUS, FIBROIDS
- URINARY TRACT INFECTION
- DORSAL FOOT PAIN (OPPOSITE SIDE)
- FINGER NUMBNESS
- GROIN/KNEE PAIN (GUIDE POINT)
- IMPOTENCE

**Manipulation:**
Insertion of 0.5 to 1.0 cun in depth. Forbidden needling during pregnancy.

**Remarks:** Treats TMJ, headaches, circulation issues, heart problems and bleeding in the groin or gynecological area.

# 66.04 Huo Zhu

(FIRE MASTER)

**Location:**
1 cun posterior to 66.03. Proximal to LIV-3.

**Overlaps or near to:** LIV-3

**Associated Channel:** Liver

**Reaction Area:** Heart

**Dao ma:** 66.03+66.04

**Indications:**
- TMJ, DEVIATION OF MOUTH AND EYE, FACIAL PARALYSIS, DIFFICULTY IN OPENING MOUTH, JAW PAIN
- DIFFICULT LABOR
- KNEE PAIN (ARTHRITIS)
- GROIN PAIN
- DORSAL FOOT PAIN
- LOWER LEG PAIN
- HEADACHE DUE TO HEART DYSFUNCTION OR HIGH BLOOD PRESSURE, DIZZINESS
- LIVER AND GASTRIC DISEASES
- NEURASTHENIA (AILMENTS FROM EMOTIONAL DISTURBANCES)
- HEART PARALYSIS, CARDIAC DISORDERS
- PAIN IN HANDS AND FEET, SWOLLEN BONES
- METRITIS AND GYNAECOLOGICAL ISSUES
- TUMORS OF THE UTERUS
- CHRONIC SORE THROAT
- EXTREME FATIGUE
- VAGINAL PAIN
- HERNIA
- STRANGURY (UTI)

- Hot flashes, night sweats
- Insomnia
- Anger/irritability
- Depression

**Manipulation:**
Insertion of 0.5 to 1.5 cun in depth. Forbidden needling during pregnancy.

**Remarks:**
Combines with 66,03, it treats an over-active heart (hypertension) or an under-active heart (poor circulation).

66.04 and 22.05 bilaterally form the Tung version of the "Four Gates".

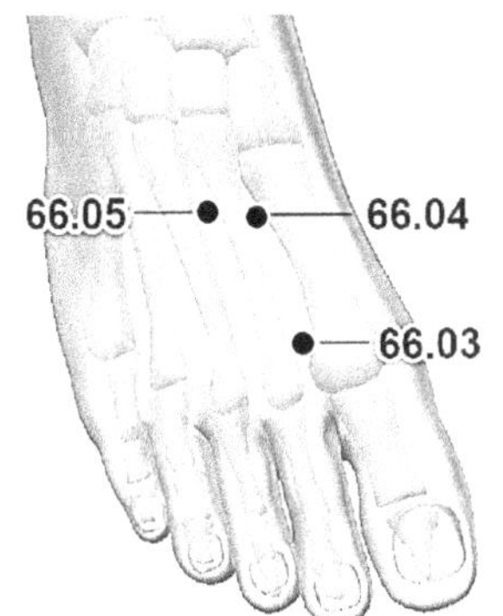


# 66.05 Men Jin
(Gold Door)

**Location:**
In the depression anterior to the junction of the 2nd and 3rd metatarsal bones. Proximal to ST-43.

**Overlaps or near to:** ST-43

**Associated Channel:** Stomach

**Reaction areas:** Stomach and Duodenum

**Indications:**
- Indigestion and bloating
- Enteritis, gastrointestinal disorders and inflammation
- Gastritis
- Abdominal distension
- Appendicitis
- Non-specific diarrhea
- Acute gastrointestinal pain
- Nasal congestion
- Migraine headache in the Tai Yang area
- Menstrual pain
- Anal prolapse
- Combine 66.05 + ST44 for: Burping
- Heavy eyelids,
- Inflammation of the uterus and ovaries

**Manipulation:**
Insertion of 0.5 to 1.0 cun in depth. Do not needle bilaterally. Avoid blood vessels.

**Remarks:** Needle for headaches and bleed for migraines.

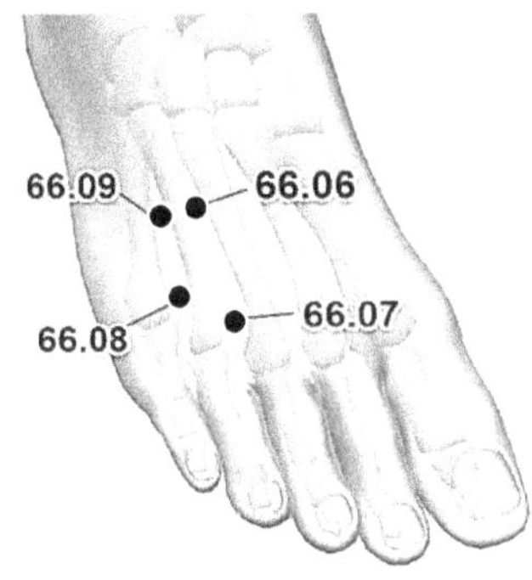


# 66.06 Mu Liu
(Wood Stay)

**Location:**
In the depression distal to the junction of the 3rd and 4th metatarsal bones, 1.5 cun from the metatarsal and phalangeal joints. 1 cun proximal to 66.07.

**Associated Channel:** Between Stomach and Gallbladder

**Reaction areas:** Liver and Spleen.

**Dao Ma:** 66.06+66.07

**Indications:**
- Middle or ring finger pain or trigger finger (opposite side)
- Neuroma (between the third and fourth metatarsal bones). Needle opposite side.
- Leukemia
- Enlargement of the Spleen
- Indigestion
- Liver disease
- Fatigue
- Gallbladder disease
- Polio
- Numbness of the whole body
- Breast cancer
- Stiff neck
- Shoulder pain
- Trigeminal nerve pain
- Ear pain
- Stiff tongue (difficulty speaking)

**Manipulation:**
Insertion of 0.5 to 1.0 cun in depth.

# 66.07 Mu Dou
(Wood Scoop)

**Location:**
Between the 3rd and 4th metatarsal bones, 0.5 cun proximal to the metatarsal and phalangeal joint.

**Associated Channel:** Between Stomach and Gallbladder

**Reaction areas:** Liver and Spleen.

**Dao Ma:** 66.06+66.07

**Indications:**
- Similar to 66.06
- Splenomegaly (lump)
- Indigestion
- Liver disease
- Fatigue
- Gallbladder disease
- Polio
- Foot nerve pain (add 66.06)

**Manipulation:**
Insertion of 0.5 to 1.0 cun in depth.

**Remarks:** 66.07+66.08 are suitable for blood diseases and numbness of the whole body.

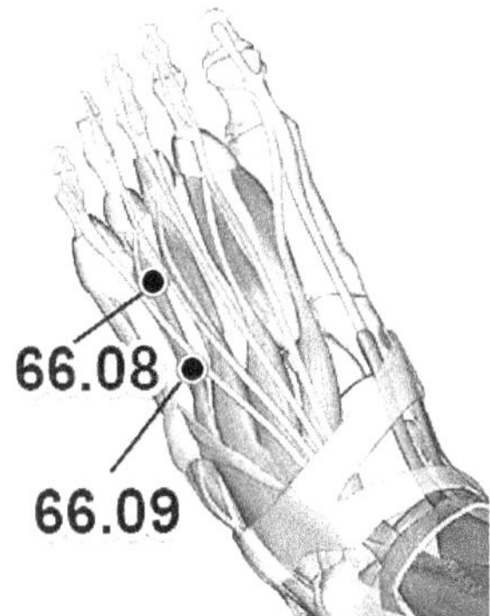


# 66.08 Liu Wan
(Sixth Finish)

**Location:**
Between the 4th and 5th metatarsal bones, 0.5 cun proximal to the metatarsal and phalangeal joint.

**Overlaps:** GB-42

**Associated Channel:** Gall bladder

**Reaction areas:** Lung and Kidney

**Dao Ma:** 66.08+66.09

**Indications:**
- Bleeding due to trauma
- Migraine (one side headache) on Shao Yang (Sanjiao) channel

- DIZZINESS
- TINNITUS.

Because of its astringent nature, this point is contraindicated for patients with asthma, cough, lung disease, excessive phlegm, as it may worsen their condition (Dr. Young, 2008).

**Manipulation:** Insert 0.3-0.5 cun deep.

**Remarks**: 66.08+66.09 treat systemic bone swelling, systemic inflammation and headaches. Use when patients complain of whole body pain.

# 66.09 Shui Qu
(WATER CURVE)

**Location:**
Located on the dorsum of the foot, between the fourth and fifth metatarsal bones, just distal to the proximal junction of the bones.1 cun posterior to 66.08. Lateral to the m. extensor digiti minimi of the foot.

**Overlaps:** GB-41

**Associated Channel:** Gallbladder

**Reaction Areas:** Lung and Kidney

**Dao Ma:** 66.08+66.09

**Indications:**
- LOW BACK/WAIST/LEG PAIN
- GB CHANNEL SCIATICA (GUIDE POINT)
- EDEMA OF LIMBS
- ABDOMINAL DISTENSION
- NECK PAIN
- MIGRAINE
- UTERINE DISORDERS
- TINNITUS
- EYE ITCHINESS
- GENERAL BONE PAIN
- RHEUMATOID ARTHRITIS
- NERVE PAIN (NEURALGIA)
- BONE PAIN OF THE HAND
- SHOULDER PAIN
- MUSCULAR ATROPHY AND NUMBNESS.
- EXTREME/LIFE-THREATENING OBESITY (USE MOXIBUSTION)

**Manipulation:**
Insertion of 0.5 to 1.0 cun in depth.

# 66.10 Huo Lian
(FIRE CONNECTION)

**Location:**
Located on the medial side of the foot, just proximal to the distal head of the first metatarsal bone, tucked into the curve.

**Overlaps:** SP-3

**Associated Channel:** Spleen

**Reaction areas:** Heart and Kidney.

**Indications:**
- DIZZINESS AND BLURRED VISION CAUSED BY HYPERTENSION
- HEART PALPITATIONS
- FATIGUE
- FRONTAL HEADACHE, MENINGITIS
- NOSE BONE PAIN
- BRAIN TUMOR
- WEAKNESS OF THE LIMBS

**Manipulation:**
Insertion along the metatarsals 0.5 to 1.0 cun in depth. One side only

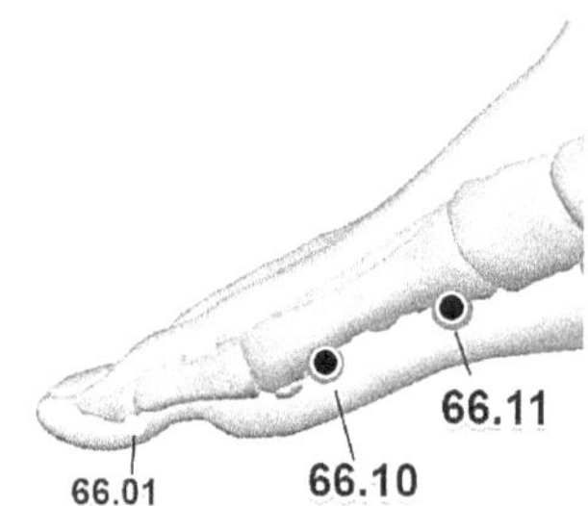


# 66.11 Huo Ju
(FIRE CHRYSANTHEMUM)

**Location:**
Locate the point on the medial side of the 1st metatarsal bone, 1.0 cun posterior to 66.10.

**Overlaps:** SP-4

**Associated Channel:** Spleen

**Reaction areas:** Heart and Kidney

**Indications:**
- GASTROINTESTINAL DISORDERS
- STOMACHACHE
- NUMBNESS OF HANDS
- HEART PALPITATION
- HIGH BLOOD PRESSURE
- DIZZINESS/VERTIGO
- LOWER LEG/FOOT PAIN
- BLURRED VISION
- SORENESS OF EYELID
- HEAVY EYELIDS
- FLOATERS
- STIFF NECK
- CERVICAL BONE SPURS
- FINGER/HAND NUMBNESS
- HEADACHE
- INABILITY TO TASTE

**Manipulation:**
Insertion 0.5 to 1.0 cun in depth.

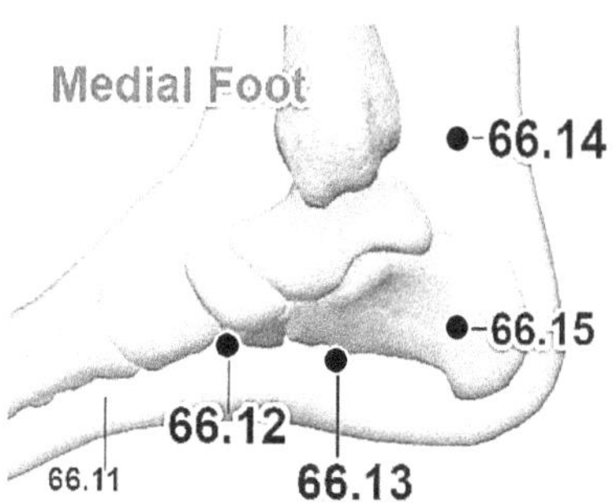


# 66.12 Huo San
(FIRE SCATTER)

**Location:**
Locate the point on the medial side of the 1st metatarsal bone, 1.0 cun proximal to 66.11 (SP-4). In the depression just below the tuberosity of the navicular bone

**Overlaps:** KID-2

**Associated Channel:** Kidney

**Reaction areas:** Heart, Kidney and Six bowels

**Indications:**
- MIGRAINE AND HEADACHE
- CANTHUS PAIN
- KIDNEY WEAKNESS
- DIZZINESS
- BLURRED VISION
- LOWER BACK PAIN FROM EXCESSIVE SEXUAL ACTIVITY
- BACK PAIN
- BRAIN TUMOR
- HIGH BLOOD PRESSURE
- HOT AND COLD FEET
- DROOLING

**Caution:** Do not needle during pregnancy.

**Manipulation:**
Insertion of 0.5 to 0.8 cun in depth.

# 66.13 Shui Jing
(WATER CRYSTAL)

**Location:**
2 cun inferior to the apex of the medial malleous.1 cun distal to KID6.

**Associated Channel:** Kidney

**Reaction area:** Uterus

**Indications:**
- SORE THROAT
- CONSTIPATION
- ABDOMINAL DISTENSION
- PELVIC PAIN

- UTERINE ENLARGEMENT, FIBROIDS, TUMORS OR INFLAMMATION
- MENOPAUSAL HOT FLASHES

**Manipulation:**
Insertion of 0.5 to 1.0 cun in depth.

# 66.14 Shui Xiang
(WATER SHAPE)

**Location:**
2 cun posterior to the medial malleous, in the depression of the anterior border of the Achilles tendon.

**Overlaps:** KID-3

**Associated Channel:** Kidney

**Reaction areas:** Kidney and Brain.

**Dao ma:** 66.14+66.15

**Indications (including traditional indications of KID-3):**
- NEPHRITIS
- EDEMA OF THE LIMBS
- PUERPERAL FEBRILE DISEASE
- CATARACT
- INSOMNIA
- AMNESIA
- NEUROSIS
- HEADACHE
- TINNITUS/DEAFNESS
- CATARACTS
- TOOTHACHE
- CHRONIC SORE THROAT
- COUGH
- ASTHMA
- EXCESSIVE URINATION
- DIABETES
- IMPOTENCE
- INFERTILITY
- LEUCORRHEA
- IRREGULAR MENSES
- NAUSEA AND VOMITING
- SPINAL BONE SPURS AND PAIN
- BACK PAIN
- LOW BACK PAIN DUE TO KIDNEY WEAKNESS
- ACHILLES TENDON PAIN.

**Manipulation:**
Insertion of 0.3 to 0.5 cun in depth or through the tendon calcaneous. Moxa to tonify Kidneys.

# 66.15 Shui Xian
(WATER FAIRY)

**Location:**
2 cun directly inferior to 66.14. 1 cun distal to KID-5.

**Associated Channel:** Kidney

**Reaction areas:** Kidney and Brain.

**Dao ma:** 66.14+66.15

**Indications:**
- NEPHRITIS
- EDEMA OF THE LIMBS
- LOW BACK PAIN DUE TO KIDNEY WEAKNESS
- VERTEBRAL PAIN
- PUERPERAL FEBRILE DISEASE
- CATARACT.

**Manipulation:**
Insertion of 0.5 cun in depth.

# ZONE 77-Lower Leg

# 77.01 Zheng Jin
(UPRIGHT TENDON)

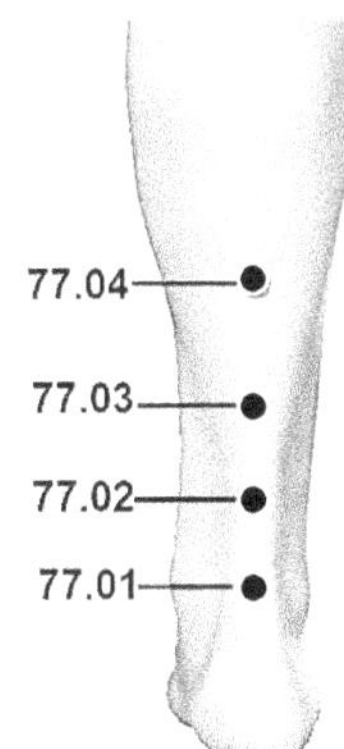


**Location:**
In the center of the tendon of calcaneus 3.5 cun superior of the base of the heel. Located on Achilles tendon between BL-60 and KID-3

**Associated Channels:**
Between Bladder and Kidney Channels

**Reaction areas:** Spine and Brain.

**Dao Ma:** 77.01+77.02 (Correct Tendons)

**Indications:**
- TWISTED BACK
- LUMBAR VERTEBRAL PAIN
- NECK PAIN AND RIGIDITY
- ANKYLOSING SPONDYLITIS
- CRANIAL ENLARGEMENT
- HYDROCEPHALUS
- BRAIN TUMOR
- SPASMS OF THE STOMACH
- LEG CRAMPS
- FOOT SPASMS
- POSTERIOR HEADACHE
- TENDON ISSUES/SPASM ("TENDON TREATS TENDON")
- UTERINE AND MENSTRUAL CRAMPS
- SPRAIN OF ACHILLES TENDON
- PLANTAR FASCIITIS
- HEEL SPURS

**Manipulation:**
Before insertion, massage the gastrocnemius muscle and Achilles tendon. Insertion of 1.0 to 2.0 cun in depth. More effective when the needle pierces through the tendon squarely and gently touches the back of the tibia (longer needles are needed). Long needle retention is more effective.

**Remarks:** Use for vertebral pain. 77.01 treats C1-C2,
77.02 treats C2-C4,
77.03 treats C4-C7/T1,
77.04 treats T1-T4.
At times, the imaging flips and the combination treats lower back pain.

**Remarks:** Useful for diseases involving the cervical spine, occipital area or cerebellum.

# 77.02 Zheng Zong
(UPRIGHT ANCESTRY)

**Location:**
2 cun superior to 77.01.

**Associated Channels:** Between Bladder and Kidney Channels

**Reaction areas:** Spine and Brain.

**Dao Ma:** 77.01+77.02

**Indications:**
- TWISTED BACK
- LUMBAR VERTEBRAL PAIN
- NECK PAIN AND RIGIDITY
- ANKYLOSING SPONDYLITIS
- CRANIAL ENLARGEMENT
- HYDROCEPHALUS
- BRAIN TUMOR
- SPASMS OF THE STOMACH
- LEG CRAMPS
- FOOT SPASMS
- POSTERIOR HEADACHE
- TENDON ISSUES/SPASM ("TENDON TREATS TENDON")
- UTERINE AND MENSTRUAL CRAMPS
- SPRAIN OF ACHILLES TENDON
- PLANTAR FASCIITIS
- HEEL SPURS

**Manipulation:**
Insertion of 1.0 to 2.0 cun in depth. More effective when the needle pierces through the tendon and touches the back of the tibia (longer needles are needed). Long needle retention is more effective.

# 77.03 Zheng Shi
(UPRIGHT SCHOLAR)

**Location:**
2 cun superior to 77.02.

**Associated Channels:** Urinary Bladder

**Reaction areas:** Spine and Lung

**Indications:**
- PAIN IN SHOULDER AND BACK
- LOWER BACK PAIN
- SCIATICA (BL CHANNEL)
- NECK PAIN

**Manipulation:**
Insertion of 0.5 to 1.0 cun in depth. Usually used with 77.04.

# 77.04 Bo Qiu
(CATCHING BALL)

**Location:**
2.5 cun superior to 77.03. 1.5 cun distal to BL-57

**Associated Channels:** Urinary Bladder

**Reaction areas:** Heart and Lung

**Indications:**
- HEMORRHOIDS
- ACUTE GASTROENTERITIS
- CHOLERA
- NOSEBLEED
- UPPER BACK PAIN
- LOWER BACK SORENESS OR PAIN
- SCIATICA (UB CHANNEL)
- LOWER LEG SPASM OR PAIN

**Manipulation:**
Insertion of 1.0 to 2.0 cun in depth.

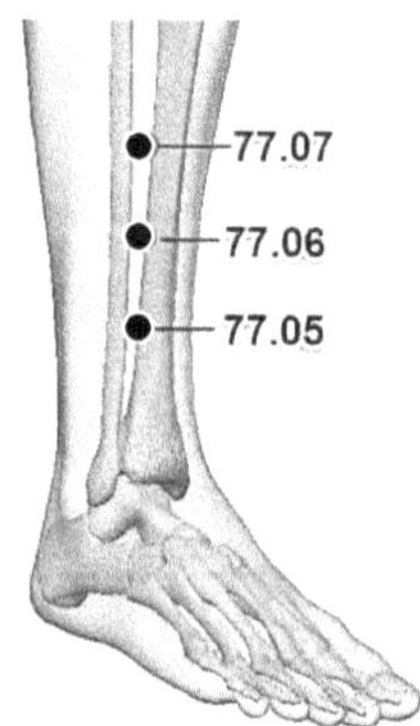


# 77.05 Yi Zhong
(FIRST WEIGHT)

**Location:**
3 cun superior to the lateral malleolus, and 1 cun anterior to the fibula bone. Anterior to GB-39.

**Near to:** GB-39

**Associated Channel:** Between Gallbladder and Stomach

**Reaction areas:** Heart, Lung, Spleen

**Dao Ma:** 77.05+77.06+77.07

**Indications:**
- HYPERTHYROIDISM
- EXOPHTHALMOS/GRAVES' DISEASE
- TONSILLITIS
- MUMPS
- BELL'S PALSY/FACIAL PARALYSIS
- TRIGEMINAL NEURALGIA
- BRAIN INJURIES
- STROKE/HEMIPLEGIA
- COMA
- MENTAL CONFUSION
- POLIO
- TMJ
- HEADACHE/MIGRAINE
- LUMPS
- LIVER DISEASES
- BLOOD DISEASES
- BREAST TUMOR
- BRAIN TUMOR
- MENINGITIS
- EYES TEAR IN THE WIND
- ENLARGED SPLEEN (RIGHT SIDE INSERTION)
- NECK PAIN (SCALENE AREA)
- SCAPULAR AND ARM PAIN
- RIB PAIN
- HIP PAIN

**Manipulation:**
Insertion of 1.0 to 2.0 cun in depth. On right side due to its spleen indications. Long needle retention if treating brain issues.

**Remarks:** This combination treats systemic stagnation or Qi deficiency. Increases blood circulation to the head.

# 77.06 Er Zhong
(SECOND WEIGHT)

**Location:**
2 cun superior to 77.05. 1 cun anterior to the fibula bone.

**Associated Channel:** Between Gallbladder and Stomach

**Reaction areas:** Heart, Lung, Spleen

**Dao Ma:** 77.05+77.06+77.07

**Indications:** See 77.05

**Manipulation:**
Insertion of 1.0 to 2.0 cun in depth.

# 77.07 San Zhong
(THIRD WEIGHT)

**Location:**
2 cun superior to 77.06. 1 cun anterior to the fibula bone.

**Associated Channel:** Between Gallbladder and Stomach

**Reaction areas:** Heart, Lung, Spleen

**Dao Ma:** 77.05+77.06+77.07

**Indications:** See 77.05

**Manipulation:**
Insertion of 1.0 to 2.0 cun in depth.

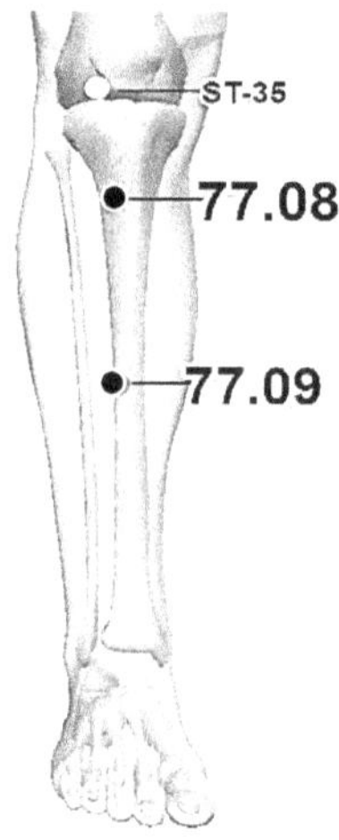


# 77.08 Si Hua Shang
(FOUR FLOWERS UPPER)

**Location:**
3 cun inferior to ST-35 on the lateral tibia.

**Near to:** ST-36

**Associated Channel:** Stomach

**Reaction areas:** Lung and Heart

**Dao Ma:** 77.08+77.09

**Indications:**
- ASTHMA
- LUNG TUMOR
- TUBERCULOSIS
- FLUID IN THE LUNGS
- TOOTHACHE
- FRONTAL HEADACHE
- FACIAL PARALYSIS/BELL'S PALSY
- HEART ISSUES (ANGINA, MYOCARDITIS, CORONARY HEART DISEASE, PALPITATIONS, TACHYCARDIA)
- CORONARY ARTERY DISEASE
- TUMOR IN THE MOUTH
- DIZZINESS

- Gastrointestinal disease
- Vomiting
- Sudden turmoil
- Epilepsy
- Hemorrhoids
- Cramp in Cholera Morbus
- Mouth ulcers/tumors
- Eye diseases
- Glaucoma
- Shoulder, arm, elbow and index finger pain
- Knee and heel spurs
- Calf spasm
- Gout
- Promotes urination

**Manipulation:**
Get as close to the tibia as possible. Insertion 2.0 to 3.0 cun in depth. 2.0 cun for asthma, 3.0 cun in depth for heart disease. Quick-prick technique to treat chronic stomach diseases and stomach ulcer. Bleeding surrounding dark vessels is highly effective.

**Remarks:** Just as ST-36 in the TCM system, 77.08 is a Top point for wind, phlegm, Qi and blood stagnation.

# 77.09 Si Hua Zhong
(Four Flowers Middle)

**Location:**
4.5 cun inferior to 77.08.  0.5 cun proximal to ST-38.

**Near to:** ST-38 and ST-37

**Associated Channel:** Stomach

**Reaction areas:** Heart, Lung and Six bowels.

**Dao Ma:** 77.08+77.09

**Indications:**
- Asthma
- Heart pain/paralysis
- Chest suffocation or discomfort
- Eye problems
- Stomach pain
- Bone inflammation and bone spurs
- Frozen shoulder
- Other indications similar to 77.08

**Manipulation:**
Insertion 2.0 to 3.0 cun in depth for asthma and eye disease. Bleeding treatment for the remaining diseases.

**Remarks:** Location is 0.5 cun above ST-38 on the Stomach channel. Use prompt prick technique to treat lung disorders. Needle same side when treating joints pain.

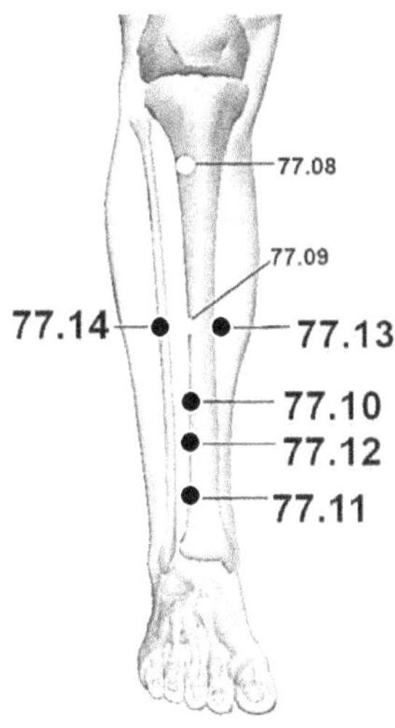


# 77.10 Si Hua Fu
(Four Flowers Append)

**Location:**
2.5 cun inferior to 77.09 or 1.0 cun distal to ST-39

**Associated channel:** Stomach

**Reaction areas:** Heart, Lung and Six bowels.

**Dao Ma:** 77.09+77.10

**Indications:**
- Asthma
- Eye disease/pain
- Migraine headache
- Heart disease
- Arteriosclerosis
- Acute stomach pain
- Frozen shoulder
- Scapular pain
- Elbow and index finger pain
- Bone inflammation and bone spurs

**Manipulation:**
Needle: 2.0-3.0 cun deep. Bleeding is useful.

# 77.11 Si Hua Xia
(Four Flowers Lower)

**Location:**
2.5 cun inferior to 77.10 or 3.5 cun proximal to ST-41.

**Associated Channel:** Stomach

**Reaction areas:** Lung, Kidney and Six bowels.

**Dao Ma:** 77.11+77.12

**Indications:**
- Intestinal inflammation
- Diarrhea
- Stomach pain

- Abdominal distension
- Chest distension
- Edema in the leg
- Teeth grinding
- Bone spurs/enlargement

**Manipulation:**
Insertion of 1.0 to 2.0 cun in depth.

**Remarks:** 77.11+77.12 are useful for gastrointestinal inflammation and acute (non-pathogenic type) diarrhea.

# 77.12 Fu Chang
(Bowel Intestine)

**Location:**
1.5 cun directly superior to 77.11

**Associated Channel:** Stomach

**Reaction areas:** Heart, Lung, Kidney and Six bowels.

**Dao Ma:** 77.11+77.12

**Indications:**
- Intestinal inflammation
- Diarrhea
- Stomach pain
- Abdominal distension
- Chest distension
- Edema in the leg
- Teeth grinding
- Bone spurs/enlargement

**Manipulation:**
Insertion of 1.0 to 2.0 cun in depth.

# 77.13 Si Hua Li
(Four Flowers Inner)

**Location:**
1.2 cun medial to 77.09 or 4.5 cun distal to ST-36, on the medial border of the tibia.

**Associated Channel:** Spleen

**Reaction areas:** Heart and Lung

**Indications:**
- Acute gastroenteritis
- Coronary artery disease
- Heart disease
- Palpitation
- Vomiting
- Knee osteoarthritis/medial knee pain (blood-letting works better)
- Bone spurs in the knee

**Manipulation:** 1.0-1.5 cun deep. Bleeding works better if there are visible veins in the area.

# 77.14 Si Hua Wai
(FOUR FLOWERS LATERAL)

**Location:**
1.5 cun lateral to 77.09. 4,5 cun distal to 77.08 or ST-36.

**Near to:** ST-40 (Gathering point of phlegm)

**Associated Channel:** Stomach

**Reaction areas:** Lung and Six Bowels

**Indications:**
- ONE SIDED BODILY DISEASES OR PAIN
- TOOTHACHE
- EAR PAIN
- MIGRAINE
- FRONTAL HEADACHE
- FACIAL PARALYSIS
- CHRONIC RHINITIS
- ASTHMA
- SHOULDER AND ARM PAIN
- INTERCOSTAL NEURALGIA
- CHEST DISTENSION
- SWOLLEN BREAST
- WAIST PAIN
- ACUTE GASTROENTERITIS
- GB CHANNEL SCIATICA
- TAIL BONE PAIN
- INSTEP/SOLE PAIN
- HYPERTENSION AND HYPERCHOLESTEROLEMIA
- CORONARY HEART DISEASE
- OBESITY
- PARKINSON'S DISEASE
- ALZHEIMER'S DISEASE
- SHINGLES
- BLEEDING 77.14 CLEARS BLOOD HEAT, DISPERSES BLOOD STAGNATION AND DISSOLVES PHLEGM.

**Manipulation:**
Insertion of 1.0 to 1.5 cun in depth. More often bled.

**Notes:** Extremely effective blood-letting area to treat chronic and difficult cases. Look for dark vessels.

# 77.15 Shang Chun
(UPPER LIP)

**Location:**
At the lower lateral ridge of the patella. Located 1.0 cun lateral to the distal apex of the patella.

**Overlaps:** ST-35

**Associated Channel:** Stomach

**Reaction area:** Lips

**Dao ma:** 77.15+77.16

**Indications:**
- LIP/MOUTH PAIN/ULCERS
- LEUKODERMA AROUND ORAL AND GENITAL AREA.
- HERPES (ORAL, ANAL AND GENITAL)

**Manipulation:**
Bleed the point until dark red blood appears.

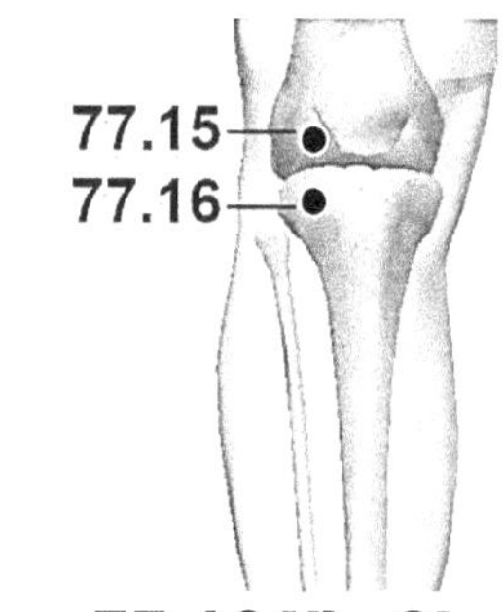


# 77.16 Xia Chun
(LOWER LIP)

**Location:**
1 cun inferior to the lateral lower patella ridge. 1 cun distal to 77.15.

**Associated Channel:** Stomach

**Reaction area:** Lower Lips

**Dao ma:** 77.15+77.16

**Indications:**
- LIP/MOUTH PAIN/ULCERS
- LEUKODERMA AROUND ORAL AND GENITAL AREA.
- HERPES (ORAL, ANAL AND GENITAL)

**Manipulation:**
Bleed the point until dark red blood appears.

# 77.17 Tian Huang
(HEAVENLY EMPEROR)

**Location:**
In the depression at the angle formed by the medial condyle of the tibia and the posterior border of the tibia.

**Overlaps:** SP-9

**Associated Channel:** Spleen

**Reaction areas:** Kidney, Heart

**Dao ma:** 77.17 and/or 77.18

**Indications:**
- FRONTAL HEADACHE
- ACID REFLUX (TO DECREASE STOMACH ACID)
- REGURGITATION

- BAD BREATH
- NEPHRITIS
- DIABETES
- HYPERCHOLESTEROLEMIA
- HEART DISEASE
- DIZZINESS
- HYPERTENSION
- RHEUMATOID ARTHRITIS
- PROTEINURIA
- TIGHTNESS OF THE NECK
- TIGHTNESS OF THORACIC SPINE AREA
- ARM/SHOULDER PAIN
- INSOMNIA

**Caution:** Contraindicated in pregnancy

**Manipulation:**
Insertion of 0.5 to 1.0 cun in depth. Moxibustion is contraindicated.

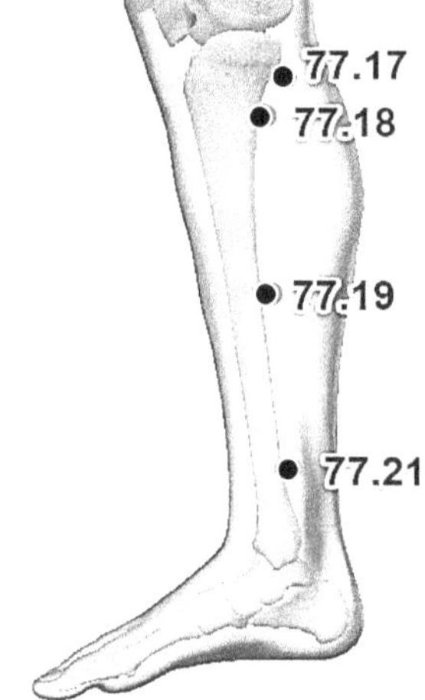


# 77.18 Tian Huang Fu
(SHEN GUAN) (KIDNEY GATE)-
TUNG'S MASTER KIDNEY POINT

**Location:**
1.5 cun inferior to 77.17 or SP-9.

**Associated Channel:** Spleen

**Reaction areas:** Heart, Kidney

**Dao Ma:** 77.17/77.18+77.19+77.21 (Lower Three Emperors)

**Indications:**
- URINARY ISSUES:
  - EDEMA
  - KIDNEY DISEASE
  - DIABETES MELLITUS
  - STRANGURY
  - INCONTINENCE
  - HEMATURIA
  - NEPHRITIS
  - PROTEINURIA
  - URINARY TRACT INFECTION

- o   DIURESIS AND NOCTURIA
- o   LOWER BACK PAIN DUE TO KIDNEY DEFICIENCY
- **GENERAL DIGESTIVE PROBLEMS:**
  - o   STOMACH DISEASE
  - o   VOMITING
  - o   ACID REFLUX
- **GYNECOLOGICAL DISORDERS:**
  - o   IRREGULAR MENSTRUATION
  - o   UTERINE TUMORS
  - o   HOT FLASHES
  - o   POSTPARTUM WEAKNESS
  - o   INFERTILITY
- **MALE GENITAL PROBLEMS:**
  - o   PROSTATE ISSUES INCL. PROSTATE ENLARGEMENT, PROSTATITIS
  - o   PREMATURE EJACULATION
  - o   IMPOTENCE
  - o   SEMINAL EMISSION
  - o   NOCTURNAL EMISSION
- **NEUROLOGICAL ISSUES**
  - o   EPILEPSY
  - o   PARKINSON'S DISEASE
  - o   FACIAL PARALYSIS
  - o   DEVIATION OF EYEBALL
  - o   TRIGEMINAL NEURALGIA
  - o   FACIAL TWITCH
  - o   DIZZINESS/VERTIGO
  - o   HEADACHE
  - o   NEUROPATHY
  - o   INSOMNIA
  - o   MENTAL DISORDERS
- **PAIN ISSUES:**
  - o   FRONTAL HEADACHE
  - o   NOSE BONE PAIN
  - o   SCIATICA
  - o   BACK PAIN
  - o   TAIL BONE PAIN
  - o   NUMBNESS AND PAIN OF THE HANDS
  - o   FROZEN SHOULDER
  - o   NECK AND SHOULDER
  - o   INABILITY TO EXTEND WRIST
- FATIGUE AND WEAKNESS
- HEART DISEASE
- ARTERIOSCLEROSIS
- HYPERTENSION
- ANEMIA
- EYE DISEASE

**Caution:** Contraindicated in low blood pressure

**Manipulation:**
Insertion of 0.5 to 1.5 cun in depth.

**Remarks:** Treats all issues from weak kidneys as defined from Western and Eastern medicine.

# 77.19 Di Huang
(EARTHLY EMPEROR)

**Location:**
In the medial tibia, 7 cun superior to the medial malleolus. Midway between 77.18 and 77.21

**Overlaps:** SP-7

**Associated Channel:** Spleen

**Reaction area:** Kidney

**Dao Ma:** 77.17/77.18+77.19+77.21 (Lower Three Emperors)

**Indications:**
- SIMILAR TO 77.18
- NEPHRITIS
- EDEMA OF THE LIMBS
- DIABETES
- STRANGURY
- IMPOTENCE
- PREMATURE EJACULATION
- NOCTURNAL EMISSION
- INVOLUNTARY EMISSION
- PROTEINURIA
- HEMATURIA
- TUMOR OF UTERUS
- IRREGULAR MENSTRUATION
- LOWER BACK PAIN DUE TO WEAK KIDNEY.

**Caution:** Contraindicated in pregnancy.

**Manipulation:**
Insertion of 1.0 to 1.5 cun in depth.

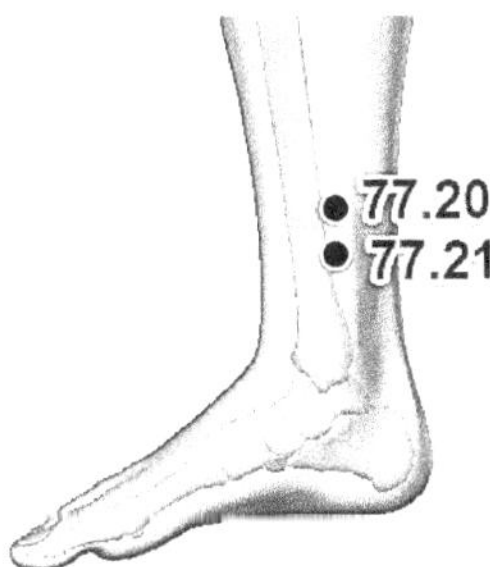


# 77.20 Si Zhi
(FOUR LIMBS)

**Location:**
3 cun below 77.19. 4 cun proximal to the tip of the medial malleolus.

**Associated Channel:** Spleen

**Reaction areas:** Heart, Kidney and Four Limbs

**Indications:**
- NECK PAIN
- ARM/ELBOW/SHOULDER PAIN
- HAND AND FOOT PAIN

- PERIPHERAL NEUROPATHY
- DIABETES

**Caution:** Contraindicated in pregnancy.

**Manipulation:**
Insertion of 0.5 to 1.5 cun in depth.

# 77.21 Ren Huang
(HUMAN EMPEROR)

**Location:**
On the posterior border of the medial tibia, 3 cun superior to the tip of medial malleolus (certain text put it as 3 cun above the top of the medial malleolus)

**Associated Channel:** Spleen

**Overlaps:** SP-6

**Reaction area:** Kidney

**Dao Ma:** 77.17/77.18+77.19+77.21

**Indications:**
- EDEMA
- KIDNEY DISEASE
- DIABETES MELLITUS
- STRANGURY
- PREMATURE EJACULATION
- IMPOTENCE
- SEMINAL EMISSION
- NOCTURNAL EMISSION
- HEMATURIA
- UTERINE TUMORS
- NEPHRITIS
- PROTEINURIA
- IRREGULAR MENSTRUATION
- INFERTILITY
- DIFFICULT LABOR
- LOWER BACK PAIN DUE TO KIDNEY DEFICIENCY
- NECK PAIN
- INCONTINENCE
- TRIGEMINAL NEURALGIA
- FATIGUE AND WEAKNESS
- CHRONIC FATIGUE SYNDROME
- INSOMNIA
- DIZZINESS
- HYPERTENSION
- GENERAL DIGESTIVE DISORDERS
- GYNECOLOGICAL DISORDERS

**Caution:** Contraindicated in low blood pressure and pregnancy

**Manipulation:**
Insertion of 0.6 to 1.2 cun in depth.

**Remarks:** Useful for sexual and reproductive issues for both men and women.

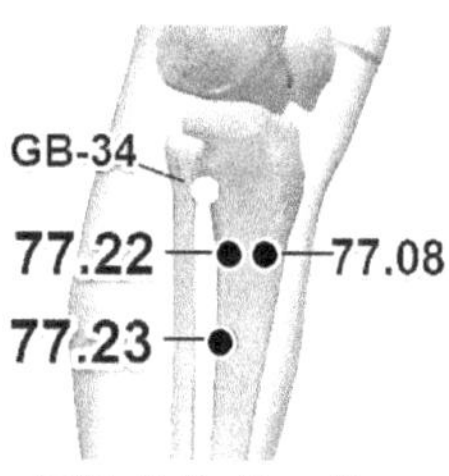



# 77.22 Ce San Li

(BESIDE THREE MILES)

**Location:**
1.5 cun lateral to 77.08 (or ST-36)

**Associated Channel:** Between Stomach and Gallbladder

**Reaction areas:** Teeth and Lung

**Dao Ma:** 77.22+77.23

**Indications:**
- TOOTHACHE
- ONE-SIDED HEADACHE
- SINUSITIS
- TRIGEMINAL NEURALGIA
- BELL'S PALSY/ FACIAL PARALYSIS
- FACIAL TICS
- WRIST PAIN
- HAND PAIN
- HEEL PAIN
- ELBOW PAIN
- NECK PAIN
- SHOULDER PAIN
- JOINT AND TENDON PROBLEMS
- ONE-SIDED MUSCULOSKELETAL PAIN OF THE BODY
- EAR PAIN
- OTITIS MEDIA
- DEAFNESS
- TINNITUS

**Manipulation:**
Insertion of 1.0 to 1.5 cun in depth.

**Remarks:** Great for headaches and issues on the face.

# 77.23 Ce Xia San Li

(LOWER BESIDE THREE MILES)

**Location:**
2 cun inferior to 77.22. On the anterior border of the fibula.

**Associated Channel:** Between Stomach and Gallbladder

**Reaction areas:** Teeth and Lung

**Dao Ma:** 77.22+77.23

**Indications:**
- TOOTHACHE
- ONE-SIDED HEADACHE
- SINUSITIS
- TRIGEMINAL NEURALGIA
- BELL'S PALSY/ FACIAL PARALYSIS
- FACIAL TICS
- WRIST PAIN
- HAND PAIN
- HEEL PAIN
- ELBOW PAIN
- NECK PAIN
- SHOULDER PAIN
- JOINT AND TENDON PROBLEMS
- ONE-SIDED MUSCULOSKELETAL PAIN OF THE BODY
- EAR PAIN
- OTITIS MEDIA
- DEAFNESS
- TINNITUS

**Manipulation:**
Insertion of 1.0 to 1.5 cun in depth.

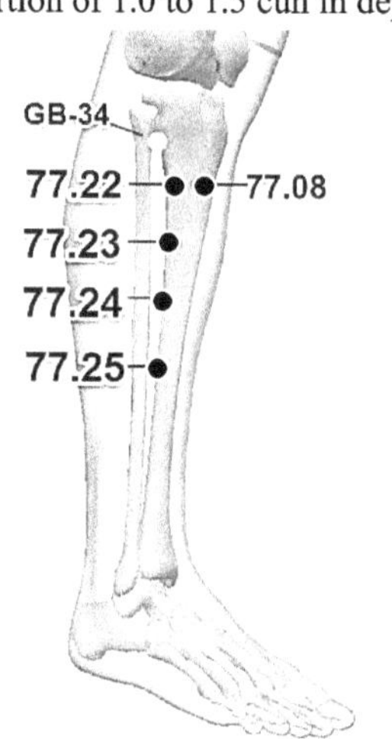



# 77.24 Zu Qian Jin

(FOOT THOUSAND GOLD)

**Location:**
0.5 cun lateral (posterior), and 2 cun inferior to 77.23.

**Associated Channel:** Between Stomach and Gallbladder

**Reaction areas:** Lung, Kidney and Thyroid gland.

**Dao Ma:** 77.24+77.25

**Indications:**
- FISH BONE STUCK IN THE THROAT
- SORE OR SWOLLEN THROAT
- THROAT ABSCESSES
- PHARYNGITIS
- TONSILLITIS
- HYPERTHYROIDISM
- GOITER (DUE TO HYPER OR HYPOTHYROIDISM)
- THYROID INFLAMMATION
- MUMPS (PAROTITIS)
- PLUM PIT QI SENSATION IN THE THROAT
- ACUTE INTESTINAL INFLAMMATION
- PAIN IN THE SHOULDER AND BACK

**Manipulation:**
Insertion of 1.0 to 1.5 cun in depth.

# 77.25 Zu Wu Jin

(FOOT FIVE GOLD)

**Location:**
2 cun directly inferior to 77.24.

**Associated Channel:** Between Stomach and Gallbladder

**Reaction areas:** Lung, Kidney and Thyroid gland.

**Dao Ma:** 77.24+77.25

**Indications:**
- FISH BONE STUCK IN THE THROAT
- SORE OR SWOLLEN THROAT
- THROAT ABSCESSES
- PHARYNGITIS
- TONSILLITIS
- HYPERTHYROIDISM
- GOITER (DUE TO HYPER OR HYPOTHYROIDISM)
- THYROID INFLAMMATION
- MUMPS (PAROTITIS)
- PLUM PIT QI SENSATION IN THE THROAT
- ACUTE INTESTINAL INFLAMMATION
- PAIN IN THE SHOULDER AND BACK

**Manipulation:**
Insertion of 1.0 to 2.0 cun in depth.

# 77.26 Qi Hu

(SEVEN TIGERS)

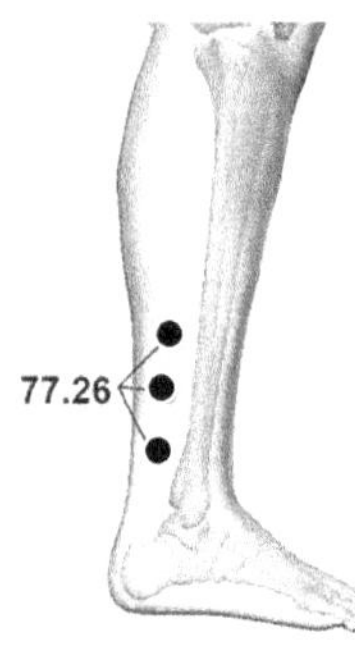



**Location:**
3 point group. Locate the first point on the longitudinal line, 1.5 cun posterior to, and 2 cun superior to, the tip of the lateral malleolus. Locate the second point 2 cun superior to the first, and the third point 2 cun superior to the second point.

**Associated Channel:** Between Urinary Bladder and Gallbladder

**Reaction areas:** Chest and Thoracic cage

**Indications:**
- STERNUM PAIN
- CLAVICLE PAIN
- RIB PAIN
- SCAPULAR PAIN
- PLEURISY

**Manipulation:**
Insertion of 0.5 to 0.8 cun in depth.

**Remarks:** Treats pain at GB-21 area and upper back pain.

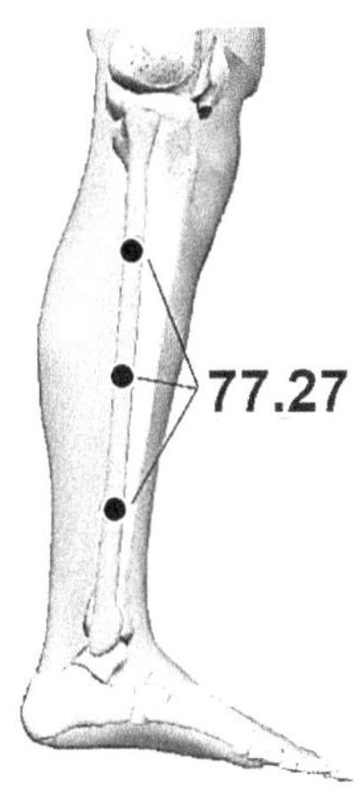


# 77.27 Wai San Guan
(OUTER THREE GATES)

**Location:**
3 points evenly distributed on the line connecting the head of the fibula and the process of the lateral malleolus.

**Associated Channel:** Gallbladder

**Reaction areas:** Lung

**Indications:**
- TONSILLITIS
- TUMOR
- CANCER (NEEDLE BILATERALLY)
- PHARYNGITIS
- PAROTITIS
- SHOULDER/ELBOW/ARM PAIN
- INABILITY TO LIFT ARM OVER THE HEAD
- HOT OR SWOLLEN HANDS
- TRIGEMINAL NEURALGIA
- SKIN CONDITIONS
- ABSCESSES

**Manipulation:**
Insertion of 1.0 to 1.5 cun in depth. Tap the tibia for the best results.

**Remarks:** Similar to 77.05-07, treats systemic stagnation, trauma, masses and tumors (including cancer)

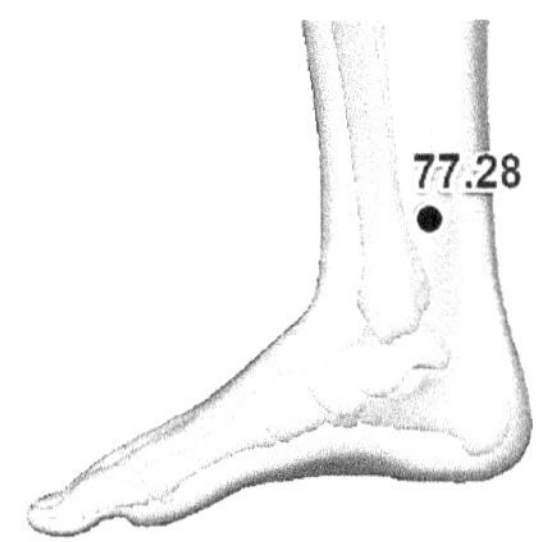


# 77.28 Guang Ming
(BRIGHT ILLUMINATION)

**Location:**
1 cun posterior to and 2 cun superior to the medial malleolus.

**Overlaps:** (anterior to) KID-7

**Associated Channel:** Kidney

**Reaction areas:** Kidney

**Indications:**
- EYE DISEASES SUCH AS ASTIGMATISM, CATARACTS, DOUBLE VISION, FLOATERS, GLAUCOMA
- ACUTE BACK STRAIN
- COUGH
- ASTHMA

**Manipulation:**
Insertion of 0.5 to 1.0 cun in depth.


# ZONE 88-Thigh

## 88.01 Tong Guan
(PENETRATING GATE)

**Location:**
On the anterior midline of the femur, 5 cun proximal to the superior border of the patella.

**Associated Channel:** Between Spleen and Stomach, closer to the Stomach meridian

**Reaction area:** Heart

**Dao Ma:** 88.01+88.02+88.03

**Indications:**
- HEART DISEASES
- PERICARDIAC PAIN
- PAIN ON BOTH SIDES OF THE HEART
- RHEUMATIC HEART DISEASE
- DIZZINESS
- VERTIGO
- HEART PALPITATIONS
- STOMACH ISSUES
- LIMB PAIN
- CEREBRAL ANEMIA

- LOWER LEG EDEMA
- SWELLING BELOW THE HEART
- VARICOSE VEINS
- RHEUMATOID ARTHRITIS
- NAUSEA AND VOMITING IN PREGNANCY

**Manipulation:**
Insertion of 0.5 to 1.0 cun in depth.

**Remarks:** This Dao Ma treats all heart issues.

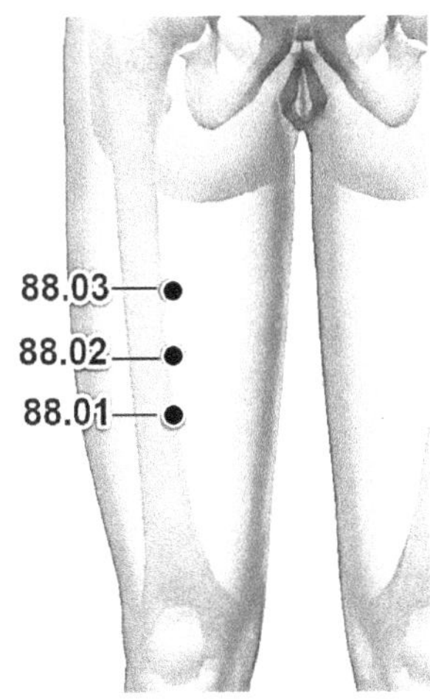


# 88.02 Tong Shan
(PENETRATING MOUNTAIN)

**Location:**
On the anterior midline of the femur, 7 cun proximal to the superior border of the patella.

**Associated Channel:** Between Spleen and Stomach, closer to the Stomach meridian

**Reaction area:** Heart

**Dao Ma:** 88.01+88.02+88.03

**Indications:**
- HEART DISEASES
- PERICARDIAC PAIN
- PAIN ON BOTH SIDES OF THE HEART
- RHEUMATIC HEART DISEASE
- DIZZINESS
- VERTIGO
- HEART PALPITATIONS
- STOMACH ISSUES
- LIMB PAIN
- CEREBRAL ANEMIA
- LOWER LEG EDEMA
- SWELLING BELOW THE HEART
- VARICOSE VEINS
- RHEUMATOID ARTHRITIS
- NAUSEA AND VOMITING IN PREGNANCY

**Manipulation:**
Insertion of 0.5 to 1.0 cun in depth.

# 88.03 Tong Tian
(PENETRATING HEAVEN)

**Location:**
On the anterior midline of the femur, 9 cun proximal to the superior border of the patella.

**Associated Channel:** Between Spleen and Stomach, closer to the Stomach meridian

**Reaction area:** Heart

**Dao Ma:** 88.01+88.02+88.03

**Indications:**
- HEART DISEASES
- PERICARDIAC PAIN
- PAIN ON BOTH SIDES OF THE HEART
- RHEUMATIC HEART DISEASE
- DIZZINESS
- VERTIGO
- HEART PALPITATIONS
- STOMACH ISSUES
- LIMB PAIN
- CEREBRAL ANEMIA
- LOWER LEG EDEMA
- SWELLING BELOW THE HEART
- VARICOSE VEINS
- RHEUMATOID ARTHRITIS
- NAUSEA AND VOMITING IN PREGNANCY

**Manipulation:**
Insertion of 0.5 to 1.0 cun in depth.

# 88.04 Jie Mei Yi
(SISTER ONE)

**Location:**
1 cun proximal and 1 cun medial to 88.02. Located 8 cun proximal, and 1.0 cun medial, to the center of the top of the patella.

**Associated Channel:** Spleen

**Reaction areas:** Kidney and Uterus

**Dao Ma:** 88.04+88.05+88.06

**Indications:**
- UTERINE/OVARIAN TUMORS/CYSTS/FIBROIDS
- UTERITIS
- HORMONAL IMBALANCE
- INFERTILITY
- IRREGULAR MENSTRUATION
- HELPS TO BRING ON MENSES
- UTERINE ITCHING
- MISCARRIAGE
- INTESTINAL PAIN
- BLEEDING PEPTIC ULCER
- VAGINAL ITCHING

- LEUKORRHEA WITH REDDISH DISCHARGE.

**Manipulation:**
Insertion of 1.0 to 2.5 cun in depth. Needle bilaterally. Needle on women only.

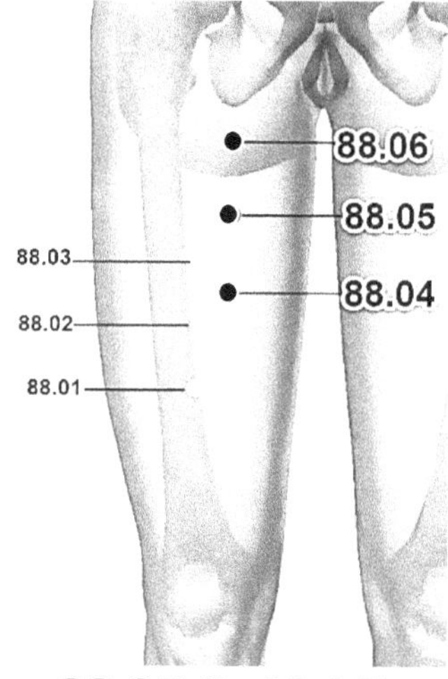


# 88.05 Jie Mei Er
(SISTER TWO)

**Location:**
2.5 cun superior to 88.04

**Associated Channel:** Spleen

**Reaction areas:** Kidney and Uterus

**Dao Ma:** 88.04+88.05+88.06

**Indications:**
- UTERINE/OVARIAN TUMORS/CYSTS/FIBROIDS
- UTERITIS
- HORMONAL IMBALANCE
- INFERTILITY
- IRREGULAR MENSTRUATION
- HELPS TO BRING ON MENSES
- UTERINE ITCHING
- MISCARRIAGE
- INTESTINAL PAIN
- BLEEDING PEPTIC ULCER
- VAGINAL ITCHING
- LEUKORRHEA WITH REDDISH DISCHARGE.

**Manipulation:**
Insertion of 1.5 to 2.5 cun in depth. Needle bilaterally. Needle on women only.

# 88.06 Jie Mei San
(SISTER THREE)

**Location:**
2.5 cun superior to 88.05

**Associated Channel:** Spleen

**Reaction areas:** Kidney and Uterus

**Dao Ma:** 88.04+88.05+88.06

**Indications:**
- UTERINE/OVARIAN TUMORS/CYSTS/FIBROIDS
- UTERITIS
- HORMONAL IMBALANCE
- INFERTILITY
- IRREGULAR MENSTRUATION
- HELPS TO BRING ON MENSES
- UTERINE ITCHING
- MISCARRIAGE
- INTESTINAL PAIN
- BLEEDING PEPTIC ULCER
- VAGINAL ITCHING
- LEUKORRHEA WITH REDDISH DISCHARGE.

**Manipulation:**
Insertion of 1.5 to 2.5 cun in depth. Needle bilaterally. Needle on women only.

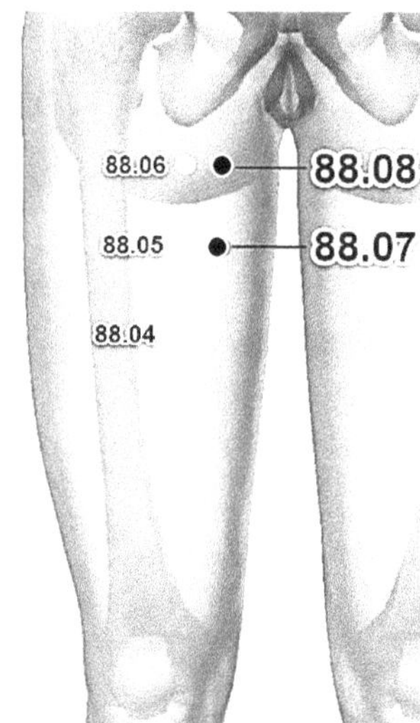


# 88.07 Gan Mao Yi
(COMMON COLD-ONE)

**Location:**
1 cun medial to 88.05. Located on the thigh, 10.5 cun proximal to the superior border of the patella, and 2.0 cun medial to the midline.

**Associated Channel:** Spleen

**Reaction areas:** Lung and Six bowels

**Dao Ma:** 88.07+88.08

**Indications:**
- CHILLS
- HIGH FEVER
- SEVERE COLD
- HEADACHE DUE TO INFLUENZA

**Manipulation:**
Insertion of 0.8 to 1.5 cun in depth. Oblique insertion.

# 88.08 Gan Mao Er
(COMMON COLD-TWO)

**Location:**
1 cun medial to 88.06 or 2.5 cun proximal to 88.07

**Associated Channel:** Spleen

**Reaction areas:** Lung and Six bowels

**Dao Ma:** 88.07+88.08

**Indications:**
- CHILLS
- HIGH FEVER
- SEVERE COLD
- HEADACHE DUE TO INFLUENZA

**Manipulation:**
Insertion of 0.8 to 1.5 cun in depth. Oblique insertion.

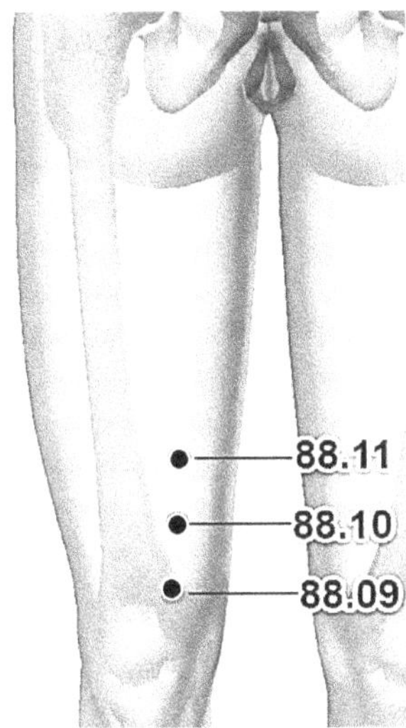


# 88.09 Tong Shen
(PENETRATING KIDNEY)

**Location:**
On the superior border of the medial kneecap. On the Spleen channel

**Associated Channel:** Spleen

**Reaction area:** Kidney

**Dao Ma:** 88.09+88.10+88.11

**Indications:**
- IMPOTENCE
- PREMATURE EJACULATION
- PAINFUL URINATION
- NEPHRITIS
- DIABETES

- DIZZINESS AND BACK PAIN DUE TO KIDNEY DEFICIENCY
- SHOULDER AND BACK PAIN
- WHOLE BODY EDEMA
- SEXUAL DISEASES
- RENAL RHEUMATISM
- UTERINE PAIN
- LEUKORRHEA WITH REDDISH DISCHARGE
- THIRST
- SORE THROAT AND DRY MOUTH
- DORSAL FOOT SWELLING
- INFLAMED INSTEP
- COLD FEET IN MEN.

**Manipulation:**
Insertion of 0.5 to 1.0 cun in depth. Suitable for bilateral needling but not necessary to use all the points.

# 88.10 Tong Wei
(PENETRATING STOMACH)

**Location:**
2 cun superior to point 88.09. On the Spleen channel.

**Overlaps:** SP-10.

**Associated Channel:** Spleen

**Reaction area:** Kidney

**Dao Ma:** 88.09+88.10+88.11

**Indications:**
- IMPOTENCE
- PREMATURE EJACULATION
- PAINFUL URINATION
- NEPHRITIS
- DIABETES
- DIZZINESS AND BACK PAIN DUE TO KIDNEY DEFICIENCY
- SHOULDER AND BACK PAIN
- WHOLE BODY EDEMA
- SEXUAL DISEASES
- RENAL RHEUMATISM
- UTERINE PAIN
- LEUKORRHEA WITH REDDISH DISCHARGE
- THIRST
- SORE THROAT AND DRY MOUTH
- DORSAL FOOT SWELLING
- INFLAMED INSTEP
- COLD FEET IN MEN
- STOMACH ISSUES

**Manipulation:**
Insertion of 0.5 to 1.0 cun in depth. Suitable for bilateral needling but not necessary to use all the points.

# 88.11 Tong Bei
(PENETRATING BACK)

**Location:**
4 cun superior to 88.09. On the Spleen channel.

**Associated Channel:** Spleen

**Reaction area:** Kidney

**Dao Ma:** 88.09+88.10+88.11

**Indications:**
- IMPOTENCE
- PREMATURE EJACULATION
- PAINFUL URINATION
- NEPHRITIS
- DIABETES
- DIZZINESS AND BACK PAIN DUE TO KIDNEY DEFICIENCY
- SHOULDER AND BACK PAIN
- WHOLE BODY EDEMA
- SEXUAL DISEASES
- RENAL RHEUMATISM
- UTERINE PAIN
- LEUKORRHEA WITH REDDISH DISCHARGE
- THIRST
- SORE THROAT AND DRY MOUTH
- DORSAL FOOT SWELLING
- INFLAMED INSTEP
- COLD FEET IN MEN
- KIDNEY STONE WITH BACK PAIN

**Manipulation:**
Insertion of 0.5 to 1.0 cun in depth. Suitable for bilateral needling but avoid using all the points.

# 88.12 Ming Huang
(BRIGHT YELLOW)

**Location:**
Center of the medial aspect of the thigh. 8 cun above the top of the patella on the medial thigh. On the Liver channel. Opposite 88.25(GB-31)

**Associated Channel:** Liver

**Reaction areas:** Kidney (superficial depth, 1 cun), Liver (middle depth, 2 cun), Heart (deep level, 3 cun)

**Dao Ma:** 88.12+88.13+88.14 (Three Upper Yellow or Three Yellows)

**Indications:**
- LIVER CIRRHOSIS
- LIVER PAIN
- HEPATITIS
- GALLBLADDER INFLAMMATION
- BODY SWELLING
- HEPATOMEGALY
- SPLENOMEGALY

- POLYCYSTIC LIVER AND KIDNEYS
- INDIGESTION
- FATIGUE
- BACK AND SPINAL PAIN/ABNORMALITIES
- ENLARGEMENT OF BONES
- BONE SPURS
- MULTIPLE SCLEROSIS
- SPINAL MENINGITIS
- CHOREA
- PARKINSON'S DISEASE
- MENIERE'S DISEASE
- DIZZINESS/VERTIGO
- BLURRED VISION
- EYE PAIN
- DRY EYES
- INDIGESTION
- LEUKEMIA
- NOSE BLEEDS
- BLEEDING GUMS

**Manipulation:**
Insertion of 1.5 to 2.5 cun in depth.

**Remarks:** Top Dao Ma useful for liver issues, fatty, depressed and stagnated livers. Also for wind and blood issues.

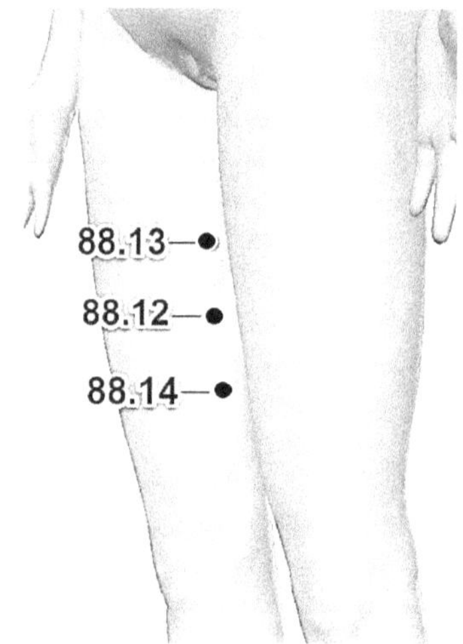


## 88.13 Tian Huang
(HEAVENLY YELLOW)

**Location:**
3 cun superior to 88.12. On the Liver channel.

**Associated Channel:** Liver

**Reaction areas:** Kidney (superficial depth, 1 cun), Liver (middle depth, 2 cun), Heart (deep level, 3 cun)

**Dao Ma:** 88.12+88.13+88.14 (Three Upper Yellow or Three Yellows)

**Indications:**
- LIVER CIRRHOSIS

- LIVER PAIN
- HEPATITIS
- GALLBLADDER INFLAMMATION
- BODY SWELLING
- HEPATOMEGALY
- SPLENOMEGALY
- POLYCYSTIC LIVER AND KIDNEYS
- INDIGESTION
- FATIGUE
- BACK AND SPINAL PAIN/ABNORMALITIES
- ENLARGEMENT OF BONES
- BONE SPURS
- MULTIPLE SCLEROSIS
- SPINAL MENINGITIS
- CHOREA
- PARKINSON'S DISEASE
- MENIERE'S DISEASE
- DIZZINESS/VERTIGO
- BLURRED VISION
- EYE PAIN
- DRY EYES
- INDIGESTION
- LEUKEMIA
- NOSE BLEEDS
- BLEEDING GUMS

**Manipulation:**
Insertion of 1.5 to 2.5 cun in depth.

## 88.14 Qi Huang
(THIS YELLOW)

**Location:**
3 cun distal to 88.12. On the Liver channel.

**Associated Channel:** Liver

**Reaction areas:** Kidney (superficial depth, 1 cun), Liver and Gallbladder (middle depth, 2 cun), Heart (deep level, 3 cun)

**Dao Ma:** 88.12+88.13+88.14 (Three Upper Yellow or Three Yellows)

**Indications:**
- JAUNDICE
- LIVER CIRRHOSIS
- LIVER PAIN
- HEPATITIS
- GALLBLADDER INFLAMMATION
- BODY SWELLING
- HEPATOMEGALY
- SPLENOMEGALY
- POLYCYSTIC LIVER AND KIDNEYS
- INDIGESTION
- FATIGUE
- BACK AND SPINAL PAIN/ABNORMALITIES
- ENLARGEMENT OF BONES

- BONE SPURS
- MULTIPLE SCLEROSIS
- SPINAL MENINGITIS
- CHOREA
- PARKINSON'S DISEASE
- MENIERE'S DISEASE
- DIZZINESS/VERTIGO
- BLURRED VISION
- EYE PAIN
- DRY EYES
- INDIGESTION
- LEUKEMIA
- NOSE BLEEDS
- BLEEDING GUMS

**Manipulation:**
Insertion of 1.5 to 2.5 cun in depth.

## 88.15 Huo Zhi
(FIRE BRANCH)

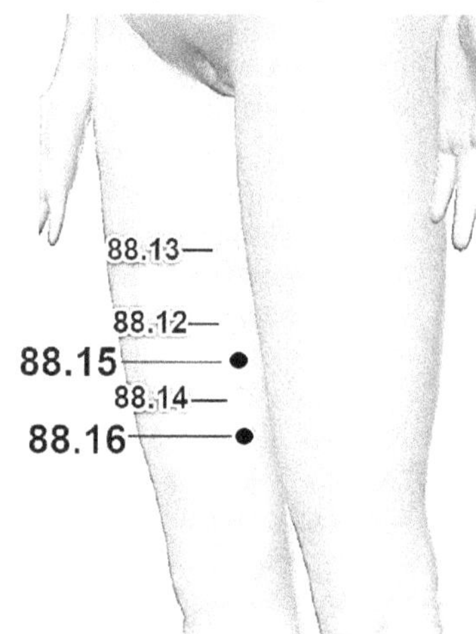


**Location:**
1.5 cun superior to point 88.14. On the Liver channel.

**Associated Channel:** Liver

**Reaction area:** Liver, Gall bladder and Heart.

**Dao Ma:** 88.14+88.15+88.16 (Gallbladder Points)

**Indications:**
- GALLBLADDER INFLAMMATION (CHOLECYSTITIS)
- HEPATITIS
- JAUNDICE
- DIZZINESS CAUSED BY JAUNDICE
- BLURRED VISION
- BACK PAIN DUE TO GALLSTONES
- EPILEPSY

**Manipulation:**
Insertion of 1.0 to 2.0 cun in depth.

# 88.16 Huo Quan
### (FIRE COMPLETE)

**Location:**
1.5 cun inferior to 88.14. On the Liver channel.

**Associated Channel:** Liver

**Reaction area:** Liver, Gall bladder and Heart.

**Dao Ma:** 88.14+88.15+88.16 (Gallbladder Points)

**Indications:**
- GALLBLADDER INFLAMMATION (CHOLECYSTITIS)
- HEPATITIS
- JAUNDICE
- DIZZINESS CAUSED BY JAUNDICE
- BLURRED VISION
- BACK PAIN DUE TO GALLSTONES
- EPILEPSY
- HEEL PAIN
- SPINE PAIN

**Manipulation:**
Insertion of 1.5 to 2.0 cun in depth.

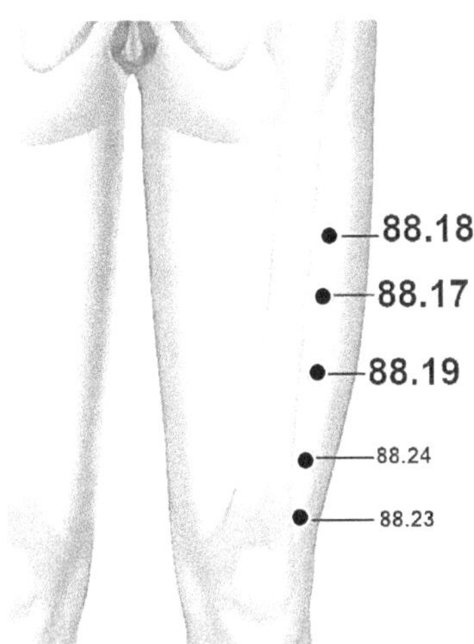


# 88.17 Si Ma Zhong
### (RAPID HORSES CENTER)

**Location:**
7 cun (8cun in certain text) superior to the outer edge of the patella. Or 3 cun anterior to GB-31. Or 1 cun proximal to ST-32. On the Stomach channel.

**Associated Channel:** Stomach

**Reaction Areas:** Liver and Lung

**Dao Ma:** 88.17+88.18+88.19 (Three Upper Horses or Four Horses)

**Indications:**
- PNEUMONIA
- TUBERCULOSIS
- PLEURISY
- COMMON COLD AND FLU
- ASTHMA AND COUGH
- RHINITIS/SINUSITIS
- ALLERGIES
- IMMUNE OR AUTOIMMUNE CONDITIONS
- THYROID PROBLEMS
- DEAFNESS/TINNITUS/OTITIS
- DERMATITIS
- PSORIASIS
- ECZEMA/URTICARIA
- SHINGLES
- SCLERODERMA
- SKIN FUNGUS
- ACNE
- FACIAL PARALYSIS/BELL'S PALSY
- CONGESTED EYES/CONJUNCTIVITIS
- BREAST PAIN - MOST EFFECTIVE
- HEMIPLEGIA
- LEG NUMBNESS, SIDE PAIN OF CHEST AND ABDOMEN, INTERCOSTAL NERVE PAIN, BOTH SIDES BACK PAIN
- SCIATICA
- BREAST PAIN/BREAST TUMOR
- MULTIPLE SCLEROSIS
- FIBROMYALGIA

**Manipulation:**
Insertion of 0.8 to 2.5 cun in depth.

**Remarks:** Another top Dao Ma, useful for all types of lung and skin issues

# 88.18 Si Ma Shang
### (RAPID HORSES UPPER)

**Location:**
2 cun superior to 88.17. On the Stomach channel.

**Associated Channel:** Stomach

**Reaction Areas:** Liver and Lung

**Dao Ma:** 88.17+88.18+88.19 (Three Upper Horses or Four Horses)

**Indications:**
- AS IN 88.17

**Manipulation:**
Insertion of 0.8 to 2.5 cun in depth.

# 88.19 Si Ma Xia
### (RAPID HORSES LOWER)

**Location:**
2 cun inferior to 88.17. On the Stomach channel.

**Associated Channel:** Stomach

**Reaction Areas:** Liver and Lung

**Dao Ma:** 88.17+88.18+88.19 (Three Upper Horses or Four Horses)

**Indications:**
- As in 88.17

**Manipulation:**
Insertion of 0.8 to 2.5 cun in depth.

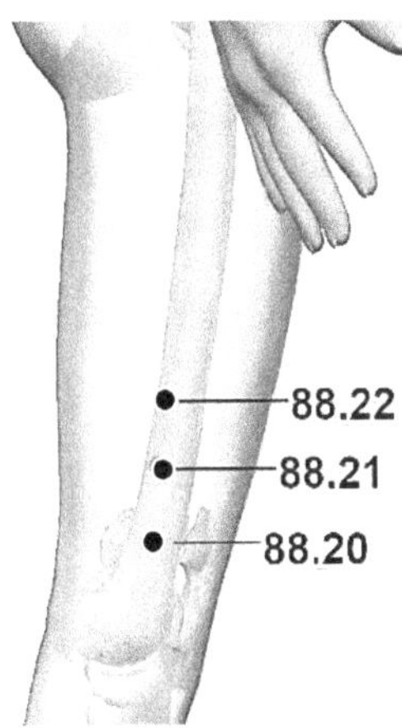


# 88.20 Xia Quan
### (LOWER FOUNTAIN)

**Location:**
2.5 cun superior to knee joint, along the medial line of the lateral thigh. On the Gallbladder channel.

**Associated Channel:** Gall bladder

**Reaction areas:** Lung and Face

**Dao Ma:** 88.20+88.21+88.22 (Three Springs)

**Indications:**
- FACIAL PARALYSIS AND NUMBNESS
- FACIAL TIC
- DEVIATED MOUTH OR EYE
- BELL'S PALSY
- TINNITUS AND POOR HEARING

**Manipulation:**
Insertion of 0.5 to 1.0 cun in depth. Touching the bone is desirable.

**Remarks:** This Dao Ma is useful for face issues.

# 88.21 Zhong Quan
### (CENTER FOUNTAIN)

**Location:**
2 cun proximal to 88.20. On the Gallbladder channel.

**Associated Channel:** Gall bladder

**Reaction areas:** Lung and Face

**Dao Ma:** 88.20+88.21+88.22 (Three Springs)

**Indications:**
- FACIAL PARALYSIS AND NUMBNESS
- FACIAL TIC
- DEVIATED MOUTH OR EYE
- BELL'S PALSY
- TINNITUS AND POOR HEARING

**Manipulation:**
Insertion of 0.5 to 1.0 cun in depth. Touching the bone is desirable.

# 88.22 Shang Quan
## (UPPER FOUNTAIN)

**Location:**
2 cun proximal to 88.21. On the Gallbladder channel.

**Associated Channel:** Gall bladder

**Reaction areas:** Lung and Face

**Dao Ma:** 88.20+88.21+88.22 (Three Springs)

**Indications:**
- FACIAL PARALYSIS AND NUMBNESS
- FACIAL TIC
- DEVIATED MOUTH OR EYE
- BELL'S PALSY
- TINNITUS AND POOR HEARING

**Manipulation:**
Insertion of 0.5 to 1.0 cun in depth. Touching the bone is desirable.

# 88.23 Jin Qian Xia
## (GOLD FRONT LOWER)

**Location:**
1 cun superior to the outer edge of the patella. On the Stomach channel.

**Associated Channel:** Stomach

**Reaction areas:** Lung and Liver

**Dao Ma:** 88.23+88.24

**Indications:**
- PROTRUSION OF THE STERNUM
- HYPOFUNCTION OF THE LUNG
- HYPOFUNCTION OF THE LIVER
- EPILEPSY
- HEADACHE
- SENSITIVE SKIN
- RABIES

**Manipulation:**
Insertion of 0.3 to 0.5 cun in depth. Needle bilaterally.

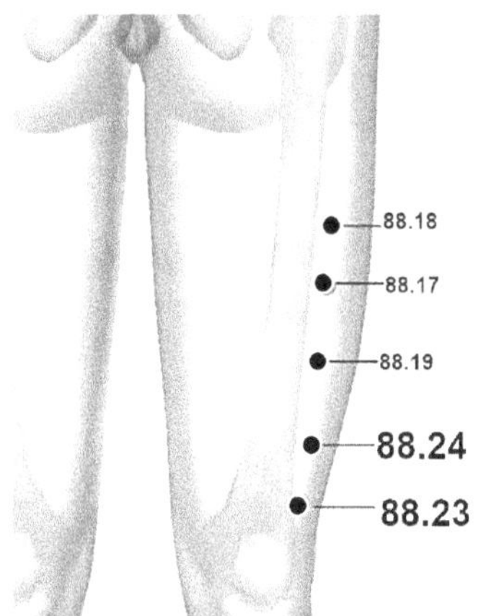


# 88.24 Jin Qian Shang
## (GOLD FRONT UPPER)

**Location:**
1.5 cun superior to 88.23. On the Stomach channel.

**Associated Channel:** Stomach

**Reaction areas:** Lung and Liver

**Dao Ma:** 88.23+88.24

**Indications:**
- PROTRUSION OF THE STERNUM
- HYPOFUNCTION OF THE LUNG
- HYPOFUNCTION OF THE LIVER
- EPILEPSY
- HEADACHE
- SENSITIVE SKIN
- RABIES

**Manipulation:**
Insertion of 0.3 to 0.5 cun in depth. Needle bilaterally.

# 88.25 Zhong Jiu Li
## (CENTER NINE MILES)

**Location:**
In the center of the median line of the lateral thigh. 7 cun (8 cun in certain text) proximal to the upper margin of the patella. On the Gallbladder channel.

**Overlaps:** GB-31

**Associated Channel:** Gall bladder

**Reaction areas:** Lung and Limbs

**Dao Ma:** 88.25+A.01 Seven Miles

**Indications:**
- MAJOR ANALGESIA AND SEDATION POINT
- ANY WIND-RELATED CONDITION
- MENTAL DISORDERS INCL. SCHIZO-PHRENIA, BIPOLAR, DEPRESSION, ETC.
- INSOMNIA
- HEADACHE AND MIGRAINE
- PAIN IN ANY OF THE FOLLOWING AREAS: UPPER, MIDDLE OR LOWER BACK; SPINE; LEG; THIGH; SOLE OF THE FOOT; EAR; EYE; BROW
- ONE-SIDED DISEASE OF GALLBLADDER CHANNEL.
- WHOLE-BODY PAIN (BILATERAL NEEDLING)
- MOVABLE PAIN
- WEAKNESS OF THE NERVOUS SYSTEM
- NUMBNESS OF THE LEGS AND BACK
- PERIPHERAL NEUROPATHY AND/OR NUMBNESS OF THE EXTREMITIES
- HEMIPLEGIA
- EPILEPSY
- FACIAL PARALYSIS
- TRIGEMINAL NEURALGIA
- VERTIGO
- DIZZINESS
- TINNITUS
- ITCHY SKIN AND WIND
- STIFF NECK
- CERVICAL SPONDYLOSIS
- BONE SPURS (MULTIPLE)
- ELBOW PAIN
- LYMPHEDEMA AS A RESULT OF BREAST CANCER SURGERY

**Manipulation:**
Insert 1.0 to 2.0 cun in depth. Gently touch the femur.

**Remarks:** Tung System's top point for systemic pain, wind, insomnia and stress.

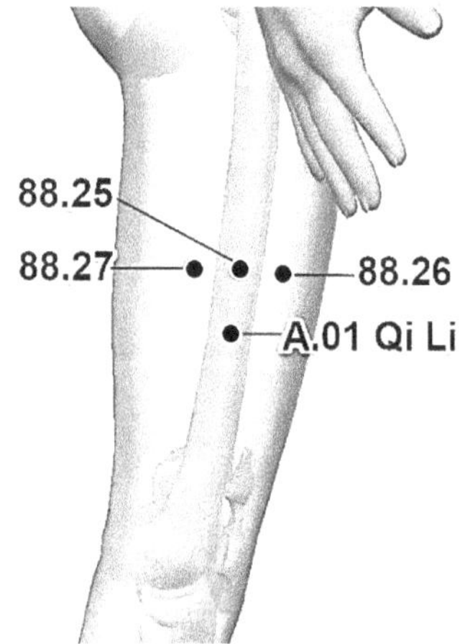


# A.01 Qi Li
## (SEVEN MILES)

**Location:**
Located 2.0 cun distal to 88.25 (GB-31)

**Overlaps:** GB-32

**Associated Channel:** Gallbladder

**Dao Ma:** 88.25+A.01 Seven Miles

**Indications:**
- HEMIPLEGIA (ESPECIALLY ARM)
- NUMBNESS OF THE HANDS OR ARMS
- NECK AND BACK PAIN
- LEG PAIN OR WEAKNESS
- NEURO-PARALYSIS
- ARTHRITIS
- ITCHING
- DIZZINESS
- VERTIGO
- DISTENDING EYES
- GALLBLADDER PAIN AND INFLAMMATION
- UPPER RIGHT QUADRANT LIVER PAIN

**Manipulation:**
Depth: 0.8-1.5 cun

## 88.26 Shang Jiu Li
(UPPER NINE MILES)

**Location:**
1.5 cun anterior to 88.25. On the Gallbladder channel.

**Associated Channel:** Gallbladder

**Reaction areas:** Heart and Kidney

**Dao Ma:** 88.25+88.26+88.27 (Three Nine Miles)

**Indications:**
- BACK, SHOULDER, HAND PAIN
- EYE PAIN
- ABDOMINAL DISTENSION DUE TO WEAK KIDNEY QI
- THIGH PAIN

**Manipulation:**
Insertion of 0.8 to 1.5 cun in depth.

## 88.27 Xia Jiu Li
(LOWER NINE MILES)

**Location:**
1.5 cun posterior to 88.25. On the Gallbladder channel.

**Associated Channel:** Gallbladder

**Reaction areas:** Back and Legs

**Dao Ma:** 88.25+88.26+88.27 (Three Nine Miles)

**Indications:**
- BACK, SHOULDER, HAND PAIN
- EYE PAIN
- ABDOMINAL DISTENSION DUE TO WEAK KIDNEY QI
- THIGH PAIN

**Manipulation:**
Insertion of 0.8 to 1.5 cun in depth.

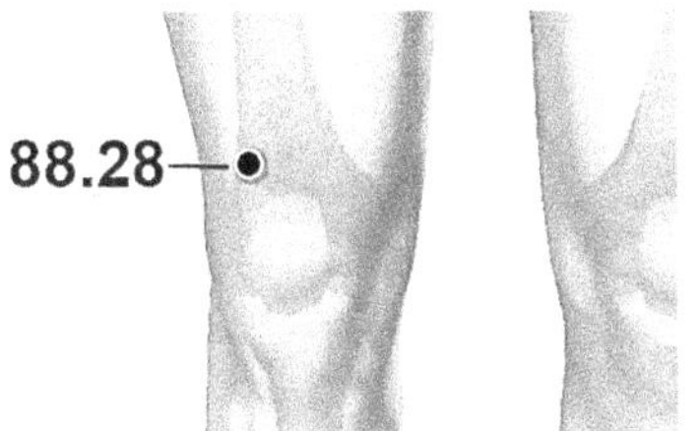


## 88.28 Jie
(RELEASE POINT)

**Location:**
1 cun superior and 0.3 cun lateral to the superior lateral corner of the patella on the Stomach Channel. 1.0 cun distal to ST-34.

**Associated Channel:** Stomach

**Reaction areas:** Heart and Blood vessels.

**Indications:**
- ACUTE TRAUMATIC/BLEEDING INJURY
- ESCAPE OF BLOOD
- SWELLING OF THE NEEDLING SITE/STUCK NEEDLE
- PAIN PRODUCED BY ACUPUNCTURE
- PAIN DUE TO INJECTION
- DIZZINESS AFTER NEEDLING
- EXTREME FATIGUE AFTER EXERTION.

**Manipulation:**
Insertion of 0.3 to 0.5 cun in depth. Short time retention for pain release. Approximately 8 minutes.

Remarks: Useful for acute situations of injury, sprains and trauma. Not useful for old/chronic injuries.

Useful when there is pain and swelling when acupuncture needle pierces a blood vessel.

## 88.29 Nei Tong Guan
(INNER PENETRATING GATE)

**Location:**
0.5 cun medial to 88.01

**Associated Channel:** Close to Stomach

**Reaction area:** Heart

**Dao Ma:** 88.29+88.30+88.31

**Indications:**
- HEMIPLEGIA
- WEAKNESS OF LIMBS DUE TO HEART WEAKNESS
- NERVOUS PARALYSIS OF LIMBS
- TRANSIENT ISCHEMIC ATTACK
- WIND-STROKE
- LOW BACK PAIN
- INABILITY TO RAISE HANDS
- RHEUMATOID ARTHRITIS OF KNEES

**Caution:** Do not needle all six points together.

**Manipulation:**
Insertion of 0.5 to 1.0 cun in depth.

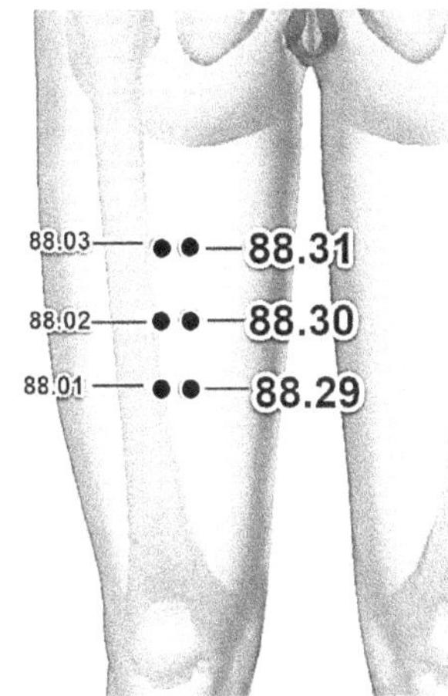


## 88.30 Nei Tong Shan
(INNER PENETRATING MOUNTAIN)

**Location:**
0.5 cun medial to 88.02. Locate 7 cun above the patella.

**Associated Channel:** Close to Stomach

**Reaction area:** Heart

**Dao Ma:** 88.29+88.30+88.31

**Indications:**
- HEMIPLEGIA
- WEAKNESS OF LIMBS DUE TO HEART WEAKNESS
- NERVOUS PARALYSIS OF LIMBS
- TIA OR CVA
- WIND-STROKE
- LOW BACK PAIN
- INABILITY TO RAISE HANDS
- RHEUMATOID ARTHRITIS OF KNEES

**Caution:** Do not needle all six points together.

**Manipulation:**
Insertion of 0.5 to 1.0 cun in depth.

## 88.31 Nei Tong Tian
(INNER PENETRATING HEAVEN)

**Location:**
0.5 cun medial to 88.03. Locate the point 0.5 cun medial to 88.03 - located 9 cun above the patella.

**Associated Channel:** Close to Stomach

**Reaction area:** Heart

**Dao Ma:** 88.29+88.30+88.31

**Indications:**

- HEMIPLEGIA
- WEAKNESS OF LIMBS DUE TO HEART WEAKNESS
- NERVOUS PARALYSIS OF LIMBS
- TIA OR CVA
- WIND-STROKE
- LOW BACK PAIN
- INABILITY TO RAISE HANDS
- RHEUMATOID ARTHRITIS OF KNEES

**Caution:** Do not needle all six points together.

**Manipulation:**
Insertion of 0.5 to 1.0 cun in depth.

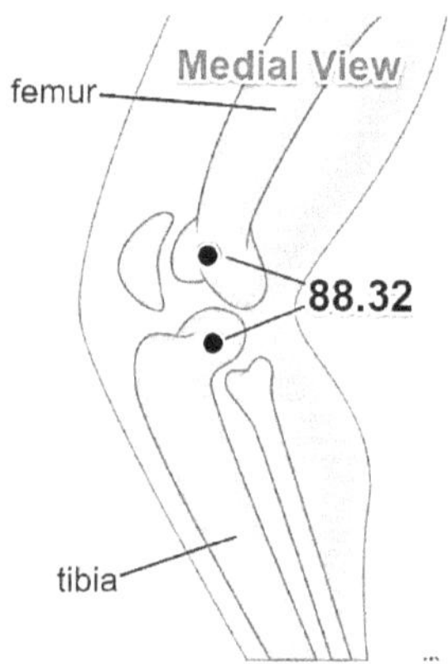


## 88.32 Shi Yin
(LOSS OF VOICE)

**Location:**
2 points group. The first point is located on the Spleen channel at the medial side of the knee joint, in line with the center of the patella. The second point is located two cun distal to the first point.

**Associated Channel:** Spleen

**Reaction areas:** Kidney and Throat.

**Indications:**
- HOARSENESS
- LOSS OF VOICE
- APHONIA
- PHARYNGITIS
- TONSILLITIS
- THYROID ENLARGEMENT
- SWOLLEN THROAT

**Manipulation:**
Insertion of 0.5 to 0.8 cun in depth.

## ZONE 99-Ear

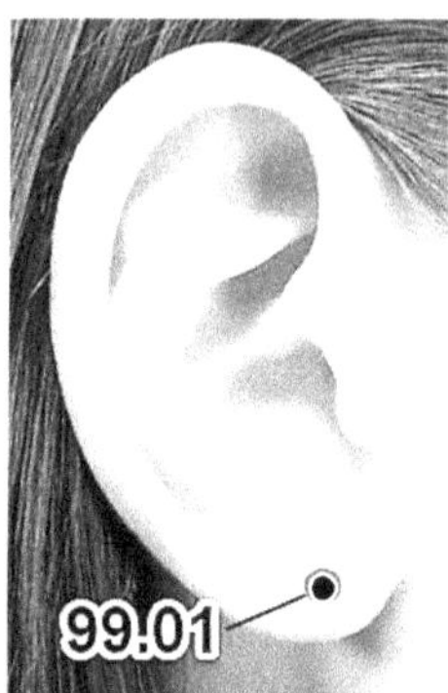


## 99.01 Er Huan
(EAR RING)

**Location:**
In the center of the ear lobe. Ear's "Eye" point.

**Reaction area:** Six bowels.

**Indications:**
- VOMITING
- INTOXICATION FROM ALCOHOL (HANGOVER)

**Manipulation:**
Insert a needle obliquely towards the face, 0.1 to 0.15 cun in depth.

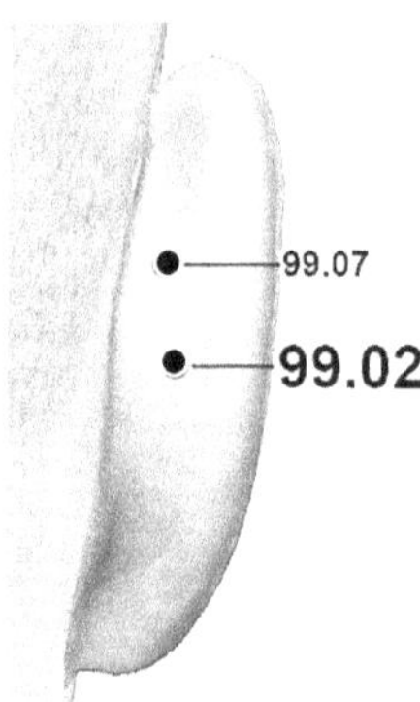


## 99.02 Mu Er
(WOOD EAR)

**Location:**
0.3 cun below the middle transverse branch of the dorsal auricular artery of the posterior aspect of the ear.

**Reaction area:** Liver

**Indications:**
- LIVER PAIN/LIVER DISEASE
- HEPATOMEGALY
- CIRRHOSIS
- FATIGUE DUE TO DEFICIENCY OF THE LIVER

- PAINFUL URINATION
- URINARY SPASMS
- Chronic gonorrhea

**Manipulation:**
Use 0.5 cun needle, insert 0.1-0.2 cun in depth. Bleed any blood vessel.

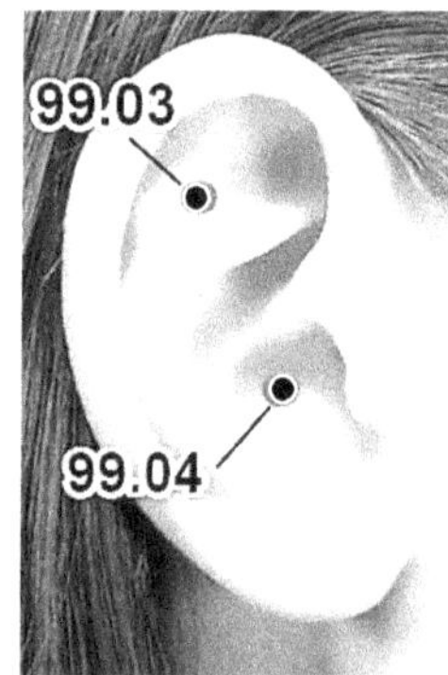


## 99.03 Huo Er
(FIRE EAR)

**Location:**
This point is on the superior crus of antihelix, at the level of the superior border of the inferior crus of antihelix, lateral to Shen Men.

**Reaction area:** Heart

**Indications:**
- HEART FAILURE
- KNEE PAIN
- LIMB PAIN

**Manipulation:**
Use 0.5 cun needle, insert 0.1 to 0.2 cun in depth.

## 99.04 Tu Er
(EARTH EAR)

**Location:**
Located on the anterior surface of the ear, in the center of the cavity of the concha.

**Reaction area:** Spleen

**Indications:**
- NEUROASTHENIA
- EXCESS OF RED BLOOD CELLS
- HIGH FEVER
- DIABETES

**Manipulation:**
Use 0.5 cun needle, insert 0.1 to 0.2 cun in depth.

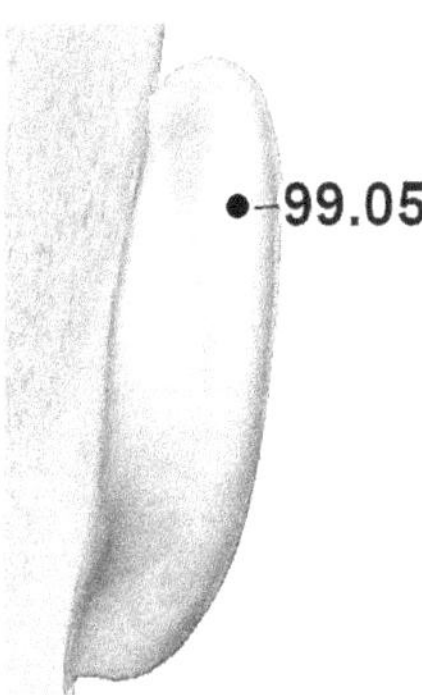


## 99.05 Jin Er
### (GOLD EAR)

**Location:**
Located on the posterior surface of the ear, on the upper third of the outer edge of the dorsal aspect of the helix. Locate a blood vessel in the area.

**Reaction area:** Lung

**Indications:**
- BL CHANNEL SCIATICA
- SCOLIOSIS
- ALLERGIC COMMON COLD

**Manipulation:**
Use 0.5 cun needle, insert 0.1 to 0.2 cun in depth.

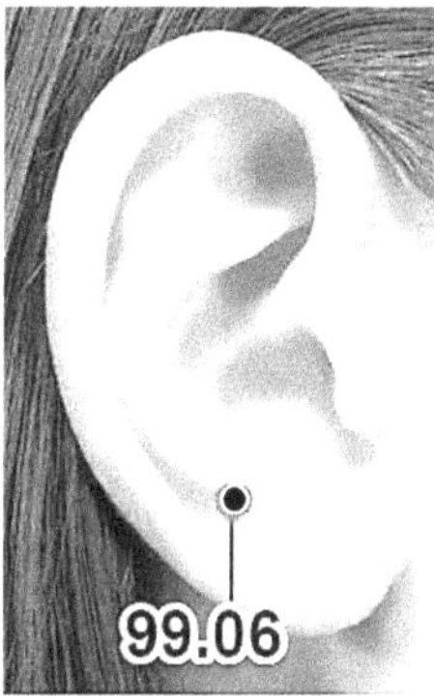


## 99.06 Shui Er
### (WATER EAR)

**Location:**
At the lower end of the outer border of the antihelix.

**Reaction area:** Kidney

**Indications:**
- DEFICIENCY OF THE KIDNEY
- KIDNEY DISEASE
- EYE ISSUES (ASTIGMATISM, NEARSIGHTEDNESS)

- DRY MOUTH
- LOW BACK PAIN (BOTH SIDES)
- ABDOMINAL DISTENSION

**Manipulation:**
Use 0.5 cun needle, insert 0.1 to 0.2 cun in depth.

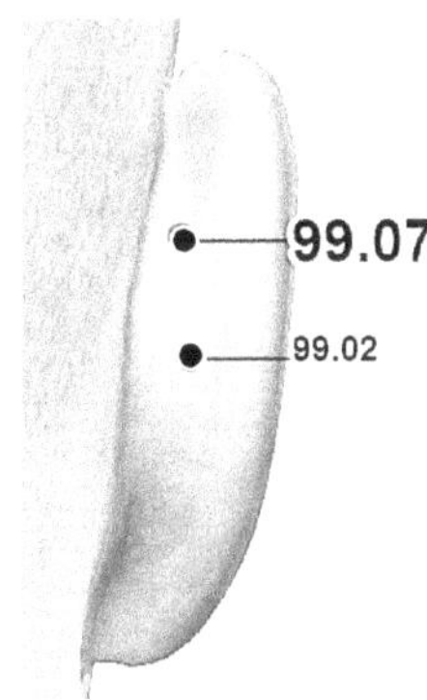


## 99.07 Er Bei
### (BACK EAR)

**Location:**
Located in the center of the upper half of the back of the ear; look for a good blood vessel.

**Reaction area:** Throat

**Indications:**
- ALLERGIES
- SYSTEMIC PAIN
- FEVER
- SHINGLES
- STYE IN THE EYE
- EYE DISEASES
- HYPERTENSION
- STRESS
- INSOMNIA
- A HANGOVER
- MOTION SICKNESS
- NIGHT SWEATS
- LOWER BACK PAIN
- COMMON COLD
- MIGRAINE HEADACHES
- HEAD ISSUES
- PHARYNGITIS
- TONSILLITIS
- TMJ
- TRIGEMINAL NEURALGIA
- FACIAL PARALYSIS
- EXCESSIVE SWEATING
- PALPITATION

**Manipulation:**
Bleed the point with a three-edged needle or lancet.

**Remarks:** Useful to bleed all the dark vessels behind the ear.

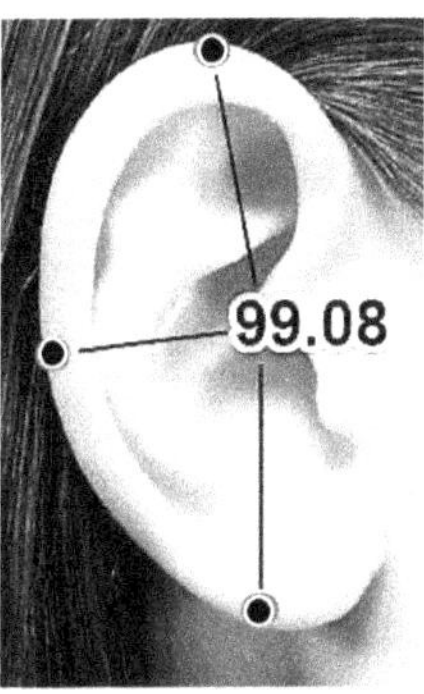


## 99.08 Er San
### (THREE EAR)

**Location:**
3 point unit. On the outer border of the helix of the ear. The upper point is at the top of the helix. The middle one is at the middle outer edge of the helix. The lowest one is at the inferior edge of the helix.

Only top point, ear apex, is commonly used.

**Reaction area:** Kidney, Lung

**Indications:**
- AS IN 99.07

**Manipulation:**
Bleed the point with a three-edged needle or lancet.

**Remarks:** Top point in the Tung system to treat allergies, hypertension, stress, sleep, systemic pain, dizziness and any head issues.

## ZONE 1010-Head and Face

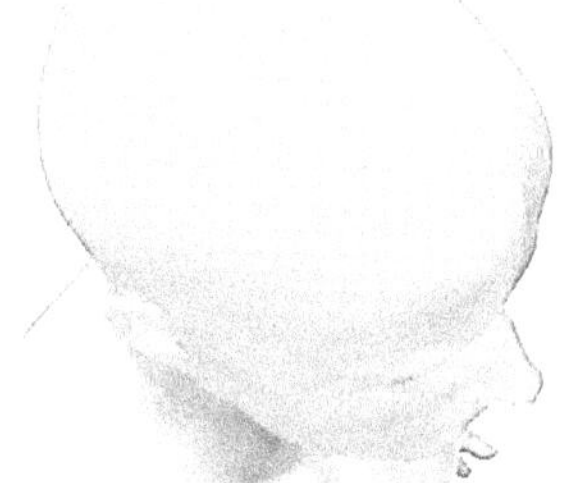


## 1010.01 Zheng Hui
### (UPRIGHTNESS MEETING)

**Location:**
In the center at the top of the head.

**Overlaps:** DU-20

**Associated Channel:** DU

**Reaction areas:** Brain, Cerebral nerve

**Indications:**

- ANXIETY OR DEPRESSION
- TREMOR OF LIMBS
- FATIGUE
- INFANTILE CONVULSION
- DEVIATION OF THE MOUTH AND EYE
- FACIAL PARALYSIS OR TICS
- STROKE/HEMIPLEGIA
- DYSFUNCTION OF THE NERVOUS SYSTEM
- CEREBRAL PALSY
- APHASIA DUE TO WIND-STROKE
- PARKINSON'S DISEASE
- APOPLEXY WITH STIFF TONGUE AND LOSS OF SPEECH.
- UNCONSCIOUSNESS OR COMA
- MENTAL RETARDATION
- EPILEPSY
- TAIL BONE PAIN
- BALL OF THE FOOT PAIN
- PROLAPSE (ANAL, UTERINE, BLADDER, HEMORRHOIDS) – CAN USE MOXIBUSTION

**Cautions:**

Not used with infants or children under the age of seven. (This ensures the fontanels are fused.)

**Manipulation:**

Insertion of 1.0 to 2.0 cun obliquely.

**Remarks:** 1010.01+1010.05, 1010.06 +1010.08 are the top points for stress.

1010.01 treats brain disorders such as stroke, tremors caused by yang rising and liver wind issues, and any type of prolapse.

# 1010.02 Zhou Yuan

(STATE ROUND)

**Location:**

1.3 cun to the left or right side of 1010.01

**Near to:** BL-7

**Associated Channel:** Urinary Bladder

**Reaction area:** Lung

**Dao Ma:** 1010.02+1010.03+1010.04

**Indications:**

- HEMIPLEGIA
- WEAKNESS OF LIMBS
- ASTHMA
- SHORTNESS OF BREATH
- SCIATICA AND BACK PAIN
- NERVOUS SYSTEM DYSFUNCTION
- TEMORS
- PARKINSON'S disease
- FATIGUE

**Manipulation:**

Insertion of 1.0 – 2.0 cun oblique insertion.

# 1010.03 Zhou Kun

(PREFECTURE ELDER BROTHER)

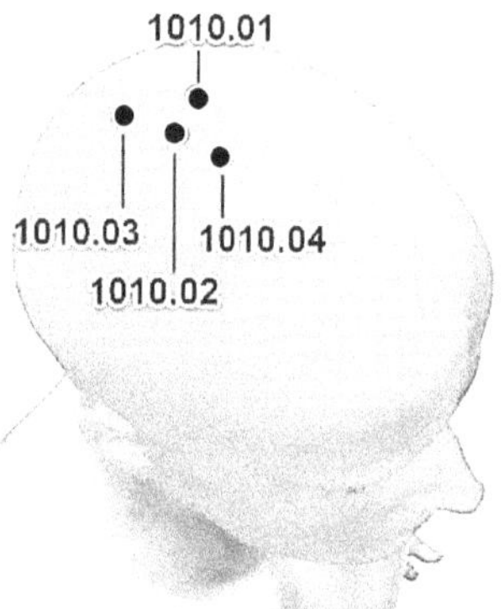


**Location:**

1.5 cun posterior to 1010.02

**Overlaps:** BL-8

**Associated Channel:** Urinary Bladder

**Reaction area:** Lung

**Dao Ma:** 1010.02+1010.03+1010.04

**Indications:**

- HEMIPLEGIA
- WEAKNESS OF LIMBS
- ASTHMA
- SHORTNESS OF BREATH
- SCIATICA AND BACK PAIN
- NERVOUS SYSTEM DYSFUNCTION
- TEMORS
- PARKINSON'S DISEASE
- FATIGUE

**Manipulation:**

Insertion of 1.0 – 2.0 cun oblique insertion

# 1010.04 Zhou Lun

(PREFECTURE MOUNTAIN)

**Location:**

1.5 cun anterior to 1010.02

**Overlaps:** BL-6

**Associated Channel:** Urinary Bladder

**Reaction area:** Lung

**Dao Ma:** 1010.02+1010.03+1010.04

**Indications:**

- HEMIPLEGIA
- TREMORS
- PARKINSON'S DISEASE
- WEAKNESS OF LIMBS
- ASTHENIA (PHYSICAL WEAKNESS)
- SHORTNESS OF BREATH

- ASTHMA
- SCIATICA AND BACK PAIN DUE TO HYPOFUNCTION OF THE LUNG
- NERVOUS SYSTEM DYSFUNCTION
- BRAIN TUMOR
- FATIGUE
- BACK PAIN
- BL CHANNEL SCIATICA

**Manipulation:**

Insertion of 1.0 – 2.0 cun oblique insertion.

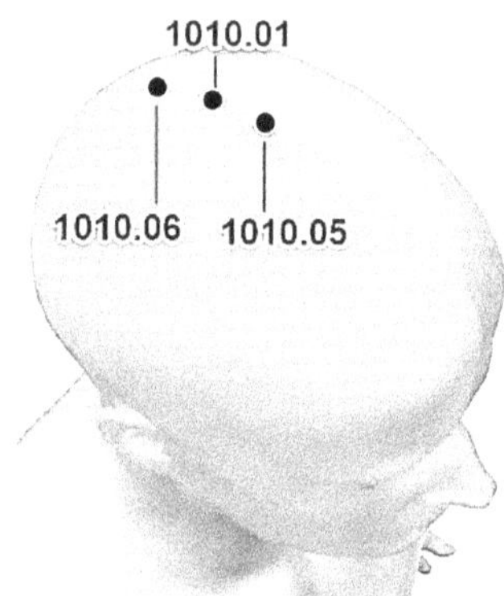


# 1010.05 Qian Hui

(ANTERIOR MEETINGS)

**Location:**

1.5 cun anterior to 1010.01

**Overlaps:** DU-21

**Associated Channel:** DU

**Reaction area:** Brain

**Indications:**

- DIZZINESS/VERTIGO
- FAINTING/UNCONSCIOUSNESS/COMA/ SHOCK
- BLURRED VISION
- SEEING SPOTS IN FRONT OF THE EYES
- BRAIN DISTENSION
- HEMIPLEGIA
- TENSION HEADACHE
- NERVOUSNESS
- ANXIETY
- DEPRESSION
- INSOMNIA
- PARKINSON'S DISEASE
- WIND DISEASES
- COCCYX PAIN

**Manipulation:**

Insertion of 1.0 – 2.0 cun oblique insertion.

# 1010.06 Hou Hui
(POSTERIOR MEETING)

**Location:** 1.6 cun longitudinally posterior to 1010.01

**Overlaps:** DU-19

**Associated Channel:** DU

**Reaction areas:** Brain and Spine

**Indications:**
- BONE TUBERCULOSIS
- MILD HEADACHE
- DIZZINESS
- SPINAL PAIN
- COCCYX PAIN
- HEEL PAIN
- NEUROPATHY
- ENCEPHALEMIA
- WIND DISEASES
- PARKINSON'S DISEASE
- APHASIA DUE TO WIND-STROKE
- HEMIPLEGIA
- NERVE PARALYSIS.

**Manipulation:** Insertion of $1.0 - 2.0$ cun oblique insertion

**Remarks:** 1010.06 combines well with 1010.01 and 1010.05 for all wind diseases.

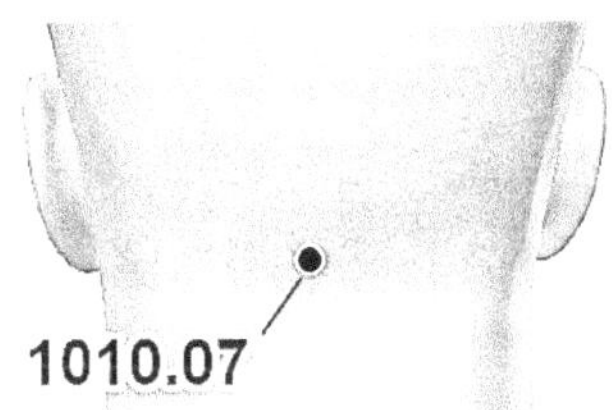

# 1010.07 Zong Shu
(TOTAL PIVOT)

**Location:**
0.8 cun above the posterior hair line. Slightly below DU-16.

**Associated Channel:** DU

**Reaction area:** Dan Tian

**Indications:**
- VOMITING
- NECK PAIN
- HEART FAILURE
- CHOLERA MORBUS
- DIARRHEA
- ACID REFLUX
- LOSS OF VOICE
- APHASIA

**Manipulation:**
Insertion of 0.1 to 0.2 cun in depth. Too deep can cause paralysis. This point is most effective when bled.

**Remarks:** Bleeding this point can stop nausea and vomiting and calm the hollow bowels.

# 1010.08 Zhen Jing
(TRANQUILITY)

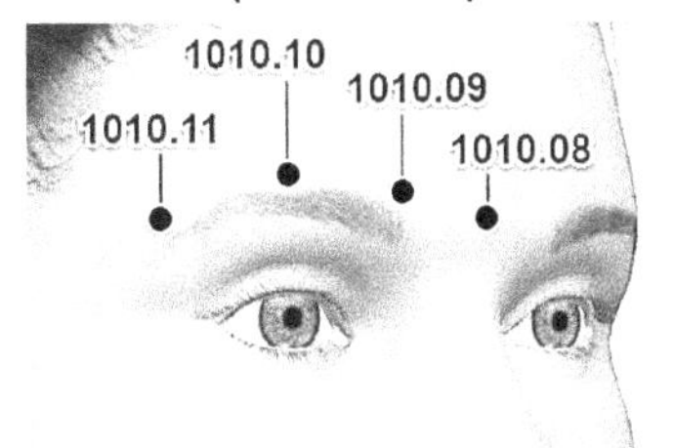


**Location:**
0.3 cun above the midpoint between the two eyebrows.

**Overlaps:** Yin Tang

**Associated Channel:** DU

**Reaction area:** Brain

**Indications:**
- MENTAL DISORDERS (STRESS, ANXIETY, DEPRESSION, MANIA)
- FRONTAL HEADACHE
- TREMOR OF LIMBS
- SORENESS AND WEAKNESS OF LEGS
- RESTLESS LEGS
- PARALYSIS OF LIMBS
- INSOMNIA
- NIGHTMARES
- FULLNESS IN THE CHEST WITH MENTAL RESTLESSNESS
- EPILEPSY

**Manipulation:**
Insert a needle subcutaneously toward the nose 0.1 to 0.2 cun in depth.

This point is can be bled.

# 1010.09 Shang Li
(UPPER MILE)

**Location:**
0.2 cun above the medial end of eyebrow. Above BL-2. On the Bladder channel.

**Associated Channel:** Urinary Bladder

**Reaction areas:** Lung and Eyes

**Dao Ma:** 1010.09+1010.10+1010.11

**Indications:**
- ACUTE HEADACHE
- DIZZINESS
- BLURRED VISION

**Manipulation:** Subcutaneous insertion 0.1 to 0.2 cun. Usually bled.

# 1010.10 Si Fu Er
(FOUR BOWELS SECOND POINT)

**Location:**
0.2 cun above the center of the eyebrow.

**Associated Channel:** Between Urinary Bladder and Sanjiao

**Reaction areas:** Lung and Eyes

**Indications:**
- ACUTE HEADACHE
- DIZZINESS/VERTIGO
- BLURRED VISION
- EYELIDS DISORDERS
- LOWER ABDOMINAL DISTENSION

**Manipulation:**
Insert a needle subcutaneously 0.1 to 0.2 cun in depth. Usually bled.

# 1010.11 Si Fu Yi
(FOUR BOWELS FIRST POINT)

**Location:**
0.2 cun above the lateral end of eyebrow. 0.2 cun above SJ-23.

**Associated Channel:** Between Urinary Bladder and Sanjiao

**Reaction areas:** Lung and Eyes

**Indications:**
- ACUTE HEADACHE
- DIZZINESS/VERTIGO
- BLURRED VISION
- EYELIDS DISORDERS
- LOWER ABDOMINAL DISTENSION

**Manipulation:**
Insert a needle subcutaneously 0.1 to 0.2 cun in depth. Usually bled.

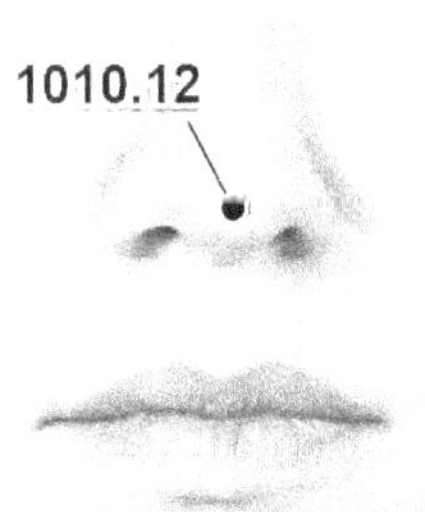


# 1010.12 Zheng Ben
(UPRIGHT SOURCE)

**Location:**
At the tip of the nose.

**Overlaps:** DU-25

**Associated Channel:** DU

**Reaction area:** Lung

**Indications:**
- ALLERGIC RHINITIS
- COMA
- PSYCHOSIS
- DECLINING BRAIN POWER
- BLEED POINT FOR ROSACEA, HYPERTROPHY OF MEMBRANE MUCOUS OF NOSE AND NASAL OBSTRUCTION
- INTOXICATION/HANGOVER

**Caution:** Do not harm nasal cartilage. Painful point.

**Manipulation:**
Insertion of 0.1 to 0.2 cun in depth. Usually bled. Feel the small cartilages on both sides of the nose tip and locate the point in the depression in between.

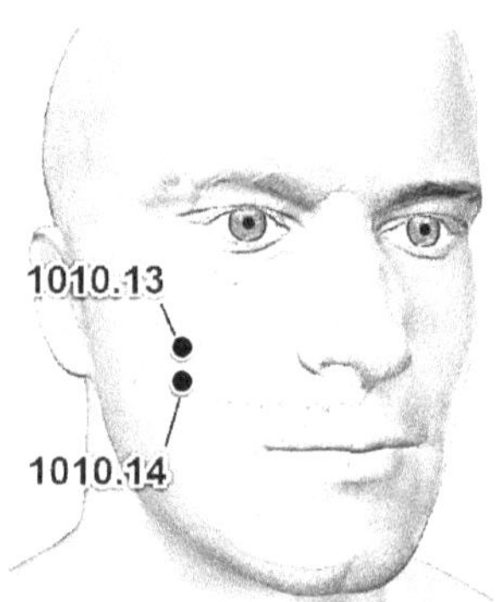


# 1010.13 Ma Jin Shui
(HORSE GOLD WATER)

**Location:**
Located directly beneath the edge of the outer canthus of the eye, just inferior to the zygomatic arch and level with LI-20 and the nasal ala.

**Overlaps:** SI-18

**Associated Channel:** Small Intestine

**Reaction areas:** Kidney and Lung

**Dao Ma:** 1010.13+1010.14

**Indications:**
- PAIN DUE TO KIDNEY STONE
- NEPHRITIS
- LUMBAR SPRAIN/LOW BACK PAIN
- PAIN IN THE CHEST DUE TO GAS
- RHINITIS/NASAL INFLAMMATION
- URETHRA PAIN
- PROSTATE DISEASES
- URINARY DISORDERS

**Manipulation:**
Insertion of 0.5 to 0.8 cun in depth.

**Remarks:** Great for all types of urinary disorders.

# 1010.14 Ma Kuai Shui
(HORSE FAST WATER)

**Location:**
0.4 cun below 1010.13. Same horizontal level as DU-26.

**Associated Channel:** Small Intestine

**Reaction areas:** Kidney and Urinary Bladder

**Dao Ma:** 1010.13+1010.14

**Indications:**
- PAIN DUE TO KIDNEY STONE
- NEPHRITIS
- LUMBAR SPRAIN/LOW BACK PAIN
- PAIN IN THE CHEST DUE TO GAS
- RHINITIS/NASAL INFLAMMATION
- URETHRA PAIN
- PROSTATE DISEASES
- URINARY DISORDERS

**Manipulation:**
Insertion of 0.5 to 0.8 cun in depth.

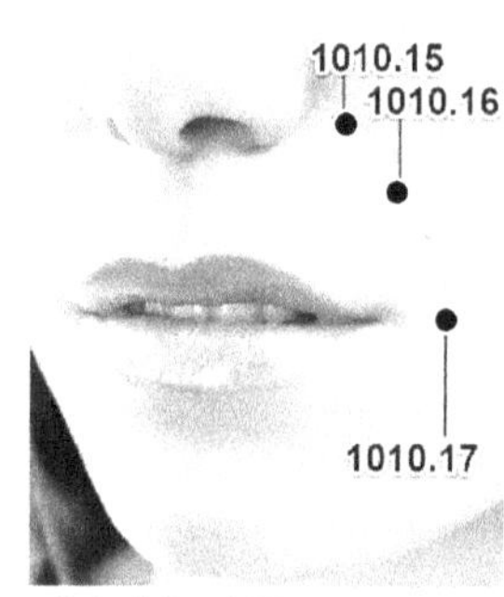


# 1010.15 Fu Kuai
(BOWELS FAST)

**Location:**
At the level of the nasal ala, lateral to the nose at the laugh line creases.

0.5 cun from the inferior lateral aspect of the ala nasi, at the level of the lower border of ala nasi.

**Near to:** LI-20

**Associated Channel:** Large Intestine

**Reaction areas:** Kidney and Six bowels.

**Indications**
- ABDOMINAL DISTENSION/PAIN
- HERNIA
- ALLERGIES, COLD AND FLU
- SINUS CONGESTION
- NASAL POLYPS
- ACNE

**Manipulation:**
Superficial insertion towards Yin Tang.

# 1010.16 Liu Kuai
(SIX FAST)

**Location:**
1.4 cun lateral to DU-26, on the laughing line.

**Associated Channel:** Close to Large Intestine

**Reaction areas:** Urinary passages

**Indications**
- URETHRA STONE
- URETHRITIS

**Manipulation:**
Insertion of 0.1 to 0.2 cun in depth.

# 1010.17 Qi Kuai
(SEVEN FAST)

**Location:**
0.5 cun lateral to the corner of the mouth.

**Overlaps:** ST-4

**Associated Channel:** Stomach

**Reaction area:** Lung

**Indications:**
- FACIAL PARALYSIS (OPPOSITE INSERTION)
- HYPOFUNCTION OF THE LUNG
- URETHRAL STONE
- URETHRA PAIN

**Manipulation:**
Insert a needle obliquely toward lateral side 0.5 to 1.5 cun in depth.

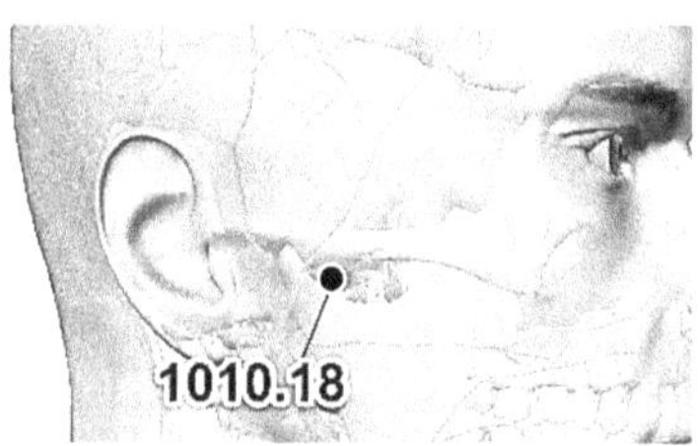


# 1010.18 Mu Zhi
(WOOD BRANCH)

**Location:**
1 cun superior and lateral from 1010.13. Located in the depression just anterior to the condyloid process

of the mandible when the mouth is wide open.

**Overlaps:** ST-7

**Associated Channel:** Stomach

**Reaction areas:** Liver and Gall bladder

**Indications:**
- DEFICIENCY IN THE LIVER OR GALLBLADDER
- PAIN DUE TO GALLSTONES AND GALLBLADDER INFLAMMATION
- NIGHT CRYING OF CHILD
- FALLING TENDENCIES OF ELDERLY DUE TO LEGS WEAKNESS

**Manipulation:**
Insertion of 0.3 to 0.5 cun in depth.

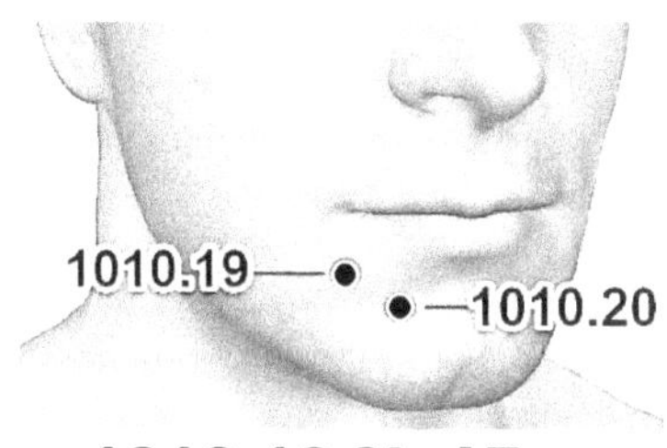


# 1010.19 Shui Tong
## (WATER THROUGH)

**Location:**
0.4 cun below the corner of the mouth.

**Overlaps:** ST-4

**Reaction area:** Kidney

**Dao Ma:** 1010.19+1010.20

**Indications:**
- LOW BACK PAIN
- ACUTE LUMBAR SPRAIN
- LEGS WEAKNESS
- DIZZINESS/VERTIGO
- FATIGUE
- DIFFICULTY BREATHING
- ASTHMA/COUGH/BRONCHITIS
- LUNG DISEASES
- PREMATURE EJACULATION
- IMPOTENCE
- PROSTATE ISSUES
- NON-STOP HICCUPS

**Manipulation:**
Insert a needle obliquely toward lateral side 0.5 to 1.0 cun in depth. Can use single through-needle from 1010.20 to 1010.19.

**Remarks:** 1010.19+1010.20 is often used with 1010.13+1010.14 for kidney and bladder problems.

Combining with 1010.20 to treat lower back pain involving the muscles of the lower back. Also any lung or breathing problem, kidney issue, cough, asthma and allergies.

# 1010.20 Shui Jin
## (WATER GOLD)

**Location:**
0.5 cun medial and inferior to 1010.19.

**Reaction area:** Kidney

**Dao Ma:** 1010.19+1010.20

**Indications:**
- LOW BACK PAIN
- ACUTE LUMBAR SPRAIN
- LEGS WEAKNESS
- DIZZINESS/VERTIGO
- FATIGUE
- DIFFICULTY BREATHING
- ASTHMA/COUGH/BRONCHITIS
- LUNG DISEASES
- PREMATURE EJACULATION
- IMPOTENCE
- PROSTATE ISSUES
- NON-STOP HICCUPS

**Manipulation:**
Insert a needle obliquely toward lateral side 0.5 to 1.0 cun in depth. Can use single needle from 1010.20 to 1010.19.

# 1010.21 Yu Huo
## (JADE FIRE)

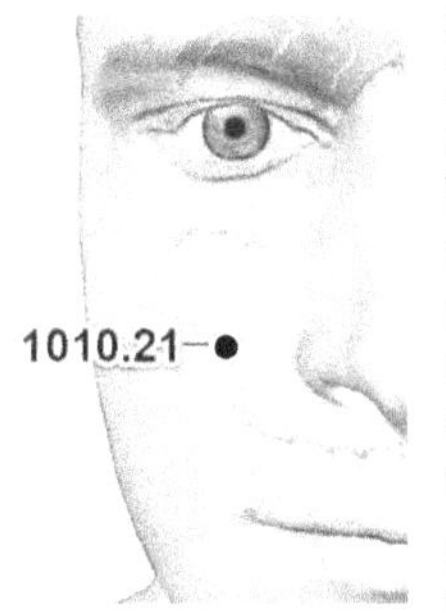


**Location:**
In the depression below the zygomatic bone on the line connecting the center of the eye.

**Overlaps:** Near ST-3 (in some text, overlaps ST-2)

**Associated Channel:** Stomach

**Reaction areas:** Heart and Liver.

**Indications:**
- SCIATICA
- SHOULDER AND ARM PAIN
- LIMB PAIN
- KNEE PAIN
- CHEEK PAIN
- UPPER JAW BONE PAIN
- PAIN DUE TO BLOOD DEFICIENCY AND EXTRAVASATED BLOOD

**Manipulation:**
Insertion of 0.1 to 0.3 cun in depth.

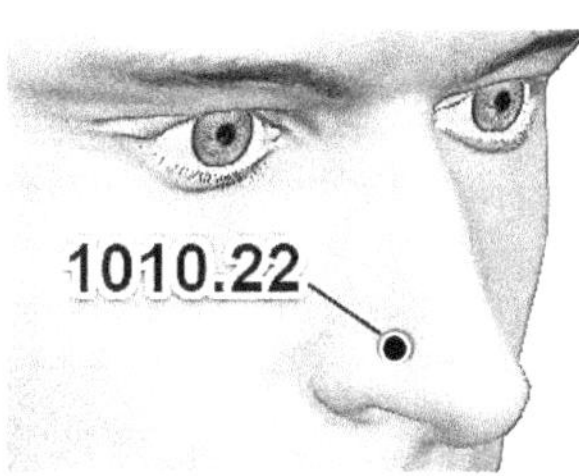


# 1010.22 Bi Yi
## (NASAL WING)

**Location:**
In the depression of the superior border of ala nasi. At the end of the curl of the nasal ala, where many cultures pierce the nose.

**Reaction areas:** Lung, Kidney and Spleen

**Indications:**
- SCIATICA DUE TO QI DEFICIENCY
- EXTREMITY PAIN DUE TO QI DEFICIENCY OR QI STAGNATION
- WHOLE-BODY PAIN DUE TO KIDNEY DEFICIENCY
- NERVE PAIN
- BONE PAIN
- EXTREME FATIGUE
- MIGRAINE
- SUPRAORBITAL PAIN
- FACIAL PARALYSIS
- HEMIPLEGIA
- DIZZINESS/VERTIGO
- BLURRED VISION
- SORE THROAT
- PAINFUL TONGUE
- SHOULDER PAIN

**Manipulation:**
Insertion of 0.1 to 0.3 cun in depth. Can go into nasal cavity but avoid the septum.

# 1010.23 Zhou Huo
## (PREFECT FIRE)

**Location:**
1.5 cun above the ear apex.

**Overlaps:** GB-8

**Associated Channel:** Gall bladder

**Reaction area:** Heart

**Indications:**
- PALPITATION
- RHEUMATIC HEART DISEASE
- WEAKNESS OF LIMBS
- LOWER BACK PAIN

**Manipulation:**
Insertion of 0.1 to 0.3 cun in depth.

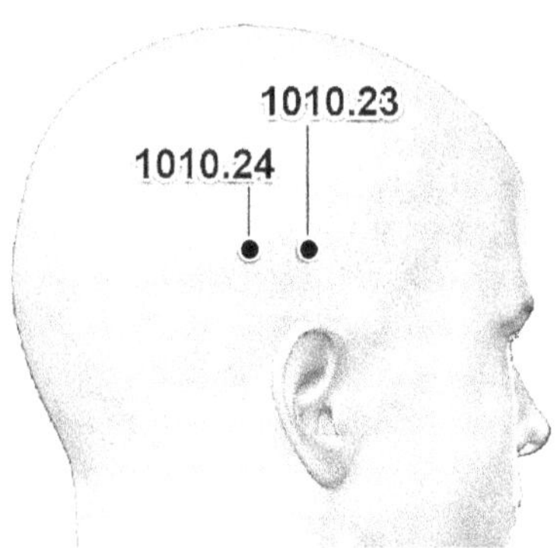

# 1010.24 Zhou Jin
(STATE GOLD)

**Location:**
1 cun posterior to 1010.23

**Associated Channel:** Gall bladder

**Reaction area:** Lung

**Indications:**
- SCIATICA DUE TO LUNG DYSFUNCTION
- RHEUMATISM DUE TO LUNG DYSFUNCTION
- LOWER BACK PAIN DUE TO LUNG DYSFUNCTION.

**Manipulation:**
Insertion of 0.2 to 0.5 cun in depth.

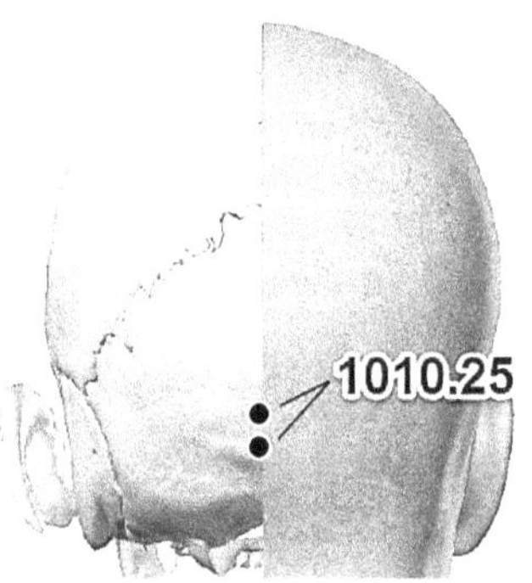

# 1010.25 Zhou Shui
(PREFECTURE WATER)

**Location:**
2-point group. The first one is located just above the external occipital protuberance and the second is 0.8 cun above the first.

**Associated Channel:** DU

**Reaction area:** Kidney

**Indications:**
- PAIN OF THE LUMBAR VERTEBRAE
- COCCYX/SACRAL PAIN
- FORAMEN NARROWING
- PARALYSIS OF THE LOWER LIMBS
- NERVOUS SYSTEM DYSFUNCTION.

**Manipulation:**
Insertion of 0.5 to 0.8 cun in depth. Oblique needling downwards from upper to lower point (threading technique).

Remarks: One of the most commonly used point for back pain, sacrum pain and pain on the DU channel.

# DT ZONE-Dorsal Torso

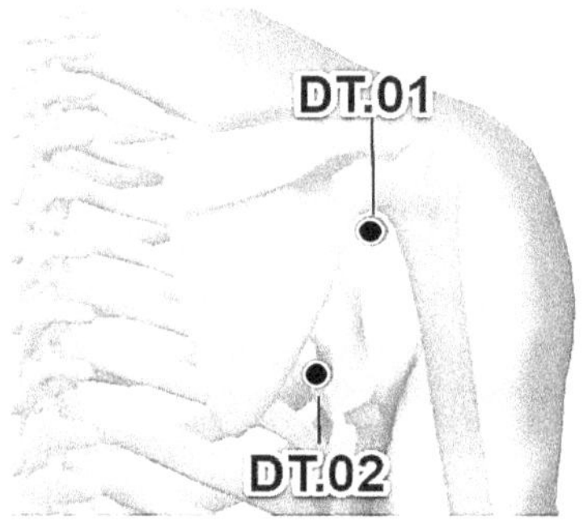

# DT.01 Fen Zhi Shang
(SEPARATE BRANCH UPPER)

**Location:**
At the inferior junction of the humerus and scapula (humero-scapular joint), on the Small Intestine channel. (At the connecting fork of the scapula and humerus)

**Associated Channel:** Small Intestine

**Reaction areas:** Liver, Endocrine Glands

**Dao Ma:** DT.01+DT.02 (Toxin Areas or Poison Points)

**Indications:**
- DRUG OR GAS POISONING
- CHEMOTHERAPY/RADIATION POISONING
- BITES BY TOXIC INSECTS OR REPTILES
- FOOD POISONING
- FOUL BREATH
- ARMPIT ODOR
- GENERALIZED/SEVERE ITCHING
- SHINGLES
- PSORIASIS
- DIABETES MELLITUS
- PAINFUL URINATION IN SEXUALLY TRANSMITTED INFECTIONS
- URINARY TRACT INFECTION
- KIDNEY FAILURE
- HEPATITIS

**Manipulation:**
More commonly dry cupped or bleed-cupped. Plum blossom applicable. Cups are positioned half on and half off the scapula.

# DT.02 Fen Zhi Xia
(SEPARATE BRANCH LOWER)

**Location:** 1.5 cun inferior and 0.5 cun medial to DT.01 on the Small Intestine channel

**Near to:** SI-9

**Associated Channel:** Small Intestine

**Reaction areas:** Breast, Lung

**Dao Ma:** DT.01+DT.02 (Toxin Areas or Poison Points)

**Indications:**
- DRUG OR GAS POISONING
- CHEMOTHERAPY/RADIATION POISONING
- BITES BY TOXIC INSECTS OR REPTILES
- FOOD POISONING
- FOUL BREATH
- ARMPIT ODOR
- GENERALIZED/SEVERE ITCHING
- SHINGLES
- PSORIASIS
- DIABETES MELLITUS
- PAINFUL URINATION IN SEXUALLY TRANSMITTED INFECTIONS
- URINARY TRACT INFECTION
- KIDNEY FAILURE
- HEPATITIS

**Manipulation:**
More commonly dry cupped or bleed-cupped. Plum blossom applicable. Cups are positioned half on and half off the scapula.

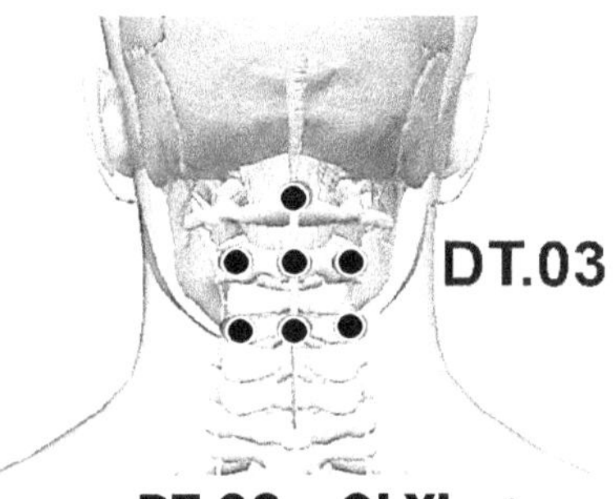

# DT.03 – Qi Xing
(SEVEN STARS)

**Location:**
Group of seven points.
Point 1- On Du Mai, 0.8 cun above posterior hairline
Point 2- 1 cun below first point
Point 3 – 2 cun below first point,

Point 4,5 – 0.8 cun lateral to second point
Point 6,7 – 1 cun below fourth and fifth points.
Start with first three points.

**Associated Channel:** DU and Urinary Bladder

**Reaction areas:** Brain, Lung

**Indications:**
- VOMITING/NAUSEA
- COMMON COLD HEADACHE
- HIGH FEVER IN CHILDREN
- INFANTILE CONVULSION
- SIMILAR INDICATIONS WITH DU-15 AND DU-16.

**Manipulation:**
Pinch up the skin and superficially bleed with lancet or bleed-cup. Gua sha applicable.

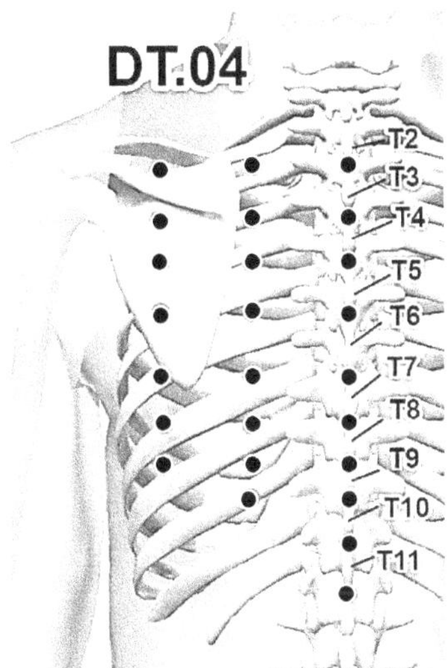

## DT.04 Wu Ling
(FIVE MOUNTAIN RANGE)

**Location:**
Group of 40 points. 15 points on each side and 10 points on mid-line.
The first line of points consists of one point below each spinal vertebra from T2 to T11; the second line of points run bilaterally 3 cun lateral to the spine, each point at the levels of T2 to T9, the third line of points run bilaterally 6 cun lateral to the spine, each point at the levels of vertebrae T2 to T8. Not necessary to needle all the points simultaneously.

**Associated Channel:** DU and Urinary Bladder

**Reaction areas:** Heart, Liver, Lung, Spleen

**Indications:**
- HIGH BLOOD PRESSURE (EMERGENCY TREATMENT)
- HEMIPLEGIA OR NUMBNESS
- HIGH FEVER (EMERGENCY TREATMENT)
- ACUTE, SEVERE HEADACHE
- SUDDEN DIZZINESS
- SEVERE COMMON COLD
- ACUTE GASTROINTESTINAL PAIN
- VOMITING DISEASES
- BACK PAIN DUE TO ARTERIOSCLEROSIS
- PERIPHERAL NEUROPATHY

**Manipulation:**
Lancet or bleed-cupping is used. One cup covers multiple points. Not necessary to bleed all points.

**Remarks:** Useful as emergency bleed points for high fever and hypertension.

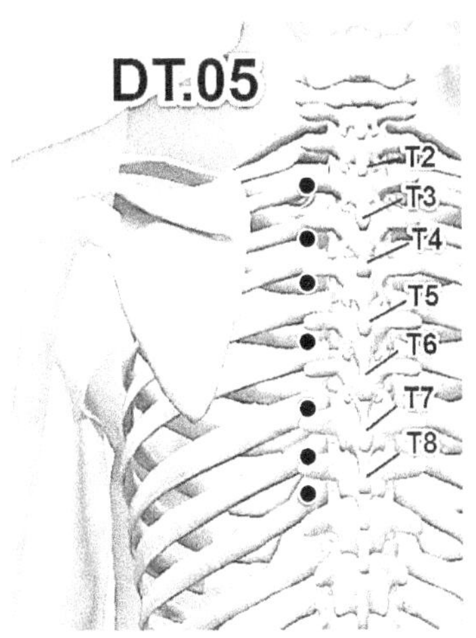

## DT.05 Shuang Feng
(DOUBLE PHOENIX)

**Location:**
Group of 14 points. 7 points on each side.
1.5 cun lateral to the DU channel, at the level of the spinous processes from T2 to T8

**Associated Channel:** Urinary Bladder

**Reaction areas:** Blood circulation

**Indications:**
- PAIN/NUMBNESS IN THE EXTREMITIES
- WHOLE BODY PAIN
- BONE SPURS

**Manipulation:**
Bleed bilaterally. Lancet or bleed-cupping is used. One cup covers multiple points

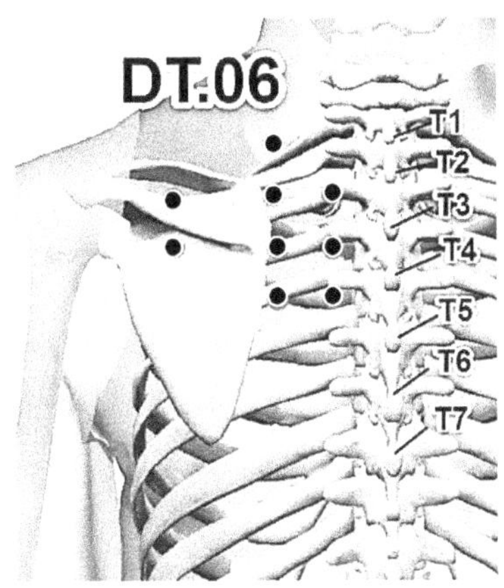

## DT.06 – Jiu Hou
(NINE MONKEYS)

**Location:**
Group of 18 points. 9 points on each side.

Located at BL-12, BL-13, BL-14, BL-41, BL-42, BL-43; also includes a point 3 cun lateral to T1, 6 cun lateral to T2, and 6 cun lateral to T3.

**Indications:**
- SCARLET FEVER
- PHLEGM STUCK IN THE BRONCHIA THAT CANNOT BE EXPELLED
- CIRCULATORY DISEASES

**Manipulation:** Lancet or bleed cupping is used. One cup covers multiple points. Bleed bilaterally.

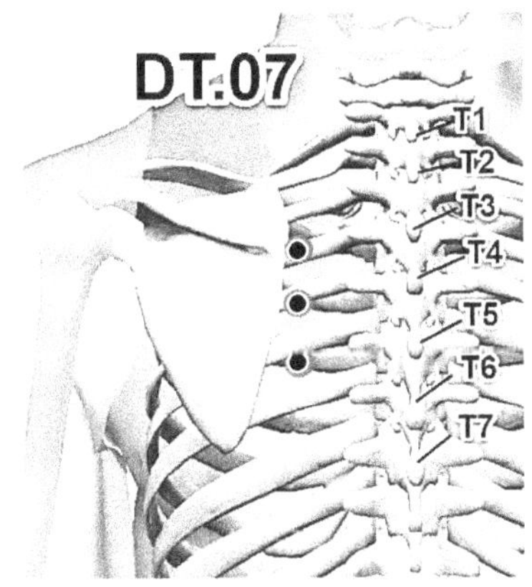

## DT.07 – San Jin
(THREE GOLD)

**Location:**
Group of 6 points. 3 points on each side.

Bilaterally, 3 cun lateral to DU channel, at the level of the spinous processes from T3 to T5.
**Equivalent** to BL-42, BL-43, BL-44

**Associated Channel:** Urinary Bladder

**Reaction areas:** Heart, Lung

**Indications:**

- DEGENERATIVE KNEE PAIN
- KNEE PAIN UNDER THE KNEE CAP
- SOFT TISSUE INFLAMMATION DUE TO BONE SPURS
- ENLARGED HEART AND HEART DISEASE

**Manipulation:**
Lancet or bleed-cupping is used. One cup covers multiple points. Bleed bilaterally or tender side.

These points are only effective for OA knee pain if the same side points are tender.

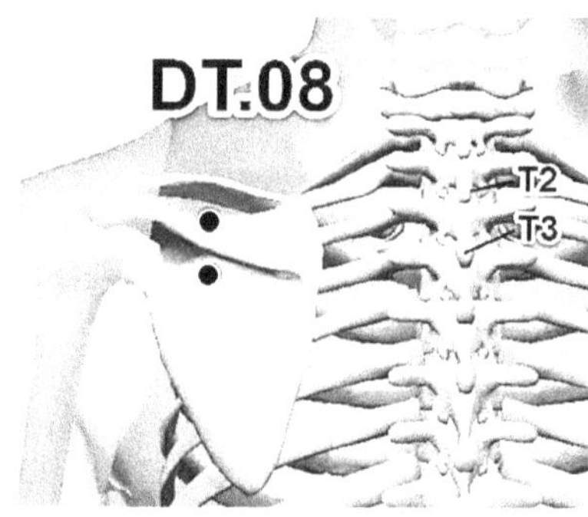

# DT.08 – Jing Zhi
(ESSENCE BRANCH)

**Location:**
Group of 4 points. 2 points on each side.

Bilaterally, 6 cun lateral to T2, and 6 cun lateral to T3.

**Associated Channel:** Small intestine and Urinary Bladder

**Reaction areas:** Kidney, Lung

**Indications:**

- GB CHANNEL SCIATICA
- SWELLING AND PAIN OF THE LOWER LEGS AND KNEE

**Manipulation:**
Lancet or bleed-cupping is used. One cup covers multiple points

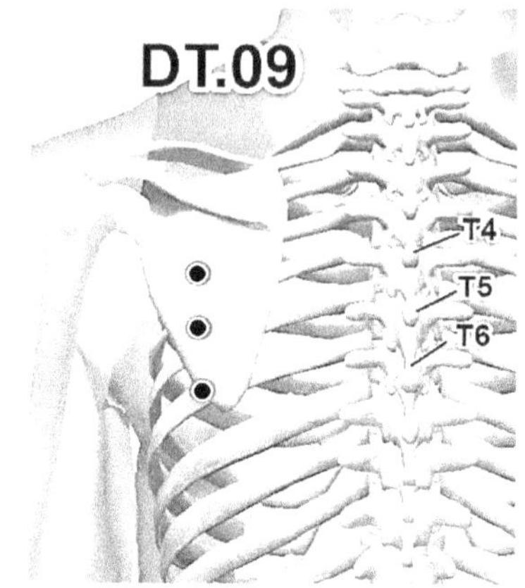

# DT.09 – Jin Lin
(GOLD FOREST)

**Location:**
Group of 6 points. 3 points on each side.

Bilaterally, 6.0 cun lateral to the space below the posterior spinous processes of T4, T5 and T6. 3 cun lateral to BL-44, BL-45, BL-46.

**Reaction areas:**
Kidney, Lung, Spleen (left side)

Kidney, Lung, Liver (right side)

**Indications:**

- SCIATICA DUE TO ARTERIOSCLEROSIS
- THIGH PAIN

**Manipulation:**
Bleed-cupping or single lancet is used. One cup covers multiple points. Bleed bilaterally. Look for tender spots.

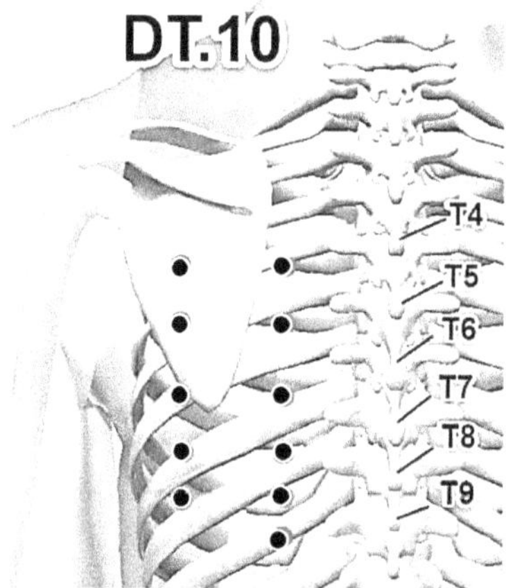

# DT.10 – Dsing Zhu
(TOP PILLAR)

**Location:**
Group of 22 points., 11 points on each side.
The first line of points run bilaterally 3 cun lateral to the spine, each point at the levels of T4 to T9, the second line of points run bilaterally 6 cun lateral to the spine, each point at the levels of vertebrae T4 to T8.

**Associated Channel:** Urinary Bladder and Small Intestine

**Reaction areas:**

Heart, Liver, Spleen (left side)

Heart, Liver, Lung (right side)

**Indications:**

- LOW BACK PAIN DUE TO ARTERIOSCLEROSIS
- WRENCHING OF THE LOW BACK.
- CHEST PAIN DUE TO GAS.
- LEG/THIGH PAIN

**Manipulation:**
Single lancet or bleed-cupping is used. One cup covers multiple points. Bleed bilaterally. Check for tender spots.

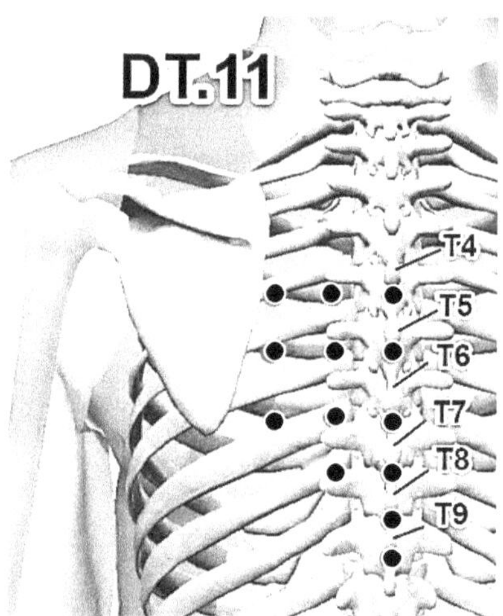

# DT.11 – Hou Xin
(POSTERIOR HEART)

**Location:**

Group of 20 points. 7 points on each side and 6 points on the mid-line.

The first line is located in the space under the spinous processes of T4 through and including T9; the second line is located bilaterally 1.5 cun lateral to T4 to T7, the third line is located bilaterally, 3 cun lateral to the spaces under T4 to T6.

**Associated Channel:** Urinary Bladder and DU

**Reaction areas:** Heart

**Indications:**

- ACNE OR BOILS
- ACUTE ERUPTIVE DISEASE
- SEVERE TOXIC HEAT
- HEART ATTACK OR CORONARY HEART DISEASE
- CIRCULATORY ISSUES
- HEMIPLEGIA
- WIND STROKE
- SEVERE COMMON COLD
- CHRONIC GASTRITIS

**Manipulation:**
Lancet of bleed-cupping is used. One cup covers multiple points. Bleed bilaterally. Check for tender spots.

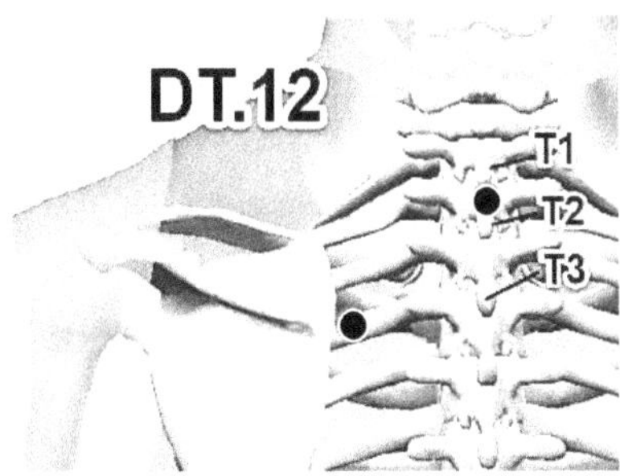


## DT.12 – Gan Mao San
(CATCH COLD THREE)

**Location:**
Group of 3 points. 1 point on each side and 1 point on mid-line.
Located at DU-13 (below T1) and bilateral BL-42(level below T3)

**Associated Channel:** Urinary Bladder and DU

**Reaction areas:** Heart

**Indications:**
- SEVERE CASES OF THE COMMON COLD
- CHEST PAIN
- COUGH
- ASTHMA

**Manipulation**:
Single lancet or bleed-cupping is used. One cup covers multiple points. Moxa applicable. Check for tender spots.

## DT.13 – Shui Zhong
(WATER CENTER)

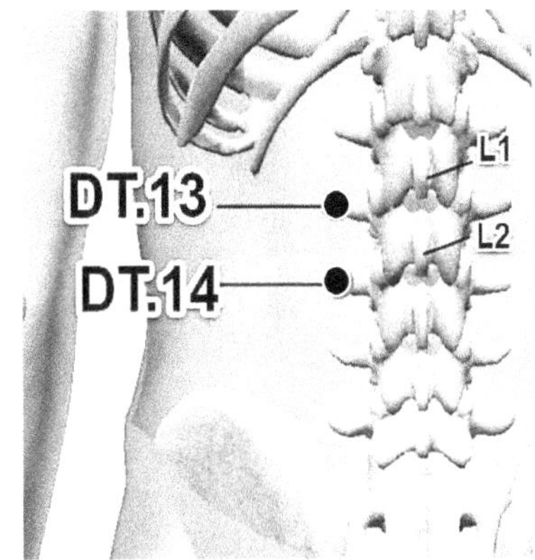


**Location:**
1.5 cun lateral to the lower border of the spinous process of the first lumbar vertebrae (L1).

**Overlaps:** BL-22

**Associated Channel:** Urinary Bladder

**Reaction areas:** Kidney

**Indications:**
- KIDNEY VACUITY PATTERNS
- KIDNEY FAILURE/STONES
- NEPHRITIS
- DYSURIA
- EDEMA
- THIRST
- SPINAL PAIN
- LUMBAR VERTEBRAE PAIN
- CONSTIPATION
- DIARRHEA
- VOMITING
- IRREGULAR MENSTRUATION

**Manipulation:** Single lancet or bleed-cupping is used. One cup covers multiple points. Moxa applicable. Check for tender spots.

## DT.14 Shui Fu
(WATER BOWELS)

**Location:**
1.5 cun lateral to the lower border of the spinous process of the second lumbar vertebrae (L2).

**Overlaps:** BL-23

**Associated Channel:** Urinary Bladder

**Reaction areas:** Kidney

**Indications:**
- KIDNEY DEFICIENCY

- NEPHRITIS
- IMPOTENCE/PREMATURE EJACULATION
- EDEMA
- RETENTION/PAINFUL URINATION
- ENURESIS
- URINARY BLADDER STONE
- BLURRED VISION
- TINNITUS/DEAFNESS
- DIZZINESS
- HEADACHE
- INSOMNIA
- DIABETES
- THIRST
- INTESTINAL INFLAMMATION
- CONSTIPATION
- RETENTION OF A DEAD FETUS
- IRREGULAR MENSTRUATION
- LEUCORRHEA
- INFERTILITY
- CHEST PAIN
- SPINAL PAIN AND RIGIDITY
- BACK PAIN

**Manipulation:**
Single lancet or bleed-cupping is used. One cup covers multiple points.

Moxa is effective and preferred. Check for tender spots.

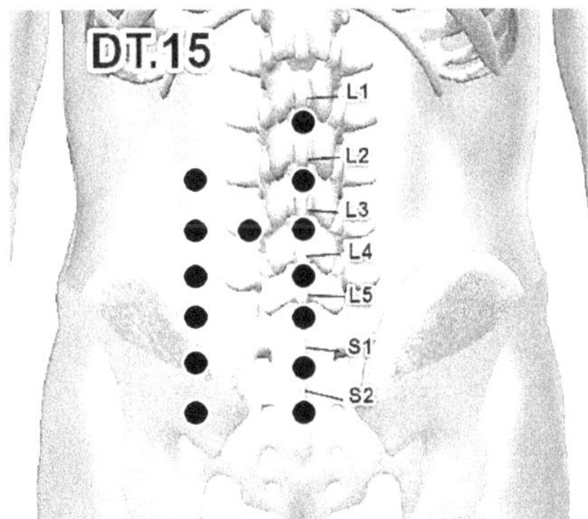


## DT.15 – San Jiang
(THREE RIVERS)

**Location:**
19 Points Group. 6 points each side and 7 points on mid-line. The first line of points consists of one point below each spinal vertebra from L1 to S2; the second line of points is located bilaterally, 3 cun lateral to the spine, with points at the levels of vertebrae L2 to S2.

**Overlapping points:**
Overlap Ming Men (Du-4), Yao Yang

Guan (Du-3), Zhi Shi (BL-52), and Bao Huang (BL-53)

**Associated Channel:** DU, Urinary Bladder

**Reaction areas:** Kidney, Six bowels

**Indications:**

- LOW BACK PAIN
- UTERINE INFLAMMATION
- AMENORRHEA
- CHEST PAIN ON BREATHING
- ACUTE INTESTINAL INFLAMMATION
- ARM PAIN
- ELBOW PAIN
- SHOULDER PAIN

**Manipulation:**

Single lancet or bleed-cupping is used. One cup covers multiple points.

**Remarks:** Because bleeding the front is not recommended, we bleed the back to treat the front.

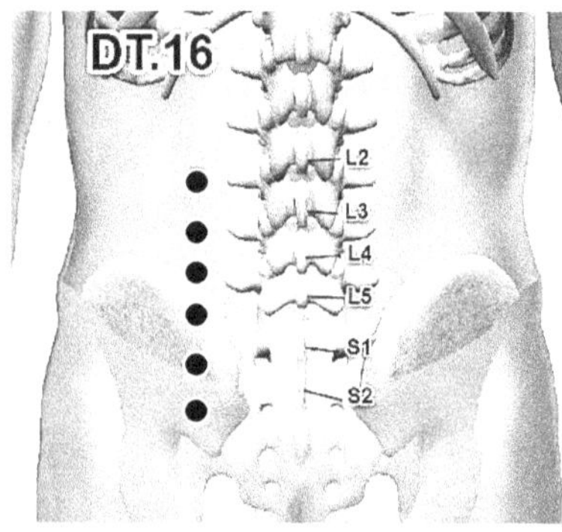

# DT.16 – Shuang He

(TWO RIVERS)

**Location:**
12 points bilaterally; each point 3 cun lateral to the spine, at the levels of L2 to S2. 6 points on each side.

**Overlapping points:** Zhi Shi (BL-52), and Bao Huang (BL-53)

**Associated Channel:** DU, Urinary Bladder

**Reaction areas:** Kidney, Six bowels

**Indications:**

- PAIN IN THE UPPER LIMBS
- PAIN AND LACK OF STRENGTH IN THE UPPER BACK AND SHOULDERS.

**Manipulation:**

Single lancet or bleed-cupping is used. One cup covers multiple points.

**Remarks:** If there is dark blood emerging, it means the treatment is effective.

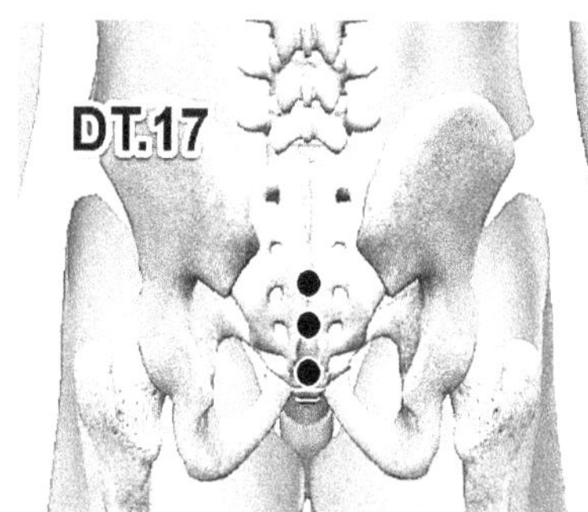

# DT.17 – Chong Xiao

(UP-SHOOTING HEAVEN)

**Location:**
Group of 3 points.

Point 1 is at the level of S3 of the sacral vertebrae. Point 2 is 1 cun inferior from Point 1. Point 3 is 1 cun inferior from Point 2.

**Associated Channel:** DU

**Reaction areas:** Cerebellum

**Indications:**

- PRESSURE OR TENSION IN HEAD AND SPINE
- DIZZINESS
- OCCIPITAL HEADACHE
- SPASMS OR CONVULSIONS
- NECK PAIN
- ARM PAIN
- ACUTE OR CHRONIC INTESTINAL DISORDERS
- OVARIAN/UTERINE DISEASE
- AMENORRHEA
- MALE OR FEMALE INFERTILITY
- ACUTE OR CHRONIC LOWER BACK PAIN

**Manipulation:**

Stretch the sacral area to check for visible veins. Bleed-cupping is used. One cup covers multiple points.

**Remarks:** Bleeding this area relieves pressure in the spine.

Bleeding the sacrum arca is a useful infertility treatment for both sexes.

# VT ZONE-Ventral Torso

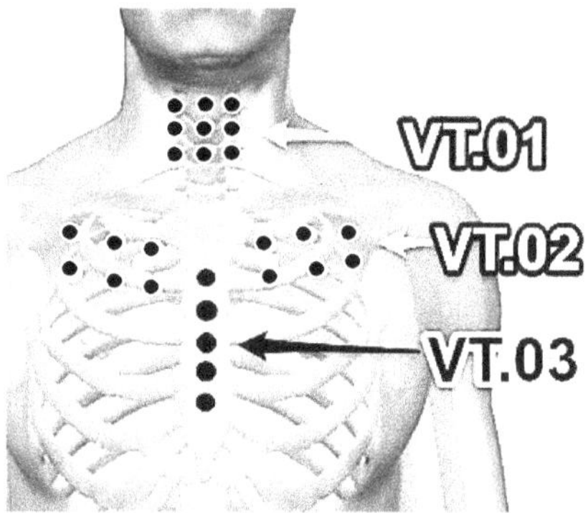

## VT.01 Hou'e Jiu

(THROAT NINE MOTHS)

**Location:**

- Point 1, or center point, is on the thyroid cartilage or over the Adam's apple.
- Points 2 and 3 are 1.5 cun lateral to Point 1, one on each side. They overlap with Renying (ST 9)
- Points 4, 5, 6 are 1 cun superior to Points 1,2,3.

**Reaction area:** Lung

**Indications:**

- SORE THROAT
- ITCHY THROAT
- TONSILITIS
- THYROIDITIS

**Manipulation:**

Pinch up the skin and carry out superficial bleeding. Do not use cupping.

## VT.02 Shierhou

(TWELVE MONKEYS)

**Location:**

12 points total

These points are arranged in 2 lines of 3 points inferior to the clavicle (6 points on each side).

The first line is 1.3 cun inferior to the clavicle, and the second line is 2.8 cun inferior to the clavicle. The 3 points are 1.5 cun apart.

8 of the points are nearby or on Kufang (ST-14), Wuyi (ST-15), Shencang (KID-25), Yuzhong (KI - 26).

**Reaction area:** Lung

**Indications:**

- SEVERE COMMON COLD
- CHOLERA
- SCARLET FEVER
- ASTHMA DUE TO ARTERIOSCLEROSIS
- FOOD POISONING WITH ABDOMINAL PAIN BUT NO VOMITING
- DIARRHEA

**Manipulation:**

These points are bled.

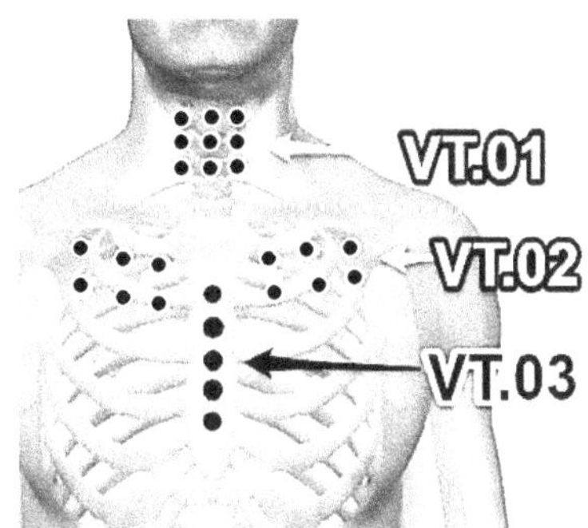


# VT.03 Jinwu
(GOLD FIVE)

**Location:**

5 points total

- The first point is on the midline of the sternum, level with the 2nd intercostal space and overlaps Zigong (REN-19).
- Each subsequent point is 1 cun inferior to the previous one, totalling 5 points.

**Reaction areas:** Heart, Trachea

**Indications:**

- Any digestive disorders, bloating, food poisoning with abdominal pain but no vomiting
- Hypochondriac pain, rib pain, flank pain
- Trachea blockage, tracheitis
- Various "Sha" syndromes

**Manipulation:**

These points are bled.

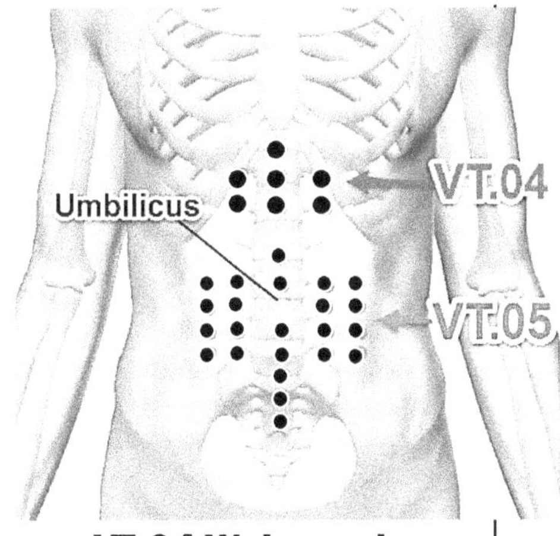


# VT.04 Weimaoqi
(STOMACH HAIR SEVEN)

**Location:**

7 points total

- Point 1 is just inferior to the tip of the xiphoid process and overlaps Zhongting (REN-16).
- Point 2 is 1 cun below Point 1.
- Point 3 is 2 cun below Point 1.
- Points 4 and 5 are 1.5 cun lateral to Point 2, one on each side
- Points 6 and 7 are 1.5 cun lateral to Point 3, one on each side

**Reaction areas:** Heart, Stomach

**Indications:**

- FEVER/HEAT STROKE
- HEART PALPITATION
- BLEEDING ULCER
- CHOLERA
- ENTERITIS
- STOMACH PAIN OR DISEASE
- WOOL-LIKE BOILS

**Manipulation:**

These points are bled.

# VT.05 Fuchaoershisan
(BOWELS NEST TWENTY-THREE)

**Location:**

23 points total

- The first 7 points are on the REN channel.
  - Points 1 and 2 are 1 cun and 2 cun superior to the umbilicus, overlapping Shuifen (REN-9) and Xiawan (REN-10).
  - Points 3-7 are all below the umbilicus, starting at 1 cun inferior. Each subsequent point is then 1 cun inferior to the previous one, totalling 5 points. They overlap with Yinjiao (REN-7), Shimen (REN-5), Guanyuan (REN-4), Zgongji (REN-3), Qugu (REN-2).

- The second set of 8 points is 1 cun lateral to the REN channel (4 points on each side).
  - Points 8 and 9 are levelled with the umbilicus.
  - Points 10 and 11 are 1 cun inferior to Points 8 and 9.
  - Points 12 and 13 are 1 cun inferior to Points 8 and 9.
  - Points 14 and 15 are 2 cun inferior to Points 8 and 9.

- The third set of 8 points is 2 cun lateral to the REN channel (4 points on each side).
  - Points 16 and 17 are levelled with the umbilicus, overlapping Tianshu (ST 25).
  - Points 18 and 19 are 1 cun superior to Points 16 and 17, overlapping Huaroumen (ST 24).
  - Points 20 and 21 are 1 cun inferior to Points 16 and 17, overlapping Wailing (ST 26).
  - Points 22 and 23 are 2 cun inferior to Points 16 and 17, overlapping Daju (ST 27).

**Indications:**

- ENTERITIS, INTESTINAL CANCER, COLON CANCER, NAVEL PAIN, FOOD POISONING WITH ABDOMINAL PAIN BUT NO VOMITING, APPENDICITIS
- PELVIC INFLAMMATORY DISEASE, UTERITIS
- NEPHRITIS, RENAL PAIN

**Manipulation:**

These points are bled.

# POINTS OF THE TRADITIONAL CHINESE MEDICINE SYSTEM

# LUNG MERIDIAN (Arm Tai Yin)

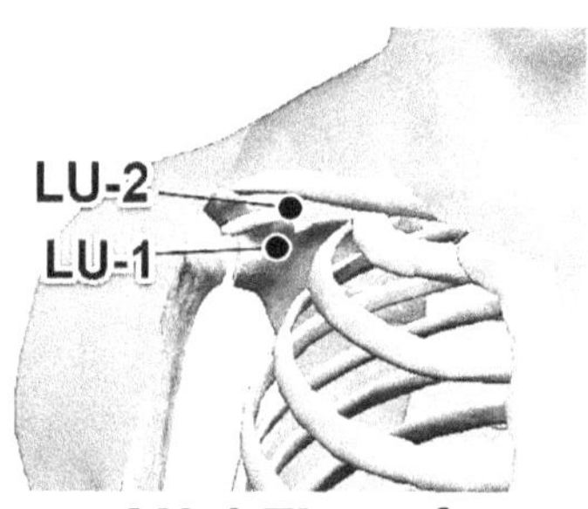


## LU-1 Zhongfu
### (MIDDLE PALACE)

FRONT MU (ALARM) POINT OF THE LU CHANNEL. ENTRY POINT. MEETING POINT OF THE LUNG AND SPLEEN CHANNELS.

**Location:**
At the level of the inter-space between the 1st and 2nd ribs, 6 cun lateral to the midline.

**Dermatome:** C4

**Main Action Areas:** Chest, Lungs, Nose, Shoulder

**Main functions:** Benefits respiration. Tonifies Lung qi. Regulates chest qi. Dispels stagnation and heat. Releases the exterior.

**Indications:**
All Lung issues, esp cough, wheezing, asthma and fullness in the chest as well as local problems such as pain in the chest, shoulder and back.

**Manipulation:** 0.5 cun laterally and horizontally.

Moxibustion applicable.

**Cautions:** Dangerous point. Do not needle deeply due to risk of pneumothorax.

## LU-2 Yun Men
### (CLOUD GATE)

**Location:**
On the antero-lateral aspect of the chest, below the lateral extremity of the clavicle, 6 cun lateral to the midline, in the centre of the hollow of the delto-pectoral triangle.

**Dermatome:** C5

**Main Action Areas:** Lungs, Upper Arm

**Main Functions:** Clears heat. Benefits the Lungs.

**Indications:**
Cough; asthma; pain in the chest, shoulder, and arm; thoracic fullness.

**Manipulation:** Needle obliquely 0.5 – 0.8 cun.

Moxibustion applicable.

**Caution:** Deep perpendicular or oblique insertion carries a substantial risk of causing a pneumothorax.

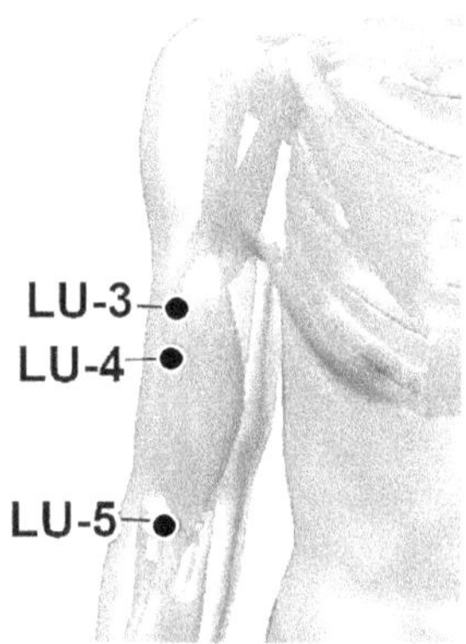


## LU-3 Tian Fu
### (PALACE OF HEAVEN)

WINDOW OF HEAVEN point

**Location:**
On the upper arm, on the lateral border of muscle biceps brachii, 3 cun inferior to the anterior axillary fold.

**Dermatome:** C5

**Main Action Areas:** Lungs, Po (Corporeal Soul), Upper Arm

**Main Functions:** Clears heat. Benefits the Lungs. Calms the Po (Corporeal Soul)

**Indications:**
Asthma; nosebleed; pain in the medial aspect of the arm.

**Manipulation:**
Needle perpendicularly 0.5-1.0 cun.

**Caution:** No moxibustion.

## LU-4 Xia Bai
### (CLASPING THE WHITE)

**Location:**
On the upper arm, on the lateral border of muscle biceps brachii, 4 cun inferior to the anterior axillary fold.

**Dermatome:** C5

**Main Action Areas:** Lungs, Heart, Chest, Arm

**Main Functions:** Regulates Qi and Blood. Benefits the Chest

**Indications:**
Cough; thoracic fullness; pain in the medial aspect of the arm.

**Manipulation:** Needle perpendicularly 0.5 – 1 cun.

Moxibustion applicable.

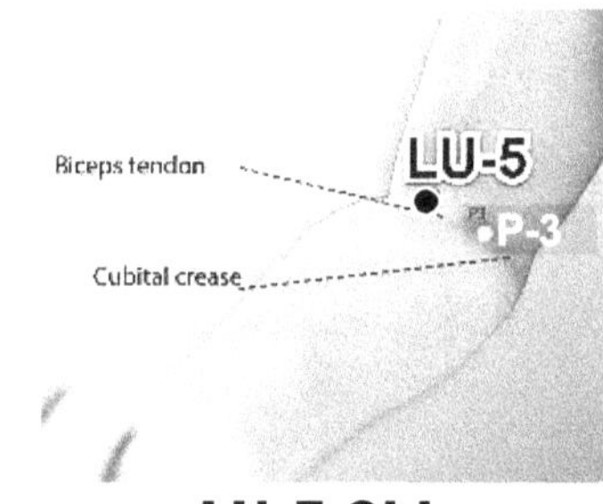


## LU-5 Chize
### (CUBIT MARSH)

HE-SEA, SEDATION, AND WATER POINT OF THE LUNG CHANNEL.

**Location:**
At the level of the elbow crease, on the lateral (radial) border of the tendon of the biceps muscle. (This tendon is better felt when the elbow is slightly flexed.)

**Shared location with Tung:** 33.16

**Dermatome:** C5/C6

**Main Action Areas:** Lungs, Chest, Upper Jiao, Elbow

**Main Functions:** Dispels phlegm. Alleviates cough. Clears the lungs. Opens the water passages

**Indications:**
Pain and swelling of elbow, arthritis of elbow, skin diseases. Cough, haemoptysis, evening fever, asthma, sore throat, fullness in the chest, infantile convulsions, spasmodic pain of the elbow and arm, mastitis.

**Manipulation:** 0.5-1.0 cun perpendicularly. Bleeding at this point is carried out for skin disorders. This is a very effective therapy for psoriasis and eczema.

**Caution:** No moxibustion.

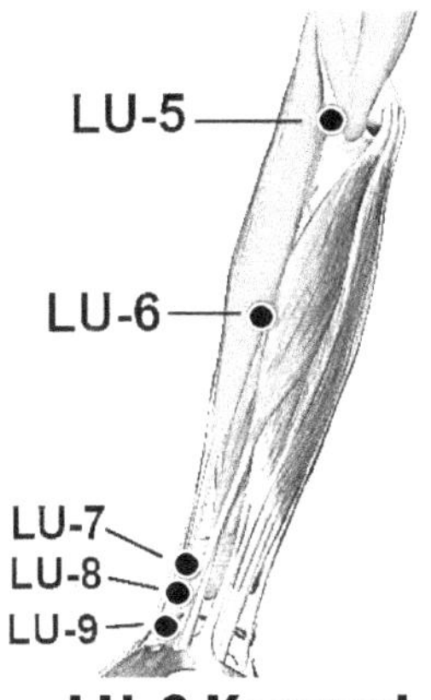



# LU-6 Kongzul

(MAXIMUM OPENING)

XI-CLEFT POINT.

**Location:**
5 cun distal to Chize [Lu.5] on the path from LU-5 to LU-9

**Dermatome:** C6

**Main Action Areas:** Nose, Lungs, Skin, Forearm

**Main Functions:** Releases the exterior. Diaphoretic. Clears heat from the upper jiao. Arrests bleeding

**Indications:**
Cough; asthma; sore throat; pain in the elbow and arm with difficulty in bending and stretching.

**Manipulation:** 0.5cun perpendicularly. Strong stimulation is carried out.

Moxibustion applicable.

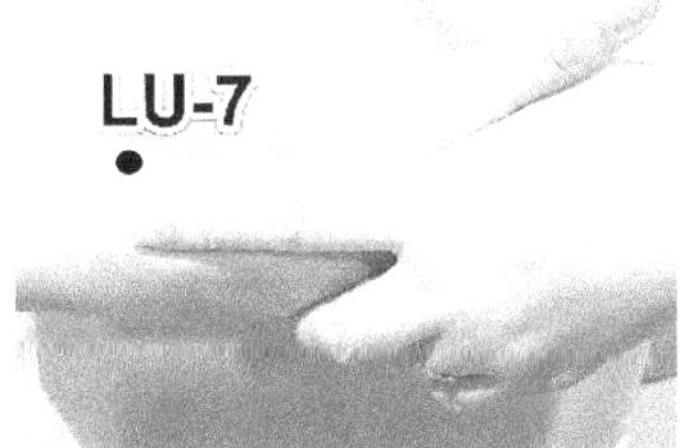



# LU-7 Lieque

(BROKEN SEQUENCE)

LUO POINT, CONFLUENT POINT OF THE CONCEPTION VESSEL, GAO WU COMMAND POINT, MA DAN-YANG HEAVENLY STAR POINT, FIVE STAR POINT. COMMAND POINT FOR HEAD AND NECK. EXIT POINT. COMMAND POINT OF THE YIN HEEL VESSEL. MASTER POINT OF THE CONCEPTION VESSEL.

**Location:**
When the index finger and the thumbs, of both hands of the patient are crossed this point is under the tip of the upper index finger. This point is best located by measuring 1.5 cun from the wrist joint crease proximally on the outer radial or lateral border of the forearm.

**Dermatome:** C6

**Main Action Areas:** Lungs, Chest, Nose, Throat, Back of the Neck, Head, Face, Bladder, Forearm

**Main Functions:** Descends and disperses Lung Qi. Releases the exterior and dispels wind. Nourishes yin and moistens fluids. Opens the conception vessel. Benefits the neck.

**Indications:**
Headache and stiffness of the neck; cough and asthma; sore throat; facial paralysis; wryness of the eyes and mouth; clenched jaws; weakness of the wrist.

**Manipulation:** 0.5 cun horizontally. The needle is inserted proximally in proximal disorders. In disorders such as arthritis of the wrist, the needle is inserted distally.

Moxibustion applicable.

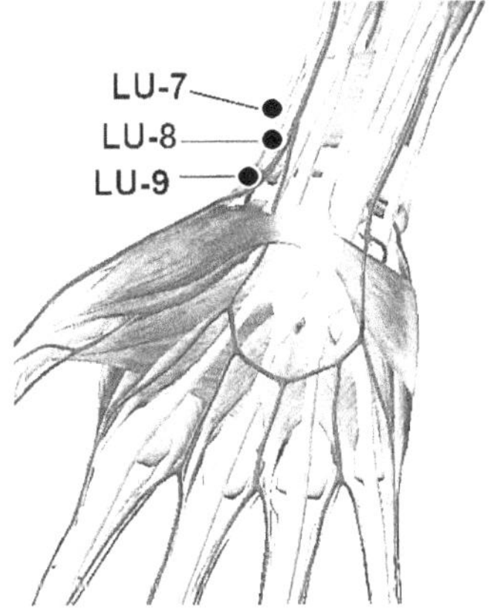



# LU-8 Jing Qu

(CHANNEL DITCH)

JING-RIVER, HORARY, AND METAL POINT OF THE LUNG CHANNEL

**Location:**
On the radial side of the forearm, 1 cun superior to the transverse wrist crease and in the depression between the radial artery and styloid process.

**Dermatome:** C6

**Main Action Areas:** Lungs, Upper Jiao

**Main Functions:** Tonifies Lung Qi. Harmonises the metal element

**Indications:** Cough; asthma; sore throat; pain in the chest and wrist.

**Manipulation:**
Insert the needle perpendicularly to a depth of 0.1–0.3 cun and stimulate until there is a sore and numb sensation in the local area radiating to the upper arm.

**Caution:** Avoid puncturing the radial artery. Moxibustion is forbidden.

# LU-9 Taiyuan

(SUPREME ABYSS)

SHU-STREAM, YUAN-SOURCE, TONIFICATION, AND EARTH POINT OF THE LUNG CHANNEL. INFLUENTIAL POINT OF THE VESSELS.

**Location:**
Outer end of the wrist crease (on the lateral side of the radial artery.

**Dermatome:** C6

**Main Action Areas:** Chest, Lungs, Blood vessels

**Main Functions:** Tonifies Chest Qi. Strengthens the breath and voice. Nourishes Lung yin. Transforms phlegm. Benefits the vessels and improves circulation

**Indications:**
Asthma; cough; expectoration of blood; sore throat; palpitations; pain in the chest and medial aspect of the forearm. Diseases of the wrist joint, arterio-sclerosis and other vascular disorders.

**Manipulation:** 0.3 cun perpendicular (avoiding artery).

Moxibustion applicable.

**Caution:** Avoid radial artery.

# LU-10 Yu Ji

(FISH BORDER)

YING-SPRING, AND FIRE POINT OF THE LUNG CHANNEL.

**Location:**
In the depression proximal to the metacarp phalangeal joint, on the radial side of the midpoint of the metacarpal bone, where the skin changes texture.

**Shared location with Tung:** 22.11

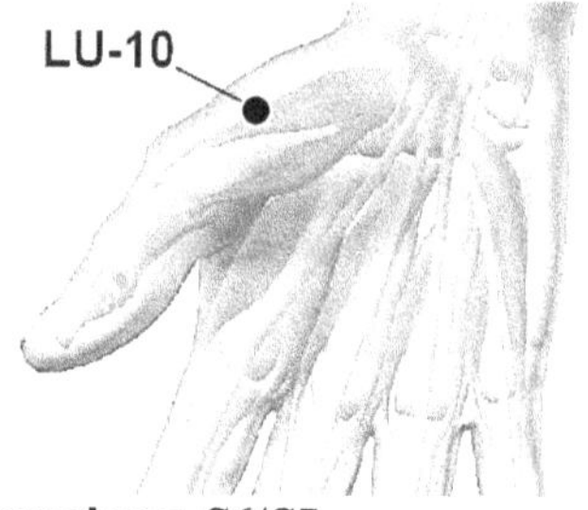



**Dermatome:** C6/C7

**Main Action Areas:** Lungs, Throat, Thumb

**Main Functions:** Clears exterior heat and phlegm-fire toxins. Benefits the throat.

**Indications:**
Cough; expectoration of blood; sore throat; fever.

**Manipulation:** 1. Insert the needle perpendicularly to a depth of 0.3–0.5 cun and stimulate until there is a distending sensation in the local area which radiates to the thumb. 2. Prick with a three-edged needle to bleed.

Moxibustion applicable.

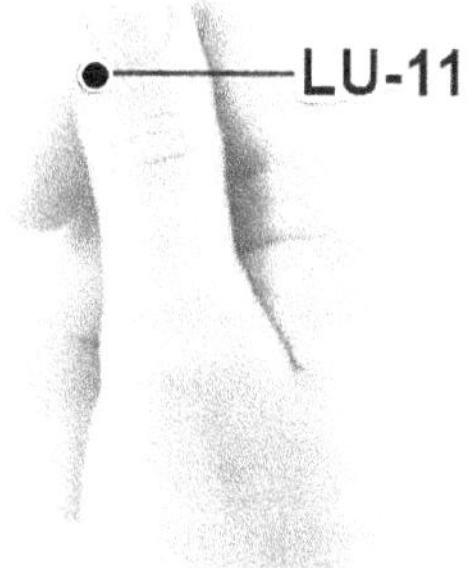



# LU-11 Shaoshang

(LESSER MERCHANT)

JING-WELL AND WOOD POINT OF THE LUNG CHANNEL. SUN SI-MIAO GHOST POINT. SECOND GHOST POINT

**Location:**
0.1 cun proximal to the outer corner of the nail of the thumb.

**Dermatome:** C6

**Main Action Areas:** Throat, Lung channel, Mind

**Main Functions:** Dispels exterior heat and wind. Restores consciousness.

**Indications:**
Hysterical attack, fainting, epileptic attack, convulsions, high fever, cardiac arrest, drowning, respiratory arrest, and other acute emergencies.

**Manipulation:** 0.1 cun perpendicularly to cause bleeding or strong acupressure to cause pain.

**Caution:** No Moxibustion.

# LARGE INTESTINE MERIDIAN (Arm Yang Ming)

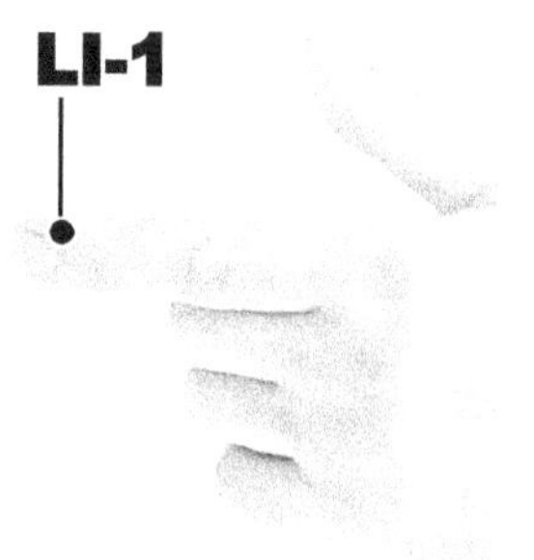



## LI-1 Shangyang

(METAL YANG)

JING-WELL, HORARY, AND METAL POINT OF THE LARGE INTESTINE CHANNEL.

**Location:**
Radial side of the index finger, 0.1 cun proximal to the corner of the nail.

**Main Action Areas:** Throat, Large intestine channel, Mind

**Main Functions:** Restores consciousness. Benefits the throat.

**Indications:**
Toothache; sore, swollen throat; swelling of the submandibular region; numbness of the fingers; heat diseases; clouding inversion.

**Manipulation:** Shallow insertion 0.1 cun, or prick the point to bleed.

**Caution:** Do not moxibustion.

## LI-2 Erjian

(SECOND POINT)

YING-SPRING POINT. SEDATION AND WATER POINT OF THE LARGE INTESTINE CHANNEL.

**Location:**
On the radial aspect of the index finger, distal to the metacarpo-phalangeal joint, at the junction of the shaft and the basis of the proximal phalanx.

**Dermatome:** C6

**Main Action Areas:** Finger, MCP joint, Throat, Teeth

**Main Functions:** Dispels wind and clears heat. Benefits the throat. Alleviates pain and swelling

**Indications:**
Blurring vision, epistaxis (nosebleed), toothache, sore throat, febrile diseases.

**Manipulation:**
Perpendicular insertion .2 - .3 cun.

Moxibustion is applicable.

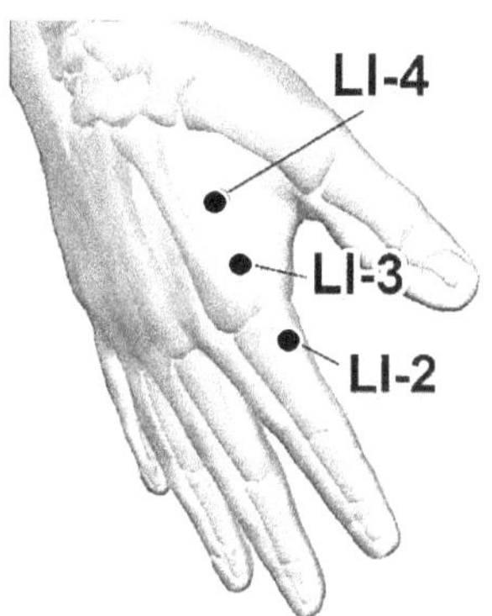



## LI-3 Sanjian

(THIRD POINT)

SHU-STREAM AND WOOD POINT OF THE LARGE INTESTINE CHANNEL.

**Location:**
On the radial aspect of the index finger, proximal to the metacarpo-phalangeal joint, at the junction of the shaft and the head of the 2nd metacarpal bone.

**Dermatome:** C6/C7

**Main Action Areas:** Throat, Teeth, Finger, Intestines

**Main Functions:** Dispels wind and clears heat. Benefits the face and throat. Alleviates regional pain

**Indications:**
Toothache, ophthalmalgia, sore throat, redness and swelling of fingers and the dorsum of the hand.

**Manipulation:**
Perpendicular insertion .5 - .8 cun.

Moxibustion is applicable.

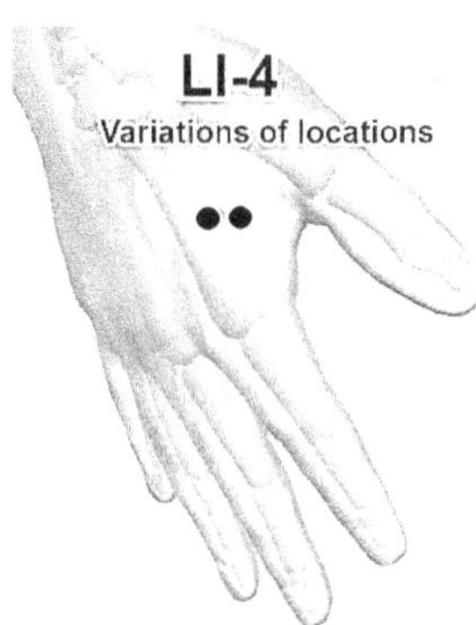


# LI-4 Hegu
## (JUNCTION VALLEY)

YUAN-SOURCE POINT OF THE LARGE INTESTINE CHANNEL. GAO WU COMMAND POINT. MA DAN-YANG HEAVENLY STAR POINT. ENTRY POINT. COMMAND POINT FOR THE FACE AND MOUTH.

**Location:**
Between the 1st and 2nd metacarpals, on the radial aspect of the middle of the 2nd metacarpal bone, at the highest spot of the muscle when the thumb and index fingers are brought close together.

There are several variations of point location for LI-4. It is recommended to palpate around for the most reactive point.

**Dermatome:** C6/C7

**Main Action Areas:** Face, Sense organs, Mouth, Teeth, Eyes, Nose, Chest, Throat, Mind, Lungs, Abdomen, Intestine, Hand.

**Main Functions:** Moves stuck Qi and dissipates fullness. Relieves pain (analgesic). Descends Yang. Clears heat. Releases the exterior. Alleviates cough

**Indications:**
a) Disorders of the thumb and forefinger and wrist joint.

b) The best analgesic point of the body both for therapy and anaesthesia.

c) Distal point for front of the head, face and special sense organs and front of neck.

d) Disorders of the large intestine.

e) Disorders of the lung.

**Manipulation:**
0.5 to 1.0 cun perpendicularly.

Moxibustion is applicable, except in pregnancy.

**Cautions:** Do not needle during pregnancy.

LI-4 is an extremely powerful point but is also one of the most common points to cause needle shock. A vaso-vagal response can lead to a sudden drop in blood pressure, shaking and even fainting.

# LI-5 Yangi
## (YANG STREAM)

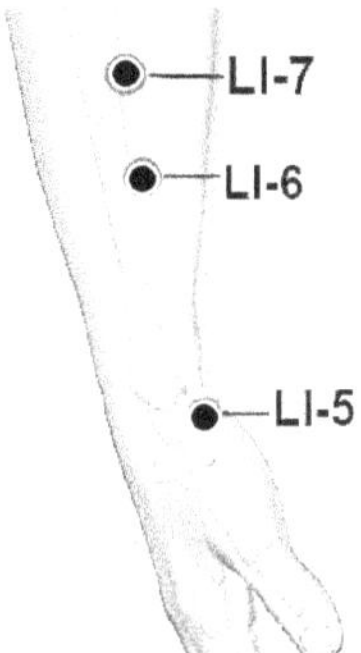


JING-RIVER AND FIRE POINT OF THE LARGE INTESTINE CHANNEL.

**Location:**
With the thumb abducted, in a depression between the tendons of the extensor pollicis longus and brevis muscles ('anatomical snuffbox'), on the radial aspect of the wrist.

**Dermatome:** C6

**Main Action Areas:** Wrist, Hand, Thumb

**Main Functions:** Alleviates pain and swelling.

**Indications:**
Headache, redness, pain and swelling of the eye, toothache, sore throat, pain of the wrist.

**Manipulation:** Perpendicular insertion .3 - .5 cun. Moxibustion is applicable.

**Cautions:** The cephalic vein is located within the anatomical snuffbox.

# LI-6 Pianli
## (DIVERGING PASSAGE)

LUO POINT OF THE LARGE INTESTINE CHANNEL.

**Location:**
3 cun proximal to LI-5, on the line connecting LI-5 and LI-11, between the abductor pollicis longus and the extensor pollicis brevis muscles, at the level of the junction between the tendon and the muscle.

**Dermatome:** C6

**Main Action Areas:** Forearm, Wrist

**Main Functions:** Alleviates pain

**Indications:**
Redness of the eye, tinnitus, deafness, epistaxis, aching of the hand and arm, sore throat, edema.

**Manipulation:** Perpendicular or oblique insertion .5 - .8 cun.

Moxibustion is applicable.

# LI-7 Wenliu
## (WARM FLOW)

XI-CLEFT POINT OF THE LARGE INTESTINE CHANNEL.

**Location:**
5 cun proximal to the anatomical snuffbox in the direction of the lateral end of the elbow crease or 1 cun distal to the midpoint of the line connecting LI-5 and LI-11.

**Dermatome:** C4

**Main Action Areas:** Forearm

**Main Functions:** Alleviates pain

**Indications:**
Headache, swelling of the face, sore throat, borborygmus, abdominal pain, aching of the shoulder and arm.

**Manipulation:** Perpendicular insertion 0.5 – 1.0 cun.

Moxibustion is applicable.

# LI-8 Xialian
## (LOWER POINT AT THE BORDER)

**Location:**
4 cun distal to the lateral end of the elbow crease in the direction of the anatomical snuffbox and on a line connecting LI-5 and LI-11.

**Dermatome:** C5/C6

**Main Action Areas:** Forearm, Elbow, Intestines

**Main Functions:** Regulates Qi and Blood and alleviates pain. Clears heat and dissipates wind. Harmonises the Yang Ming.

**Indications:**
Abdominal pain, borborygmus, pain in the elbows and arm, motor impairment of the upper limbs.

**Manipulation:** Perpendicular insertion 0.5 – 1.0 cun.

Moxibustion is applicable.

## LI-9 Shanglian

(UPPER POINT AT THE BORDER)

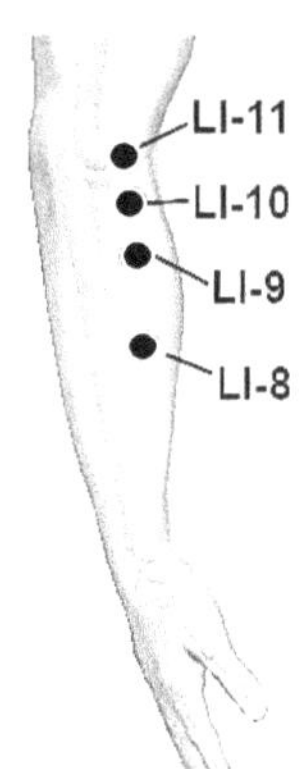


**Location:**
3 cun distal to the lateral end of the elbow crease in the direction of the anatomical snuffbox, on the line connecting LI-5 and LI-11.

**Dermatome:** C5/C6

**Main Action Areas:** Forearm, Elbow, Intestines

**Main Functions:** Regulates Qi and Blood and alleviates pain.  Clears heat and dissipates wind. Harmonises the Yang Ming.

**Indications:**
Aching of the shoulder and arm, motor impairment of the upper limbs, numbness of the hand and arm, borborygmus, abdominal pain.

**Manipulation:** Perpendicular insertion 0.5 – 1.0 cun.

Moxibustion is applicable.

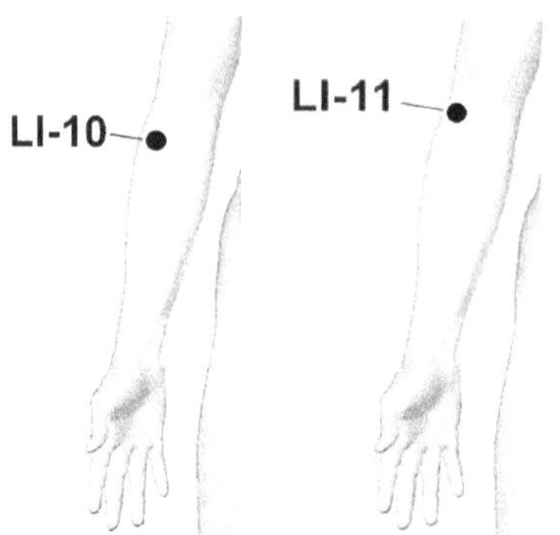


## LI-10 Shousanli

(ARM THREE MILES)

**Location:**
On the lateral aspect of the forearm, 2 cun below Quchi (LI-11.).

**Shared location with Tung:** 33.07

**Dermatome:** C5

**Main Action Areas:** Forearm and Elbow, Entire Upper Limb, Shoulder, Stomach, Intestines

**Main Functions:** Strengthens the upper limbs. Alleviates pain. Harmonises the Yang Ming

**Indications:**
Tennis elbow, arthritis of elbow, pain, tremor or paralysis of the forearm as in stroke, paraesthesia. Abdominal pain, diarrhea, toothache, swelling of the cheek.

**Manipulation:** 1.0 - 1.5 cun perpendicularly.

Moxibustion applicable.

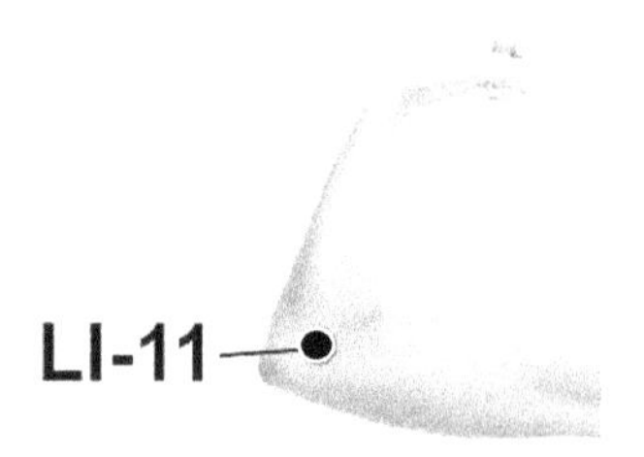


## LI-11 Quchi

(POND AT THE BEND)

HE-SEA, TONIFICATION, AND EARTH POINT OF THE LARGE INTESTINE CHANNEL.

**Location:**
a) At the outer end of the elbow crease when the elbow is semiflexed.

b) It is midway between chize (LU-5), and lateral epicondyle of the humerus, when the elbow is semiflexed.

**Dermatome:** C5

**Main Action Areas:** Elbow, Forearm, Throat, Face (nose, eyes, mouth, ears), Lungs, Abdomen, Intestines

**Main Functions:** Clears heat and damp heat. Descends rising Yang. Regulates Qi. Dispels stasis

**Indications:**
Disorders of the elbow, tennis elbow, paralysis of the arm, fever, high blood pressure, skin diseases. This is the best homeostatic point of the body.

**Manipulation:** 1-0 to 1.5 cun perpendicularly.

Moxibustion applicable.

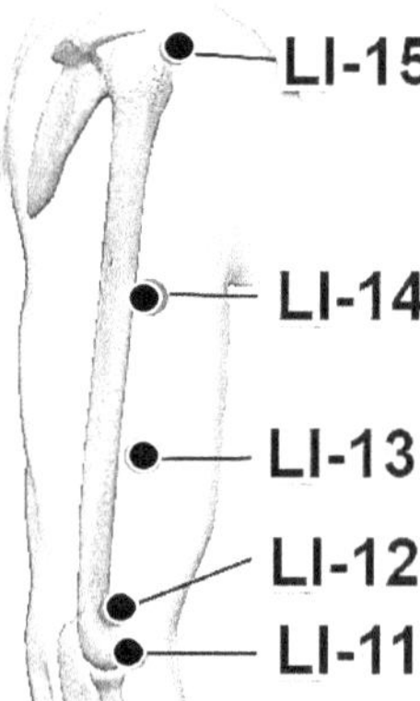


## LI-12 Zhouliao

(ELBOW BONE HOLE)

**Location:**
1 cun proximal to the lateral end of the elbow crease LI-11, on the anterior border of the humerus.

**Dermatome:** C5

**Main Action Areas:** Elbow

**Main Functions:** Regulates Qi and Blood. Alleviates pain.

**Indications:**
Pain, numbness and contracture of the elbow and arm.

**Manipulation:** Perpendicular insertion 0.5 – 1.0 cun.

Moxibustion is applicable.

## LI-13 Shouwuli

(ARM FIVE MILES)

**Location:**
On the lateral aspect of the upper arm, 3 cun proximal to the lateral end of the elbow crease LI-11, in the direction of the head of the humerus.

**Shared location with Tung:** 44.08

**Dermatome:** C5

**Main Action Areas:** Elbow, Shoulder, Arm, Chest

**Main Functions:** Regulates Qi and Blood. Alleviates pain. Benefits the chest and alleviates cough.

**Indications:**
Pain in the shoulder and arm, rigidity of the neck, scrofula.

**Manipulation:** Perpendicular insertion 0.5 – 1.0 cun.

Moxibustion is applicable.

**Cautions:** Avoid Artery.

## LI-14 Binao

(UPPER ARM PROMINENCE)

MEETING POINT OF THE LARGE INTESTINE CHANNEL WITH THE SMALL INTESTINE AND BLADDER CHANNELS

**Location:**
On the lateral aspect of the upper arm, on a line connecting LI-11 and LI-15, 7 cun proximal to LI-11 and slightly superior to the pointed insertion of the deltoid muscle.

**Dermatome:** C4/C5

**Main Action Areas:** Arm, Shoulder

**Main Functions:** Regulates Qi and Blood. Alleviates pain

**Indications:**
Pain in the shoulder and arm, rigidity of the neck, scrofula.

**Manipulation:** 0.8 to 1.5 cun perpendicularly or oblique.

Moxibustion applicable.

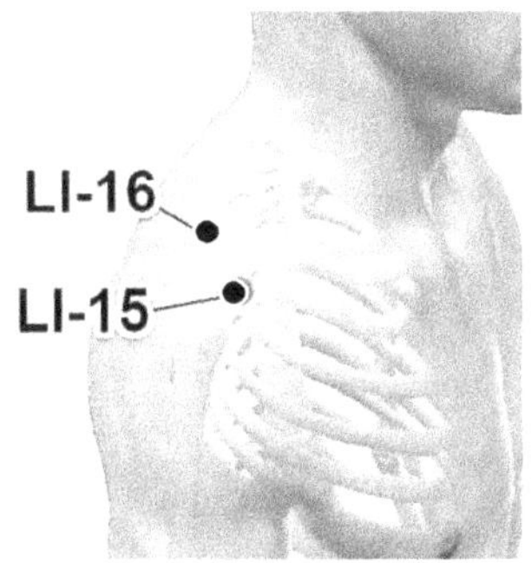


## LI-15 Jianyu
(Shoulder and Clavicle)

Meeting point of the Large Intestine channel with the Yang Heel vessel.

**Location:**
At the anterior depression lateral to the tip of the acromion process.

**Dermatome:** C3

**Main Action Areas:** Shoulder

**Main Functions:** Regulates Qi and Blood. Dispels stasis. Alleviates pain

**Indications:**
Disorders of the shoulder and the surrounding tissue, e.g., periarthritis of the shoulder (frozen shoulder), paralysis of the arm.

**Manipulation:** 0.5 to 1.0 cun perpendicularly.

Moxibustion applicable.

## LI-16 Jugu
(Large Bone-Acromion)

Meeting point of the Large Intestine channel with the Yang Heel vessel.

**Location:**
In a depression between the acromial extremity of the clavicle and the junction of the scapular spine and the acromion.

**Shared location with Tung:** 44.07

**Dermatome:** C3

**Main Action Areas:** Shoulder, Chest

**Main Functions:** Regulates Qi and Blood. Dispels stasis. Alleviates pain. Opens the chest

**Indications:**
Pain and motor impairment of the upper extremities, pain in the shoulder and back.

**Manipulation:** Perpendicular or slightly oblique laterally downwards insertion .5 - .7 cun. Moxibustion is applicable.

**Cautions:** Deep medial insertion may penetrate the Lung.

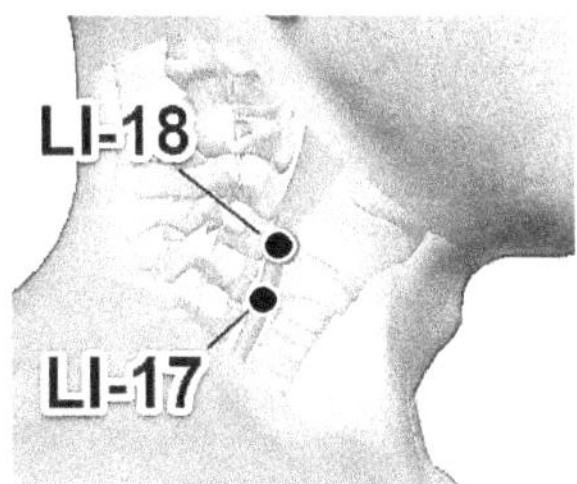


## LI-17 Tianding
(Head's Tripod)

**Location:**
On the posterior border of the sternocleidomastoid muscle, 1 cun below the laryngeal prominence

**Dermatome:** C3

**Main Action Areas:** Throat, Ear

**Main Functions:** Regulates Qi and Blood. Dispels stasis. Alleviates pain. Opens the chest.

**Indications:**
Sudden loss of voice, sore throat, scrofula, goiter.

**Manipulation:** Perpendicular insertion .3 - .5 cun. Moxibustion is applicable.

**Cautions:** The carotid artery and jugular vein are in this area.

## LI-18 Neck-Futu
(Beside the Prominence)

Window of the Heaven point

**Location:** 3 cun lateral to the prominence of the thyroid cartilage [Adams apple].

**Dermatome:** C3

**Main Action Areas:** Throat

**Main Functions:** Alleviates swelling and pain

**Indications:**
Cough, excessive sputum, sore throat, thyroid enlargement, insufficiency of the thyroid gland.

**Manipulation:** Perpendicular insertion 0.3 - 0.5 cun.

Moxibustion is applicable.

**Remarks:** This is a *Dangerous point* [vulnerable point] as the great vessels of the neck, vagus nerve, sympathetic trunk are situated in this area.

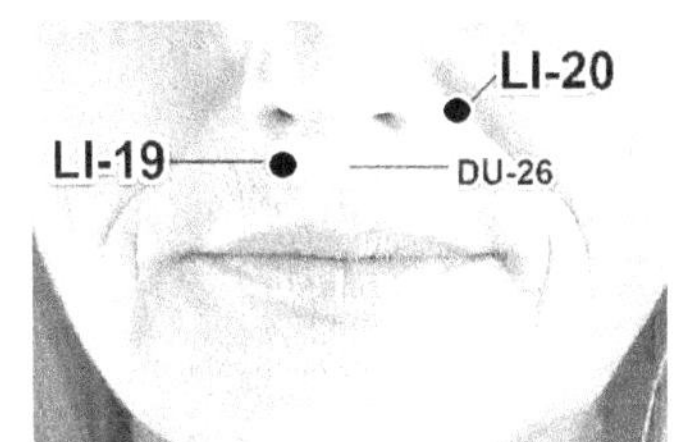


## LI-19 Nose-Heliao
(Mouth Grain Hole)

**Location:**
0.5 cun lateral to point Renzhong [DU-26.]. On the maxilla, slightly below the lateral margin of the nostril.

**Dermatome:** Trigeminal nerve (maxillary branch)

**Main Action Areas:** Nose, Upper Lip, Eyes, Brain

**Main Functions:** Opens the nose. Regulates Qi and Blood. Clears the brain and dispels wind. Similar to LI-20

**Indications:**
Bleeding from nose (epistaxis), nasal obstruction, facial paralysis, trigeminal neuralgia, headache.

**Manipulation:** 0.3 to 0.5 cun obliquely, directed medially

**Caution:** No Moxibustion.

## LI-20 Yingxiang
(Receiving Fragrance)

Intersection of the Stomach on the Large Intestine channel

**Location:**
In the nasolabial groove, on the level of the midpoint of the lateral border of the ala nasi.

**Shared location with Tung:** 1010.15

**Dermatome:** Trigeminal nerve (maxillary branch)

**Main Action Areas:** Nose, Eyes, Cheek and Mouth

**Main Functions:** Improves breathing and smell. Clears heat and dissipates wind. Regulates Qi

**Indications:**
Rhinitis, nose bleeding (epistaxis), blocking of the nose due to inflammation, sinusitis, facial paralysis, trigeminal neuralgia, toothache, loss of sense of smell, ear problems incl loss of hearing.

**Manipulation:** 0.3- to 0.5 cun obliquely and directed medially.

**Caution:** No Moxibustion.

# STOMACH MERIDIAN (Leg Yang Ming)

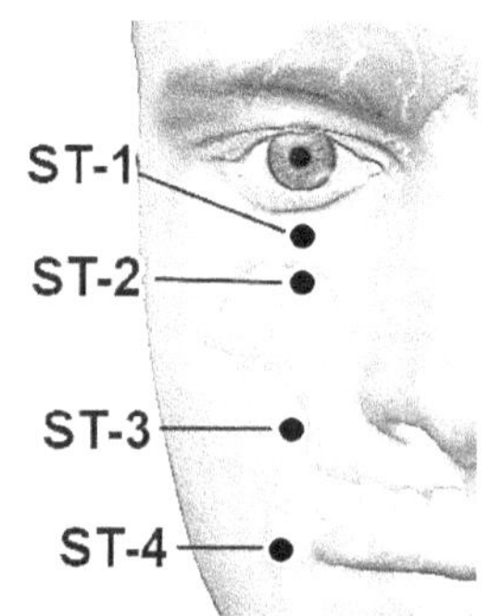


# ST-1 Chengqi
(TEAR CONTAINER)

ENTRY POINT

**Location:**
Below the eyeball at the midpoint of the lower margin of the orbit.

**Dermatome:** Trigeminal nerve

**Main Action Areas:** Eyes and area below

**Main Functions:** Benefits the eyes and area below. Improves vision. Dispels wind and clears heat. Improves appearance

**Indications:**
Redness, swelling and pain of the eye, lacrimation, night blindness, twitching of eyelids, facial paralysis.

**Manipulation:** 0-3 to 0.5 cun perpendicularly. Insert needle along floor of orbit with patient's eyeball turned upwards.

**Caution:** All points located in the orbit are Dangerous points.

No Moxibustion.

# ST-2 Sibai
(FOUR DIRECTION BRIGHTNESS)

**Location:**
0.7 cun below Chengqi [ST-1], in the infra-orbital foramen.

**Shared location with Tung:** 1010.21

**Dermatome:** Trigeminal nerve

**Main Action Areas:** Eye, Area below eye, Cheek, Nose

**Main Functions:** Dispels wind and clears heat. Stops excessive lacrimation. Improves appearance

**Indications:**
Eye diseases, facial paralysis, trigeminal neuralgia.

**Manipulation:** 0.3 cun perpendicularly into the infra-orbital foramen.

**Cautions:** Deep insertion may injure the eyeball or infraorbital nerves. Manipulation is contra-indicated.

Contra-indicated for moxibustion.

# ST-3 Juliao
(LARGE BONE HOLE)

MEETING POINT OF THE STOMACH WITH THE YANG HEEL VESSEL. MUSCLE MERIDIAN MEETING POINT OF THE 3 LEG YANG.

**Location:**
Directly below Sibai [ST-2.], at the level of the lower border of the ala nasi.

**Dermatome:** Trigeminal nerve

**Main Action Areas:** Cheeks and centre of the face, Nose, Sinuses, Eyes, Gums and Teeth

**Main Functions:** Dispels wind and clears heat. Opens the nose. Alleviates pain

**Indications:**
Facial paralysis, trigeminal neuralgia, rhinitis, toothache.

**Manipulation:** 0-3 to 0 5 cun obliquely.

**Caution:** No moxibustion

# ST-4 Dicang
(EARTH GRANARY)

MEETING POINT OF THE STOMACH AND LARGE INTESTINE CHANNELS WITH THE YANG HEEL AND CONCEPTION VESSELS.

**Location:**
0.4 cun lateral to the corner of the mouth.

**Shared location with Tung:** 1010.17

**Dermatome:** Trigeminal nerve

**Main Action Areas:** Mouth, Lips, Front of Cheek

**Main Functions:** Depresses appetite

**Indications:**
Facial paralysis, trigeminal neuralgia, increased salivation, cheilosis, speech difficulties, mutism, disorders of upper teeth, anaesthesia for extraction of upper teeth.

**Manipulation:** Oblique or subcutaneous insertion .5 - .8 cun; or puncture towards ST-6.

Moxibustion is applicable.

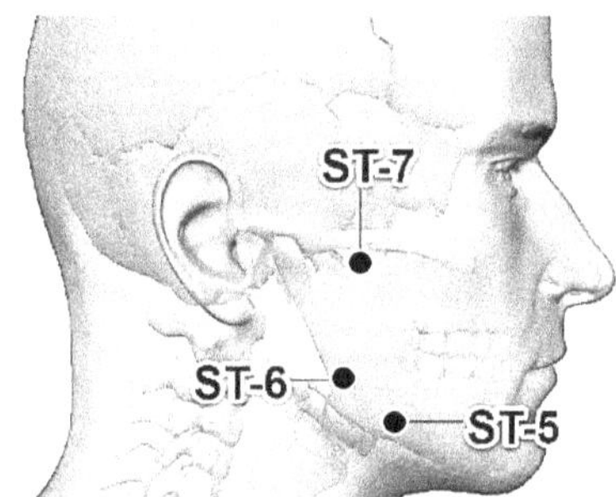


# ST-5 Daying
(LARGE RECEPTACLE – FACIAL ARTERY)

**Location:**
At the lowest point of the anterior border of the masseter muscle.

**Dermatome:** Trigeminal nerve

**Main Action Areas:** Cheek, Gums, Jaw, Teeth

**Main Functions:** Regulates Qi and Blood. Dispels stasis. Alleviates pain

**Indications:**
Facial paralysis, trigeminal neuralgia, toothache, parotitis.

**Manipulation:** Oblique or subcutaneous insertion .3 - .5 cun.

Moxibustion is applicable.

**Cautions:** The facial artery and vein are in this area.

# ST-6 Jiache

(JAW BONE)

SEVENTH GHOST POINT

**Location:**
Most prominent point of the masseter muscle felt on clenching the jaws.

**Dermatome:** Trigeminal nerve

**Main Action Areas:** Jaw, TMJ, Teeth, Cheek, Head, Mind

**Main Functions:** Benefits the jaw. Dispels stasis. Alleviates pain. Calms the mind

**Indications:**
Facial paralysis, trigeminal neuralgia, toothache, parotitis, spasm of masseter, trismus.

**Manipulation:** 0.3 cun perpendicularly or horizontally toward ST-4.

Moxibustion applicable.

# ST-7 Xiaguan

(BELOW THE ARCH)

INTERSECTION OF THE GALLBLADDER ON THE STOMACH CHANNEL

**Location:**
In the depression on the lower border of the zygomatic arch.

**Shared location with Tung:** 1010.18

**Dermatome:** Trigeminal nerve

**Main Action Areas:** Jaw, TMJ, Ear, Cheek, Teeth

**Main Functions:** Dissipates stasis. Alleviates pain and swelling. Benefits the TMJ

**Indications:**
Facial paralysis, trigeminal neuralgia, toothache, arthritis of mandibular joint. Important local/trigger point.

**Manipulation:** 0.5 cun perpendicularly or oblique.

No Moxibustion.

# ST-8 Touwei

(HEAD CORNER)

MEETING POINT OF THE STOMACH AND GALL BLADDER CHANNELS WITH THE YANG LINKING VESSEL.

**Location:**
0.5 cun lateral to the corner of the anterior hairline. 0.5 cun within the anterior hairline and 4.5 cun lateral to

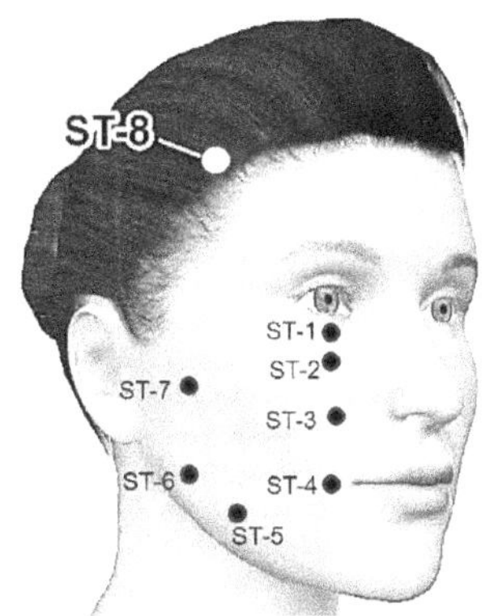


the anterior midline (DU-24), directly above ST-7 and GB-3.

**Dermatome:** Trigeminal nerve

**Main Action Areas:** Head, Eyes, Mind

**Main Functions:** Dispels wind and dampness. Benefits the head, brain and eyes. Stops lacrimation

**Indications:**
Migraine, ophthalmoplegia, increased lacrimation

**Manipulation:** 0.5 cun horizontally directed posteriorly. For headache anteriorly for eye disorders.

**Caution:** No Moxibustion.

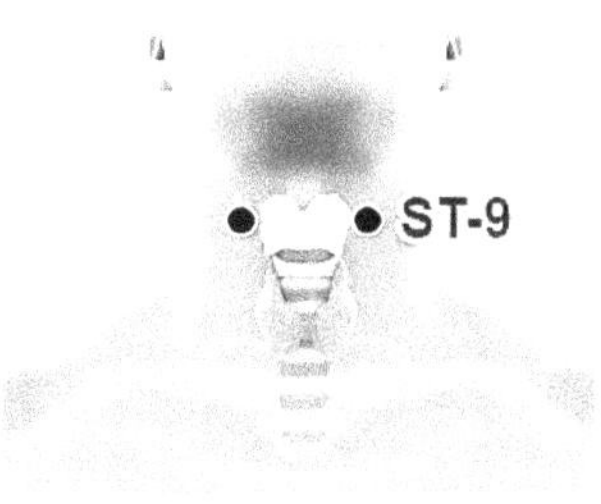


# ST-9 Renying

(MAN'S PROGNOSIS – CAROTID ARTERY)

MEETING POINT OF THE STOMACH AND GALL BLADDER CHANNELS. WINDOW OF HEAVEN POINT, POINT OF THE STAR OF QI.

**Location:**
1.5 cun lateral to the anterior midline, on the level of the laryngeal prominence and at the anterior border of the sternocleidomastoid muscle.

**Dermatome:** C3

**Main Action Areas:** Throat, Thyroid gland, Face, Head, Brain, Heart, Blood vessels

**Main Functions:** Descends rising Yang. Clears heat. Calms the mind and body. Increases PSNS activity. Lowers heart rate and output. Lowers blood pressure. Benefits the throat and thyroid.

**Indications:**
Sore throat, asthma, goiter, dizziness, flushing of the face.

**Manipulation:** Perpendicular insertion .3 - .5 cun. Manual pressure of the ST-9 helps excessive rising of Yang Qi.

**Cautions:** Dangerous point. Requires skill in needling. The carotid artery lies deep to this point, and must be held laterally while needling this point.

No moxibustion.

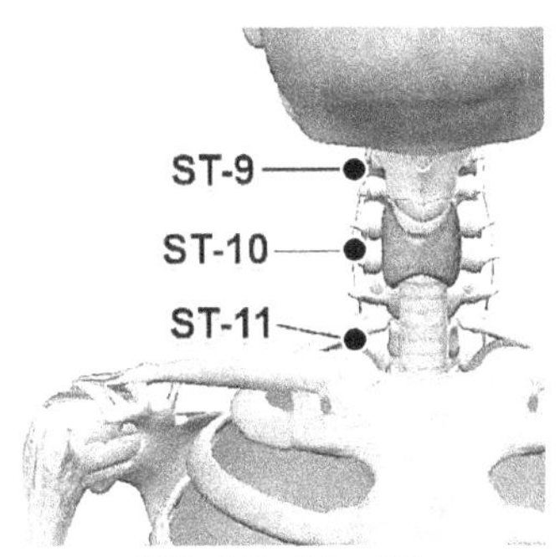


# ST-10 Shuitu

(LIQUID PASSAGE)

**Location:**
On the anterior border of the sternocleidomastoid muscle, at the midpoint of a line connecting ST-9 and ST-11.

**Dermatome:** C3

**Main Action Areas:** Throat, Thyroid gland

**Main Functions:** Benefits the throat

**Indications:**
Sore throat, asthma, cough.

**Manipulation:** Perpendicular insertion .3 - .5 cun.

**Cautions:** The carotid artery lies deep to this point, and must be held laterally while needling this point.

No moxibustion.

# ST-11 Qishe

(RESIDENCE OF THE BREATH QI)

**Location:**
On the upper border of the clavicle, between the tendons of the sternal and clavicular heads of the sternocleido-mastoid muscle.

**Dermatome:** C3

**Main Action Areas:** Throat, Thyroid gland

**Main Functions:** Benefits the throat

**Indications:**
Sore throat, pain and rigidity of the neck, asthma, hiccup, goiter.

**Manipulation:** Perpendicular insertion .3 - .5 cun. Under the points from ST-11 to ST-18, there are important organs and a main artery.

Moxibustion is applicable.

**Cautions:** Deep insertion may penetrate the Lung.

# ST-12 Quepen
(EMPTY BASIN)

MEETING POINT OF THE STOMACH, LARGE INTESTINE, SMALL INTESTINE, TRIPLE ENERGIZER (SANJIAO), AND GALL BLADDER CHANNELS.

**Location:**
In the supraclavicular fossa, superior to the midpoint of the clavicle, approximately 4 cun lateral to the anterior midline.

**Dermatome:** C3

**Main Action Areas:** Chest, Lungs, Shoulder

**Main Functions:** Descends rising Qi. Lowers blood pressure. Clears heat

**Indications:**
Cough, asthma, sore throat, pain in the supraclavicular fossa.

**Manipulation:** Perpendicular or oblique insertion .3 - .5 cun.

Moxibustion is applicable.

**Cautions:** Deep or posterior insertion may penetrate the Lung or subclavian vessels. Contraindicated during pregnancy and heavy menstruation.

# ST-13 Qihu
(DOOR OF THE BREATH)

**Location:**
At the midpoint of the clavicle and on its inferior border, 4 cun lateral to the anterior midline.

**Dermatome:** C4

**Main Action Areas:** Clavicle, Shoulder, Chest

**Main Functions:** Alleviates pain and stiffness. Benefits the breathing

**Indications:**
Fullness in the chest, asthma, cough, hiccup, pain in the chest, hypochondrium.

**Manipulation:** Oblique or subcutaneous insertion .3 - .5 cun.

Moxibustion is applicable.

**Cautions:** Deep or perpendicular insertion may penetrate the Lung or subclavian vessels.

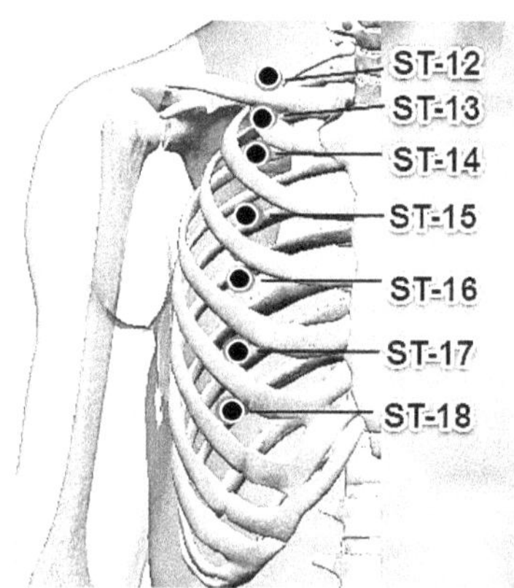


# ST-14 Kufang
(BREATH STOREROOM)

**Location:**
On the midclavicular line, in the first intercostal space, 4 cun lateral to the anterior midline.

**Dermatome:** T2

**Main Action Areas:** Chest, Breast

**Main Functions:** Alleviates pain and swelling. Benefits the breast and Lungs

**Indications:**
Sensation of fullness and pain in the chest, cough.

**Manipulation:** Oblique or subcutaneous insertion 0.3 - 0.5 cun.

Moxibustion is applicable.

**Cautions:** Deep or perpendicular insertion may penetrate the Lung.

# ST-15 Wuyi
(HIDING THE BREATH)

**Location:**
In the 2nd intercostal space, on the midclavicular line, 4 cun lateral to the anterior midline.

**Dermatome:** T2/T3

**Main Action Areas:** Chest, Lungs, Breast

**Main Functions:** Alleviates pain and swelling. Benefits the breast and Lungs

**Indications:**
Fullness and pain in the chest and the costal region, cough, asthma, mastitis.

**Manipulation:** Oblique or subcutaneous insertion 0.3 - 0.5 cun.

Moxibustion is applicable.

**Cautions:** Deep or perpendicular insertion may penetrate the Lung.

# ST-16 Yingchuang
(BREAST WINDOW)

**Location:**
In the 3rd intercostal space, on the midclavicular line, 4 cun lateral to the anterior midline.

**Dermatome:** T3

**Main Action Areas:** Breast

**Main Functions:** Alleviates pain and swelling

**Indications:**
Fullness and pain in the chest and hypochondrium, cough, asthma, mastitis.

**Manipulation:** Oblique or subcutaneous insertion 0.3 - 0.5 cun.

Moxibustion is applicable.

**Cautions:** Deep or perpendicular insertion may penetrate the Lung.

# ST-17 Ruzhong
(BREAST CENTRE – NIPPLE)

**Location:**
In the centre of the nipple.

**Indications:**
This point serves only as a landmark for locating points on the chest and abdomen.

**Manipulation:** No needling. No moxibustion.

# ST-18 Rugen
(BREAST ROOT)

**Location:** On the nipple-line, in the 5th intercostal space, on the infra mammary line.

**Dermatome:** T4/T5

**Main Action Areas:** Breasts, Lungs, Chest, Liver

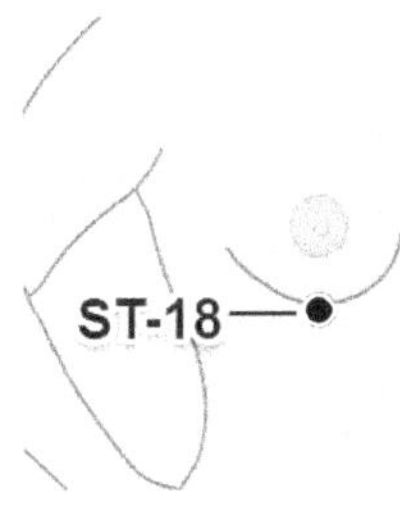


**Main Functions:** Dispels stasis. Benefits the breasts

**Indications:** Mastitis, deficient lactation, chest pain, cough, dyspnoea, angina pectoris and other heart disorders.

**Manipulation:** Oblique or subcutaneous insertion 0.3 - 0.5 cun.

Moxibustion is applicable.

**Cautions:** Deep or perpendicular insertion may penetrate the Lung.

# ST-19 Burong
(NOT CONTAINED)

**Location:**
2 cun below the sternocostal angle and 2 cun lateral to the anterior midline.

**Dermatome:** T6/T7

**Main Action Areas:** Stomach, Abdomen, Heart

**Main Functions:** Harmonises the middle jiao

**Indications:**
Abdominal distensions, vomiting, gastric pain, anorexia.

**Manipulation:** Perpendicular insertion .5 - .8 cun.

Moxibustion is applicable.

**Cautions:** Deep insertion may penetrate an enlarged Heart or Liver.

# ST-20 Chengman
(RECEIVING FULLNESS)

**Location:**
3 cun below the sternocostal angle (or 5 cun above the umbilicus) and 2 cun lateral to the anterior midline.

**Dermatome:** T8

**Main Action Areas:** Stomach, Abdomen, Heart

**Main Functions:** Harmonises the middle jiao

**Indications:**
Gastric pain, abdominal distension, vomiting, anorexia.

**Manipulation:** Perpendicular insertion .5 – 1.0 cun.

Moxibustion is applicable.

**Cautions:** Deep insertion may penetrate the peritoneal cavity or an enlarged Liver.

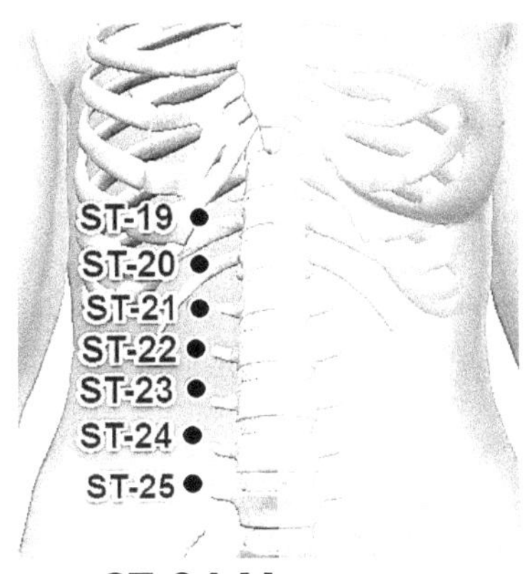


# ST-21 Liangmen
(GRAIN GATE – EPIGASTRIUM)

**Location:**
4 cun vertically above Tianshu (ST-25) or 2 cun lateral to the anterior midline (REN-12), 4 cun above the umbilicus (or 4 cun below the subcostal angle).

**Dermatome:** T9

**Main Action Areas:** Epigastrium, Abdomen, Heart

**Main Functions:** Descends rebellious Qi. Relieves stagnation. Harmonises the Stomach

**Indications:**
Acute and chronic gastritis, peptic ulcer, nausea, vomiting, (i.e. upper abdominal disorders).

**Manipulation:** 0.5 - 1.0 cun perpendicularly on the left side or obliquely on the right side as it is over the gall bladder.

Moxibustion applicable.

**Cautions:** This point on the patients' right is a Dangerous point, as it overlies the gall-bladder.

# ST-22 Guanmen
(SHUTTING THE GATE – PYLORUS)

**Location:**
3 cun above the umbilicus (or 5 cun inferior to the sternocostal angle) and 2 cun lateral to the anterior midline.

**Dermatome:** T9/T10

**Main Action Areas:** Epigastrium, Abdomen, Chest

**Main Functions:** Regulates Stomach Qi

**Indications:**
Abdominal distension and pain, anorexia, borborygmus, diarrhea, edema

**Manipulation:** Perpendicular insertion .8 - 1.0 cun.

Moxibustion is applicable.

**Cautions:** Deep needling may penetrate the peritoneal cavity.

# ST-23 Taiyi
(GREAT UNITY)

**Location:**
2 cun above the umbilicus and 2 cun lateral to the anterior midline.

**Dermatome:** T9/T10

**Main Action Areas:** Stomach, Heart

**Main Functions:** Harmonises the middle jiao. Soothes the Heart and calms the mind.

**Indications:**
Gastric pain, irritability, mania, indigestion.

**Manipulation:** Perpendicular insertion .7 - 1.0 cun.

Moxibustion is applicable.

**Cautions:** Deep needling may penetrate the peritoneal cavity.

# ST-24 Huaroumen
(CHIME GATE)

**Location:**
1 cun above the umbilicus and 2 cun lateral to the anterior midline.

**Dermatome:** T10

**Main Action Areas:** Stomach, Abdomen, Heart

**Main Functions:** Harmonises the Stomach and intestines. Calms the mind

**Indications:**
Gastric pain, vomiting, mania.

**Manipulation:** Perpendicular insertion .7 - 1.0 cun.

Moxibustion is applicable.

**Cautions:** Deep needling may penetrate the peritoneal cavity.

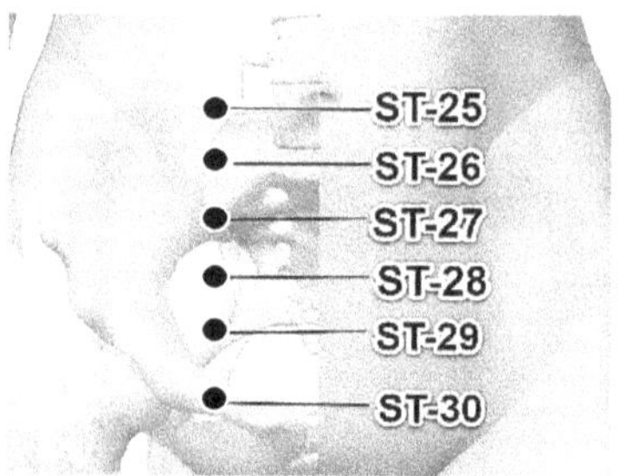



# ST-25 Tianshu

(HEAVEN'S PIVOT)

FRONT-MU POINT OF THE LARGE INTESTINE

**Location:**
2 cun lateral to the umbilicus.

**Dermatome:** T10

**Main Action Areas:** Intestines, Umbilicus, Abdomen, Uterus

**Main Functions:** Clears dampness and heat. Regulates Qi in the lower jiao. Benefits the intestines

**Indication:**
Acute and chronic gastro-enteritis, diarrhoea, constipation, acute appendicitis, intestinal paralysis (paralytic ileus), paralysis of muscles of the abdominal wall (i.e., all abdominal disorders).

**Manipulation:** 0-5 - 1.0 cun perpendicularly.

Moxibustion is applicable except during pregnancy.

**Cautions:** Deep needling may penetrate the peritoneal cavity. Use with caution in pregnancy.

# ST-26 Wailing

(OUTER MOUND)

**Location:**
1 cun below the umbilicus and 2 cun lateral to the anterior midline.

**Dermatome:** T10/T11

**Main Action Areas:** Intestines, Abdomen

**Main Functions:** Regulates the lower jiao

**Indications:** Abdominal pain, hernia, dysmenorrhea.

**Manipulation:** 0.7 - 1.0 cun perpendicularly.

Moxibustion is applicable except during pregnancy.

**Cautions:** Deep needling may penetrate the peritoneal cavity. Use with caution in pregnancy.

# ST-27 Daju

(GREAT BULGE)

**Location:**
2 cun below the umbilicus and 2 cun lateral to the anterior midline.

**Dermatome:** T11

**Main Action Areas:** Abdomen

**Main Functions:** Regulates the lower jiao

**Indications:**
Lower abdominal distension, dysuria, hernia, seminal emission, premature ejaculation.

**Manipulation:** 0.7 - 1.0 cun perpendicularly.

Moxibustion is applicable except during pregnancy.

**Cautions:** Deep needling may penetrate the peritoneal cavity. Use with caution in pregnancy.

# ST-28 Shuidao

(WATERWAY)

**Location:**
3 cun below the umbilicus or 2 cun above the upper border of the pubic symphysis and 2 cun lateral to the anterior midline.

**Dermatome:** T11

**Main Action Areas:** Urogenital system, Uterus

**Main Functions:** Clears dampness and heat. Regulates Qi in the lower jiao. Benefits menstruation. Increases libido and fertility

**Indications:**
Lower abdominal distension, retention of urine, edema, hernia, dysmenorrhea, sterility.

**Manipulation:** 0.7 - 1.0 cun perpendicularly.

Moxibustion is applicable except during pregnancy.

**Cautions:** Deep needling may penetrate the peritoneal cavity or a full bladder. Use with caution in pregnancy.

# ST-29 Guilai

(RESTORING POSITION)

**Location:**
4 cun vertically below ST-25

**Dermatome:** T12

**Main Action Areas:** Lower Abdomen, Uterus, Genitals

**Main Functions:**
Regulates the lower jiao

**Indications:**
Pelvic disorders; dysmenorrhoea, hernia: epididymitis, impotence.

**Manipulation:** 0.7 - 1.0 cun perpendicularly.

Moxibustion is applicable except during pregnancy.

**Cautions:** Deep needling may penetrate the peritoneal cavity or a full bladder. Use with caution in pregnancy.

# ST-30 Qichong

(QI SURGE)

MEETING POINT OF THE STOMACH CHANNEL WITH THE PENETRATING VESSEL. SEA OF NOURISHMENT.

**Location:**
2 cun lateral to the upper border of the pubic symphysis and medial to the femoral artery and vein, approximately 1 cun superior to the inguinal groove.

**Dermatome:** T12

**Main Action Areas:** Reproductive organs, Uterus, Testicles, Bladder, Intestines, Lower Abdomen

**Main Functions:** Benefits the lower jiao. Regulates Qi and Blood. Benefits menstruation. Improves sexual function. Increases fertility.

**Indications:**
Pain and swelling of the external genitalia; hernia; menstrual disorders.

**Manipulation:** 0.5 - 1.0 cun perpendicularly.

Moxibustion is applicable except during pregnancy.

**Cautions:** Deep needling may penetrate the peritoneal cavity or a full bladder. Use with caution in pregnancy.

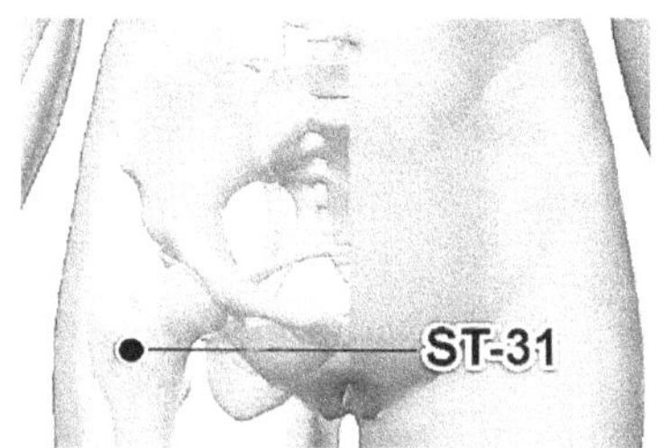


# ST-31 Biguan
(THIGH GATE)

**Location:**
The meeting point of the vertical line from the anterior superior iliac spine and the horizontal line from the upper border of the pubic symphysis.

**Dermatome:** L1

**Main Action Areas:** Hips, Lower Limbs

**Main Functions:** Dissipates stasis and alleviates pain and stiffness. Dispels wind and dampness

**Indications:**
Paralysis of lower limbs as in hemiplegia, osteoarthritis of the hip, numbness of the lower limb.

**Manipulation:** 1-5 cun perpendicularly.

Moxibustion applicable.

# ST-32 Femur Futu
(CROUCHING RABBIT)

**Location:**
a) 6 cun above the midpoint of the superior border of the patella.

b) With patient seated, place contralateral wrist crease of the acupuncturist on middle of knee cap and the fingers along the thigh. This point is located at the tip of the middle finger.

**Dermatome:** L2

**Main Action Areas:** Thigh

**Main Functions:** Dispels wind, dampness and cold. Alleviates pain

**Indications:**
Paralysis of lower extremities, arthritis of the knee, wasting and weakness of the quadriceps. This is a motor point.

**Manipulation:** 1-5 cun perpendicularly piercing along the lateral border of the femur, or 2.0 - 3.0 cun obliquely in a proximal direction.

Moxibustion applicable.

# ST-33 Yinshi
(YIN MARKET)

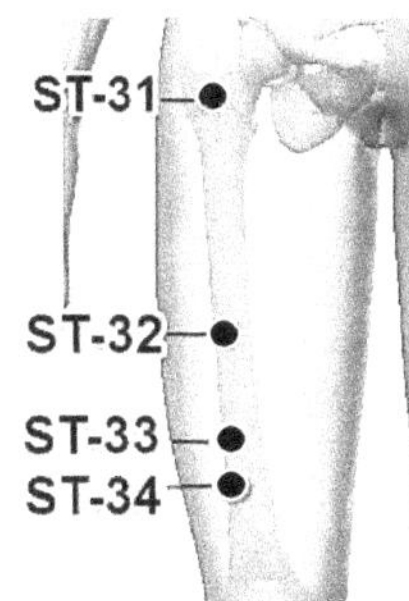


**Location:**
On a line joining the lateral patellar border and the anterior superior iliac spine, 3 cun superior to the upper lateral border of the patella.

**Dermatome:** L2/L3

**Main Action Areas:** Thigh

**Main Functions:** Dispels wind, dampness and cold. Alleviates pain.

**Indications:**
Numbness, soreness, motor impairment of the leg and knee, motor impairment of the lower extremities.

**Manipulation:**
Perpendicular insertion .7 - 1.0 cun.

Moxibustion is applicable.

# ST-34 Liangqiu
(RIDGE MOUND)

Xi-Cleft point.

**Location:**
2 cun above the lateral end of the upper border of the patella.

**Shared location with Tung:** 88.28

**Dermatome:** L3

**Main Action Areas:** Stomach, Epigastrium, Lower Limbs, Knees

**Main Functions:** Pacifies the Stomach. Descends rebellious Qi. Alleviates pain

**Indications:**
Disorders of the knee, acute gastro-intestinal disorders.

**Manipulation:** 0.5 - 1.0 cun perpendicularly.

Moxibustion is applicable.

**Remarks:** This is the Xi-Cleft point of the Stomach Channel. In acute gastric and intestinal disorders the pain and colic are rapidly relieved with this point.

# ST-35 Dubi
(CALF'S NOSE)

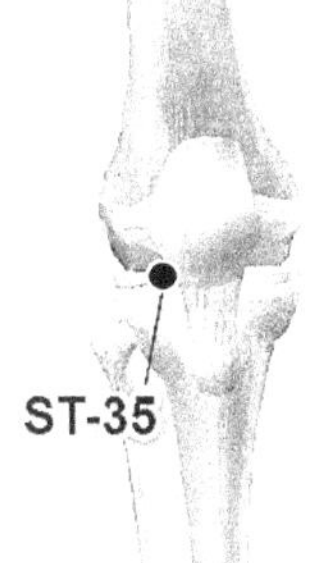


(Also known as lateral-Xiyan.)
**Location:**
This is in the depression (below the patella) on the lateral side of the ligamentum patellae. It is best located with the knee slightly bent.

**Dermatome:** L3

**Main Action Areas:** Knees

**Main Functions:** Alleviates pain, stiffness and swelling. Strengthens the knees

**Indications:**
Arthritis of knee, sprain/strain of knee.

**Manipulation:**

a) 1 to 2 cun perpendicular insertion, angled slightly medially towards the centre of the knee joint, or BL-40.

b) 1 to 1.5 cun horizontal insertion, through or under the patellar ligament to connect with the Nei Xiyan (EX-LE-4)

c) 1 to 2 cun oblique superior medial insertion under the patella.

Moxibustion is applicable.

**Cautions:** Strictly observe clean needle technique to avoid causing infection within the knee joint capsule.

# ST-36 Zusanli
(LEG THREE MILES)

HE-SEA, HORARY, AND EARTH POINT OF THE STOMACH CHANNEL. COMMAND POINT OF THE ABDOMEN. SEA OF NOURISHMENT POINT. LOWER HE-SEA POINT, GAO WU COMMAND POINT, MA DAN-YANG HEAVENLY STAR POINT.

**Location:**
One finger breadth lateral to the inferior end of the tibial tuberosity. 3 cun below the knee crease.

**Shared location with Tung:** 77.08

**Dermatome:** L5

**Main Action Areas:** Entire body, Abdomen, Chest, Mind, Stomach and

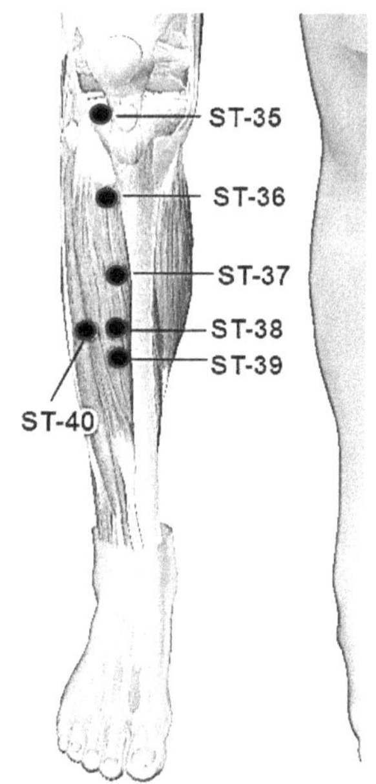

Spleen, Digestive system, Lower Limb, Knee

**Main Functions:** Tonifies and lifts Qi and Yang. Nourishes Blood, fluids and Yin. Boosts the immune system. Benefits the Stomach and Spleen. Regulates Qi. Calms the mind.

**Indication:**
Gastritis, nausea, vomiting, enteritis, diarrhoea, obesity, constipation, appendicitis and other diseases of the digestive tract, paralysis of lower limb, polyneuropathy of the lower limb.

**Manipulation:** 0.5 - 1.5 cun perpendicularly.

Moxibustion applicable.

# ST-37 Shangjuxu
(UPPER GREAT EMPTINESS)

LOWER HE SEA POINT OF THE LARGE INTESTINE. SEA OF BLOOD POINT.

**Location:**
3 cun below to Zusanli (St. 36), one finger breadth lateral to the anterior margin of the tibia.

**Dermatome:** L5

**Main Action Areas:** Large Intestine, Digestive system, Abdomen

**Main Functions:** Regulates the Large Intestine. Dispels dampness. Alleviates pain and diarrhoea

**Indications:**
Diarrhoea, acute appendicitis, paralysis of lower limb.

**Manipulation:** 0.5 - 1.5 cun perpendicularly.

Moxibustion applicable.

# ST-38 Tiaokou
(LINES OPENING)

**Location:**
5 cun below Zusanli (St. 36.) one finger breadth lateral to the anterior border of the tibia.

**Shared location with Tung:** 77.09

**Dermatome:** L5

**Main Action Areas:** Shoulder, Digestive system

**Main Functions:** Dispels wind, dampness and cold. Alleviates pain. Benefits the shoulder

**Indication:**
Numbness, soreness and pain of the knee and leg, weakness and motor impairment of the shoulder, abdominal pain.

**Manipulation:** 1-5 cun perpendicularly., or penetrate through to Chengshan (BL- 57),

Moxibustion applicable.

**Remarks:** In a frozen shoulder this point could be manually stimulated while the patient mobilizes the shoulder joint to obtain an increased range of movement.

# ST-39 Xiajuxu
(LOWER GREAT VOID)

LOWER HE-SEA OF THE SMALL INTESTINE. SEA OF BLOOD POINT.

**Location:**
3 cun below to ST-37. 1 cun distal to ST-38 and 1 finger-breath lateral to the anterior crest of the tibia.

**Dermatome:** L5

**Main Action Areas:** Small Intestine, Digestive system, Alleviates pain

**Main functions:** Regulates the intestines. Alleviates pain.

**Indications:**
Lower abdominal pain, backache referring to the testis, mastitis, numbness and paralysis of the lower extremities.

**Manipulation:** 1.0 cun perpendicularly, Moxibustion applicable.

# ST-40 Fenglong
(ABUNDANT BULGE)

LUO-CONNECTING POINT.

**Location:**
One finger breadth lateral to Tiaokou (ST-38).

**Shared location with Tung:** 77.14

**Dermatome:** L5

**Main Action Areas:** Small Intestine, Digestive system, Abdomen

**Main Functions:** Regulates the intestines. Alleviates pain

**Indications:**
Cough, excessive sputum, epilepsy.

**Manipulation:** 1-5 cun perpendicularly.

Moxibustion applicable.

**Remarks:** According to traditional Chinese medicine, epilepsy is related to excessive sputum.

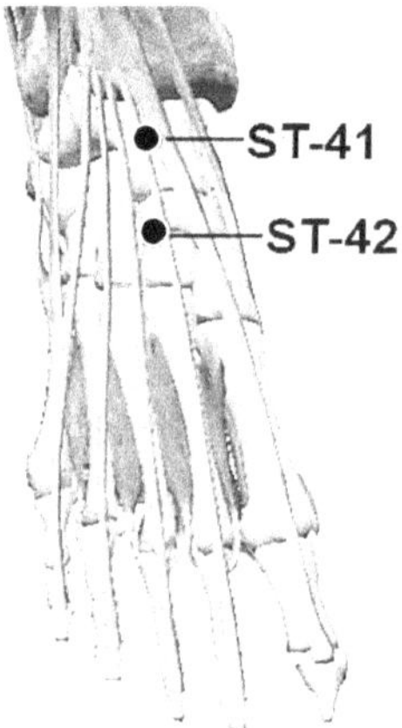

# ST-41 Jiexi
(STREAM DIVIDE)

JING-RIVER, TONIFICATION, AND FIRE POINT OF THE STOMACH CHANNEL.

**Location:**
On the front ankle crease midway between the tips of the malleoli. On the ankle, on the level of the highest prominence of the lateral malleolus, in the depression between the tendons of the extensor digitorum and the extensor hallucis longus.

**Dermatome:** L5

**Main Action Areas:** Ankle, Foot, Stomach, Head

**Main Functions:** Alleviates pain. Clears heat

**Indications:**
Disorders of the ankle joint and soft tissues of the area, paralysis of the leg, foot drop, hemiplegia, varicose veins, chronic ulcers of the ankle area.

**Manipulation:** 0.5cun perpendicularly.

# ST-42 Chongyang
## (RUSHING YANG)

YUAN-SOURCE POINT OF THE STOMACH CHANNEL. EXIT POINT.

**Location:**
On the highest point of the dorsum of the foot, between the tendons of the extensor hallucis longus and the extensor digitorum longus, directly lateral to the point where the dorsalis pedis artery may be palpated. The point is bordered proximally by the 2nd and 3rd metatarsal bones and distally by the 2nd and 3rd cuneiform bones.

**Alternative location:** Sometimes, this point may be located lateral to the medial portion of the extensor digitorum longus tendon (joining the 2nd toe).

**Dermatome:** L5

**Main Action Areas:** Stomach, Middle jiao, Foot, Mind

**Main Functions:** Tonifies Qi and Yang. Alleviates swelling and pain

**Indications:**
Pain of the upper teeth, redness and swelling of the dorsum of the foot, facial paralysis, muscular atrophy and motor impairment of the foot.

**Manipulation:** Perpendicular insertion .2 - .5 cun.

Moxibustion is applicable.

**Cautions:** The dorsalis pedis artery lies deep to this point.

# ST-43 Xiangu
## (SUNKEN VALLEY)

SHU-STREAM AND WOOD POINT OF THE STOMACH CHANNEL.

**Location:**
In the depression between the bases of the 2nd and 3rd metatarsals.

**Shared location with Tung:** 66.05

**Dermatome:** L5

**Main Action Areas:** Foot

**Main Functions:** Regulates Qi and Blood. Alleviates swelling and pain

**Indications:**
Being the best analgesic point of leg, it is used for surgery of lower limb and brain.

**Manipulation:** 0.5 cun perpendicularly. Strong stimulation is used.

Moxibustion applicable.

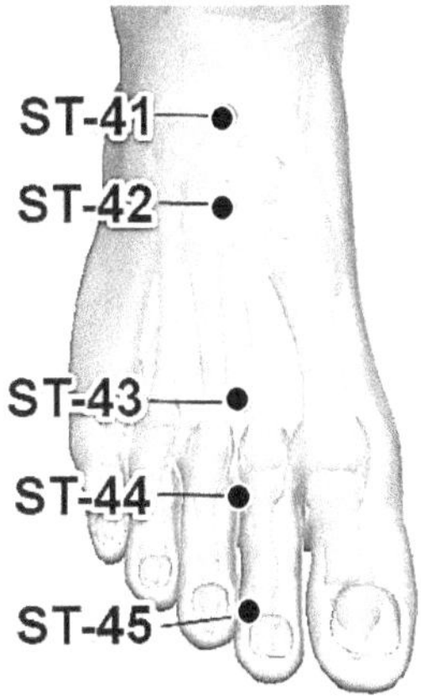


# ST-44 Neiting
## (INNER COURT)

YING-SPRING AND WATER POINT OF THE STOMACH CHANNEL. MA DAN-YANG HEAVENLY STAR POINT.

**Location:**
0.5 cun proximal to the web margin between the 2nd and 3rd toes.

**Dermatome:** L5

**Main Action Areas:** Stomach, Digestive system, Face, Mouth, Eyes, Head, MTP joints and Toes

**Main Functions:** Clears heat and damp heat. Benefits the digestive system. Alleviates swelling and pain

**Indications:**
Distal point for toothache, headache, best analgesic point of lower limb and can be used for relief of pain of the lower limb, in arthritis of joints of toes and feet.

**Manipulation:** 0.3 cun perpendicularly or obliquely.

Moxibustion applicable.

**Remarks:** This is the best analgesic point of the leg for therapy. It is also one of the Bafeng (Ex. 36.) points.

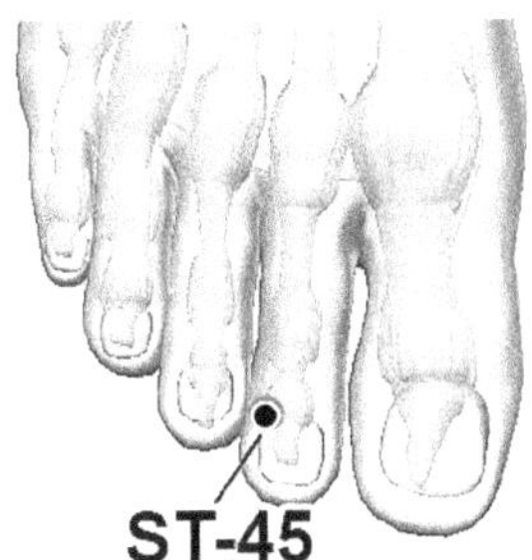


# ST-45 Lidui
## (STRICT EXCHANGE)

JING-WELL, SEDATION, AND METAL POINT OF THE STOMACH CHANNEL.

**Location:**
On the 2nd toe, 0.1 cun from the lateral corner of the nail.

**Dermatome:** L5

**Main Action Areas:** Face, Eyes, Mouth, Stomach, Stomach channel, Mind

**Main Functions:** Resuscitates

**Indications:**
Facial swelling, deviation of the mouth, epistaxis, toothache, sore throat and hoarse voice, abdominal distension, coldness in the leg and foot, febrile diseases, dream-disturbed sleep, mania.

**Manipulation:** Subcutaneous insertion .1 cun. Moxibustion is applicable.

# SPLEEN MERIDIAN (Leg Tai Yin)

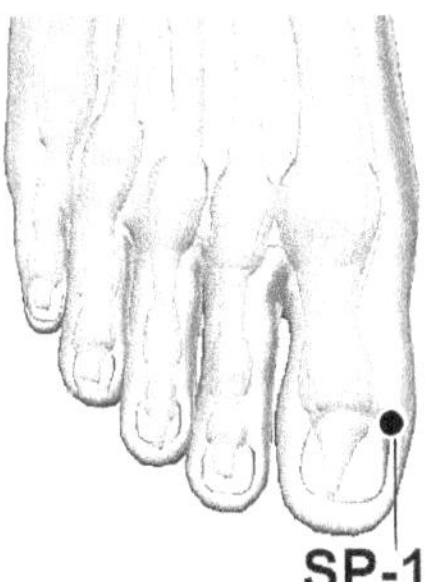


# SP-1 Yinbai
## (HIDDEN WHITE)

JING-WELL AND WOOD POINT OF THE SPLEEN CHANNEL. ENTRY POINT. SUN SI-MIAO GHOST POINT.

**Location:**
On the big toe, 0.1 cun from the medial corner of the nail.

**Shared location with Tung:** 66.01

**Dermatome:** L5

**Main Action Areas:** Uterus, Blood vessels, Mind

**Main Functions:** Arrests bleeding. Lifts Qi. Calms and clears the mind

**Indications:**
Abdominal distension, bloody stools, menorrhagia, uterine bleeding, mental disorders, dream-disturbed sleep, convulsion.

**Manipulation:** Subcutaneous insertion 0.1 cun.

Moxibustion is applicable.

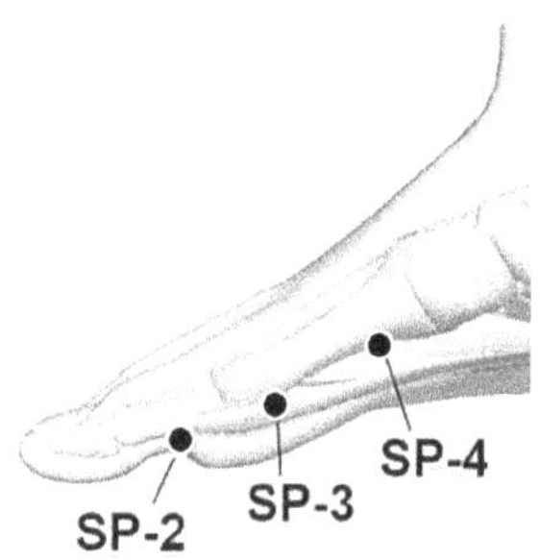


# SP-2 Dadu

(GREAT METROPOLIS)

YING-SPRING, TONIFICATION AND FIRE POINT OF THE SPLEEN CHANNEL.

**Location:**
On the medial aspect of the big toe, at the junction of the shaft and the base of the proximal phalanx, distal to the 1st metatarsophalangeal joint.

**Dermatome:** L5

**Main Action Areas:** MTP joint, Toe, Digestive system

**Main Functions:** Clears dampness and heat

**Indications:**
Abdominal distension, gastric pain, constipation, febrile diseases with anhidrosis.

**Manipulation:** Subcutaneous insertion 0.1 cun.

Moxibustion is applicable.

# SP-3 Taibai

(SUPREME WHITE)

SHU-STREAM, YUAN-SOURCE, HORARY POINT, AND EARTH POINT OF THE SPLEEN CHANNEL.

**Location:**
On the medial aspect of the foot, in the depression proximal to the head of the 1st metatarsal bone, at the border of the red and white skin.

**Shared location with Tung:** 66.10

**Dermatome:** L5

**Main Action Areas:** Digestive system, Intestines, Urinary system, Muscles, Mind

**Main Functions:** Transforms dampness. Tonifies Spleen Qi and Yang

**Indications:**
Gastric pain, abdominal distension, constipation, dysentery, vomiting, diarrhea, borborygmus, sluggishness, beriberi.

**Manipulation:** Perpendicular insertion 0.3 – 0.5 cun.

Moxibustion is applicable

# SP-4 Gongsun

(GRANDFATHER GRANDSON)

LUO POINT OF THE SPLEEN CHANNEL. CONFLUENT POINT OF THE PENETRATING VESSEL. COMMAND POINT OF THE YIN LINKING VESSEL. MASTER POINT OF THE CHONG VESSEL.

**Location:**
On the medial side of the foot in the depression below the base of the 1st metatarsal bone, at the junction of the two colours of the skin on the medial border of the foot.

**Shared location with Tung:** 66.10

**Dermatome:** L5

**Main Action Areas:** Stomach, Abdomen, Uterus, Heart, Mind

**Main Functions:** Opens the Chong Mai. Tonifies the Spleen and Stomach. Nourishes Blood. Regulates Qi. Dispels Blood stasis. Benefits menstruation

**Indications:**
Gastric pain, vomiting, abdominal pain and distension, diarrhea, dysentery, borborygmus.

**Manipulation:**
0.5-0.8 cun perpendicularly.

Moxibustion applicable.

**Remarks:** Useful for digestive system, gynaecology. Also regulates the heart and calm the mind.

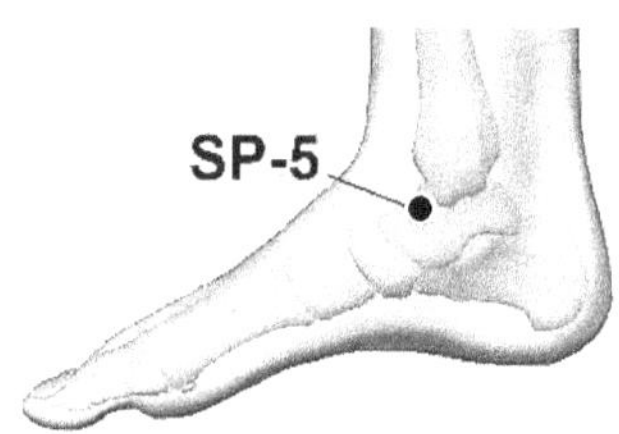


# SP-5 Shangqiu

(SHANG MOUND)

JING-RIVER, SEDATION, AND METAL POINT OF THE SP CHANNEL.

**Location:**
In the depression at the junction of a vertical line drawn along the anterior border and a horizontal line drawn along the lower border of the medial malleolus. Or: In the depression halfway between the highest prominence of the medial malleolus and the tubercle of the navicular bone.

**Dermatome:** L4/L5

**Main Action Areas:** Ankle, Abdomen

**Main Functions:** Regulates Qi and Blood. Dries dampness. Benefits the lower jiao

**Indications:**
Abdominal distension, constipation, diarrhea, borborygmus, pain and rigidity of the tongue, pain in the foot and ankle, hemorrhoid.

**Manipulation:**
0.2-0.3 cun perpendicularly.

Moxibustion applicable.

# SP-6 Sanyinjiao

(THREE YIN INTERSECTION)

MEETING POINT OF THE SPLEEN, LIVER, AND KIDNEY CHANNELS. GROUP LOU POINT FOR THE 3 LEG YIN.

**Location:**
3 cun proximal to the highest prominence of the medial malleolus, on the posterior border of the medial crest of the tibia.

**Shared location with Tung:** 77.21

**Dermatome:** L4

**Main Action Areas:** Entire body, Abdomen, Uterus, Liver, Spleen, Kidney

**Main Functions:** Boosts the Spleen and Stomach. Transforms dampness. Nourishes Blood and Yin. Calms the mind. Dispels stasis. Benefits menstruation. Promotes labour

**Indications:**
Gastro-intestinal disorders, genito-urinary disorders, lower limb disorders, skin disorders, All three Yin Channels of the leg meet at this point and it is therefore used in disorders of the Liver, Spleen and Kidney.

**Manipulation:** Perpendicular insertion .5 - 1.0 cun.

Moxibustion is applicable.

**Cautions:** Contraindicated during pregnancy.

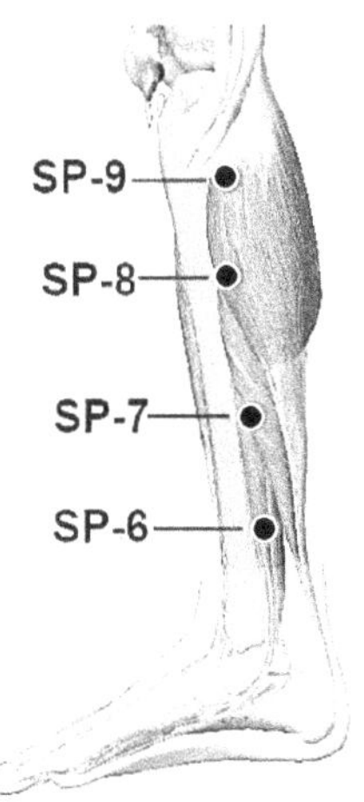

# SP-7 Lougu
(DRIPPING VALLEY)

**Location:**
6 cun proximal to the highest prominence of the medial malleolus, on the posterior border of the medial crest of the tibia.

**Shared location with Tung:** 77.19

**Dermatome:** L4

**Main Functions:** Fortifies the Spleen and harmonizes the stomach, disinhibits damp and disperses swelling, frees the channels and quickens the connecting vessels, regulates Qi and blood.

**Indications:** Abdominal distension, borborygmus, coldness, numbness and paralysis of the knee and leg.

**Manipulation:** Perpendicular insertion .5 - 1.0 cun.

Moxibustion is applicable.

# SP-8 Diji
(EARTH PIVOT)

XI-CLEFT POINT OF THE SPLEEN CHANNEL.

**Location:**
3 cun distal to the junction of the shaft and the medial condyle of the tibia, at the posterior border of the medial crest of the tibia.

**Dermatome:** L4

**Main Action Areas:** Uterus, Abdomen, Knee

**Main Functions:** Invigorates Blood. Dispels stasis. Regulates menstruation

**Indications:**
Abdominal pain and distension, diarrhea, edema, dysuria, nocturnal emission, irregular menstruation, dysmenorrhea.

**Manipulation:**
Perpendicular insertion 0.5 - 1.0 cun. Moxibustion is applicable.

# SP-9 Yinlingquan
(YIN MOUND SPRING)

HE-SEA AND WATER POINT OF THE SPLEEN CHANNEL.

**Location:**
At the level of the lower border of the tibial tuberosity at the depression below the lower border of the medial condyle.

Located at same level with GB-34 but on opposite sides.

**Shared location with Tung:** 77.17

**Dermatome:** L5

**Main Action Areas:** Lower jiao, Urogenital system, Intestines, Abdomen, Knee

**Main Functions:** Drains dampness. Regulates the lower jiao. Alleviates pain

**Indications:**
Abdominal pain and distension, diarrhea, dysentery, edema, jaundice, dysuria, enuresis, incontinence of urine, genital pain, dysmenorrhea, knee pain.

**Manipulation:**
Perpendicular insertion .5 - 1.0 cun. Moxibustion is applicable.

**Remarks:** Effective for intestinal and urogenital systems.

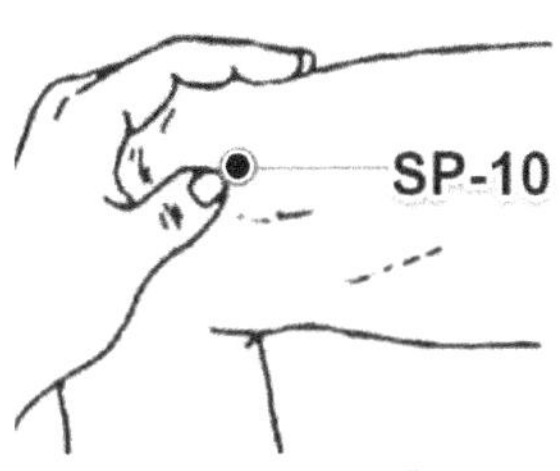


# SP-10 Xuehai
(SEA OF BLOOD)

**Location:** With the knee flexed, SP-10 is located 2 cun proximal and slightly medial to the medial superior border of the patella, in a depression on the vastus medialis muscle.

**Shared location with Tung:** 88.10

**Dermatome:** L3

**Main Action Areas:** Skin, Gynaecological system, Genitals

**Main Functions:** Invigorates and cools Blood. Alleviates itching. Dispels dampness

**Indications:**
Irregular menstruation, dysmenorrhea, uterine bleeding, amenorrhea, urticarial, eczema, erysipelas, pain in the medial aspect of the thigh.

**Manipulation:**
Perpendicular insertion 0.5 - 1.0 cun.

Moxibustion is applicable

# SP-11 Jimen
(WINNOWING GATE)

**Location:**
6 cun proximal to SP-10 or 8 cun proximal to the medial upper border of the patella, at the midpoint of the femur between the sartorius and vastus lateralis muscles.

**Dermatome:** L2/L3

**Main Action Areas:** Medial thigh, Knee, Inguinal area, Genitourinary system, Lower Abdomen

**Main Functions:** Activates the channel and strengthens the lower limbs. Alleviates pain. Opens the genito-urinary area. Drains dampness and clears heat

**Indications:**
Dysuria, enuresis, pain and swelling in the inguinal region, muscular atrophy, motor impairment, pain and paralysis of the lower extremities.

**Manipulation:** Perpendicular insertion .5 - 1.0 cun.

Moxibustion is applicable.

**Cautions:** Femoral artery lies deep to this point.

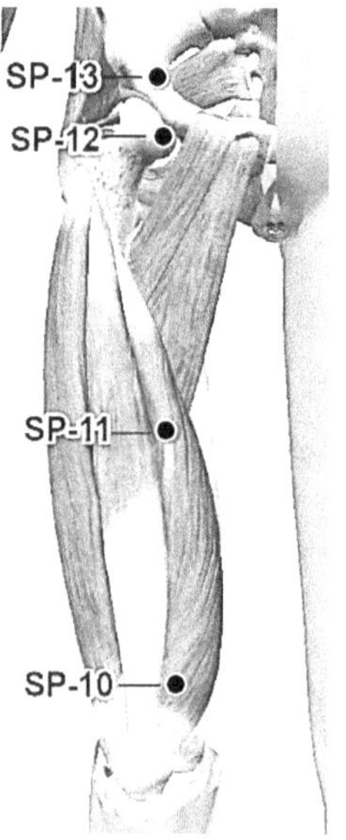


# SP-12 Chongmen

(RUSHING GATE)

**Location:**
3.5 cun lateral to the midline, at the level of the upper border of the pubic symphysis, lateral to the femoral artery.

**Dermatome:** L1

**Main Action Areas:** Lower limbs, Groin, Blood vessels

**Main Functions:** Improves Qi and Blood circulation. Dispels cold from the channels. Alleviates pain.

**Indications:**
Abdominal pain, hernia, dysuria.

**Manipulation:** Perpendicular insertion .5 - 1.0 cun.

Moxibustion is applicable.

**Cautions:** Femoral artery lies deep to this point.

# SP-13 Fushe

(ABODE OF THE FU)

MEETING POINT OF THE SPLEEN AND LIVER CHANNELS WITH THE YIN LINKING VESSEL.

**Location:**
4 cun lateral to the anterior midline and 0.7 cun superior to the upper border of the pubic symphysis.

**Dermatome:** T12

**Main Action Areas:** Lower abdomen, Groin, Intestine

**Main Functions:** Regulates Qi in the intestines

**Indications:**
Lower abdominal pain, hernia.

**Manipulation:** Perpendicular insertion .5 - 1.0 cun.

Moxibustion is applicable.

**Cautions:** In thin patients, deep needling may penetrate the peritoneal cavity.

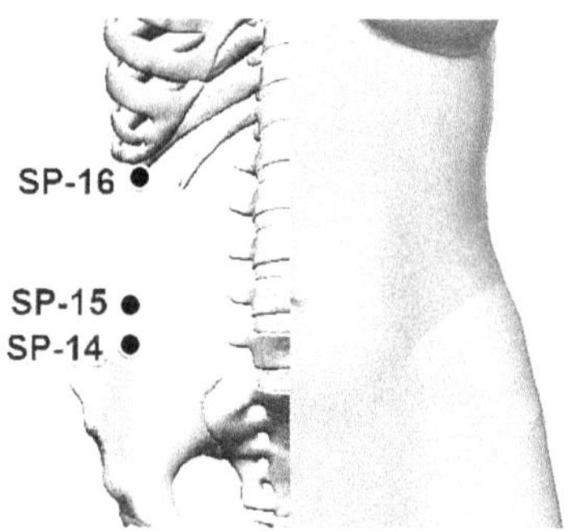


# SP-14 Fujie

(ABDOMEN KNOT)

**Location:**
4 cun lateral to the anterior midline, on the mamillary line, 3 cun superior to SP-13 or 1.3 cun inferior to SP-15.

**Dermatome:** T10/T11

**Main Action Areas:** Intestines, Abdomen

**Main Functions:** Regulates Qi in the intestines. Descends rebellious Qi.

**Indications:**
Pain around the umbilical region, abdominal distension, hernia, diarrhea, constipation.

**Manipulation:** Perpendicular insertion .5 - 1.0 cun.

Moxibustion is applicable.

**Cautions:** In thin patients, deep needling may penetrate the peritoneal cavity.

# SP-15 Daheng

(GREAT HORIZONTAL)

MEETING POINT OF THE SPLEEN CHANNEL WITH THE YIN LINKING VESSEL.

**Location:**
4 cun lateral to the umbilicus (on the nipple-line)

**Dermatome:** T10

**Main Action Areas:** Intestines, Abdomen

**Main Functions:** Tonifies the Spleen. Regulates the intestines. Treats constipation

**Indications:**
Constipation, diarrhoea, intestinal paralysis, intestinal parasitosis, dyspepsia, abdominal distension.

**Manipulation:** Perpendicular insertion .7 - 1.2 cun.

Moxibustion is applicable.

**Cautions:** In thin patients, deep needling may penetrate the peritoneal cavity or an enlarged spleen or liver.

# SP-16 Fuai

(ABDOMEN SORROW)

MEETING POINT OF THE SPLEEN CHANNEL WITH THE YIN LINKING VESSEL.

**Location:**
3 cun above the centre of the umbilicus and 4 cun lateral to the anterior midline, on the mamillary line.

**Dermatome:** T8/T9

**Main Action Areas:** Hypochondrium, Abdomen

**Main Functions:** Harmonises the Spleen and Large Intestine

**Indications:**
Abdominal pain, indigestion, constipation, dysentery.

**Manipulation:** Perpendicular insertion 0.5 - 1.0 cun.

Moxibustion is applicable.

**Cautions:** In thin patients, deep needling may penetrate the peritoneal cavity or an enlarged spleen.

# SP-17 Shidou

(FOOD CAVITY)

**Location:**
In the 5th intercostal space, 6 cun lateral to the anterior midline (in male patients, 2 cun lateral to the nipple).

**Dermatome:** L5

**Main Action Areas:** Chest, Ribs, Breast

**Main Functions:** Regulates Qi and Blood.

**Indications:** Fullness and pain in the chest and hypochondriac region.

**Manipulation:** Oblique or subcutaneous insertion toward the lateral direction .3 - .5 cun.

Moxibustion is applicable.

**Cautions:** Do not needle perpendicularly, especially in thin patients, due to risk of pneumo-thorax.

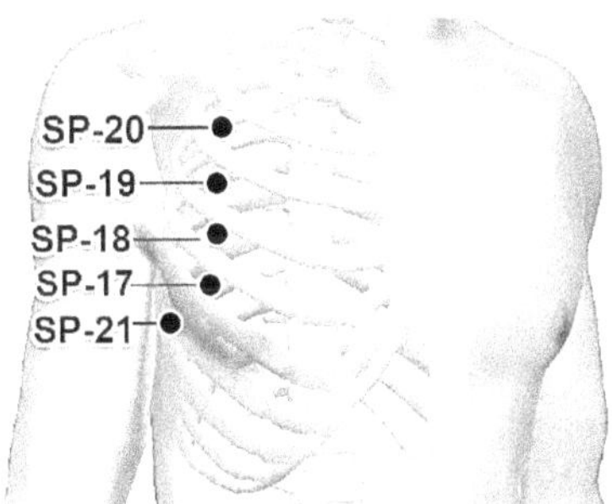


## SP-18 Tianxi

(HEAVENLY STREAM)

**Location:**
In the 4th intercostal space, 6 cun lateral to the anterior midline or 2 cun lateral to the midclavicular line.

**Dermatome:** T4

**Main Action Areas:** Chest, Ribs, Breast

**Main Functions:** Regulates Qi and Blood.

**Indications:**
Fullness and pain in the chest and hypochondrium, cough, hiccup, mastitis, insufficient lactation.

**Manipulatrion:** Oblique or subcutaneous insertion toward the lateral direction .3 - .5 cun.

Moxibustion is applicable.

**Cautions:** Do not needle perpendicularly, especially in thin patients, due to risk of pneumothorax

## SP-19 Xiongxiang

(CHEST VILLAGE)

**Location:**
In the 3rd intercostal space, 6 cun lateral to the anterior midline or 2 cun lateral to the mid-clavicular line.

**Dermatome:** T3

**Main Action Areas:** Chest, Ribs, Breast

**Main Functions:** Regulates Qi and Blood

**Indications:**
Fullness and pain in the chest and hypochondriac region.

**Manipulation:** Oblique or subcutaneous insertion toward the lateral direction .3 - .5 cun.

Moxibustion is applicable.

**Cautions:** Do not needle perpendicularly, especially in thin patients, due to risk of pneumothorax

## SP-20 Zhourong

(ENCICLING GLORY)

**Location:**
In the 2nd intercostal space, 6 cun lateral to the anterior midline or 2 cun lateral to the mid-clavicular line.

**Dermatome:** T2

**Main Action Areas:** Chest, Ribs, Breast

**Main Functions:** Regulates Qi and Blood.

**Indications:**
Fullness in the chest and hypochondriac region, cough, hiccough.

**Manipulatrion:** Oblique or subcutaneous insertion toward the lateral direction .3 - .5 cun.

Moxibustion is applicable.

**Cautions:** Do not needle perpendicularly, especially in thin patients, due to risk of pneumothorax.

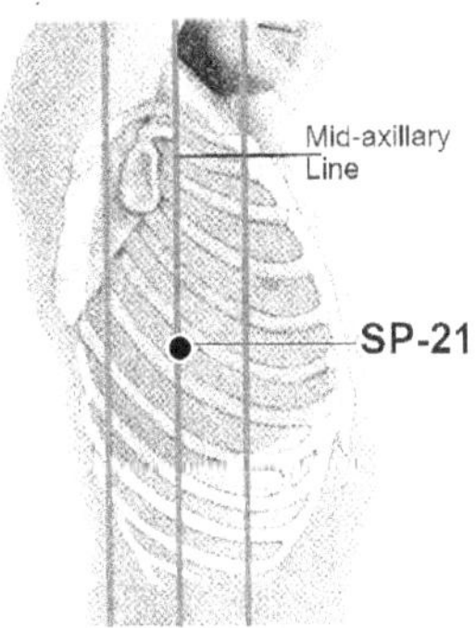


## SP-21 Dabao

(GREAT WRAPPING)

GREAT LUO OF THE SPLEEN. EXIT POINT

**Location:**
On the midaxillary line, in the 6th intercostal space.

Note: According to some texts, this point is located in the 7th intercostal space.

**Dermatome:** T6

**Main Action Areas:** Ribs, Thorax, Breast, Entire Body.

**Main Functions:** Invigorates Blood and dispels stasis. Dispels cold and warms the body. Alleviates pain.

**Indications:**
Pain in the chest and hypochondriac region, asthma, general aching and weakness.

**Manipulatrion:** Oblique or subcutaneous insertion toward the lateral direction .3 - .5 cun.

Moxibustion is applicable.

**Cautions:** Do not needle perpendicularly, especially in thin patients, due to risk of pneumothorax

## HEART MERIDIAN (Arm Shao Yin)

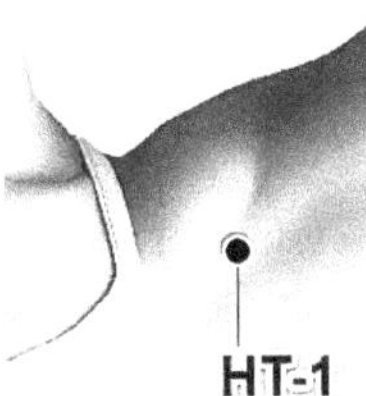


## HT-1 Jiquan

(SUMMIT SPRING)

ENTRY POINT

**Location:**
With the arm abducted, in the centre of the axilla, medial to the axillary artery.

**Dermatome:** T1/T2

**Main Action Areas:** Axilla, Shoulder, Chest, Heart

**Main Functions:** Clears heat. Regulates sweat. Regulates Heart Qi

**Indications:**
Pain in the costal and cardiac regions, scrofula, cold pain of the elbow and arm, dryness of the throat.

**Manipulation:** Perpendicular or oblique insertion 0.3 -0.5 cun. Needle with arm lifted above the head.

Moxibustion is applicable.

**Cautions:** Avoid the axillary artery.

## HT-2 Qingling
### (Green Spirit)

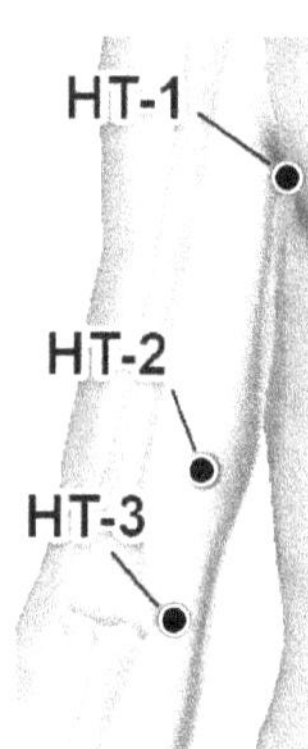


**Location:** 3 cun proximal to the cubital crease, on the medial border of the biceps brachii muscle.

**Dermatome:** C8/T1

**Main Action Areas:** Shoulder, Arm, Chest, Lungs

**Main Functions:** Regulates Qi. Alleviates pain.

**Indications:**
Pain in the cardiac and hypochondriac regions, shoulder and arm.

**Manipulation:** Perpendicular insertion 0.3 -0.5 cun.

Moxibustion is applicable.

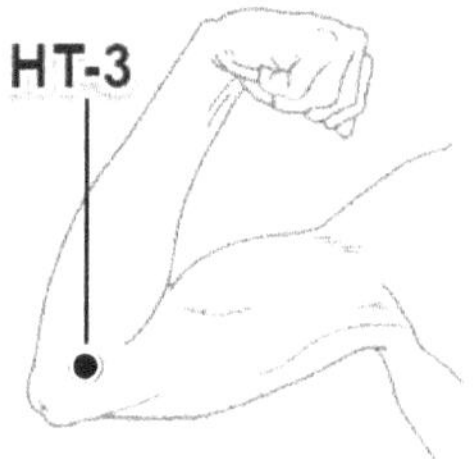


## HT-3 Shaohai
### (Lesser Sea)

Five Star, He-Sea, and Water point of the Heart channel.

**Location:**
Midway between the elbow crease and medial epicondyle of the humerus when elbow is fully flexed.

**Dermatome:** C8/T1

**Main Action Areas:** Elbow, Chest, Heart

**Main Functions:** Clears heat. Transforms phlegm. Soothes the Heart

**Indications:**
Cardiac pain, spasmodic pain and numbness of the hand and arm, tremor of the hand, scrofula, pain in the axilla and hypochondriac region.

**Manipulation:** Perpendicular insertion 0.5 -1.0 cun.

Moxibustion is applicable.

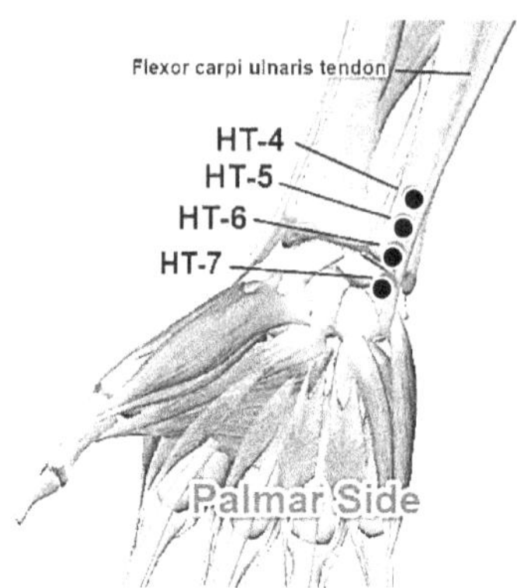


## HT-4 Lingdao
### (Spirit Path)

River and Metal point of the Heart channel.

**Location:**
1.5 cun proximal to the transverse wrist crease, on the radial side of the tendon of the flexor carpi ulnaris muscle.

**Dermatome:** C8

**Main Action Areas:** Forearm, Wrist, Heart

**Main Functions:** Regulates Qi and Blood. Alleviates pain. Calms the mind.

**Indications:**
Cardiac pain, spasmodic pain of the elbow and arm, sudden loss of voice.

**Manipulation:** Perpendicular insertion 0.3 -0.5 cun.

Moxibustion is applicable.

## HT-5 Tongli
### (Penetrating the Interior)

Luo point of the Heart channel, Ma Dan-yang Heavenly Star point.

**Location:**
1 cun proximal to Shenmen (HT-7) on the radial side of the tendon of the flexor carpi ulnaris.

**Dermatome:** C8

**Main Action Areas:** Heart, Tongue, Bladder, Wrist

Main Functions: **Regulates and tonifies** Heart Qi. Calms the mind. Benefits the tongue. Regulates speech

**Indications:**
Palpitations, dizziness, blurring of vision, sore throat, sudden loss of voice, aphasia with stiffness of the tongue, stuttering, pain in the wrist and elbow.

**Manipulation:** Perpendicular insertion 0.3 -0.5 cun.

Moxibustion is applicable.

## HT-6 Yinxi
### (Yin Cleft)

Xi-Cleft point of the Heart channel.

**Location:**
0.5 cun proximal to Shenmen (HT-7)

**Dermatome:** C8

**Main Action Areas:** Exterior, Heart, Mind, Wrist

**Main Functions:** Clears heat and fire. Calms the mind. Secures sweat

**Indications:**
Angina pectoris, palpitation, excessive sweating.

**Manipulation:** Perpendicular insertion 0.3 -0.5 cun.

Moxibustion is applicable.

## HT-7 Shenmen
### (Spirit Gate)

Yuan-Source, Shu-Stream, Sedation and Earth point of the Heart channel

**Location:**
On the radial side of the tendon of flexor carpi ulnaris muscle, at the wrist crease. medial end of distal most wrist crease.

HT-7 is level with the proximal border of the pisiform bone when the wrist is flexed. Falls on the distal wrist flexion crease, about same level as LU-9.

**Dermatome:** C8

**Main Action Areas:** Heart, Mind, Wrist

**Main Functions:** Calms the mind. Nourishes Heart Blood. Soothes the Heart. Clears heat

**Indication:**
Cardiac pain, irritability, palpitation hysteria, amnesia, insomnia, mania, epilepsy, dementia, pain in the hypochondriac region, feverish sensation in the palm, yellowish sclera.

**Manipulation:** Perpendicular insertion 0.3 -0.5 cun.

Moxibustion is applicable.

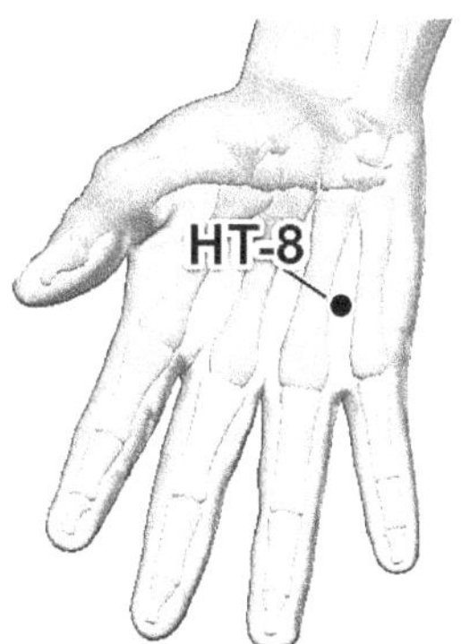


## HT-8 Shaofu

### (LESSER PALACE)

YING-SPRING, HORARY AND FIRE POINT OF THE HEART CHANNEL.

**Location:**
In the Palmar surface of the hand, between the tips of the ring finger and little finger on lightly clenching the fist.

**Shared location with Tung:** 22.10

**Dermatome:** C7/C8

**Main Action Areas:** Hand, Heart, Mind

**Main Functions:** Clears Heart fire. Cools and calms the Heart. Benefits the palms

**Indications:**
Palpitations, pain in the chest, spasmodic pain of the little finger, feverish sensation in the palm, enuresis, dysuria, pruritus of the external genitalia.

**Manipulation:** Perpendicular insertion 0.3 -0.5 cun.

Moxibustion is applicable

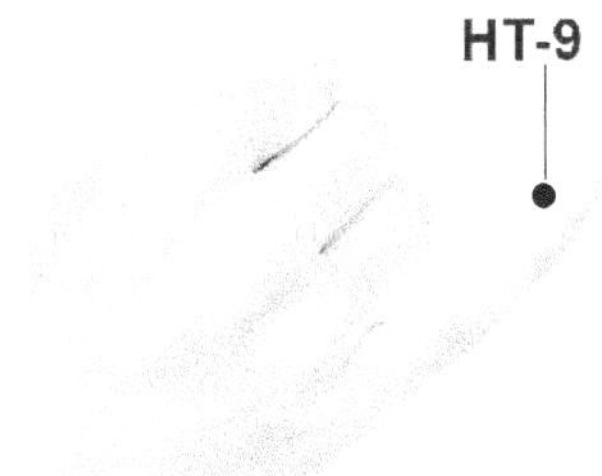


## HT-9 Shaochong

### (LESSER RUSHING)

JING-WELL, TONIFICATION, WOOD AND EXIT POINT OF THE HEART CHANNEL.

**Location:**
0.1 cun proximal to radial corner of the nail of the little finger.

**Dermatome:** C8

**Main Action Areas:** Mind, Heart, Chest

**Main Functions:** Resuscitates consciousness. Regulates Heart Qi

**Indications:**
Palpitation, pain in the chest, apoplexy, and other acute emergencies.

**Manipulation:** 0.1 cun perpendicularly to cause bleeding or acupressure in emergencies if a needle is not available.

# SMALL INTESTINE MERIDIAN (Arm Tai Yang)

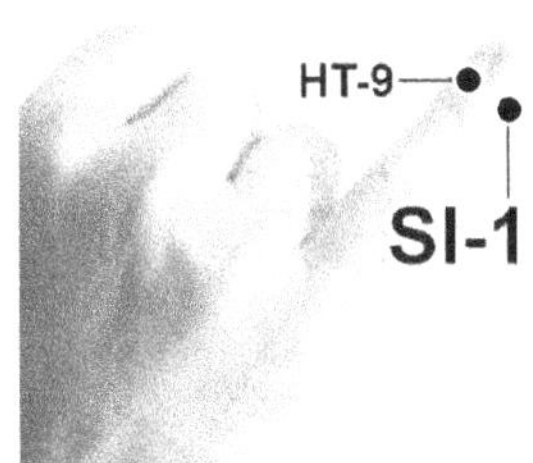


## SI-1 Shaoze

### (LESSER MARSH)

JING-WELL AND METAL POINT OF THE SMALL INTESTINE CHANNEL. ENTRY POINT.

**Location:**
On the little finger, 0.1 cun from the ulnar corner of the nail.

**Shared location with Tung:** 11.16

**Dermatome:** C8

**Main Action Areas:** Breast, Mind

**Main Functions:** Promotes lactation. Restores consciousness. Releases the exterior

**Indications:**
Headache, febrile diseases, loss of consciousness, redness of the eye, cloudiness of the cornea.

**Manipulation:** Subcutaneous insertion .1 cun or prick to bleed.

Moxibustion is applicable.

## SI-2 Qiangu

### (FRONT VALLEY)

**Location:**
On the ulnar aspect of the little finger, distal to the metacarpo-phalangeal

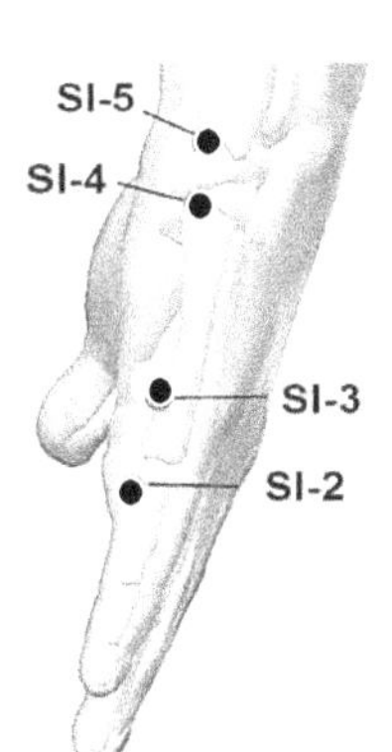


joint, at the junction of the shaft and the base of the pro-ximal phalanx.

**Dermatome:** C8

**Main Action Areas:** Shoulder, Arm, Chest, Lungs

**Main Functions:** Regulates Qi. Alleviates pain.

**Indications:**
Numbness of the fingers, febrile diseases, tinnitus, headache, reddish urine.

**Manipulation:** Perpendicular insertion 0.3 -0.5 cun.

Moxibustion is applicable.

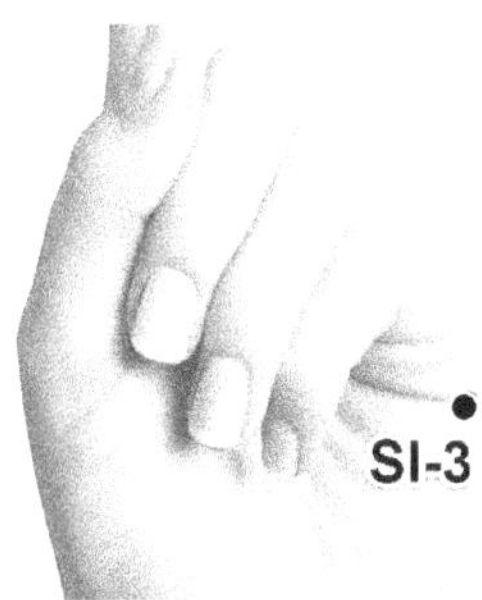


## SI-3 Houxi

### (BACK STREAM)

SHU-STREAM, TONIFICATION, AND WOOD POINT OF THE SMALL INTESTINE CHANNEL. CONFLUENT POINT AND MASTER POINT OF THE GOVERNING VESSEL. COMMAND POINT OF THE YANG LINKING VESSEL.

**Location:**
At the medial end of the main transverse crease of the palm on clenching the fist.

**Shared location with Tung:** 22.06

**Dermatome:** C8

**Main Action Areas:** Hand, Neck, Spine, Sense organs, Mind, Brain, Nervous system, Heart

**Main Functions:** Descends Yang. Clears heat. Opens the Governor Vessel. Benefits the spine

**Indication:**
Pain and rigidity of the neck, tinnitus, deafness, sore throat, mania, malaria,

acute lumbar sprain, night sweating, febrile diseases, contracture and numbness of the fingers, pain in the shoulder and elbow.

**Manipulation:** Perpendicular insertion 0.5 -0.7 cun.

Moxibustion is applicable.

# SI-4 Wangu
(WRIST BONE)

YUAN-SOURCE POINT OF THE SMALL INTESTINE CHANNEL.

**Location:**
On the ulnar border of the hand, between the 5th metacarpal bone and the carpal bones, on the border of the red and white skin.

**Dermatome:** C8

**Main Action Areas:** Wrist, Hand

**Main Functions:** Alleviates swelling and pain

**Indications:**
Febrile diseases with anhidrosis, headache, rigidity of the neck, contracture of the fingers, pain in the wrist, jaundice.

**Manipulation:** Perpendicular insertion 0.3 -0.5 cun.

Moxibustion is applicable.

# SI-5 Yanggu
(YANG VALLEY)

JING-RIVER, HORARY, AND FIRE POINT OF THE SMALL INTESTINE CHANNEL

**Location:**
On the ulnar aspect of the wrist, at the level of the lateral joint space.

**Dermatome:** C8

**Main Action Areas:** Wrist, Hand

**Main Functions:** Alleviates swelling and pain

**Indications:**
Swelling of the neck and submandibular region, pain of the hand and wrist, febrile diseases.

**Manipulation:** Perpendicular insertion 0.3 -0.5 cun.

Moxibustion is applicable.

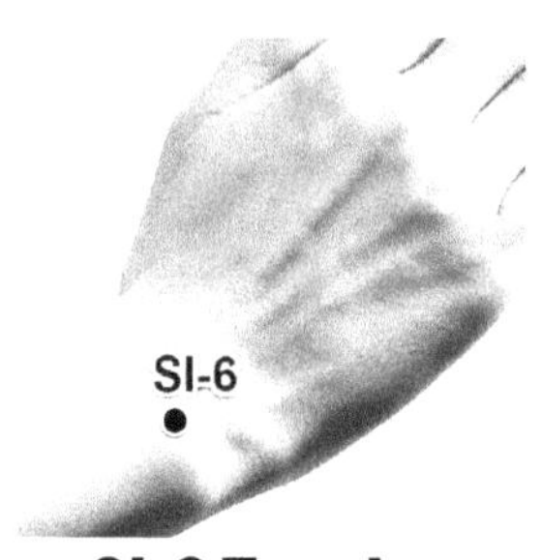


# SI-6 Tanglao
(SUPPORT THE AGED)

XI-CLEFT POINT.

**Location:**
Dorsal to the head of the ulna in the body cleft on the radial side of the styloid process, found with the palm facing the chest.position.

**Dermatome:** C8

**Main Action Areas:** Arm, Wrist, Shoulder

**Main Functions:** Regulates Qi and Blood. Alleviates pain

**Indication:**
Blurring of vision, pain in the shoulder, elbow and arm. Effective to stop pain along the SI Channel.

**Manipulation:** Perpendicular insertion 0.3 -0.5 cun.

Moxibustion is applicable.

# SI-7 Zhizheng
(BRANCH OF THE UPRIGHT)

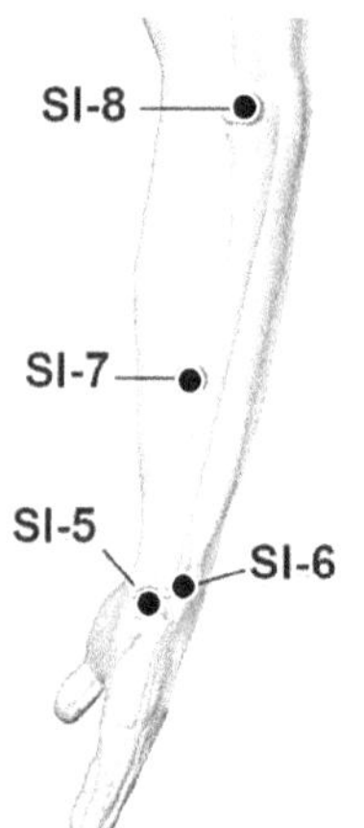


LUO POINT OF THE SMALL INTESTINE CHANNEL.

**Location:**
5 cun proximal to the wrist joint, on the line connecting the ulnar wrist joint space with the ulnar sulcus of the elbow (SI-5 to SI-8) or 1 cun distal to the midpoint of this line.

**Dermatome:** C8

**Main Action Areas:** Forearm, Hand, Head

**Main Functions:** Releases the exterior. Clears heat. Calms the Shen. Regulates Qi and Blood. Alleviates pain.

**Indications:**
Neck rigidity, headache, dizziness, spasmodic pain in the elbow and fingers, febrile diseases, mania.

**Manipulation:** Perpendicular insertion 0.3 -0.5 cun.

Moxibustion is applicable.

**Cautions:** The ulnar nerve lies deep to this point.

# SI-8 Xiaohai
(SMALL SEA)

**Location:**
With the elbow flexed, in the depression between the olecranon process of the ulna and the medial epicondyle of the humerus.

**Dermatome:** C8

**Main Action Areas:** Elbow, Forearm, Ulnar nerve

**Main Functions:** Regulates Qi and Blood. Alleviates pain

**Indications:**
Headache, swelling of cheek, pain in nape, shoulder, arm and elbow, epilepsy.

**Manipulation:** Perpendicular insertion 0.3 -0.5 cun.

Moxibustion is applicable.

**Cautions:** The ulnar nerve lies deep to this point.

# SI-9 Jianzhen
(TRUE SHOULDER)

**Location:**
With the arm adducted, 1 cun superior to the posterior axillary fold, on the lower border of the deltoid muscle.

**Dermatome:** C5

**Main Action Areas:** Shoulder, Scapula, Arm

**Main Functions:** Regulates Qi and Blood. Alleviates pain

**Indications:**
Frozen shoulder, sprains and strains of the shoulder muscles, paralysis of the upper limb.

**Manipulation:** Perpendicular insertion 0.5 -1.0 cun.

Moxibustion is applicable.

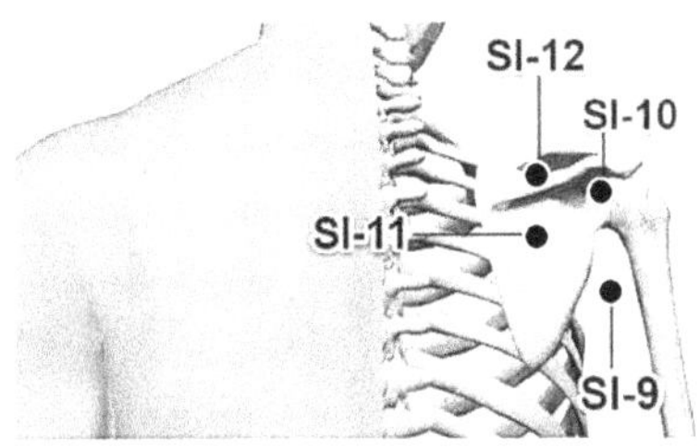

# SI-10 Naoshu

(UPPER ARM SHU)

MEETING POINT OF THE SMALL INTESTINE AND BLADDER CHANNELS WITH THE YANG LINKING AND YANG HEEL VESSELS.

**Location:**
With the arm adducted, on an imaginary line extending in a superior direction from the posterior axillary fold, on the lower border of the scapular spine.

**Shared location with Tung:** 44.17

**Dermatome:** C4/C5

**Main Action Areas:** Shoulder, Scapula, Arm

**Main Functions:** Regulates Qi and Blood. Alleviates pain

**Indications:**
Swelling of the shoulder, aching and weakness of the shoulder and arm.

**Manipulation:** Perpendicular insertion 0.5 -1.0 cun.

Moxibustion is applicable.

# SI-11 Tianzong

(HEAVENLY GATHERING)

**Location:**
On the scapula, in a depression on the infraspinatus muscle, one third of the distance from the midpoint of the scapular spine and the inferior angle of the scapula.

**Dermatome:** T2

**Main Action Areas:** Shoulder, Scapula, Arm, Chest

**Main Functions:** Regulates Qi and Blood. Alleviates pain. Relaxes the chest.

**Indications:**
Pain in the scapular region, pain in the lateroposterior aspect of the elbow and arm, asthma.

**Manipulation:** Perpendicular or oblique insertion 0.5 -1.0 cun.

Moxibustion is applicable.

# SI-12 Bingfeng

(GRASPING THE WIND)

MEETING POINT OF THE SMALL INTESTINE, LARGE INTESTINE, TRIPLE ENERGIZER, AND GALL BLADDER CHANNELS.

**Location:**
Directly above S.I-11, in the centre of the supraspinous fossa.

**Dermatome:** C4

**Main Action Areas:** Scapula, Supraspinatus

**Main Functions:** Regulates Qi and Blood. Alleviates pain.

**Indications:**
Pain in the scapular region, numbness and aching of the upper extremities, motor impairment of the shoulder and arm.

**Manipulation:** Perpendicular or oblique insertion 0.5 - 0.7 cun.

Moxibustion is applicable.

**Cautions:** Deep needling may penetrate the Lung.

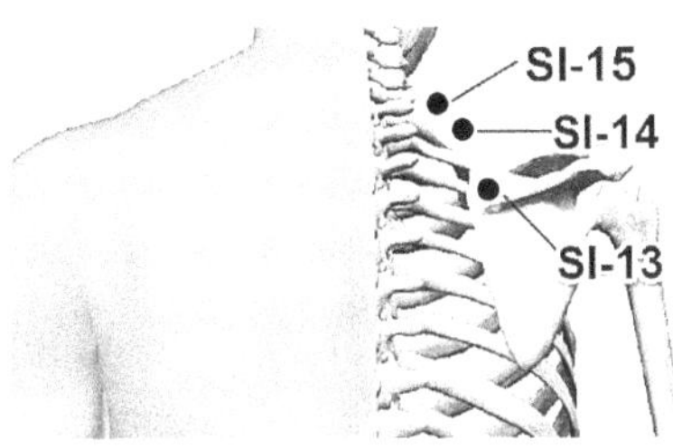

# SI-13 Quyuan

(CROOKED WALL)

**Location:**
At the medial end of the supraspinous fossa.

**Dermatome:** C4

**Main Action Areas:** Scapula, Supraspinatus

**Main Functions:** Regulates Qi and Blood. Alleviates pain.

**Indications:**
Pain and stiffness of the scapular region.

**Manipulation:** Perpendicular or oblique insertion 0.3 - 0.5 cun.

Moxibustion is applicable.

**Cautions:** Deep needling may penetrate the Lung.

# SI-14 Jianwaishu

(OUTER SHOULDER SHU)

**Location:**
3 cun lateral to the lower border of the spinous process of the 1st thoracic vertebra, at the insertion of the levator scapulae muscle.

**Dermatome:** C4

**Main Action Areas:** Shoulder, Neck, Levator scapulae muscle

**Main Functions:** Regulates Qi and Blood. Alleviates pain.

**Indications:**
Aching of the shoulder and back, pain and rigidity of the neck.

**Manipulation:** Oblique insertion 0.3 - 0.7 cun.

Moxibustion is applicable.

**Cautions:** Improper needling may penetrate the Lung

# SI-15 Jianzhongshu

(MIDDLE SHOULDER SHU)

**Location:**
2 cun lateral to the lower border of the spinous process of the 7th thoracic vertebra.

**Dermatome:** C3/C4

**Main Action Areas:** Neck, Shoulder, Chest

**Main Functions:** Regulates Qi and Blood. Alleviates pain. Relaxes the chest.

**Indications:**
Cough, asthma, pain in the shoulder and back, haemoptysis.

**Manipulation:** Oblique insertion 0.3 - 0.6 cun.

Moxibustion is applicable.

**Cautions:** Improper needling may penetrate the Lung

# SI-16 Tianchuang

(HEAVENLY WINDOW)

WINDOW OF HEAVEN POINT

**Location:**
Approximately 3.5 cun lateral to the anterior midline, at the level of the laryngeal prominence, on the posterior border of the sternocleidomastoid muscle. Posterior to LI-18.

**Dermatome:** C3

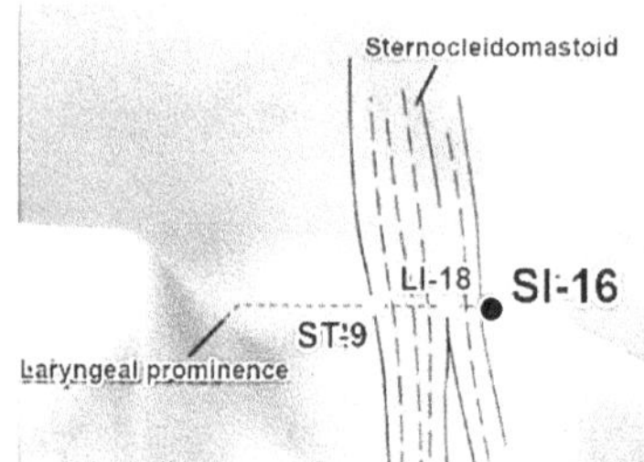



**Main Action Areas:** Throat, Neck, Ears, Shoulder

**Main Functions:** Regulates Qi and Blood. Alleviates pain. Relieves swelling.

**Indications:** Sore throat, sudden loss of voice, deafness, tinnitus, stiffness and pain of the neck.

**Manipulation:** Perpendicular insertion 0.3 - 0.7 cun.

Moxibustion applicable.

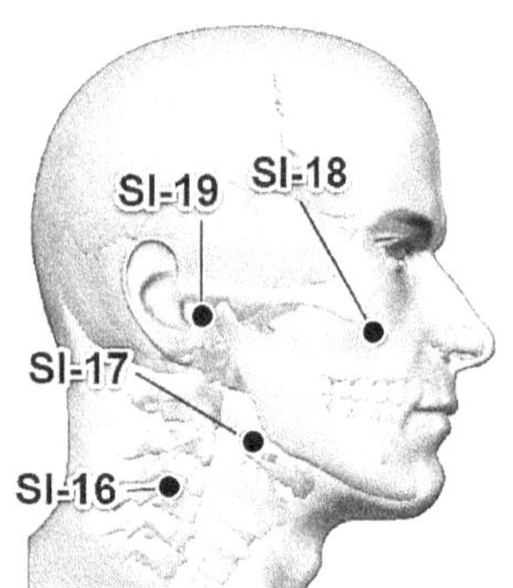



## SI-17 Tianrong

(HEAVENLY APPEARANCE)

**Location:** On the anterior border of the sternocleidomastoideus at the level of the angle of the jaw.

**Dermatome:** C3

**Main Action Areas:** Throat, Ears

**Main Functions:** Regulates Qi and Blood. Alleviates pain. Relieves swelling

**Indications:** Deafness, tinnitus, sore throat, swelling of the cheek, foreign body sensation in the throat, goiter.

**Manipulation:** Perpendicular insertion 0.5 - 0.7 cun.

Moxibustion applicable.

**Cautions:** This point is a Dangerous point as it is situated near the great vessels of the neck. The needle should be directed towards the tonsils and not backwards to avoid the carotid body.

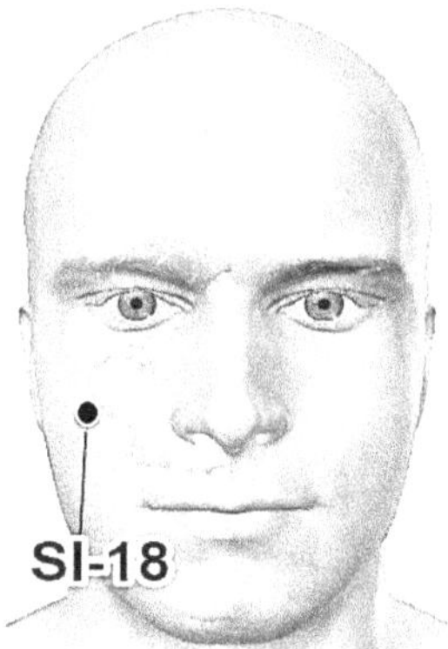



## SI-18 Quanliao

(CHEEKBONE CREVICE)

MEETING POINT OF THE SMALL INTESTINE AND TRIPLE ENERGIZER CHANNELS. MUSCLE MERIDIAN MEETING POINT OF THE 3 LEG YANG.

**Location:**
In the depression below the zygomatic bone on a vertical line downwards from the outer canthus of the eye.

**Shared location with Tung:** 1010.13

**Dermatome:** Facial nerve

**Main Action Areas:** Cheeks, Face

**Main Functions:** Clears heat. Dissipates cold. Tonifies the cheeks

**Indications:**
Facial paralysis, twitching of eyelids, pain in the face, toothache, swelling of the cheek, yellowish sclera.

**Manipulation:** 0.3 - 0.5 cun perpendicularly.

Caution: If inserted too deep, needle may enter the mouth cavity and cause bleeding.

**Remarks:** This is an effective analgesic point in the head region.

## SI-19 Tinggong

(PALACE OF HEARING)

MEETING POINT OF THE SMALL INTESTINE, TRIPLE ENERGIZER, AND GALL BLADDER CHANNELS. EXIT POINT.

**Location:**
In the depression felt between the tragus and the mandibular joint when the mouth is slightly open.

**Dermatome:** Facial nerve

**Main Action Areas:** Ears, Temple, Jaw

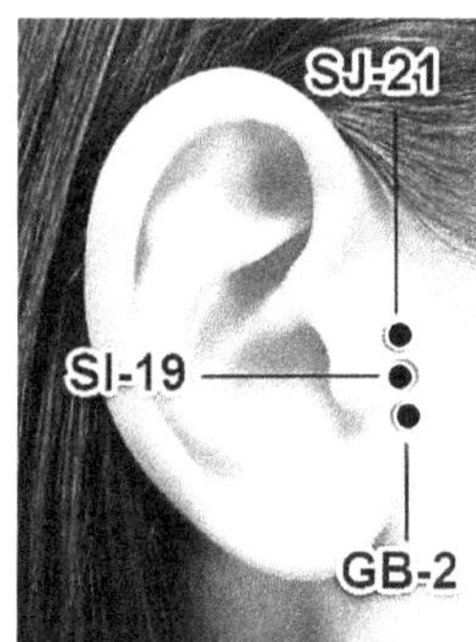



**Main Functions:** Improves hearing and benefits the ears. Regulates Qi and Blood. Alleviates pain. Clears heat

**Indications:**
Ear disorders, e.g., deafness, tinnitus, vertigo, Meniere's disease, ear infections.

**Manipulation:** 0.5cun perpendicularly. It is more usual however to puncture through the points Ermen (SJ-21), Tinggong (SI-19) and Tinghui (GB-2) horizontally downwards. This is known as the puncturing - through technique.

## URINARY BLADDER MERIDIAN (Leg Tai Yang)

## BL-1 Jingming

(BRIGHT EYES)

MEETING POINT OF THE BLADDER, SMALL INTESTINE, STOMACH, GALL BLADDER, AND TRIPLE ENERGIZER CHANNELS WITH THE GOVERNING, YIN HEEL AND YANG HEEL VESSELS, ENTRY POINT.

**Location:**
0.1 cun medial and superior to the inner canthus of the eye near the medial border of the orbit.

**Dermatome:** Facial nerve

**Main Action Areas:** Eyes

**Main Functions:** Clears and brightens the eyes. Improves vision. Dispels wind and clears heat. Alleviates pain. Nourishes Yin. Improves appearance

**Indications:**
Redness, swelling and pain of the eye, itching of the canthus, lacrimation, night blindness, color blindness, blurring of vision.

**Manipulation:** As this is a Dangerous point, puncture superficially 0.2 cun, or insert slowly (without any attempt at manipulation), 0.5-1.0 cun along the medial wall of the orbit.

**Caution:** No moxibustion

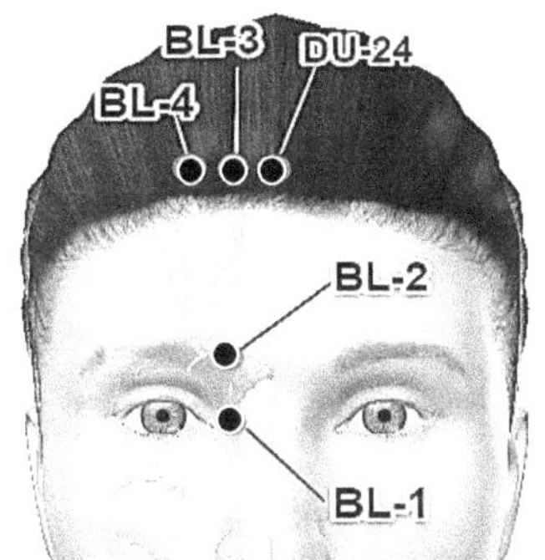


# BL-2 Zanzhu
### (GATHERED BAMBOO)

**Location:**
In the depression at the medial end of the eyebrow, directly above the inner canthus of the eye.

**Shared location with Tung:** 1010.09

**Dermatome:** Trigeminal nerve

**Main Action Areas:** Eyes, Forehead

**Main Functions:** Regulates Qi and Blood. Alleviates pain. Dispels wind. Clears heat

**Indications:**
Headache, blurring or failing of vision, pain in the supra-orbital region, lacrimation, redness, swelling and pain of the eye, twitching of eyelids, glaucoma.

**Manipulation:** 0-3 - 0.5 cun horizontally or laterally. Can prick to bleed.

**Caution:** No moxibustion

# BL-3 Meichong
### (EYEBROWS' POURING)

**Location:**
0.5 cun within the anterior hairline, vertically above the medial canthus of the eye.

**Dermatome:** Trigeminal nerve

**Main Action Areas:** Head

**Main Functions:** Dispels wind. Clears heat. Alleviates pain.

**Indications:**
Excessive lacrimation, headache, giddiness, epilepsy, nasal obstruction.

**Manipulation:** Subcutaneous insertion 0.3 - 0.5 cun.

**Caution:** No Moxibustion

# BL-4 Qucha
### (CROOKED CURVE)

**Location:**
0.5 cun superior to the anterior hairline and 1.5 cun lateral to the midline (or one third of the distance between DU-24 and ST-8).

**Dermatome:** Trigeminal nerve

**Main Action Areas:** Nose, Head

**Main Functions:** Dispels wind. Clears heat. Alleviates pain.

**Indications:**
Headache, nasal obstruction, epistaxis, blurring and failing of vision.

**Manipulation:** Subcutaneous insertion 0.3 - 0.5 cun.

Moxibustion applicable.

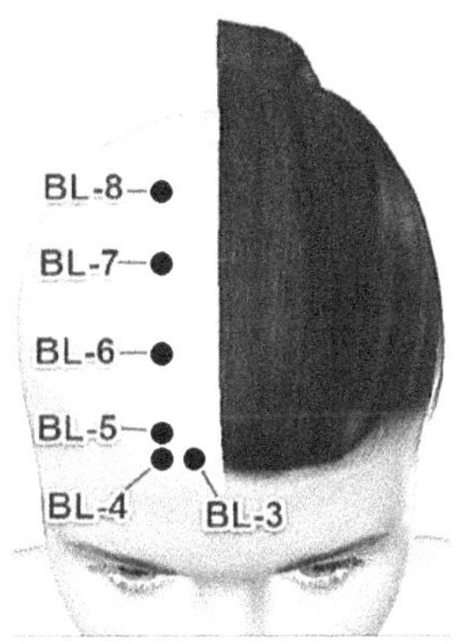


# BL-5 Wuchu
### (FIFTH PLACE)

**Location:**
1 cun superior to the anterior hairline and 1.5 cun lateral to the midline or one third of the distance between DU-24 and ST-8.

**Dermatome:** Trigeminal nerve, C2

**Main Action Areas:** Head, Eyes, Nose

**Main Functions:** Subdues interior wind, restores consciousness.

**Indications:**
Headache, blurring of vision, epilepsy, convulsion.

**Manipulation:** Subcutaneous insertion 0.3 - 0.5 cun.

Moxibustion applicable.

# BL-6 Chengguan
### (RECEIVING LIGHT)

**Location:**
2.5 cun superior to the anterior hairline and 1.5 cun lateral to the midline or one third of the distance between DU-24 and ST-8.

**Shared location with Tung:** 1010.04

**Dermatome:** C2

**Main Action Areas:** Head, Eyes, Nose

**Main Functions:** Clears heat and eliminates vexation, brightens the eyes and opens the portals.

**Indications:**
Headache, blurring of vision, nasal obstruction.

**Manipulation:** Subcutaneous insertion 0.3 - 0.5 cun.

**Caution:** No Moxibustion

# BL-7 Tongtian
### (HEAVENLY CONNECTION)

**Location:**
1.5 cun lateral to the midline and 4 cun superior to the anterior hairline or 1 cun anterior to DU-20.

**Shared location with Tung:** 1010.02

**Dermatome:** C2

**Main Action Areas:** Head, Eyes, Nose

**Main Functions:** Subdues wind, clears the nose, brightens the eyes, stops convulsions, opens the orifices.

**Indications:**
Headache, giddiness, nasal obstruction, epistaxis, rhinorrhea.

**Manipulation:** Subcutaneous insertion 0.3 - 0.5 cun.

Moxibustion applicable.

# BL-8 Luoque
### (DECLINING CONNECTION)

**Location:**
1.5 cun lateral to the midline and 5.5 cun superior to the anterior hairline or 0.5 cun posterior to DU-20.

**Shared location with Tung:** 1010.03

**Dermatome:** C2

**Main Action Areas:** Head, Eyes, Nose

**Main Functions:** Dissipates wind and clears heat, clears the head and brightens the eyes.

**Indications:**
Dizziness, blurring of vision, tinnitus, mania.

**Manipulation:** Subcutaneous insertion 0.3 - 0.5 cun.

**Caution:** No Moxibustion

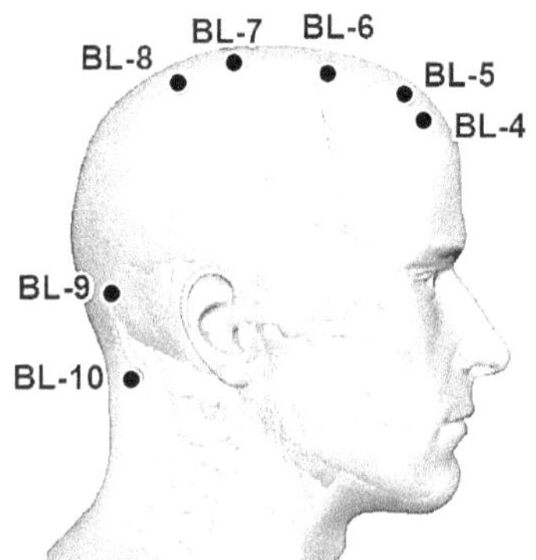


# BL-9 Yuzhen
(JADE PILLOW)

**Location:**
2.5 cun superior to the posterior hairline and 1.3 cun lateral to the midline or DU-17 (directly superior to the external occipital protuberance).

**Dermatome:** C2

**Main Action Areas:** Head, Eyes, Sense organs

**Main Functions:** Dispels wind and quickens connecting vessels, frees the portals and brightens eyes.

**Indications:**
Headache and neck pain, dizziness, ophthalmalgia, nasal obstruction.

**Manipulation:** Subcutaneous insertion 0.3 - 0.5 cun.

Moxibustion applicable.

# BL-10 Tianzhu
(HEAVENLY PILLAR)

WINDOW OF HEAVEN POINT

**Location:**
In the lower border of the occiput, between the transverse processes of the first and second cervical vertebrae 1.3 cun lateral to the midline. (1.3 cun lateral to Yamen (DU-15).

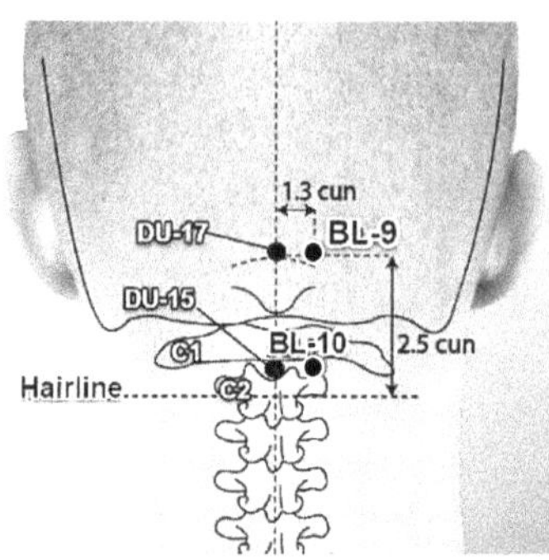


**Dermatome:** C3

**Main Action Areas:** Neck, Head, Tai Yang area, Entire body

**Main Functions:** Expels wind, clears the brain, opens the orifices, soothes the sinews, removes obstructions from the channel, brightens the eyes, invigorates the lower back.

**Indications:**
Headache, nasal obstruction, sore throat, neck rigidity, pain in shoulder and back.

**Manipulation:** Perpendicular or oblique insertion .5 - .8 cun.

**Cautions:** Do not insert the needle deeply medially upwards to avoid injuring the medulla oblongata.

No moxibustion.

# BL-11 Dashu
(GREAT SHUTTLE)

MEETING POINT OF THE BLADDER, SMALL INTESTINE, TRIPLE HEATER, AND GALL BLADDER AND THE GOVERNING VESSEL, INFLUENTIAL POINT OF BONES, SEA OF BLOOD.

**Location:** 1.5 cun lateral to the lower border of the spinous process of the first thoracic vertebra.

**Dermatome:** C5/C6

**Main Action Areas:** Bones, Chest, Lungs, Neck

**Main Functions:** Releases the exterior. Regulates Lung Qi and alleviates cough. Nourishes Blood. Benefits the bones

**Indications:** Pain in the shoulder girdle area, arthritis of the joints. Used in all bone and cartilage disorders.

**Manipulation:** 0.3 cun perpendicularly or obliquely downwards.

Moxibustion applicable.

**Cautions:** Risk of pneumothorax.

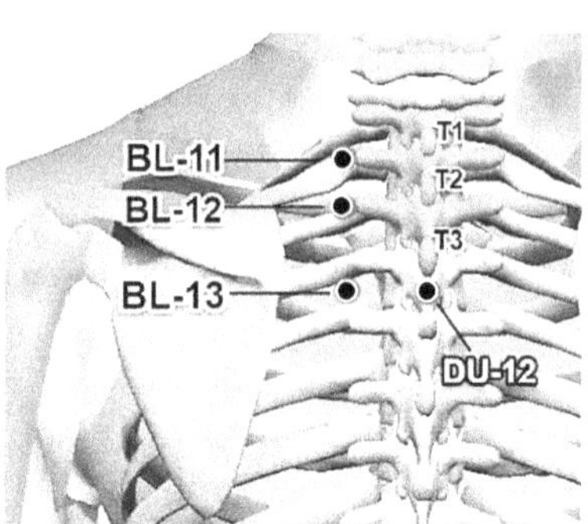


# BL-12 Fengmen
(WIND GATE)

MEETING POINT OF THE BLADDER CHANNEL WITH THE GOVERNING VESSEL

**Location:**
1.5 cun lateral to the posterior midline, on the level of the lower border of the spinous process of the 2nd thoracic vertebra (T2).

**Dermatome:** C5/T1

**Main Action Areas:** Lungs, Chest, Exterior, Upper back

**Main Functions:** Expels and prevents exterior wind, releases the exterior, stimulates the Lung dispersing function, regulates nutritive and defensive Qi.

**Indications:**
Common cold, cough, fever and headache, neck rigidity, backache.

**Manipulation:** Oblique insertion 0.5 - 0.7 cun.

Moxibustion is applicable.

**Cautions:** Risk of pneumothorax.

# BL-13 Feishu
(LUNG SHU)

BACK-SHU POINT OF THE LUNG.

**Location:**
1.5 cun lateral to the lower border of the spinous process of the third thoracic vertebra.

**Dermatome:** T3

**Main Action Areas:** Lungs, Chest, Exterior, Upper back

**Main Functions:** Tonifies and regulates Lung Qi. Releases the exterior. Nourishes Yin

**Indications:**
Lung disease, nose disorders, disorders of the skin (Lung is connected to the skin), lesions of the soft tissue of the dorsal spine area.

**Manipulation:** 0.3 - 0.5 cun perpendicularly or obliquely downwards.

Moxibustion applicable.

**Cautions:** Risk of pneumothorax

**Remarks:** Widely used for lung disorders. Also helps release stuck emotional states such as grief and sadness.

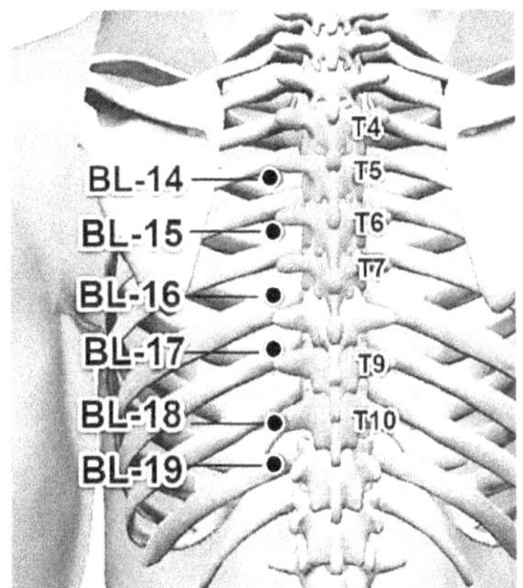


# BL-14 Jueyinshu

(ABSOLUTE YIN SHU)

BACK-SHU POINT OF THE PERICARDIUM.

**Location:**
1.5 cun lateral to the lower border of the spinous process of the fourth thoracic vertebra.

**Dermatome:** T4

**Main Action Areas:** Chest, Heart

**Main Functions:** Regulates Chest Qi. Benefits the Heart and Liver

**Indications:**
Heart disease, brain disorders, cough and thoracic oppression. As a local point, can be used for upper back pain.

**Manipulation:** 0.3 - 0.5 cun perpendicularly or obliquely downwards or medially.

Moxibustion is applicable.

**Cautions:** Risk of pneumothorax.

# BL-15 Xinshu

(HEART SHU)

BACK-SHU POINT OF THE HEART.

**Location:** 1.5 cun lateral to the lower border of the spinous process of the fifth thoracic vertebra.

**Dermatome:** T5

**Main Action Areas:** Chest, Heart

**Main Functions:** Regulates Qi and Blood in the Chest. Tonifies Heart Qi. Calms the mind

**Indications:** Heart disease, neurasthenia, hysteria, epilepsy, schizophrenia, insomnia, anxiety.

**Manipulation:** 0.3 - 0.5 cun perpendicularly or obliquely downwards.

Moxibustion is applicable.

**Cautions:** Risk of pneumothorax.

# BL-16 Dushu

(GOVERNING SHU)

**Location:**
1.5 cun lateral to the posterior midline, on the level of the lower border of the spinous process of the 6th thoracic vertebra (T6).

**Dermatome:** T6

**Main Action Areas:** Chest, Abdomen, Spine, Skin

**Main Functions:** Regulates Qi and Blood in the chest and abdomen. Dispels stasis and pain

**Indications:**
Cardiac pain, abdominal pain.

**Manipulation:** 0.3 - 0.5 cun perpendicularly or obliquely downwards.

Moxibustion is applicable.

**Cautions:** Risk of pneumothorax.

# BL-17 Geshu

(DIAPHRAGM SHU)

INFLUENTIAL POINT FOR BLOOD. BACK-SHU POINT OF THE DIAPHRAGM.

**Location:**
1.5 cun lateral to the lower border of spinous process of the seventh thoracic vertebra (at the level of the lower border of the scapula).

**Dermatome:** T7

**Main Action Areas:** Diaphragm, Chest, Abdomen, Entire body

**Main Functions:** Nourishes Blood. Invigorates Blood and dispels stasis. Clears Blood heat. Relaxes the diaphragm. Benefits the skin

**Indications:**
Paralysis of diaphragm, hiccough, anorexia nervosa, anaemia, chronic haemorrhagic diseases.

**Manipulation:** 0.3 - 0.5 cun perpendicularly or obliquely down wards.

Moxibustion is applicable.

**Cautions:** Risk of pneumothorax.

# BL-18 Ganshu

(LIVER SHU)

BACK-SHU POINT OF THE LIVER.

**Location:**
1.5 cun lateral to the lower border of the spinous process of the ninth thoracic vertebra.

**Dermatome:** T9

**Main Action Areas:** Liver, Hypochondrium, Abdomen, Eyes

**Main Functions:** Regulates Liver Qi. Dispels stasis. Nourishes Blood. Clears heat and dampness. Benefits the eyes

**Indications:**
Jaundice, pain in the hypochondriac region, redness of the eye, blurring of vision, night blindness, mental disorders, epilepsy, backache, spitting of blood, epistaxis.

**Manipulation:** 0.5 - 0.7 cun perpendicularly or obliquely down wards.

Moxibustion is applicable.

**Cautions:** Risk of pneumothorax.

# BL-19 Danshu

(GALLBLADDER SHU)

BACK-SHU POINT OF THE GALL BLADDER.

**Location:** 1.5 cun lateral to the lower border of the spinous process of the tenth thoracic vertebra.

**Dermatome:** T10

**Main Action Areas:** Gallbladder, Liver, Hypochondrium, Abdomen

**Main Functions:** Regulates Gallbladder and Liver Qi. Dispels stasis. Alleviates pain. Clears dampness and heat. Dispels ShaoYang pathogens

**Indications:** Jaundice, bitter taste of the mouth, pain in the chest and hypochondriac region, pulmonary tuberculosis, afternoon fever.

98

**Manipulation:** 0.5 - 0.7 cun perpendicularly or obliquely downwards.

Moxibustion is applicable.

**Cautions:** Risk of pneumothorax.

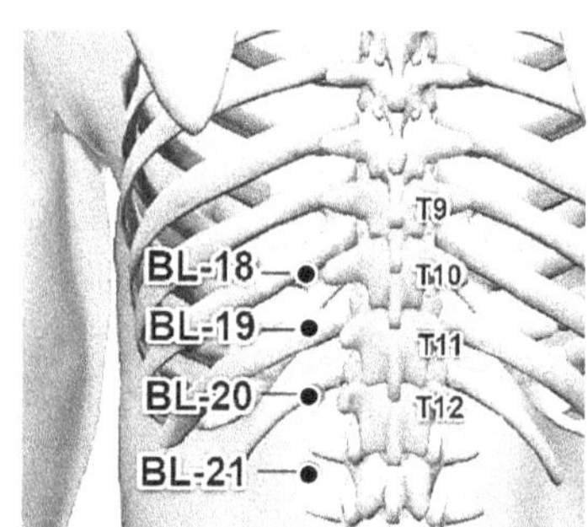


# BL-20 Pishu

(SPLEEN SHU)

Back-Shu point of the Spleen.

**Location:**
1.5 cun lateral to the lower border of the spinous process of the eleventh thoracic vertebra.

**Dermatome:** T11

**Main Action Areas:** Spleen, Stomach, Intestines, Digestive system, Muscles, Entire body, Lower thoracic area

**Main Functions:** Boosts Spleen and Stomach Qi. Boosts transformation and movement. Clears dampness

**Indications:**
Gastro-intestinal disorders, oedema, allergic disorders, soft tissue disorders.

**Manipulation:** 0.5 - 0.7 cun perpendicularly or obliquely downwards.

Moxibustion is applicable.

**Cautions:** Risk of pneumothorax.

# BL-21 Weishu

(STOMACH SHU)

BACK-SHU POINT OF THE STOMACH.

**Location:**
1.5 cun lateral to the lower border of the spinous process of the twelfth thoracic vertebra.

**Dermatome:** T10

**Main Action Areas:** Digestive system, Stomach

**Main Functions:** Regulates Stomach Qi. Benefits the digestion. Descends rebellious Qi

**Indications:**
Pain in the chest and hypochondriac and epigastric regions, anorexia, abdominal distension, borborygmus, diarrhea, nausea, vomiting.

**Manipulation:** 0.5 - 0.7 cun perpendicularly or obliquely downwards.

Moxibustion is applicable.

**Cautions:** Risk of pneumothorax.

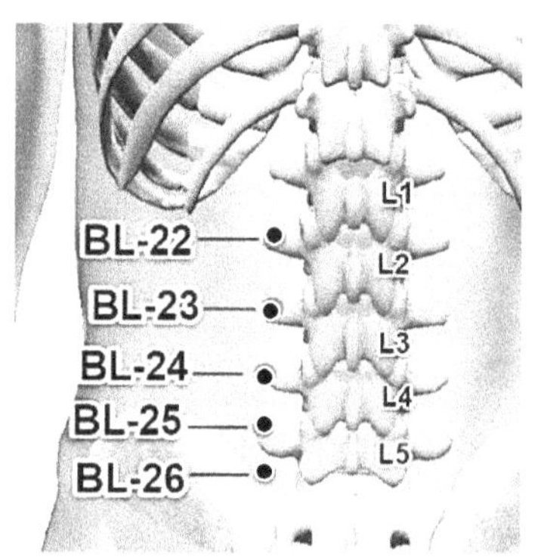


# BL-22 Sanjiaoshu

(SANJIAO SHU)

BACK-SHU POINT OF THE SANJIAO

**Location:**
1.5 cun lateral to the lower border of the spinous process of the first lumbar vertebra.

**Shared location with Tung:** DT.13

**Dermatome:** T12/L1

**Main Action Areas:** Urinary system

**Main Functions:** Resolves dampness. Opens the water passages. Harmonises the Triple Energizer

**Indications:**
Abdominal distension, flatulence, loss of appetite, incontinence of urine, local disorders of the spine.

**Manipulation:** Perpendicular insertion .5 - 1.0 cun.

Moxibustion is applicable.

**Cautions:** Deep perpendicular needling may cause Kidney injury.

# BL-23 Shenshu

(KIDNEY SHU)

BACK-SHU POINT OF THE KIDNEY.

**Location:**
1.5 cun lateral to the lower border of the spinous process of the second lumbar vertebra (at the level of the lower border of the rib cage.)

**Shared location with Tung:** DT.14

**Dermatome:** T10

**Main Action Areas:** Kidneys, Lumbar area, Abdomen, Genitourinary system, Entire body

**Main Functions:** Boosts the Kidneys. Tonifies Yang and warms the lower jiao. Nourishes Yin and cools empty heat. Resolves dampness. Benefits urination. Alleviates pain

**Indications:**
Genito-urinary dis-orders, ear disease, bone disorders, alopecia, local disorders of the spine.

**Manipulation:** 1.0 cun perpendicularly or obliquely towards the vertebral column.

Moxibustion is applicable.

**Cautions:** Deep perpendicular needling may cause Kidney injury.

# BL-24 Qihaishu

(SEA OF QI)

SEA OF QI SHU

**Location:**
1.5 cun lateral to the posterior midline, on the level of the lower border of the spinous process of the 3rd lumbar vertebra (L3).

**Dermatome:** L2/L3

**Main Action Areas:** Lumbar area

**Main Functions:** Regulates Qi and Blood. Alleviates pain.

**Indications:**
Lower back pain, irregular menstruation, dysmenorrhea, asthma.

**Manipulation:** Perpendicular insertion .5 - 1.0 cun.

Moxibustion is applicable.

# BL-25 Dachangshu

(LARGE INTESTINE SHU)

BACK-SHU POINT OF THE LARGE INTESTINE.

**Location:**
1.5 cun lateral to the lower border of the spinous process of the fourth lumbar vertebra (at the level of the upper border of the iliac crest.)

**Dermatome:** L2/L3

**Main Action Areas:** Intestines, Lumbar area

**Main Functions:** Alleviates constipation and diarrhoea. Regulates Qi and alleviates pain

**Indications:**
Diarrhoea, constipation, low backache, sciatica, paralysis the lower extremities.

**Manipulation:** 1.0 - 1.5 cun perpendicularly.

Moxibustion applicable.

# BL-26 Guanyuanshu

(GATE OF ORIGIN SHU)

GATE OF ORIGIN SHU

**Location:**
1.5 cun lateral to the posterior midline, on the level of the lower border of the spinous process of the 5th lumbar vertebra (L5).

**Dermatome:** L2/L3

**Main Action Areas:** Lumbosacral joint, Genitourinary system

**Main Functions:** Benefits the urinary system. Clears dampness and heat. Regulates Qi and alleviates pain.

**Indications:**
Lower back pain, abdominal distension, diarrhea, enuresis, sciatica, frequent urination.

**Manipulation:** 1.0 - 1.5 cun perpendicularly.

Moxibustion applicable.

# BL-27 Xiaochangshu

(SMALL INTESTINE SHU)

BACK-SHU POINT OF THE SMALL INTESTINE.

**Location:**
1.5 cun lateral to the midline, level with the first posterior sacral foramen, in the depression over the sacro-iliac joint.

**Dermatome:** S1

**Main Action Areas:** Small Intestine, Sacroiliac joint, Urinary system

**Main Functions:** Benefits the urinary system. Clears dampness and heat. Regulates Qi and alleviates pain

**Indications:**
Lower abdominal pain and distension, dysentery, nocturnal emission, haematuria, enuresis, morbid leukorrhea, lower back pain, sciatica.

**Manipulation:** 1.0-1.5 cun perpendicularly, or 2 to 3 cun obliquely towards BL-25.

Moxibustion applicable.

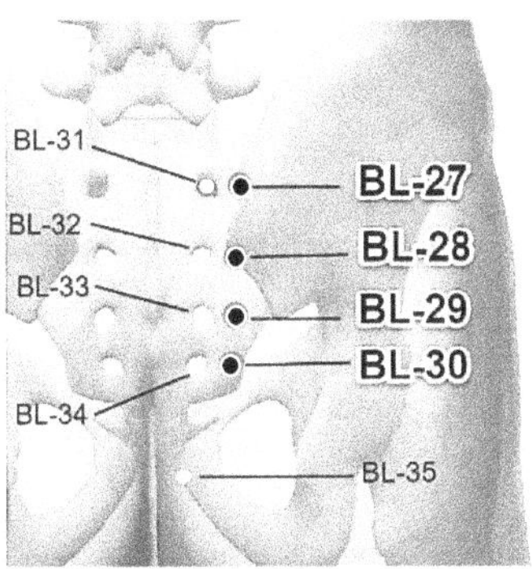


# BL-28 Pangguangshu

(BLADDER SHU)

BACK-SHU POINT OF THE URINARY BLADDER.

**Location:**
1.5 cun lateral to the midline, level with the second posterior sacral foramen, in the depression just over the sacro-iliac joint.

**Dermatome:** S2

**Main Action Areas:** Bladder, Sacroiliac joint, Urinary system

**Main Functions:** Regulates the Bladder. Benefits the urinary system. Clears dampness and heat. Alleviates pain

**Indications:**
Retention of urine, enuresis, frequent urination, diarrhea, constipation, stiffness and pain of the lower back.

**Manipulation:** 0.5 - 1.0 cun perpendicularly.

Moxibustion applicable.

# BL-29 Zhonglushu

(MID SPINE SHU)

**Location:**
1.5 cun lateral to the posterior mid-line, on the level of the 3rd sacral foramen.

**Dermatome:** S3

**Main Action Areas:** Sacrum

**Main Functions:** Strengthens the lumbar spine, warms yang and dissipates cold.

**Indications:**
Dysentery, hernia, stiffness and pain of the lower pain.

**Manipulation:** 0.8 - 1.2 cun perpendicularly.

Moxibustion applicable.

# BL-30 Bai Huan Shu

(WHITE RING SHU)

**Location:**
1.5 cun lateral to the posterior midline, on the level of the 4th sacral foramen.

**Dermatome:** S3/S4

**Main Action Areas:** Sacrum, Anus, Genitals

**Main Functions:** Regulates Qi and Blood. Alleviates pain. Benefits the anus.

**Indications:**
Enuresis, pain due to hernia, morbid leukorrhea, irregular menstruation, dysuria, cold sensation, pain of lower back, constipation, tenesmus, prolapse of the rectum.

**Manipulation:** 0.8 - 1.2 cun perpendicularly.

**Caution:** No Moxibustion

# BL-31 Shangliao

(UPPER CREVICE)

MEETING POINT OF THE BLADDER AND GALL BLADDER channels.

**Location:**
Over the 1st sacral foramen

**Dermatome:** S1

**Main Action Areas:** Sacrum, Genitals

**Main Functions:** Regulates Qi and Blood. Alleviates pain.

**Indications:**
Lower back pain, dysuria, constipation, irregular menstruation, morbid leukorrhea, prolapse of the uterus.

**Manipulation:** 0.8 - 1.2 cun perpendicularly.

Moxibustion applicable.

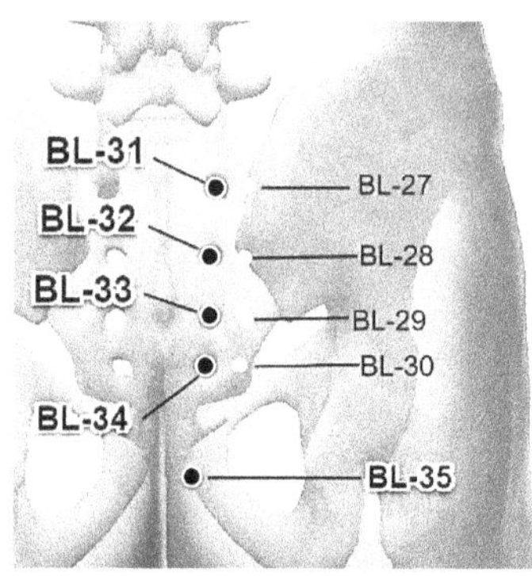

# BL-32 Ciliao
(SECOND CREVICE)

MEETING POINT OF THE BLADDER AND GALL BLADDER CHANNELS.

**Location:** On the second sacral foramen.

**Dermatome:** S2

**Main Action Areas:** Sacrum, Uterus, Genitals

**Main Functions:** Regulates Qi and Blood. Alleviates pain. Induces labour

**Indications:** Lower back pain, hernia, irregular menstruation, leukorrhea, dysmenorrhea, nocturnal emission, impotence, enuresis, dysuria, muscular atrophy, pain, numbness and motor impairment of the lower extremities.

**Manipulation:** 0.8 - 1.2 cun perpendicularly.

Moxibustion applicable.

# BL-33 Zhongliao
(MIDDLE CREVICE)

MEETING POINT OF THE BLADDER AND GALL BLADDER CHANNELS.

**Location:** On the third sacral foramen.

**Dermatome:** S3

**Main Action Areas:** Sacrum, Uterus, Genitals

**Main Functions:** Regulates Qi and Blood. Alleviates pain. Induces labour.

**Indications:** Lower back pain, constipation, diarrhea, dysuria, irregular menstruation, morbid leukorrhea.

**Manipulation:** 0.8 - 1.2 cun perpendicularly.

Moxibustion applicable.

# BL-34 Xialiao
(LOWER CREVICE)

MEETING POINT OF THE BLADDER AND GALL BLADDER CHANNELS.

**Location:** On the 4th sacral foramen.

**Dermatome:** S4

**Main Action Areas:** Sacrum, Uterus, Genitals

**Main Functions:** Regulates Qi and Blood. Alleviates pain. Induces labour.

**Indications:** Lower back pain, lower abdominal pain, dysuria, constipation, morbid leukorrhea.

**Manipulation:** 0.8 - 1.2 cun perpendicularly.

Moxibustion applicable.

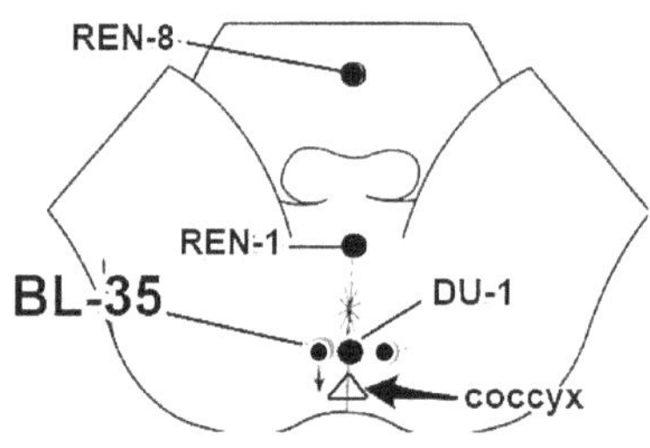


# BL-35 Huiyang
(MEETING OF YANG)

**Location:** 0.5 cun lateral to the posterior midline, on the level of the tip of the coccyx.

**Dermatome:** S5

**Main Action Areas:** Coccyx, Anus, Genitals

**Main Functions:** Clears and discharges Lower Energizer damp-heat.

**Indications:** Dysentery, bloody stools, diarrhea, hemorrhoids, impotence, morbid leukorrhea.

**Manipulation:** 0.5 - 1.0 cun perpendicularly.

Moxibustion applicable.

**Remarks:** Useful for local disorders.

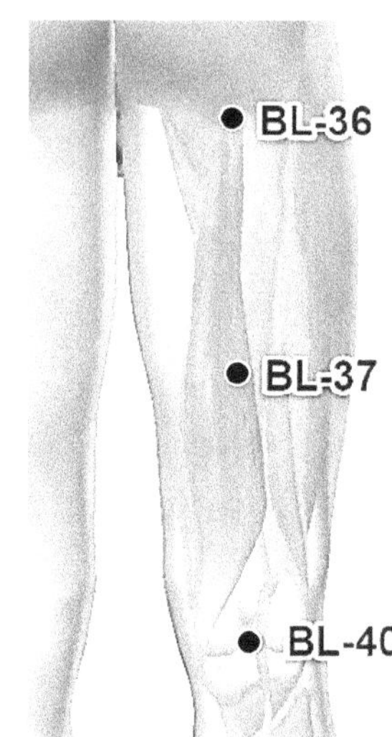


# BL-36 Chengfu
(HOLD AND SUPPORT)

**Location:** In the middle of the gluteal fold.

**Dermatome:** S2

**Main Action Areas:** Buttock, Thigh, Lower Limb, Sciatic Nerve

**Main Functions:** Regulates Qi and Blood. Alleviates pain

**Indications:** Sciatica, paralysis of lower limb, haemorrhoids.

**Manipulation:** 1.0 - 1.5 cun perpendicularly.

Moxibustion applicable.

# BL-37 Yinmen
(GATE OF ABUNDANCE)

**Location:** Midpoint on a line joining Chengfu (BL-36) and Weizhong (BL-40), or 6 cun below Chengfu (BL-36)

**Dermatome:** S2

**Main Action Areas:** Thigh, Lower Limb

**Main Functions:** Regulates Qi and Blood. Alleviates pain and sciatica

**Indications:** Sciatica, lumbo-sacral disorders, paralysis of lower limb.

**Manipulation:** 1.0-2.0 cun perpendicularly.

Moxibustion applicable.

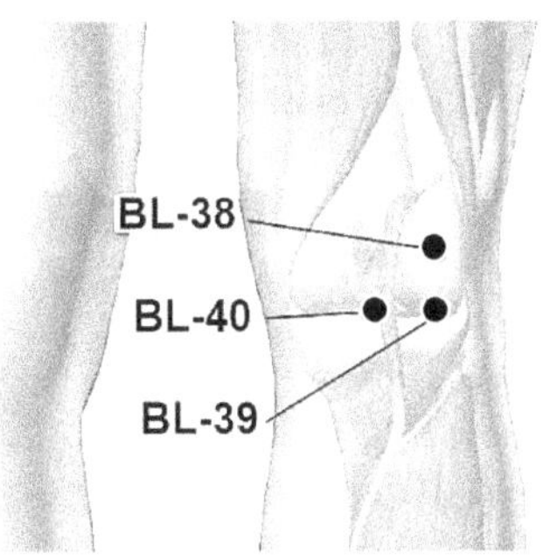


# BL-38 Fuxi

### (FLOATING CLEFT)

**Location:**
On the laterodorsal aspect of the knee, 1 cun superior and lateral to the centre of the popliteal crease (BL-40), medial to the biceps femoris muscle, or 1 cun proximal to BL-39.

**Dermatome:** L2/L3

**Main Action Areas:** Knee

**Main Functions:** Soothes the sinews and quickens the connecting vessels, quickens the blood and relieves pain, clears and disinhibits the Lower Energizer.

**Indications:**
Numbness of the gluteal and femoral regions, contracture of the tendons in the popliteal fossa.

**Manipulation:** 0.5 - 1.0 cun perpendicularly.
Moxibustion applicable.

# BL-39 Weiyang

### (OUTSIDE OF THE CROOK)

LOWER HE-SEA POINT OF TRIPLE ENERGIZER.

**Location:**
At the lateral end of the popliteal crease, on the medial side of the tendon of the long head of the biceps femoris muscle, 1 cun lateral to BL-40 (in the centre of the popliteal crease).

**Dermatome:** L5

**Main Action Areas:** Knee, Lower Limbs, Urinary system

**Main Functions:** Regulates urination and opens the water passages. Regulates Qi and alleviates pain.

**Indications:**
Stiffness and pain of the lower back, distension and fullness of the lower abdomen, edema, dysuria, cramp of the leg and foot.

---

**Manipulation:** 0.5 - 1.0 cun perpendicularly.
Moxibustion applicable.

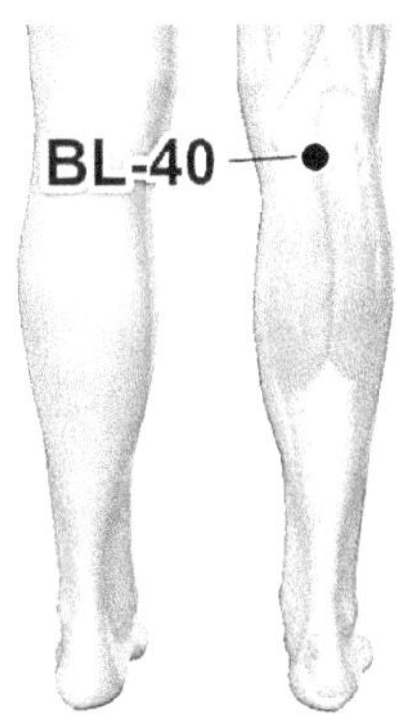


# BL-40 Weizhong

### (MIDDLE OF THE CROOK)

HE-SEA, AND COMMAND POINT OF THE BACK, EARTH POINT, MA DAN-YANG HEAVENLY STAR POINT.

**Location:**
At the midpoint of the popliteal transverse crease.

**Dermatome:** L5-S2

**Main Action Areas:** Lower back, Knee, Lower limbs, Urinary system, Skin

**Main Functions:** Clears heat, resolves damp, relaxes the sinews, removes obstructions from the channel, cools blood, eliminates stasis of blood, clears summer heat. Alleviates itching

**Indication:**
Sciatica, lumbago, paralysis of the lower limb, genitourinary disorders, disorders of the knee joint, skin diseases.

**Manipulation:** 0.5 - 1.0 perpendicularly or prick to bleed with three-edged needle.

**Caution:** No Moxibustion.

# BL-41 Fufen

### (ATTACHED BRANCH)

MEETING POINT OF THE BLADDER AND SMALL INTESTINE CHANNELS.

**Location:**
3 cun lateral to the posterior midline, on the level of the lower border of the spinous process of the 2nd thoracic vertebra (T2).

**Dermatome:** T2

---

**Main Action Areas:** Shoulder, Upper back, Lungs

**Main Functions:** Courses wind and dissipates cold, soothes the sinews and quickens the connecting vessels.

**Indications:**
Stiffness and pain of the shoulder, back and neck, numbness of the elbow and arm.

**Manipulation:** 0.3 - 0.5 cun perpendicularly or obliquely.

Moxibustion is applicable.

**Cautions:** Risk of pneumothorax.

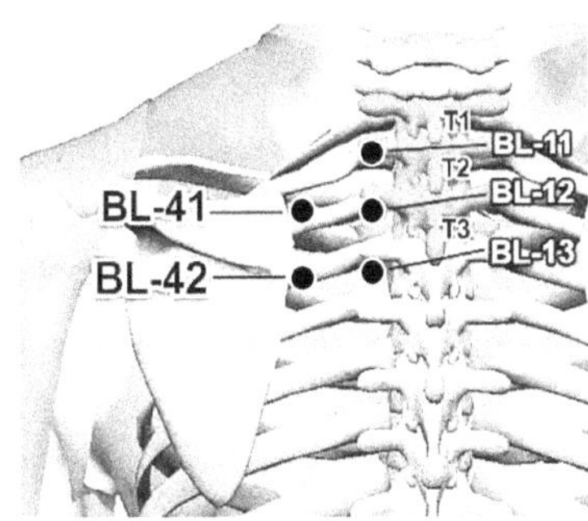


# BL-42 Pohu

### (DOOR OF THE CORPOREAL SOUL)

**Location:** 3 cun lateral to the posterior midline, on the level of the lower border of the spinous process of the 3rd thoracic vertebra (T3).

**Dermatome:** T3

**Main Action Areas:** Chest, Upper back, Lungs, Mind

**Main Functions:** Stimulates the descending of Lung Qi, regulates Qi, clears heat, stops cough and asthma, subdues rebellious Qi.

**Indications:** Pulmonary tuberculosis, hemoptysis, cough, asthma, neck rigidity, pain in the shoulder and back.

**Manipulation:** 0.3 - 0.5 cun obliquely.

Moxibustion is applicable.

**Cautions:** Risk of pneumothorax.

# BL-43 Gaohuang

### (VITAL REGION SHU)

**Location:**
3 cun lateral to the posterior midline, on the level of the lower border of the spinous process of the 4th thoracic vertebra (T4).

**Dermatome:** T4

**Main Action Areas:** Chest, Lungs, Heart, Upper back

**Main Functions:** Regulates chest Qi. Strengthens the Lungs and Heart. Alleviates pain

**Indications:**
Pulmonary tuberculosis, cough, asthma, spitting of blood, night sweating, poor memory, nocturnal emission.

**Manipulation:** 0.3 - 0.5 cun perpendicularly or obliquely.

Moxibustion is applicable.

**Cautions:** Risk of pneumothorax.

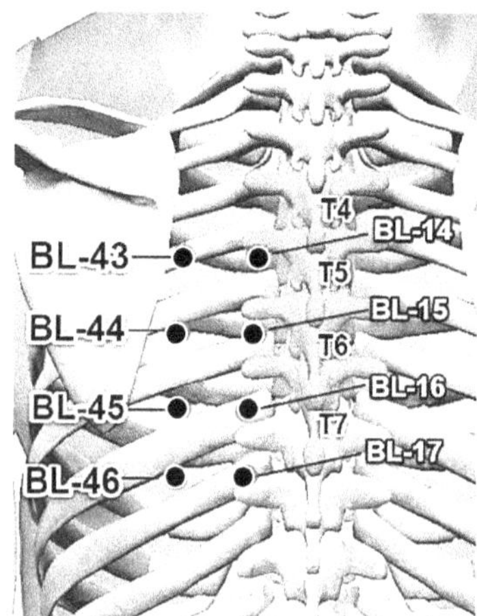


# BL-44 Shentang
(SPIRIT HALL)

**Location:**
3 cun lateral to the posterior midline, on the level of the lower border of the spinous process of the 5th thoracic vertebra (T5).

**Dermatome:** T5

**Main Action Areas:** Chest, Heart, Upper back

**Main Functions:** Regulates chest Qi. Benefits the Heart. Balances the mind. Alleviates pain.

**Indications:**
Asthma, cardiac pain, palpitation, stuffy chest, cough, stiffness and pain of the back.

**Manipulation:** 0.3 - 0.5 cun obliquely.

Moxibustion is applicable.

**Cautions:** Risk of pneumothorax.

# BL-45 Yixi
(CRY OF PAIN)

**Location:**
3 cun lateral to the posterior midline, on the level of the lower border of the spinous process of the 6th thoracic vertebra (T6).

**Dermatome:** T6

**Main Action Areas:** Chest, Back

**Main Functions:** Resolves the exterior and clears heat, diffuses the Lung and rectifies Qi, frees the channels and quickens the connecting vessels.

**Indications:**
Cough, asthma, pain of the shoulder and back.

**Manipulation:** 0.3 - 0.5 cun obliquely downward.

Moxibustion is applicable.

**Cautions:** Risk of pneumothorax.

# BL-46 Geguan
(DIAPHRAGM'S GATE)

**Location:**
3 cun lateral to the posterior midline, on the level of the lower border of the spinous process of the 7th thoracic vertebra (T7).

**Dermatome:** T7

**Main Action Areas:** Diaphragm, Back

**Main Functions:** Regulates Qi and Blood. Alleviates pain.

**Indications:**
Dysphagia, hiccup, vomiting, belching, pain and stiffness of the back.

**Manipulation:** 0.3 - 0.5 cun obliquely.

Moxibustion is applicable.

**Cautions:** Risk of pneumothorax.

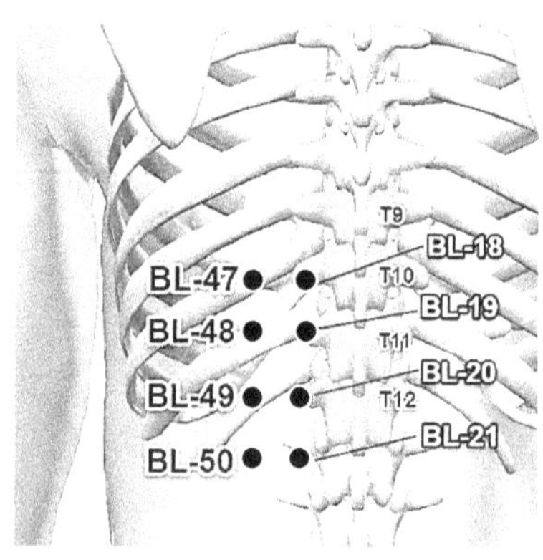


# BL-47 Hunmen
(GATE OF THE ETHEREAL SOUL)

**Location:**
3 cun lateral to the posterior midline, on the level of the lower border of the spinous process of the 9th thoracic vertebra (T9).

**Dermatome:** T8/T9

**Main Action Areas:** Hypochondrium, Abdomen, Liver

**Main Functions:** Regulates Qi and Blood. Balances the Ethereal Soul,

**Indications:**
Pain in the chest and hypochondriac region, back pain, vomiting, diarrhea.

**Manipulation:** 0.3 - 0.5 cun obliquely.

Moxibustion is applicable.

**Cautions:** Risk of pneumothorax.

# BL-48 Yanggang
(YANG'S KEY LINK)

**Location:**
3 cun lateral to the posterior midline, on the level of the lower border of the spinous process of the 10th thoracic vertebra (T10).

**Dermatome:** T9/T10

**Main Action Areas:** Gallbladder, Spleen, Digestive system

**Main Functions:** Clears heat and dampness. Regulates Qi in the middle jiao.

**Indications:**
Borborygmus, abdominal pain, diarrhea, pain in the hypochondriac region, jaundice.

**Manipulation:** 0.3 - 0.5 cun obliquely.

Moxibustion is applicable.

**Cautions:** Risk of pneumothorax.

# BL-49 Yishe
(ABODE OF THOUGHT)

**Location:**
3 cun lateral to the posterior midline, on the level of the lower border of the spinous process of the 11th thoracic vertebra (T11).

**Dermatome:** T10/T11

**Main Action Areas:** Spleen, Mind

**Main Functions:** Boosts the Spleen. Improves concentration and thinking.

**Indications:**
Abdominal distension, borborygmus,

vomiting, diarrhea, difficulty in swallowing.

**Manipulation:** 0.3 - 0.5 cun obliquely.

Moxibustion is applicable.

**Cautions:** Risk of pneumothorax.

# BL-50 Weicang
(STOMACH GRANARY)

**Location:**
3 cun lateral to the posterior midline, on the level of the lower border of the spinous process of the 12th thoracic vertebra (T12).

**Dermatome:** T12/L1

**Main Action Areas:** Stomach

**Main Functions:** Tonifies Stomach Qi. Descends rebellious Qi.

**Indications:**
Abdominal distension, pain in the epigastric region and back, infantile indigestion.

**Manipulation:** 0.3 - 0.5 cun obliquely.

Moxibustion is applicable.

**Cautions:** Risk of pneumothorax.

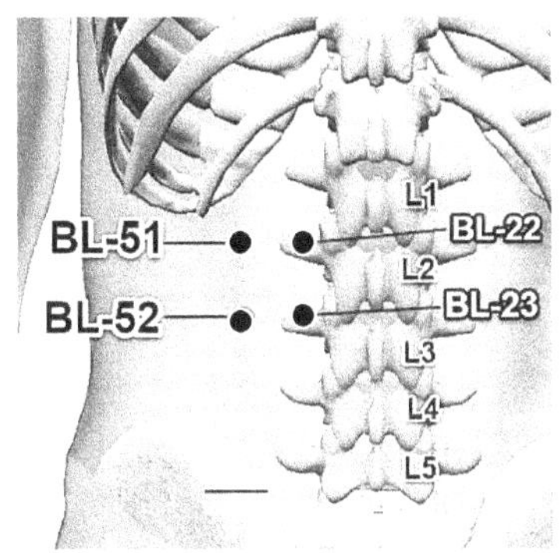


# BL-51 Huangmen
(VITALS GATE)

**Location:**
3 cun lateral to the posterior midline, on the level of the lower border of the spinous process of the 1st lumbar vertebra (L1).

**Dermatome:** T12/L1

**Main Action Areas:** Abdomen, Epigastrium

**Main Functions:** Regulates Qi in the Chest and Abdomen.

**Indications:**
Abdominal pain, constipation, abdominal mass.

**Manipulation:** 0.3 - 0.5 cun obliquely.

Moxibustion is applicable.

**Cautions:** Risk of kidney injury.

# BL-52 Zhishi
(RESIDENCE OF THE WILL)

**Location:**
3 cun lateral to the posterior midline, on the level of the lower border of the spinous process of the 2nd lumbar vertebra (L2).

**Dermatome:** L1/L2

**Main Action Areas:** Kidneys, Lumbar area, Lower Jiao

**Main Functions:** Boosts the Kidneys. Increases vitality. Strengthens the willpower.

**Indications:**
Nocturnal emission, impotence, enuresis, frequency of urination, dysuria, irregular menstruation, pain in the back and knee, edema.

**Manipulation:** 0.5 - 0.8 cun obliquely.

Moxibustion is applicable.

**Cautions:** Risk of kidney injury.

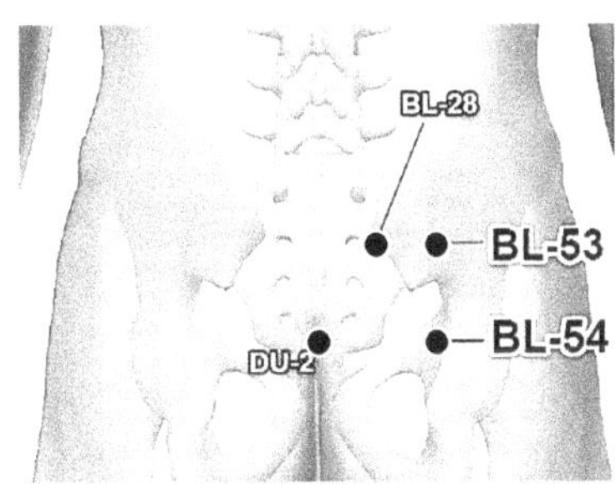


# BL-53 Baohuang
(BLADDER VITALS)

**Location:**
3 cun lateral to the posterior midline, on the level of the 2nd sacral foramen.

**Dermatome:** S1/S2

**Main Action Areas:** Sacrum, Buttock, Genitourinary system

**Main Functions:** Regulates Qi and Blood in the lower jiao. Alleviates pain.

**Indications:**
Borborygmus, abdominal distension, pain in the lower back, anuria.

**Manipulation:** Perpendicular insertion .8 - 1.2 cun.

Moxibustion is applicable.

# BL-54 Zhibian
(ORDER'S LIMIT)

**Location:**
At the level of the fourth sacral foramen, 3.0 cun lateral to the midline.

**Dermatome:** S3

**Main Action Areas:** Sacrum, Buttock, Lower Limbs, Anus

**Main Functions:** Regulates Qi and Blood in the lower jiao. Alleviates pain.

**Indication:**
Pain in the lumbosacral region, muscular atrophy, motor impairment of the lower extremities, dysuria, swelling around external genitalia, hemorrhoids, constipations, beriberi.

**Manipulation:** Perpendicular insertion 1.0 – 2.0 cun.

Moxibustion is applicable.

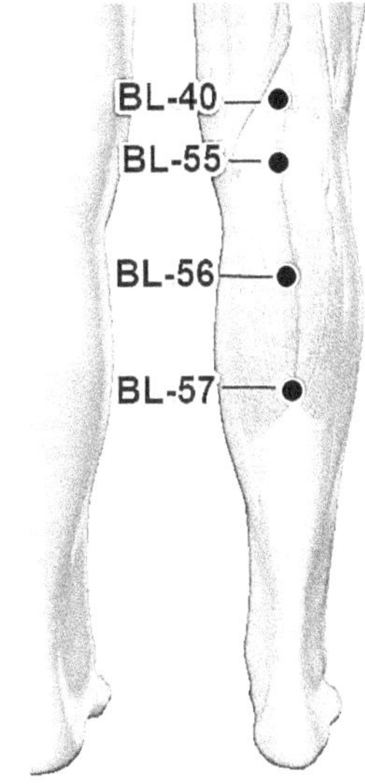


# BL-55 Heyang
(CONFLUENCE OF YANG)

**Location:**
2 cun inferior to the midpoint of the popliteal crease, in a depression between the two bellies of the gastrocnemius muscle.

**Dermatome:** L4-S1

**Main Action Areas:** Calf, Knee, Genitals

**Main Functions:** Strengthens the lumbus and boosts the Kidney, soothes the sinews and quickens the connecting vessels, regulates the Penetrating and Conception vessels.

**Indications:**
Lower back pain, pain and paralysis of the lower extremities.

**Manipulation:** Perpendicular insertion .7 - 1.0 cun.

Moxibustion is applicable.

# BL-56 Chengjin
(SUPPORT THE SINEWS)

**Location:**
5 cun inferior to the midpoint of the popliteal crease, between the two bellies of the gastrocnemius muscle.

**Dermatome:** L4-S1

**Main Action Areas:** Anus, Calf and leg

**Main Functions** Soothes the sinews and quickens the connecting vessels.

**Indications:**
Spasm of the gastrocnemius muscle, hemorrhoids, acute lower back pain.

**Manipulation:** Perpendicular insertion .8 - 1.2 cun.

Moxibustion is applicable.

# BL-57 Chengshan
(SUPPORTING MOUNTAIN)

MA DAN-YANG HEAVENLY STAR POINT

**Location:**
At the level where the two bellies of the gastrocnemius unite to form the tendo Achilles, 8 cun below Weizhong (BL-40), or half way between Weizhong (BL-40) and the bottom of the heel.

**Shared location with Tung:** 77.04

**Dermatome:** L4-S1

**Main Action Areas:** Anus, Calf and Leg

**Main Functions:** Regulates Qi and Blood. Alleviates pain. Treats haemorrhoids

**Indications:**
Sciatica, cramps of the calf muscles, pain in the sole of foot. paralysis of lower limb, haemorrhoids.

**Manipulation:** Perpendicular insertion .8 - 1.2 cun.

Moxibustion is applicable.

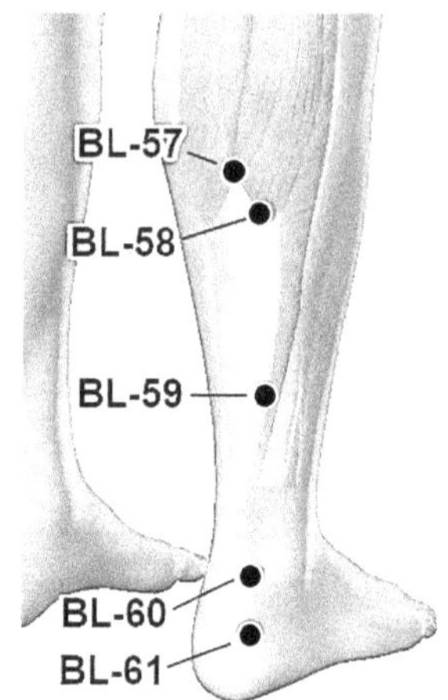


# BL-58 Feiyang
(SOARING UPWARD)

LUO-CONNECTING POINT.

**Location:**
7 cun directly above Kunlun (BL-60), on the lateral aspect of the calf muscle.

**Dermatome:** S1

**Main Action Areas:** Lower limbs, Anus, Tai Yang area, Lower Back

**Main Functions:** Dispels wind, dampness and heat. Clears the Tai Yang. Regulates Qi and Blood. Alleviates pain

**Indications:**
Ophthalmoplegia. Headache, blurring of vision, nasal obstruction, epistaxis, back pain, hemorrhoids, weakness of the leg.

**Manipulation:** Perpendicular insertion .7 - 1.0 cun.

Moxibustion is applicable.

# BL-59 Fuyang
(INSTEP YANG)

XI-CLEFT OF THE YANG HEEL VESSEL.

**Location:**
On the lateral aspect of the lower leg, 3 cun superior to BL-60 (in the depression between the highest prominence of the lateral malleolus and the Achilles tendon).

**Dermatome:** S1

**Main Action Areas:** Calf, Head

**Main Functions:** Dispels wind and dampness. Clears the Tai Yang. Alleviates pain.

**Indications:**
Heavy sensation of the head, headache, lower back pain, redness and swelling of the external malleolus, paralysis of the lower extremities.

**Manipulation:** Perpendicular insertion 0.5 - 1.0 cun.

Moxibustion is applicable.

# BL-60 Kunlun
(KUNLUN MOUNTAINS)

JING-RIVER AND FIRE POINT OF THE BLADDER CHANNEL, MA DAN-YANG HEAVENLY STAR POINT

**Location:**
Midway between the tip of the lateral malleolus and the lateral border of the tendo Achilles.

**Dermatome:** S1

**Main Action Areas:** Tai Yang area, Lower Limb, Ankle, Lumbus, Spine, Neck, Head, Uterus

**Main Functions:** Clears the Tai Yang and expels exterior pathogens. Descends rising Yang, subdues wind and clears heat. Regulates Qi and Blood and dispels stasis from the lower jiao. Promotes labour. Alleviates pain

**Indications:**
Painful disorders of the ankle (arthritis, Achilles tendinitis), sciatica, lumbago, paralysis of the lower limb. Headache, blurring of vision, neck rigidity, epistaxis, pain in the shoulder, back and arm, swelling and pain of the heel, difficult labor, epilepsy.

**Manipulation:** 0.5 - 0.8 cun perpendicularly.

Moxibustion is applicable.

**Caution:** Contra-indicated during pregnancy.

# BL-61 Pucan
(SERVANT'S RESPECT)

JING-RIVER AND FIRE POINT OF THE BLADDER CHANNEL, MA DAN-YANG HEAVENLY STAR POINT

**Location:**
On the lateral aspect of the heel, 1.5 cun inferior to BL-60 (in the depression between the highest prominence of the lateral malleolus

and the Achilles tendon), in a depression on the calcaneus.

**Dermatome:** S1

**Main Action Areas:** Ankle, Heel

**Main Functions:** Frees channels and quickens the connecting vessels, disperses swelling, relieves pain.

**Indications:** Muscular atrophy and weakness of the lower extremities, pain in the heel.

**Manipulation:** Perpendicular insertion 0.3 – 0.5 cun.

Moxibustion is applicable.

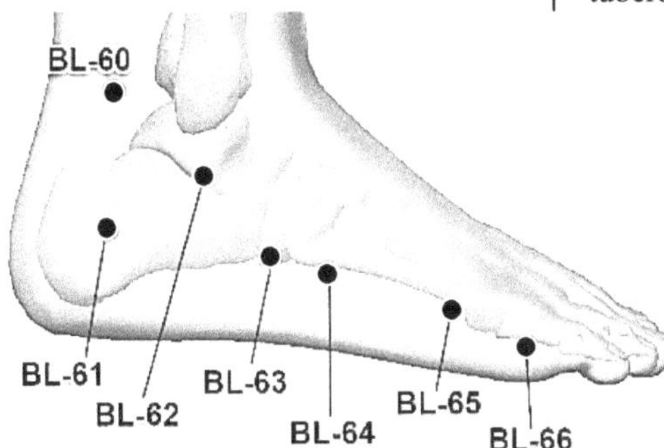


# BL-62 Shenmai

(Extending Vessel)

Confluent point of the Yang Heel vessel, Sun Si-miao Ghost point. Command point of the Governing vessel. Master point of the Yang Heel vessel.

**Location:** 0.5 cun inferior to the tip of the lateral malleolus.

**Dermatome:** S1

**Main Action Areas:** Head, Spine, Lower limb, Ankle

**Main Functions:** Descends rising Yang and clears heat. Subdues interior wind. Clears the head. Calms the mind. Alleviates pain

**Indications:** Convulsions, epilepsy, apoplexy, mental disorders, drug addictions, foot drop.

**Remarks:** this is the most important sedative and tranquilizer point of the lower limb.

**Manipulation:** Perpendicular insertion 0.3 -0.5 cun.

Moxibustion is applicable.

# BL-63 Jinmen

(Golden Gate)

Xi-Cleft of the Bladder channel, meeting point of the Bladder channel with the Yang Linking vessel.

**Location:** On the lateral aspect of the foot, proximal to the tuberosity of the 5th metatarsal bone, in a depression anterior and inferior to BL-62 between the calcaneus and the cuboid bone. Note: Some authors locate BL-63 between the cuboid bone and the tuberosity of the 5th metatarsal; the more tender point should be selected.

**Dermatome:** S1

**Main Action Areas:** Bladder channel, Spine and Lumbar region, Lower Limbs

**Main Functions:** Regulates Qi and Blood. Alleviates pain.

**Indications:** Mania, epilepsy, infantile convulsion, backache, pain in the external malleolus, motor impairment and pain of the lower extremities.

**Manipulation:** Perpendicular insertion 0.3 -0.5 cun.

Moxibustion is applicable.

# BL-64 Jinggu

(Capital Bone)

Yuan-Source point of the BL channel.

**Location:** On the lateral aspect of the foot, distal to the tuberosity of the 5th metatarsal bone.

**Dermatome:** S1

**Main Action Areas:** Head, Eyes, Bladder channel

**Main Functions:** Dispels wind and clears heat. Calms the mind. Alleviates pain.

**Indications:** Headache, neck rigidity, pain in the lower back and thigh, epilepsy.

**Manipulation:** Perpendicular insertion 0.3 -0.5 cun.

Moxibustion is applicable.

# BL-65 Shugu

(Restraining Bone)

Sedation, wood, and Shu-Stream point of the Bladder channel.

**Location:** On the lateral aspect of the foot, in the depression proximal to the head of the 5th metatarsal bone.

**Dermatome:** S1

**Main Action Areas:** Foot, Metatarsal, Head

**Main Functions:** Dispels wind and clears heat. Alleviates pain

**Indications:** Mania, headache, neck rigidity, blurring of vision, backache, pain in the lower extremities.

**Manipulation:** Perpendicular insertion 0.3 -0.5 cun.

Moxibustion is applicable.

# BL-66 Zutonggu

(Foot Connecting Valley)

Horary, water, Ying-Spring point of the Bladder channel.

**Location:** At the lateral border of the foot, in the depression distal to the metatarsophalangeal joint of the little toe.

**Dermatome:** S1

**Main Action Areas:** MTP joint, Toe, Head

**Main Functions:** Dispels wind and clears heat. Alleviates pain.

**Indications:** Headache, neck rigidity, blurring of vision, epistaxis, mania.

**Manipulation:** Perpendicular insertion 0.2 -0.3 cun.

Moxibustion is applicable.

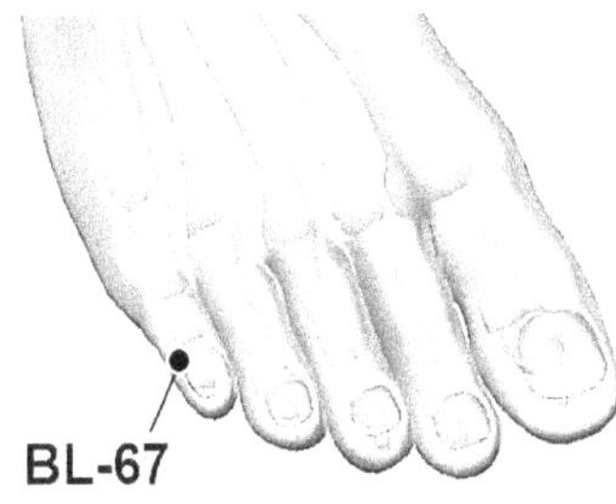

# BL-67 Zhiyin
(REACHING YIN)

JING-WELL, TONIFICATION, AND METAL POINT OF THE BLADDER CHANNEL. EXIT POINT.

**Location:**
0.1 cun proximal to the lateral end of the proximal border of the little toe.

**Dermatome:** S1

**Main Action Areas:** Uterus, Head

**Main Functions:** Corrects position of the foetus. Dispels exterior pathogens and clears the Tai Yang

**Indications:**
Headache, nasal obstruction, epistaxis, ophthalmalgia, malposition of fetus, difficult labor, retention of afterbirth, feverish sensation in the sole. This point helps to reinforce uterine contractions and expedite delivery at full term. (Abortion may be caused in the earlier months of pregnancy.)

**Manipulation:** Superficial insertion 0.1 cun. Use moxibustion for malposition of fetus.

Moxibustion is applicable.

**Cautions:** Contra-indicated during early pregnancy.

# KIDNEY MERIDIAN (Leg Shao Yin)

## KID-1 Yongquan
(GUSHING SPRING)

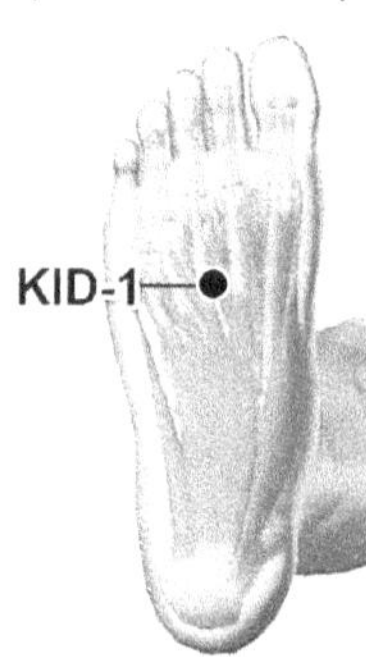


JING-WELL, SEDATION AND WOOD POINT OF THE KIDNEY CHANNEL. ENTRY POINT

**Location:**
In the-sole of the foot, on a line drawn posteriorly between the 2nd and 3rd toes, in the depression formed between the anterior one-third and posterior two-third parts of the sole when the toes are plantar flexed.

**Dermatome:** L5

**Main Action Areas:** Head, Mind, Entire body, Sole of the foot

**Main Functions:** Clears fire. Sedates interior wind. Calms the mind. Resuscitates.

**Indications:**
This is the most effective Jing-Well point for needling and is used in fainting, coma, shock,hysteria, epileptic attack, infantile convulsions, cyclical vomiting, severe morning sickness and other acute emergency conditions. It is also indicated in plantar farcitis, plantar warts, and excessive sweating of sole of the foot.

**Manipulation:** Perpendicular insertion 0.3 -0.5 cun.

Moxibustion is applicable.

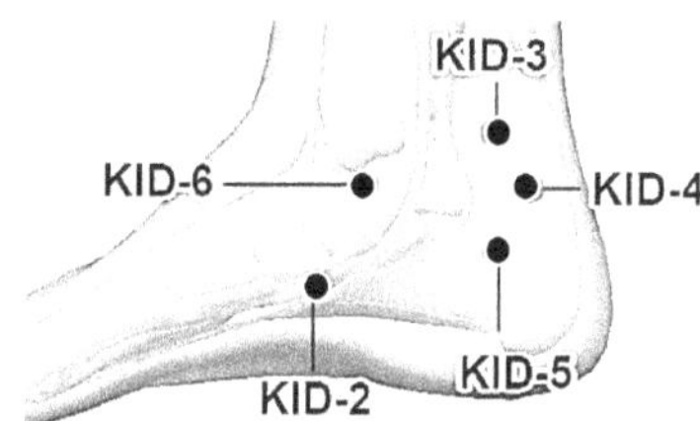


## KID-2 Rangu
(BLAZING VALLEY)

YING-SPRING AND FIRE POINT OF THE KIDNEY CHANNEL.

**Location:**
At the medial border of the foot, in a depression at the anterior border of the navicular bone, at the border of the 'red and white' skin.

**Shared location with Tung:** 66.12

**Dermatome:** L5

**Main Action Areas:** Kidneys, Spine, Entire body

**Main Functions:** Clears empty fire. Nourishes Kidney Yin. Benefits the genitourinary system.

**Indications:**
Pruritus vulvae, prolapse of uterus, irregular menstruation, nocturnal emission, hemoptysis, thirst, diarrhea, swelling and pain of the dorsum of foot, acute infantile omphalitis.

**Manipulation:** Perpendicular insertion 0.3 -0.5 cun.

Moxibustion is applicable.

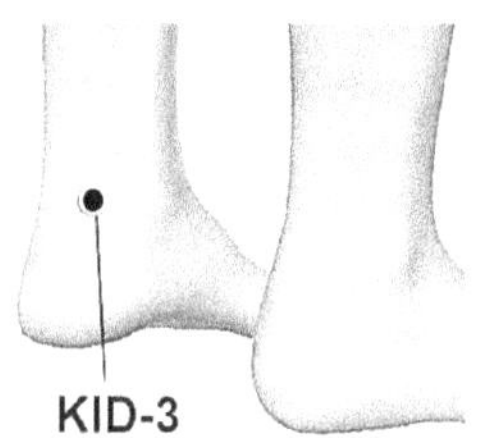


## KID-3 Taixi
(SUPREME STREAM)

SHU-STREAM, YUAN-SOURCE, AND EARTH POINT OF THE KIDNEY CHANNEL.

**Location:**
Midway between the tip of the medial malleolus and the medial border the tendo Achilles.

**Shared location with Tung:** 66.14

**Dermatome:** S1

**Main Action Areas:** Kidneys, Spine, Entire body

**Main Functions:** Augments Kidney Yin and Yang. Tonifies yuan Qi. Benefits the genitourinary system. Increases fertility

**Indications:**
Genital and urinary disorders, impotence, low back ache, disorders of the ankle. In acute asthma or in cases of frequent asthmatic attacks, stimulation of this point may be usefully carried out (excess of Lung), teeth disorders.

**Manipulation:** Up to 1.0 cun perpendicularly, or towards Kunlun (BL-60).

Moxibustion applicable.

## KID-4 Dazhong
(GREAT BELL)

LUO POINT OF THE KIDNEY CHANNEL.

**Location:**
Anterior to the medial border of the Achilles tendon, superior to its insertion at the calcaneus.

**Dermatome:** S1

**Main Action Areas:** Mind, Kidneys, Lungs

**Main Functions:** Reinforces the Kidneys. Strengthens willpower. Harmonises the Kidney and Lung.

**Indications:**
Spitting of blood, asthma, stiffness and

pain of the lower back, dysuria, constipation, pain in the heel, dementia.

**Manipulation:** Perpendicular insertion 0.3 -0.5 cun.

Moxibustion is applicable.

## KID-5 Shuiquan
(WATER SPRING)

XI-CLEFT POINT

**Location:**
1.0 cun below Taixi (K. 3.), on the medial surface of the calcaneum.

**Shared location with Tung:** 66.15

**Dermatome:** L4

**Main Action Areas:** Lower jiao, Gynaecological and urinary system, Eyes

**Main Functions:** Benefits urination, promotes blood circulation, stops abdominal pain, regulates uterus.

**Indications:**
Amenorrhea, irregular menstruation, dysmenorrhea, prolapse of uterus, dysuria, blurring of vision. Renal colic.

**Manipulation:** Perpendicular insertion 0.3 -0.5 cun.

Moxibustion is applicable.

## KID-6 Zhahoai
(SHINING SEA)

CONFLUENT POINT AND MASTER POINT OF THE YIN HEEL VESSEL. COMMAND POINT OF THE CONCEPTION VESSEL.

**Location:**
In the depression 1.0 cun directly below the tip of the medial malleolus.

**Shared location with Tung:** 66.13

**Dermatome:** L4

**Main Action Areas:** Head, Eyes, Ears, Throat, Mind, Lower jiao, Uterus, Entire body

**Main Functions:** Nourishes Yin. Cools empty heat. Regulates the Yin Qiao Mai

**Indications:**
Gento-urinary disorders, oedema of the ankle.

**Manipulation:** Perpendicular insertion 0.3 -0.5 cun.

Moxibustion is applicable.

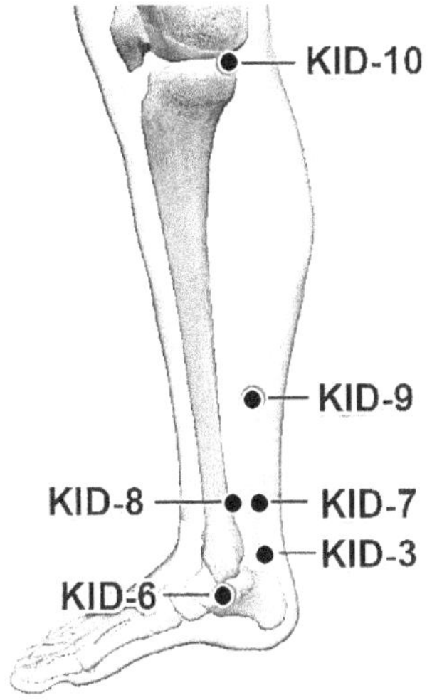


## KID-7 Fuliu
(RETURNING CURRENT)

JING-RIVER, TONIFICATION, AND METAL POINT OF THE KIDNEY CHANNEL.

**Location:**
2 cun proximal to Taixi (KID-3) on the medial border of the tendo calcaneus.

**Shared location with Tung:** 77.28

**Dermatome:** L4

**Main Action Areas:** Water passages. Lower jiao.

**Main Functions:** Tonifies the Kidneys, resolves damp, eliminates edema, strengthens the lower back, regulates sweating.

**Indications:**
Edema, abdominal distension, diarrhca, borborygmus, muscular atrophy of the leg, night sweating, spontaneous/excessive sweating, febrile diseases without sweating.

**Manipulation:** Perpendicular insertion 0.5 -0.7 cun.

Moxibustion is applicable.

## KID-8 Jiaoxin
(EXCHANGE BELIEF)

XI-CLEFT POINT OF THE YIN HEEL VESSEL

**Location:**
2 cun proximal to the highest prominence of the medial malleolus, posterior to the medial border of the tibia.

**Dermatome:** L4

**Main Action Areas:** Genitourinary system

**Main Functions:** Removes obstructions from the channel, stops abdominal pain, removes masses, regulates menses.

**Indications:**
Irregular menstruation, dysmenorrhea, uterine bleeding, prolapse of uterus, diarrhea, constipation, pain and swelling of testes.

**Manipulation:** Perpendicular insertion 0.5 -0.7 cun.

Moxibustion is applicable.

## KID-9 Zhubin
(GUESTHOUSE)

XI-CLEFT OF THE YIN LINKING VESSEL.

**Location:**
5 cun proximal to the highest prominence of the medial malleolus, 2 cun posterior to the medial border of the tibia.

**Dermatome:** L4

**Main Action Areas:** Heart, Mind, Lower jiao

**Main Functions:** Clears and calms the Heart and mind. Regulates Qi.

**Indications:**
Mental disorders, pain in the foot and lower leg, hernia.

**Manipulation:** Perpendicular insertion 0.5 -0.7 cun.

Moxibustion is applicable.

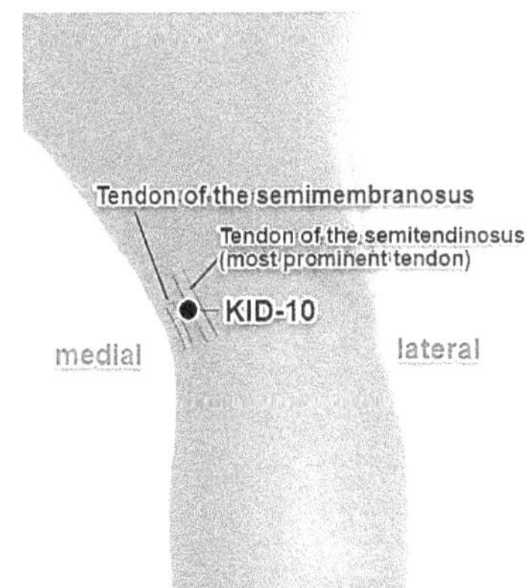


## KID-10 Yingu
(YIN VALLEY)

HE-SEA, HORARY AND WATER POINT OF THE KIDNEY CHANNEL.

**Location:**
At the medial end of the popliteal crease, between the tendons of the semimembranosus and semi-

tendinosus muscles, on the level of the knee joint space.

**Dermatome:** L3

**Main Action Areas:** Lower jiao, Genito-urinary system

**Main Functions:** Nourishes Yin and cools lower jiao heat. Transforms dampness.

**Indications:**
Impotence, hernia, uterine bleeding, dysuria, pain in the knee and popliteal fossa, mental disorders.

**Manipulation:** Perpendicular insertion 0.8 -1.0 cun.

Moxibustion is applicable.

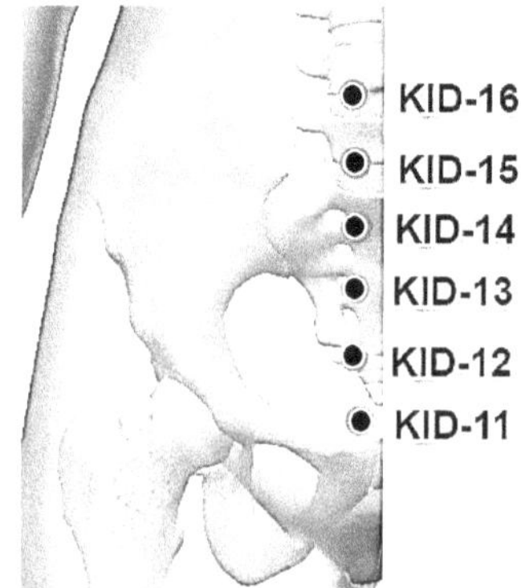


# KID-11 Henggu
## (PUBIC BONE)

MEETING POINT OF THE KIDNEY CHANNEL WITH THE PENETRATING VESSEL.

**Location:**
At the upper border of the pubic symphysis, 0.5 cun lateral to the anterior midline.

**Dermatome:** T12/L1

**Main Action Areas:** Bladder, Genitals, Lower jiao

**Main Functions:** Benefits the lower jiao. Improves sexual function and fertility.

**Indications:**
Fullness and pain of the lower abdomen, dysuria, enuresis, nocturnal emission, impotence, pain of genitalia.

**Manipulation:** Perpendicular insertion .5 - 1.0 cun.

Moxibustion is applicable.

**Cautions:** Deep insertion will penetrate a full bladder.

# KID-12 Dahe
## (GREAT LUMINANCE)

MEETING POINT OF THE KIDNEY CHANNEL WITH THE PENETRATING VESSEL.

**Location:**
1 cun superior to the upper border of the pubic symphysis, 0.5 cun lateral to the anterior midline.

**Dermatome:** T12

**Main Action Areas:** Bladder, Genitals, Uterus, Lower jiao

**Main Functions:** Benefits the lower jiao.

**Indications:**
Nocturnal emission, impotence, morbid leukorrhea, pain in the external genitalia, prolapse of uterus.

**Manipulation:** Perpendicular insertion .5 - 1.0 cun.

Moxibustion is applicable.

**Cautions:** Deep insertion will penetrate a full bladder.

# KID-13 Qixue
## (QI CAVE)

MEETING POINT OF THE KIDNEY WITH THE PENETRATING VESSEL.

**Location:**
2 cun superior to the upper border of the pubic symphsis, 0.5 cun lateral to the anterior midline.

**Dermatome:** T11

**Main Action Areas:** Uterus, Lower jiao, Emotional panic and anxiety

**Main Functions:** Benefits the lower jiao. Consolidates Qi in the lower jiao.

**Indications:**
Irregular menstruation, dysmenorrhea, dysuria, abdominal pain, diarrhea.

**Manipulation:** Perpendicular insertion .5 - 1.0 cun.

Moxibustion is applicable.

**Cautions:** Deep insertion will penetrate a full bladder.

# KID-14 Siman
## (FOUR FULLNESSES)

MEETING POINT OF THE KIDNEY WITH THE PENETRATING VESSEL.

**Location:**
2 cun inferior to the umbilicus, 0.5 cun lateral to the anterior midline.

**Dermatome:** T11

**Main Action Areas:** Large intestine, Lower jiao

**Main Functions:** Supplements Kidney Qi, regulates the Penetrating and Conception vessels, promotes free flow through the waterways.

**Indications:**
Abdominal pain and distension, diarrhea, nocturnal emission, irregular menstruation, dysmenorrhea, postpartum abdominal pain.

**Manipulation:** Perpendicular insertion .5 - 1.0 cun.

Moxibustion is applicable.

**Cautions:** Deep insertion may penetrate the peritoneal cavity.

# KID-15 Zhongzhu
## (MIDDLE FLOW)

MEETING POINT OF THE KIDNEY WITH THE PENETRATING VESSEL.

**Location:**
1 cun inferior to the umbilicus, 0.5 cun lateral to the anterior midline.

**Dermatome:** T11

**Main Action Areas:** Intestines, Lower jiao

**Main Functions:** Nourishes the Kidney channel, regulates the Penetrating and Conception vessels, disinhibits the Lower Energizer.

**Indications:**
Irregular menstruation, abdominal pain, constipation.

**Manipulation:** Perpendicular insertion .5 - 1.0 cun.

Moxibustion is applicable.

**Cautions:** Deep insertion may penetrate the peritoneal cavity.

# KID-16 Huangshu
## (VITALS SHU)

MEETING POINT OF THE KIDNEY WITH THE PENETRATING vessel.

**Location:**
0.5 cun lateral to the centre of the umbilicus.

**Dermatome:** T10

**Main Action Areas:** Umbilicus, Abdomen, Intestines

**Main Functions:** Warms the abdomen. Regulates intestinal Qi. Alleviates pain.

**Indications:**
Abdominal pain and distention, vomiting, constipation, diarrhea.

**Manipulation:** Perpendicular insertion .5 - 1.0 cun.

Moxibustion is applicable.

**Cautions:** Deep insertion may penetrate the peritoneal cavity.

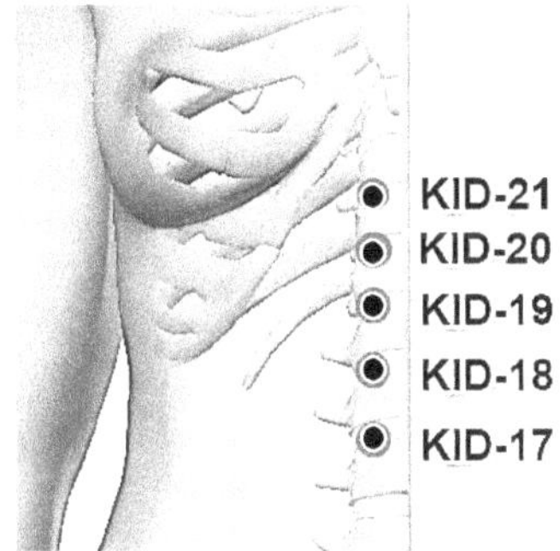


# KID-17 Shangqu

(SHANG BEND)

MEETING POINT OF THE KIDNEY WITH THE PENETRATING VESSEL.

**Location:**
2 cun superior to the umbilicus, 0.5 cun lateral to the anterior midline.

**Dermatome:** T8/T9

**Main Action Areas:** Abdomen, Epigastrium

**Main Functions:** Regulates Qi. Benefits the abdomen. Alleviates pain.

**Indications:**
Abdominal pain, diarrhea, constipation.

**Manipulation:** Perpendicular insertion .5 - 1.0 cun.

Moxibustion is applicable.

**Cautions:** Deep insertion may penetrate the peritoneal cavity.

# KID-18 Shiguan

(STONE GATE)

MEETING POINT OF THE KIDNEY WITH THE PENETRATING VESSEL.

**Location:**
3 cun superior to the umbilicus, 0.5 cun lateral to the anterior midline.

**Dermatome:** T7/8

**Main Action Areas:** Epigastrium, Stomach

**Main Functions:** Harmonises the Stomach. Descends rebellious Qi. Alleviates pain

**Indications:**
Vomiting, abdominal pain, constipation, postpartum abdominal pain, sterility.

**Manipulation:** Perpendicular insertion .5 - 1.0 cun.

Moxibustion is applicable.

**Cautions:** Deep insertion may penetrate the peritoneal cavity.

# KID-19 Yindu

(YIN METROPOLIS)

MEETING POINT OF THE KIDNEY WITH THE PENETRATING VESSEL.

**Location:**
Midway between the sternocostal angle and the centre of the umbilicus, 0.5 cun lateral to the anterior mid-line.

**Dermatome:** T7

**Main Action Areas:** Epigastrium, Stomach

**Main Functions:** Harmonises the Stomach. Descends rebellious Qi. Alleviates pain.

**Indications:**
Borborygmus, abdominal pain, epigastric pain, constipation, vomiting.

**Manipulation:** Perpendicular insertion .5 - 1.0 cun.

Moxibustion is applicable.

**Cautions:** Deep insertion may penetrate the peritoneal cavity.

# KID-20 Futonggu

(ABDOMEN CONNECTING VALLEY)

MEETING POINT OF THE KIDNEY WITH THE PENETRATING VESSEL.

**Location:**
5 cun superior to the umbilicus or 3 cun inferior to the sternocostal angle, 0.5 cun lateral to the anterior midline.

**Dermatome:** T6/T7

**Main Action Areas:** Epigastrium, Stomach

**Main Functions:** Harmonises the Stomach. Descends rebellious Qi. Alleviates pain.

**Indications:**
Abdominal pain and distension, vomiting, indigestion.

**Manipulation:** Perpendicular insertion .5 - 1.0 cun.

Moxibustion is applicable.

**Cautions:** Deep insertion may penetrate the peritoneal cavity.

# KID-21 Youmen

(HIDDEN GATE)

MEETING POINT OF THE KIDNEY WITH THE PENETRATING VESSEL.

**Location:**
2 cun inferior to the sternocostal angle, 0.5 cun lateral to the anterior midline.

**Dermatome:** T6/T7

**Main Action Areas:** Epigastrium, Chest

**Main Functions:** Harmonises the Stomach. Clears heat.

**Indications:**
Courses the Liver and rectifies Qi, fortifies the Spleen and harmonizes the Stomach, clears abdominal heat.

**Manipulation:** Perpendicular insertion 0.3 – 0.7 cun.

Moxibustion is applicable.

**Cautions:** Deep insertion may penetrate the peritoneal cavity or liver.

# KID-22 Bulang

(WALKING CORRIDOR)

EXIT POINT

**Location:**
In the 5th intercostal space (ICS), 2 cun lateral to the anterior midline.

**Dermatome:** T5

**Main Action Areas:** Chest, Epigastrium

**Main Functions:** Regulates Qi. Descends rebellious Qi

**Indications:**
Cough, asthma, distension and fullness in the chest and hypochondriac region, vomiting, anorexia.

**Manipulation:** Oblique or subcutaneous insertion .3 - .5 cun.

Moxibustion is applicable.

**Cautions:** Deep needling may penetrate the Liver, Lung, or Heart.

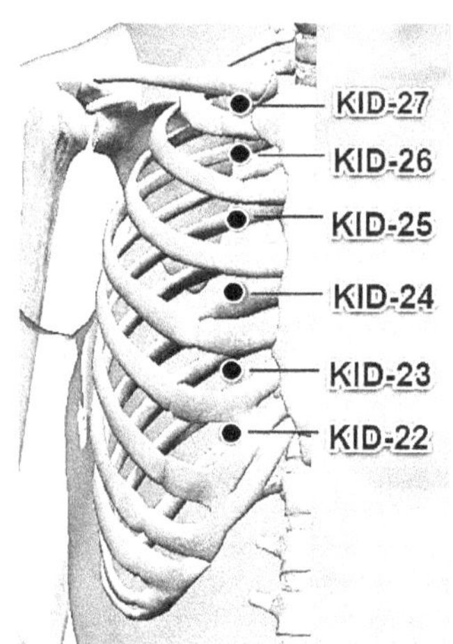



## KID-23 Shenfeng

(SPIRIT SEAL)

**Location:**
In the 4th intercostal space (ICS), 2 cun lateral to the anterior midline.

**Dermatome:** T4

**Main Action Areas:** Chest, Lungs, Breast, Stomach

**Main Functions:** Descends rebellious Qi. Opens and relaxes the chest. Benefits the breast.

**Indications:**
Cough, asthma, fullness in the chest and hypochondriac region, mastitis.

**Manipulation:** Oblique or subcutaneous insertion .3 - .5 cun.

Moxibustion is applicable.
**Cautions:** Deep needling may penetrate the Lung.

## KID-24 Lingxu

(SPIRIT RUIN)

**Location:**
In the 3rd intercostal space (ICS), 2 cun lateral to the anterior midline.

**Dermatome:** T3

**Main Action Areas:** Chest, Lungs, Breast

**Main Functions:** Descends rebellious Qi. Opens and relaxes the chest. Benefits the breast.

**Indications:**
Cough, asthma, fullness in the chest and hypochondria region, mastitis.

**Manipulation:** Oblique or subcutaneous insertion .3 - .5 cun.

Moxibustion is applicable.
**Cautions:** Deep needling may penetrate the Lung.

## KID-25 Shencang

(SPIRIT STOREHOUSE)

**Location:**
In the 2nd intercostal space (ICS), 2 cun lateral to the anterior midline.

**Dermatome:** T2

**Main Action Areas:** Chest, Lungs, Heart

**Main Functions:** Benefits respiration. Regulates Chest Qi.

**Indications:**
Cough, asthma, chest pain.

**Manipulation:** Oblique or subcutaneous insertion .3 - .5 cun.

Moxibustion is applicable.
**Cautions:** Deep needling may penetrate the Lung.

## KID-26 Yuzhong

(COMFORTABLE CHEST)

**Location:**
In the 1st intercostal space (ICS), 2 cun lateral to the anterior midline.

**Dermatome:** C4

**Main Action Areas:** Epigastrium, Chest

**Main Functions:** Harmonises the Stomach. Clears heat

**Indications:**
Cough, asthma, accumulation of phlegm, fullness in the chest and hypochondriac region.

**Manipulation:** Oblique or subcutaneous insertion .3 - .5 cun.

Moxibustion is applicable.
**Cautions:** Deep needling may penetrate the Lung.

## KID-27 Shufu

(SHU MANSION)

**Location:**
At the lower border of the clavicle, 2 cun lateral to the anterior Midline.

**Dermatome:** C4

**Main Action Areas:** Chest, Throat

**Main Functions:** Descends rebellious Qi. Regulates Chest Qi

**Indications:**
Cough, asthma, chest pain.

**Manipulation:** Oblique or subcutaneous insertion .3 - .5 cun.

Moxibustion is applicable.
**Cautions:** Deep needling may penetrate the Lung.

# PERICARDIUM MERIDIAN (Arm Jue Yin)

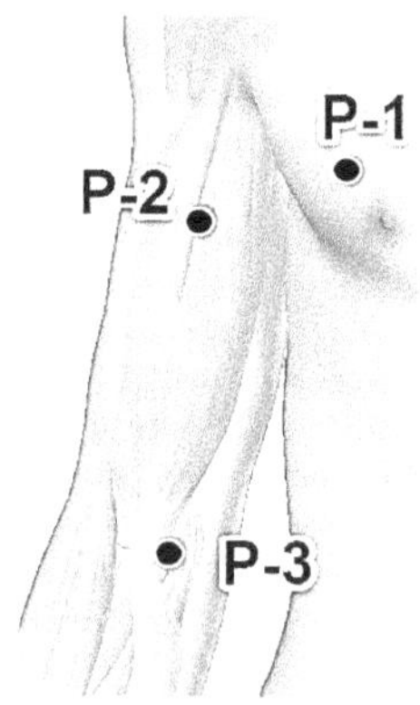



## P-1 Tianchi

(HEAVENLY POND)

MEETING POINT OF THE PERICARDIUM, GALL BLADDER, LIVER AND TRIPLE ENERGIZER CHANNELS, WINDOW OF HEAVEN POINT, ENTRY POINT.

**Location:**
In the 4th intercostal space (ICS), 1 cun lateral to the nipple.

**Dermatome:** T4

**Main Action Areas:** Breast, Chest, Ribs, Heart

**Main Functions:** Regulates Qi. Dispels stasis and unbinds the chest. Benefits the breast.

**Indications:**
Suffocating sensation in the chest, pain in the hypochondriac region, swelling and pain of the axillary region.

**Manipulation:** Oblique or subcutaneous insertion .2 - .4 cun.

Moxibustion is applicable.

**Cautions:** Do not puncture the mammary glands.

## P-2 Tianquan
### (HEAVENLY SPRING)

**Location:**
Between the two heads of the biceps brachii muscle, 2 cun inferior to the axillary fold.

**Dermatome:** At junction of C5/T2

**Main Action Areas:** Chest, Breast, Arm

**Main Functions:** Opens the chest and rectifies Qi, nourishes the Heart and calms the spirit, quickens the blood, transforms stasis, relieves pain.

**Indications:**
Cardiac pain, distension of the hypochondriac region, cough, pain in the chest, back and the medial aspect of the arm.

**Manipulation:** Perpendicular insertion 0.5 - 0.7 cun.

Moxibustion is applicable.

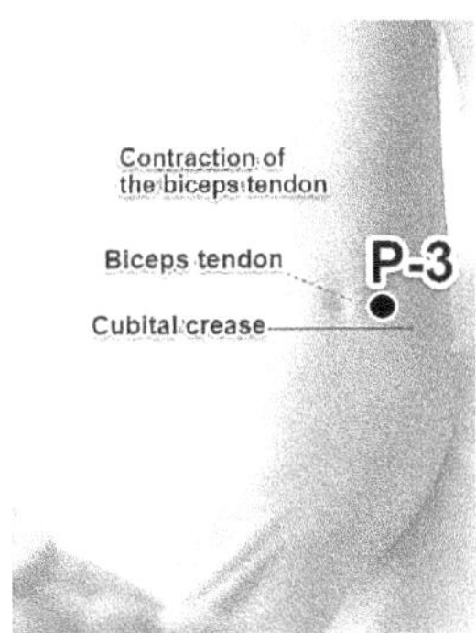


## P-3 Quze
### (MARSH AT THE CROOK)

HE-SEA, WATER POINT OF THE PERICARDIUM CHANNEL.

**Location:**
In the ante-cubital crease, on the medial (ulnar) border of the biceps tendon.

**Dermatome:** C8/T1

**Main Action Areas:** Chest, Heart, Stomach, Elbow

**Main Functions:** Clears heat. Dispels stasis. Descends rebellious Qi

**Indications:**
Angina pectoris, palpitation, anxiety.

**Manipulation:** 1.0 cun perpendicularly. In cases of fever of chronic skin diseases prick to bleed with three-edged needle.

**Cautions:** The brachial artery and veins lie deep to this point.

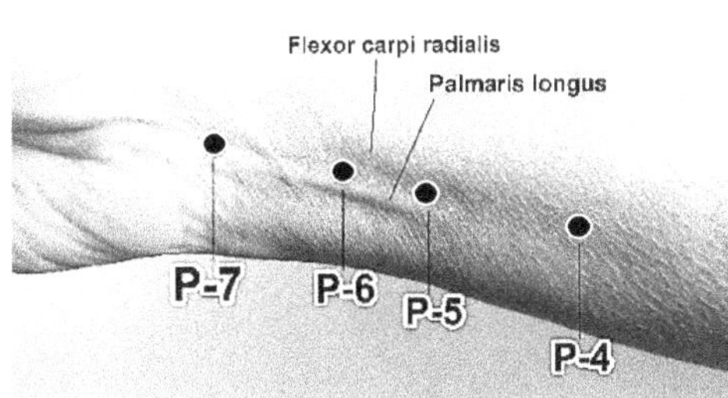


## P-4 Ximen
### (XI CLEFT GATE)

XI-CLEFT POINT OF THE PERICARDIUM CHANNEL.

**Location:**
5 cun proximal to the midpoint of the wrist crease between the tendons of the palmaris longus and flexor carpi radialis.

**Dermatome:** C6-C8

**Main Action Areas:** Heart, Mind, Forearm

**Main Functions:** Cools Blood. Dispels stasis. Regulates Heart Qi. Calms the mind

**Indications:**
As it is the Xi-Cleft point of the Pericardium Channel, it can be used to treat acute heart diseases e.g.,angina pectoris, pericarditis, tachycardia and other disorders of cardiac rythm; acute depression and hysteria.

**Manipulation:** 0.5-1.0 cun perpendicularly.

Moxibustion applicable.

## P-5 Jianshi
### (INTERMEDIARY MESSENGER)

JING-RIVER, METAL, AND TONIFICATION POINT OF THE PERICARDIUM CHANNEL. GROUP LOU POINT FOR THE 3 ARM YIN.

**Location:**
3 cun proximal to the anterior wrist joint space ('most distal wrist crease'), between the tendons of the palmaris longus and flexor carpi radialis muscles.

**Dermatome:** C6-C8

**Main Action Areas:** Chest, Wrist, Heart, Stomach

**Main Functions:** Regulates Chest Qi. Resolves phlegm. Calms the mind. Descends rebellious Qi.

**Indications:**
Cardiac pain, palpita-tion, stomach ache, vomiting, febrile diseases, irritability, malaria, mental disorders, epilepsy, swelling of axilla, contracture of elbow and arm.

**Manipulation:** 0.5-1.0 cun perpendicularly.

Moxibustion applicable.

## P-6 Neiguan
### (INNER GATE)

LUO POINT OF THE PC CHANNEL, COMMAND POINT FOR THE CHONG VESSEL. MASTER POINT FOR THE YIN LINKING VESSEL.

**Location:**
2 cun proximal to the midpoint of the wrist crease, between the tendons of the palmaris longus and flexor carpi radialis muscles.

**Dermatome:** C6-C8

**Main Action Areas:** Chest, Heart, Mind, Stomach, Wrist, Forearm, Neck

**Main Functions:** Regulates Qi and Blood. Dispels stasis. Relaxes the chest. Benefits the breasts. Calms the mind. Descends rebellious Qi. Harmonises the Stomach

**Indications:**
Cardiac pain, palpitation, stuffy chest, pain in the hypochon-driac region, stomach ache, nausea, vomiting, hiccups, mental disorders, epilepsy, insomnia, febrile diseases, irritability, malaria, contracture and pain in the elbow and arm.

**Manipulation:** 1.0 cun perpendicularly, or through to Waiguan (SJ-5).

Moxibustion is applicable.

**Cautions:** The median nerve lies directly beneath this point.

## P-7 Daling
### (GREAT MOUND)

SHU-STREAM, YUAN-SOURCE, SEDATION AND EARTH POINT OF THE PERICARDIUM CHANNEL. SUN SI-MIAO GHOST POINT.

**Location:**
At the midpoint of the wrist crease between the tendons of the palmaris longus and flexor carpi radialis.

**Dermatome:** C7

**Main Action Areas:** Wrist, Chest, Heart, Stomach

**Main Functions:** Regulates Qi and Blood. Alleviates pain. Relaxes the chest. Calms the mind. Descends rebellious Qi.

**Indications:**
Diseases of the wrist joint, early median carpal compression without positive neurological signs.

**Manipulation:** 0.3-0.5 cun perpendicularly.

Moxibustion is applicable.

**Cautions:** The median nerve lies directly beneath this point.

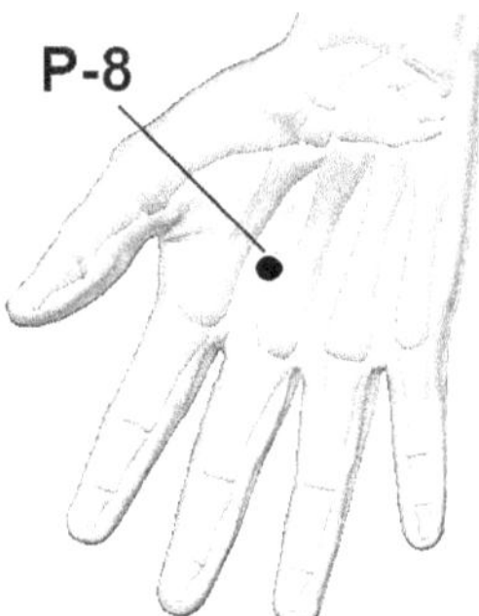

# P-8 Laogong
### (PALACE OF TOIL)

YING-SPRING, HORARY, EXIT, AND FIRE POINT OF THE PERICARDIUM CHANNEL. SUN SI-MIAO GHOST POINT.

**Location:**
At the centre of the palm, in the depression between the second and third metacarpal bones, on the radial side of the third metacarpal.

**Dermatome:** C7

**Main Action Areas:** Palm, Chest, Heart, Mind

**Main Functions:** Clears heat. Restores consciousness. Calms the mind. Descends rebellious Qi. Focuses Qi in Qigong therapy

**Indications:**
Disorders of the palm, rheumatic arthritis of carpal joints, Dupuytrens contracture, excessive sweating of the palm. Cardiac pain, mental disorders, epilepsy, gastritis, foul breath, fungus infection of the hand and foot, vomiting, nausea.

**Manipulation:** 0.3-0.5 cun perpendicularly.

Moxibustion is applicable.

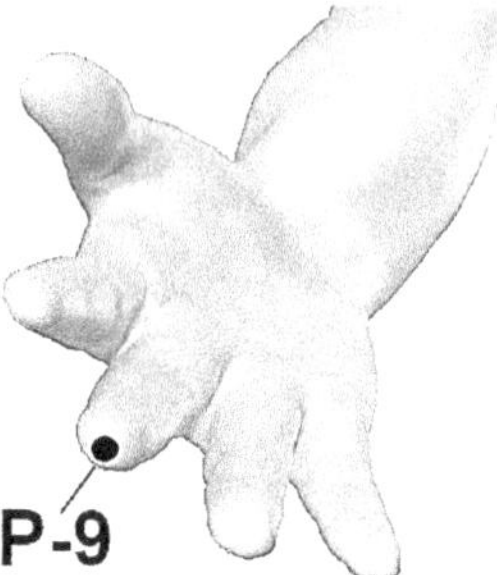

# P-9 Zhongchong
### (MIDDLE RUSHING)

JING-WELL, TONIFICATION, AND WOOD POINT OF THE PERICARDIUM CHANNEL.

**Location:**
On the most distal point of the middle finger.

**Dermatome:** C8

**Main Action Areas:** Heart, Mind

**Main Functions:** Restores consciousness. Opens the orifices. Opens the chest.

**Indications:**
Cardiac pain, palpitation, loss of consciousness, aphasia with stiffness and swelling of tongue, febrile diseases, heat stroke, convulsion, feverish sensation in the palm.

**Manipulation:** Superficial insertion .1 cun, or prick to cause bleeding.

Moxibustion is applicable.

# SANJIAO (Triple Energizer) MERIDIAN (Arm Shao Yang)

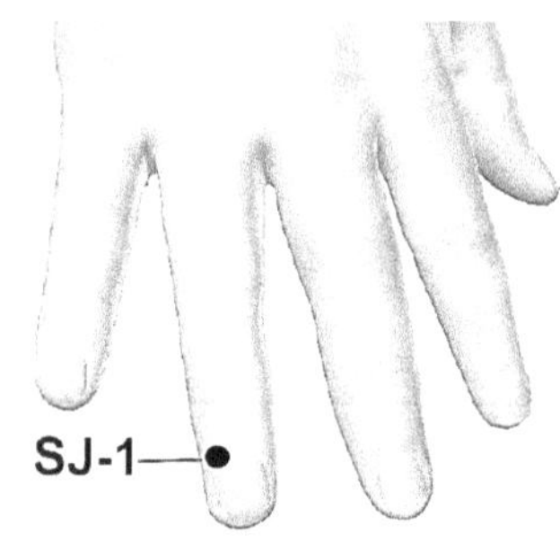

# SJ-1 Guanchong
### (RUSHING PASS)

JING-WELL AND METAL POINT OF THE TRIPLE ENERGIZER (SANJIAO) CHANNEL. ENTRY POINT.

**Location:**
On the ring finger, 0.1 cun from the ulnar corner of the nail.

**Dermatome:** C7

**Main Action Areas:** Mind, Ears, Triple Energizer channel

**Main Functions:** Clears heat. Benefits the ears. Resuscitates consciousness.

**Indications:**
Headache, redness of eyes, sore throat, stiff tongue, febrile diseases, irritability.

**Manipulation:** Superficial insertion 0.1 cun, or prick to cause bleeding.

Moxibustion is applicable.

**Remarks:** As in other jing-well points, SJ-1 helps restore consciousness in cases of coma or fainting.

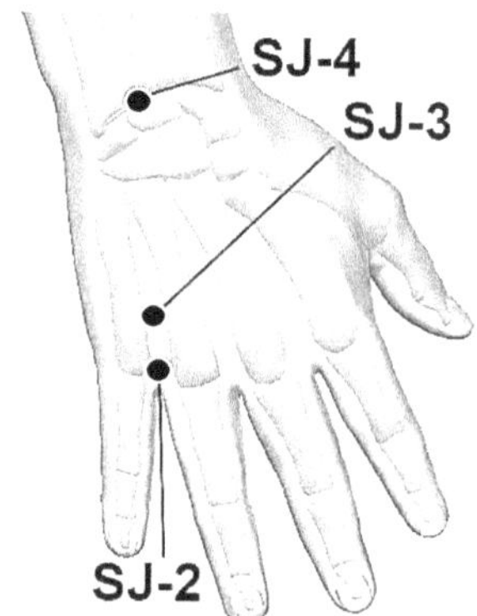

# SJ-2 Yemen
### (FLUID GATE)

YING-SPRING AND WATER POINT OF THE TRIPLE ENERGIZER (SANJIAO) CHANNEL.

**Location:**
Between the little finger and ring finger, proximal to the margin of the web.

**Dermatome:** C7

**Main Action Areas:** Ears, MCP joint

**Main Functions:** Dissipates wind and clears heat. Benefits the ears. Alleviates pain.

**Indications:**
Headache, redness of the eyes, sudden deafness, sore throat, malaria, pain in arm.

**Manipulation:** Oblique insertion .3 - .5 cun. towards the interspace of the metacarpal bones.

Moxibustion is applicable.

# SJ-3 Zhongzhu

(CENTRAL ISLET)

SHU-STREAM, WOOD AND TONIFICATION POINT OF THE TRIPLE ENERGIZER CHANNEL (SANJIAO).

**Location:**
On the dorsum of the hand, in the depression between the heads of the 4th and 5th metacarpal bones. This point is best located by clenching the fist.

**Shared location with Tung:** 22.06

**Dermatome:** C7

**Main Action Areas:** MCP joints, Triple Energizer channel, Ears

**Main Functions:** Clears heat, expels wind, benefits ears, lifts the mind, removes obstructions from the channel, regulates Qi.

**Indications:**
Headache, redness of the eyes, deafness, tinnitus, sore throat, febrile diseases, pain in the elbow and arm, motor impairment of fingers.

**Manipulation:** 0.3- 0.5 cun perpendicularly.

Moxibustion applicable.

# SJ-4 Yangghi

(YANG POOL)

YUAN-SOURCE POINT OF THE TRIPLE ENERGIZER (SANJIAO) CHANNEL.

**Location:**
On the dorsum of the wrist (above the wrist joint space, 'dorsal wrist crease'), in the gap between the tendons of the extensor digitorum (on the ulnar aspect) and the extensor digiti minimi muscles (on the radial aspect).

**Dermatome:** C7

**Main Action Areas:** Wrist, Triple Energizer channel, Ears

**Main Functions:** Regulates the Triple Energizer. Alleviates pain. Tonifies yuan Qi.

**Indications:**
Pain in the arm, shoulder and wrist, malaria, deafness, thirst.

**Manipulation:** 0.3- 0.5 cun perpendicularly.

Moxibustion applicable.

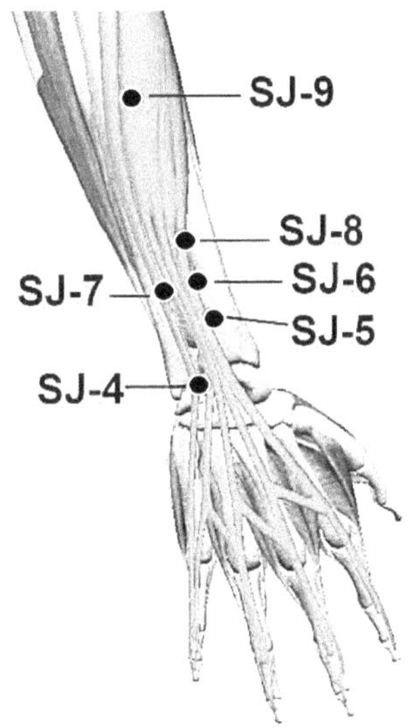


# SJ-5 Waiguan

(OUTER PASS)

LUO POINT OF THE TRIPLE ENERGIZER (SANJIAO) CHANNEL. CONFLUENT POINT AND MASTER POINT OF THE YANG LINKING VESSEL. COMMAND POINT OF THE BELT VESSEL.

**Location:**
2 cun proximal to the midpoint of the dorsal transverse crease of the wrist, between the radius and the ulna.

**Dermatome:** C7

**Main Action Areas:** Lungs, Liver, Ears, Head, Eyes, Forearm and wrist, Triple Energizer channel

**Main Functions:** Releases the exterior and dispels wind. Dispels stasis and smooths the Liver. Clears interior and exterior heat. Descends excessive Yang. Alleviates pain

**Indications:**
Paralysis of upper limb, temporal headache, ear disorders, stiff neck.

**Manipulation:** 0.5- 1.0 cun perpendicularly.

Moxibustion applicable.

# SJ-6 Zhigou

(BRANCHING DITCH)

JING-RIVER, FIRE, AND HORARY POINT OF THE TRIPLE ENERGIZER CHANNEL (SANJIAO)

**Location:**
1 cun proximal to Waiguan (SJ-5).

**Shared location with Tung:** 33.04

**Dermatome:** C7

**Main Action Areas:** Chest, Sides, Abdomen, Large intestine, Ears, Throat

**Main Functions:** Chest heat. Dispels stasis. Releases the exterior

**Indications:**
Tinnitus, deafness, pain in the hypochondriac region, vomiting, constipation, febrile diseases, aching and heavy sensation of the shoulder and back, sudden hoarseness of voice.

**Manipulation:** 0.8- 1.2 cun perpendicularly.

Moxibustion applicable.

# SJ-7 Huizong

(ANCESTRAL MEETING)

XI-CLEFT POINT OF THE TRIPLE ENERGIZER CHANNEL (SANJIAO)

**Location:**
3 cun proximal to the dorsal wrist joint space ('dorsal wrist crease') and 0.5 cun ulnar to the centre of the forearm.

**Dermatome:** C6-C8 border

**Main Action Areas:** Upper limb, Ears

**Main Functions:** Dispels stasis and alleviates pain. Clears heat.

**Indications:**
Deafness, pain in the ear, epilepsy, pain of the arm.

**Manipulation:** 0.5- 1.0 cun perpendicularly.

Moxibustion applicable.

# SJ-8 Sanyangluo

(THREE YANG CONNECTION)

GROUP LOU FOR THE 3 ARM YANG.

**Location:**
1.0 cun proximal to Zhigou (SJ-6)

**Dermatome:** C6/C7

**Main Action Areas:** Forearm, Arm, Ears, Throat

**Main Functions:** Clears heat, removes obstructions from the channels.

**Indications:**
Deafness, sudden hoarseness of voice, pain in the chest and hypochondriac region, pain in the hand and arm, toothache.

**Manipulation:** 0.5- 1.0 cun perpendicularly.

Moxibustion applicable.

**Cautions:** Some texts contraindicate this point for needling and moxibustion. Consider using laser instead.

# SJ-9 Sidu
(FOUR RIVERS)

**Location:**
7 cun proximal to the dorsal wrist joint space ('dorsal wrist crease'), between the radius and the ulna.

**Dermatome:** C6

**Main Action Areas:** Forearm, Elbow

**Main Functions:** Alleviates stiffness and pain. Releases the exterior.

**Indications:**
Deafness, toothache, migraine, sudden hoarseness of voice, pain in the forearm.

**Manipulation:** 0.5- 1.0 cun perpendicularly.

Moxibustion applicable.

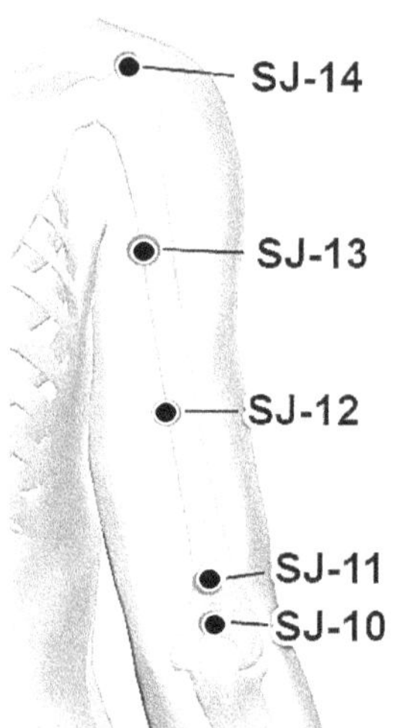


# SJ-10 Tianjing
(HEAVENLY WELL)

HE-SEA, SEDATION, AND EARTH POINT OF THE TRIPLE ENERGIZER CHANNEL.

**Location:**
On the lateral aspect of the upper arm, with the elbow flexed in a depression approximately 1 cun proximal to the olecranon.

**Dermatome:** C7

**Main Action Areas:** Elbow, Arm, Triple Energizer channel

**Main Functions:** Regulates Qi and Blood. Alleviates pain and swelling.

**Indications:**
Migraine, pain in the neck, shoulder and arm, epilepsy, scrofula, goiter.

**Manipulation:** 0.3- 0.5 cun perpendicularly.

Moxibustion applicable.

# SJ-11 Qinglengyuan
(CLEAR COLD ABYSS)

**Location:**
On the lateral aspect of the upper arm, with the elbow flexed 1 cun proximal to SJ-10 or 2 cun proximal to the olecranon, on the triceps brachii muscle.

**Dermatome:** C7

**Main Action Areas:** Elbow, Arm, Triple Energizer channel.

**Main Functions:** Frees the channel and connecting vessel, clears heat and drains fire.

**Indications:**
Motor impairment and pain of the shoulder and arm, migraine.

**Manipulation:** 0.3- 0.5 cun perpendicularly.

Moxibustion applicable.

# SJ-12 Xiaoluo
(DISPERSING LUO RIVER)

**Location:**
4 cun proximal to SJ-10 (with the elbow flexed in a depression superior to the olecranon) or 5 cun proximal to the olecranon on a line connecting the olecranon and the lateral extremity of the acromion (location of SJ-14).

**Dermatome:** C5-T1

**Main Action Areas:** Upper arm, shoulder and elbow, Triceps brachii muscle

**Main Functions:** Alleviates stiffness and pain. Drains dampness and treats swelling.

**Indications:**
Headache, neck rigidity, motor impairment and pain of the arm.

**Manipulation:** 0.5- 0.7 cun perpendicularly.

Moxibustion applicable.

# SJ-13 Naohui
(UPPER ARM MEETING)

MEETING POINT OF THE TRIPLE ENERGIZER CHANNEL AND THE YANG LINKING VESSEL.

**Location:**
3 cun distal to the lateral extremity of the acromion (location of SJ-14), on a line connecting SJ-14 and the olecranon, at the junction of this line with the margin of the deltoid muscle.

**Dermatome:** C5-T1

**Main Action Areas:** Upper arm and shoulder

**Main Functions:** Alleviates stiffness and pain.

**Indications:**
Goiter, pain in the shoulder and arm.

**Manipulation:** 0.5- 0.8 cun perpendicularly.

Moxibustion applicable.

# SJ-14 Jianliao
(SHOULDER CREVICE)

**Location:**
Inferior to the lateral extremity of the acromion between the acromial and spinal portions of the deltoid muscle or, with the arm abducted, in the posterior of the two depressions on the shoulder joint.

**Dermatome:** C4

**Main Action Areas:** Shoulder

**Main Functions:** Regulates Qi and Blood. Alleviates pain and reduces stiffness

**Indications:**
Frozen shoulder, pain in the arm, paralysis of the arm.

**Manipulation:** 1.0 cun perpendi-cularly towards Jiquan (HT-1).

Moxibustion applicable.

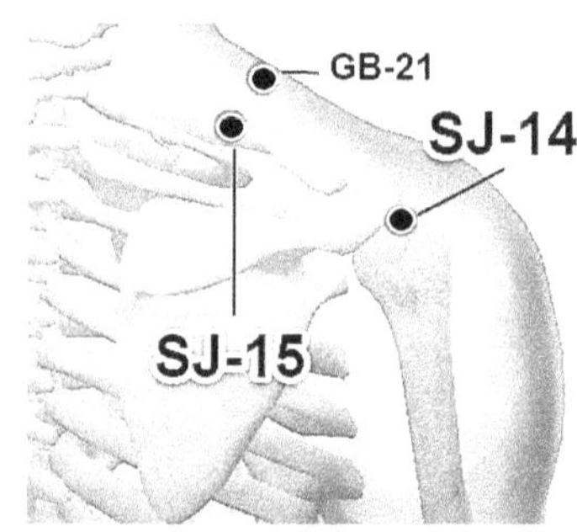

## SJ-15 Tianliao

(HEAVENLY CREVICE)

MEETING POINT OF THE TRIPLE ENERGIZER AND GALL BLADDER CHANNELS AND THE YANG LINKING VESSEL.

**Location:**
1 cun posterior to GB-21.

**Dermatome:** C4

**Main Action Areas:** Shoulder, Chest

**Main Functions:** Regulates Qi and Blood. Alleviates pain and stiffness.

**Indications:**
Pain in the shoulder and elbow, stiffness of the neck.

**Manipulation:** 0.3- 0.5 cun perpendicularly.

Moxibustion applicable.

**Cautions:** Perpendicular needling may penetrate the Lung.

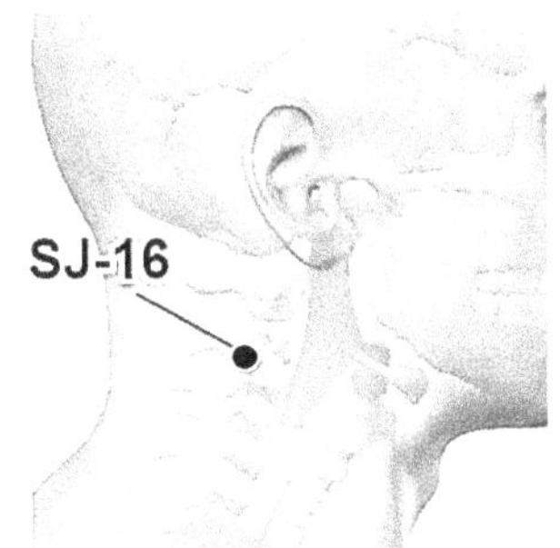

## SJ-16 Tianyou

(WINDOW OF HEAVEN)

WINDOW OF HEAVEN POINT.

**Location:**
At the posterior border of the sternocleidomastoid muscle, directly inferior to the mastoid process, on the level of the mandibular angle.

**Dermatome:** C3

**Main Action Areas:** Throat and neck, Ears

**Main Functions:** Regulates Qi and Blood. Alleviates pain. Transforms dampness and reduces swelling. Dispels wind and clears heat.

**Indications:**
Headache, neck rigidity, facial swelling, blurring of vision, sudden deafness.

**Manipulation:** 0.3- 0.5 cun perpendicularly.

Moxibustion applicable.

## SJ-17 Yifeng

(WIND SCREEN)

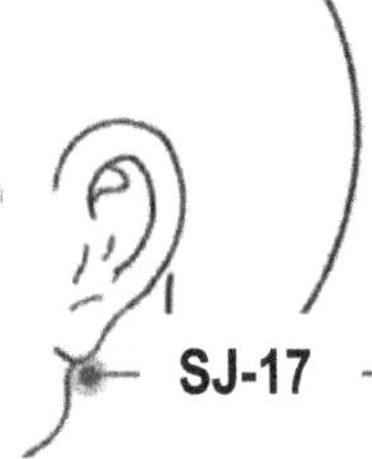


MEETING POINT OF THE TRIPLE ENERGIZER AND THE GALL BLADDER CHANNELS.

**Location:**
In the highest point of the depression behind the ear lobe, between the angle of the jaw and the mastoid process.

**Dermatome:** C2/C3

**Main Action Areas:** Ears, Face, Throat, Neck

**Main Functions:** Benefits the ear. Alleviates pain. Clears heat. Dispels wind. Treats the facial nerve.

**Indications:**
Tinnitus (avoid excessive stimulation), ear disorders, dizziness, facial paralysis, parotitis, throat pain.

**Manipulation:** 0.5- 1.0 cun perpendicularly and anteriorly.

This point should be needled with the patient's mouth slightly open.

Moxibustion applicable.

**Caution:** This point is close to the facial nerve, therefore no deep needling.

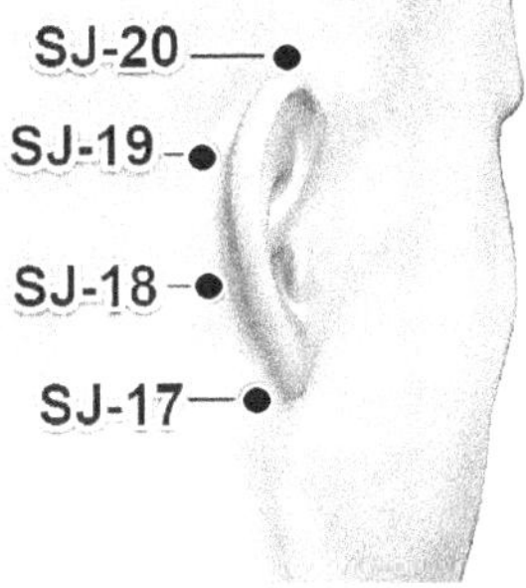


## SJ-18 Qimai

(SPASM VESSEL)

**Location:**
Posterior to the ear, in a well-defined depression in the centre of the mastoid.

**Dermatome:** C2/C3

**Main Action Areas:** Ear, Mastoid area, Head

**Main Functions:** Benefits the ears. Dredges the channel and alleviates

pain. Dispels exterior wind. Subdues interior wind. Calms the mind.

**Indications:**
Headache, tinnitus, deafness, infantile convulsion.

**Manipulation:** Subcutaneous insertion .3 - .5 cun, or prick to cause bleeding.

Moxibustion is applicable.

## SJ-19 Luxi

(SKULL'S REST)

**Location:**
Posterior to the ear, in a well-defined depression superior to the centre of the ear.

**Dermatome:** C2/C3

**Main Action Areas:** Head, Brain, Temple

**Main Functions:** Calms the mind. Dredges the channels and alleviates pain.

**Indications:**
Headache, tinnitus, deafness, infantile convulsion.

**Manipulation:** Oblique insertion .3 - .5 cun. Moxibustion is applicable.

**Cautions:** Avoid artery.

## SJ-20 Jiaosun

(MINUTE ANGLE)

MEETING POINT OF THE TRIPLE ENERGIZER, SMALL INTESTINE, AND GALL BLADDER CHANNELS.

**Location:**
Directly superior to the apex of the ear. Fold the ear forward, and locate the point on the scalp 0.3 cun above the hairline next to the top of the ear.

**Dermatome:** C2/C3 but also crossover to trigeminal nerve

**Main Action Areas:** Ear, Mouth

**Main Functions:** Regulates Qi and Blood. Alleviates pain and swelling.

**Indications:**
Tinnitus, redness, pain and swelling of the eye, swelling of the gum, toothache, parotitis.

**Manipulation:** Subcutaneous insertion .3 - .5 cun towards the eye.

Moxibustion is applicable.

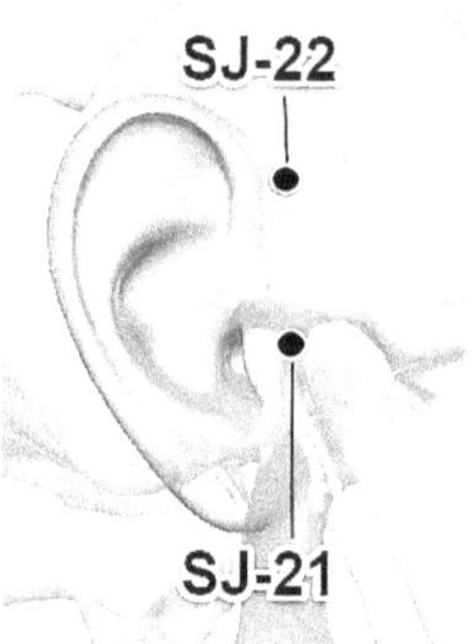



## SJ-21 Ermen

(EAR GATE)

**Location:**
In the depression in front of the supra-tragic notch. It is easier to locate when the mouth is slightly open.

**Dermatome:** Trigeminal nerve

**Main Action Areas:** Ears, Temple, Jaw

**Main Functions:** Improves hearing and benefits the ears. Regulates Qi and Blood. Alleviates pain. Clears heat

**Indications:**
Tinnitus, deafness, otorrhea, toothache, stiffness of the lip.

**Manipulation:** 0.5 cun perpendicularly or more usually, horizontally downwards through Tinggong (SI-19) to Tinghui (GB-2) (puncturing-through technique).

Moxibustion applicable.

If pus discharge from the ear, moxibustion is contra-indicated.

## SJ-22 Erheliao

(EAR HARMONY CREVICE)

MEETING POINT OF THE TRIPLE ENERGIZER, GALL BLADDER AND SMALL INTESTINE CHANNELS. EXIT POINT.

**Location:**
In a depression at the border of the circumauricular temporal hairline, anterior to and on the level of the root of the auricle.

**Dermatome:** Trigeminal nerve

**Main Action Areas:** Ears

**Main Functions:** Dredges the channels and alleviates pain. Dispels wind. Benefits the ears

**Indications:**
Migraine, tinnitus, lockjaw.

**Manipulation:** Transversely (subcutaneously) 0.5 cun.

Moxibustion applicable.

**Caution:** Superficial temporal artery.

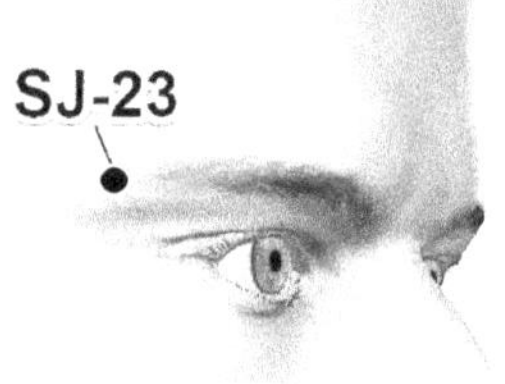



## SJ-23 Sizhukong

(SILKEN BAMBOO HOLLOW)

**Location:**
In the depression at the lateral end of the eyebrow.

**Shared location with Tung:** 1010.11

**Dermatome:** Trigeminal nerve

**Main Action Areas:** Eyes, Temple

**Main Functions:** Regulates Qi and Blood. Alleviates pain. Dispels wind and clears heat. Clears the eyes.

**Indications:**
Headache, redness and pain of the eye, blurring of vision, twitching of the eyelid, toothache, facial paralysis.

**Manipulation:** 0.5 cun horizontally and posteriorly in the direction of Shuaigu (GB-8).

**Caution:** No moxibustion.

# GALL BLADDER MERIDIAN (Leg Shao Yang)

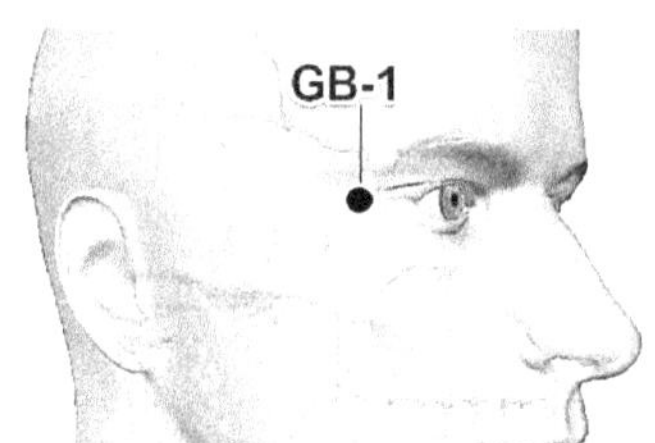



## GB-1 Tongziliao

(PUPIL CREVICE)

MEETING POINT OF THE GALL BLADDER, SMALL INTESTINE AND TRIPLE ENERGIZER CHANNELS. ENTRY POINT.

**Location:**
0.5 cun lateral to the outer canthus of the eye. In a bony depression on the lateral aspect of the orbital margin, on the level of the outer canthus of the eye.

**Dermatome:** Trigeminal nerve

**Main Action Areas:** Eyes, Outer canthus

**Main Functions:** Benefits the eyes and improves vision. Dispels wind and heat. Regulates Qi and Blood

**Indications:**
Eye diseases, facial paralysis, headache, trigeminal neuralgia.

**Manipulation:** 0.5 cun horizontally and posteriorly.

**Caution:** No moxibustion

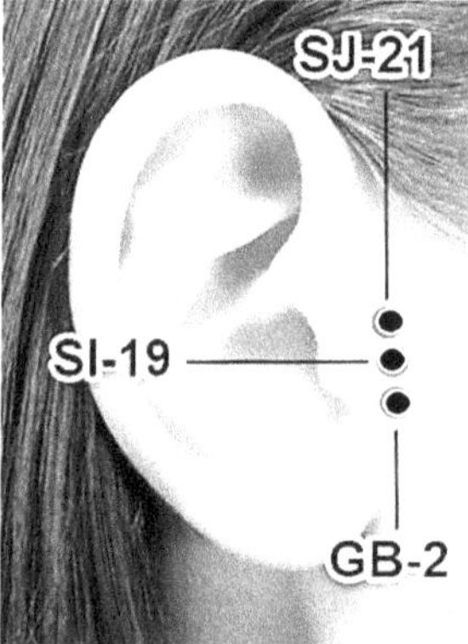



## GB-2 Tinghui

(MEETING OH HEARING)

MEETING POINT OF THE GALL BLADDER, TRIPLE ENERGIZER, STOMACH, AND LARGE INTESTINE CHANNELS.

**Location:**
In the depression immediately in front of the intertragic notch when the mouth is open.

**Dermatome:** Trigeminal nerve

**Main Action Areas:** Ears, Temple, Jaw

**Main Functions:** Improves hearing and benefits the ears. Regulates Qi and Blood. Alleviates pain. Dispels wind and clears heat.

**Indications:**
Ear disorders, jaw pain, chronic infections of the auditory canal and the external ear, arthritis of the mandible, trismus, facial paralysis, trigeminal neuralgia.

**Manipulation:** 1.0 cun perpendicularly or use the puncturing through technique (see Ermen (SJ-21)) with mouth open.

Moxibustion applicable.

# GB-3 Shangguan

(ABOVE THE JOINT)

MEETING POINT OF THE GALL BLADDER, TRIPLE ENERGIZER, AND STOMACH CHANNELS.

**Location:**
In a depression on the upper border of the zygomatic arch, approximately 1 cun anterior to the root of the ear, superior to ST-7.

**Dermatome:** Trigeminal nerve

**Main Action Areas:** Temple, Jaw, Ears

**Main Functions:** Regulates Qi and Blood. Alleviates pain. Clears heat. Improves hearing.

**Indications:**
Headache, deafness, tinnitus, diplacusis, deviation of the eye and mouth, toothache, facial neuralgia.

**Manipulation:** Perpendicular insertion .3 - .5 cun.

Moxibustion is applicable.

**Cautions:** Do not deep insertion.

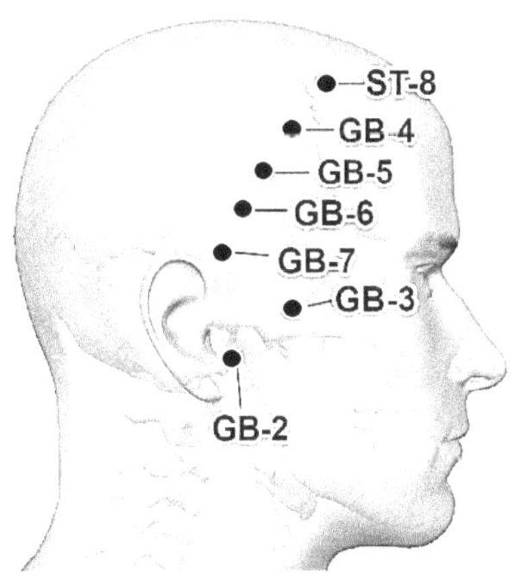


# GB-4 Hanyan

(JAW SERENITY)

**Location:**
At the junction of the upper quarter and the second quarter of a line connecting ST-8 and GB-7.

**Dermatome:** Trigeminal nerve

**Main Action Areas:** Temple, Jaw, Ears

**Main Functions:** Regulates Qi and Blood. Alleviates pain.

**Indications:**
Migraine, vertigo, tinnitus, pain in the outer canthus, toothache, convulsion, epilepsy.

**Manipulation:** Subcutaneous insertion 0.3 - 0.5 cun.

Moxibustion is applicable.

# GB-5 Xuanlu

(SUSPENDED SKULL)

MEETING POINT OF THE GALL BLADDER, TRIPLE ENERGIZER, STOMACH, AND LARGE INTESTINE CHANNELS.

**Location:**
At the junction of the 2nd and 3rd quarter of an imaginary line connecting ST-8 and GB-7.

**Dermatome:** Trigeminal nerve

**Main Action Areas:** Temple, Jaw, Ears

**Main Functions:** Regulates Qi and Blood. Alleviates pain.

**Indications:**
Temporal headache, migraine, trigeminal neuralgia, tooth pain.

**Manipulation:** Subcutaneous insertion 0.3 - 0.5 cun.

Moxibustion is applicable.

# GB-6 Xuanli

(SUSPENDED HAIR)

MEETING POINT OF THE GALL BLADDER, TRIPLE ENERGIZER, STOMACH, AND LARGE INTESTINE CHANNELS.

**Location:**
At the junction of the lower quarter and the upper three quarters of a line connecting ST-8 and GB-7.

**Dermatome:** Trigeminal nerve

**Main Action Areas:** Temple, Jaw, Ears

**Main Functions:** Regulates Qi and Blood. Alleviates pain.

**Indications:**
Temporal headache, migraine, trigeminal neuralgia, tooth pain, tinnitus, frequent sneezing.

**Manipulation:** Subcutaneous insertion 0.3 - 0.5 cun.

Moxibustion is applicable.

# GB-7 Qubin

(CROOK OF THE TEMPLE)

MEETING POINT OF THE GALL BLADDER AND BLADDER CHANNELS.

**Location:**
In a depression on the level of the apex of the ear, within the circum-auricular temporal hairline, approximately at the junction of a horizontal line through the apex of the ear and a vertical line along the posterior border of the temple anterior to the ear.

On the temple, approximately one finger-width anterior to SJ-20, level with the apex of the auricle.

**Dermatome:** Trigeminal nerve

**Main Action Areas:** Temple, Ear, Cheek

**Main Functions:** Regulates Qi and Blood. Alleviates pain.

**Indications:**
Headache, swelling of cheek, trismus, pain in temporal region, infantile convulsion.

**Manipulation:** Subcutaneous insertion 0.3 - 0.5 cun.

Moxibustion is applicable.

# GB-8 Shuaigu

(LEADING VALLEY)

MEETING POINT OF THE GALL BLADDER AND BLADDER CHANNELS.

**Location:**
Directly above the apex of the ear, 1.5 cun above the hairline. (The apex of the ear may be conveniently located by folding the ear over forwards on itself.)

1 cun directly above SJ-20.

**Dermatome:** Trigeminal nerve, C2/C3

**Main Action Areas:** Temple, Ear, Brain

**Main Functions:** Regulates Qi and Blood. Alleviates pain. Relieves poisoning

**Indications:**
Migraine, ear disease, dizziness, vertigo.

**Manipulation:** Subcutaneous insertion 0.3 - 0.5 cun.

Moxibustion is applicable.

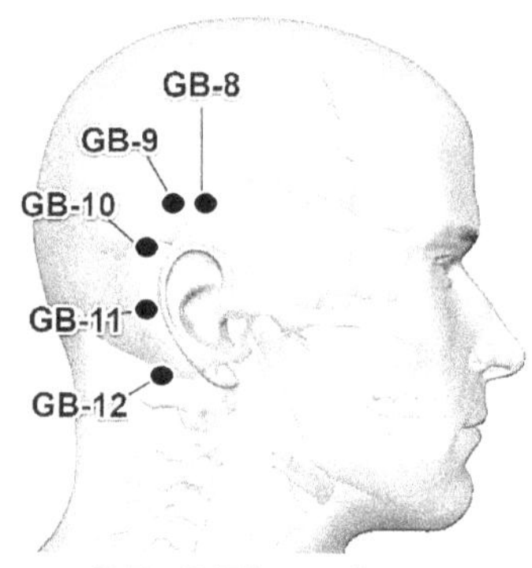

# GB-9 Tianchong

(HEAVENLY RUSHING)

MEETING POINT OF THE GALL BLADDER AND BLADDER CHANNELS.

**Location:**
1.5 cun directly superior to the apex of the ear (SJ-20) and 0.5 cun posterior to GB-8. Approximately superior to the posterior margin of the ear.

**Dermatome:** C2/C3

**Main Action Areas:** Head, Brain, Mind, Ear

**Main Functions:** Regulates Qi and Blood. Alleviates pain. Calms the mind.

**Indications:**
Headache, epilepsy, swelling and pin of the gums, convulsion.

**Manipulation:** Subcutaneous insertion 0.3 - 0.5 cun.

**Caution:** No Moxibustion.

# GB-10 Fubai

(FLOATING WHITE)

MEETING POINT OF THE GALL BLADDER AND BLADDER CHANNELS.

**Location:**
Posterior to the ear, at the junction of the upper third with the two lower thirds of the curved line connecting GB-9 and GB-12.

**Dermatome:** C2/C3

**Main Action Areas:** Side of head, Ear, Brain

**Main Functions:** Regulates Qi and Blood. Alleviates pain.

**Indications:**
Headache, deafness, tinnitus.

**Manipulation:** Subcutaneous insertion 0.3 - 0.5 cun.

Moxibustion is applicable.

# GB-11 Touqiaoyin

(HEAD PORTAL YIN)

MEETING POINT OF THE GALL BLADDER, TRIPLE ENERGIZER, BLADDER, AND SMALL INTESTINE CHANNELS.

**Location:**
Posterior to the ear, at the junction of the lower third with the two upper thirds of the curved line connecting GB-9 and GB-12.

**Dermatome:** C2/C3

**Main Action Areas:** Side of head, Eye, Ear, Brain

**Main Functions:** Regulates Qi and Blood. Alleviates pain.

**Indications:**
Pain in the head and neck, tinnitus, deafness, pain in the ears.

**Manipulation:** Subcutaneous insertion 0.3 - 0.5 cun.

Moxibustion is applicable.

# GB-12 Wangu

(MASTOID PROCESS)

MEETING POINT OF THE GALL BLADDER AND BLADDER CHANNELS.

**Location:**
In a depression directly posterior and inferior to the mastoid process.

**Dermatome:** C2/C3

**Main Action Areas:** Neck, Head, Ears, Throat

**Main Functions:** Relaxes the body and calms the mind. Dissipates stasis and relieves swelling. Alleviates pain. Benefits the throat.

**Indications:**
Headache, insomnia, swelling of the cheek, retro-auricular pain, deviation of eye and mouth, toothache.

**Manipulation:** Oblique insertion 0.3 - 0.5 cun.

Moxibustion is applicable.

# GB-13 Benshen

(SPIRIT ROOT)

MEETING POINT OF THE GALL BLADDER CHANNEL WITH THE YANG LINKING VESSEL. MUSCLE MERIDIAN MEETING POINT OF THE 3 ARM YANG.

**Location:** 3 cun lateral to DU-24 (on the midline, 0.5 cun superior to the anterior hairline).

**Dermatome:** Trigeminal nerve

**Main Action Areas:** Head, Mind

**Main Functions:** Calms the mind, eliminates wind, gathers essence to the head, clears the brain.

**Indications:** Headache, insomnia, vertigo, epilepsy.

**Manipulation:** Subcutaneous insertion 0.3 - 0.5 cun.

Moxibustion is applicable.

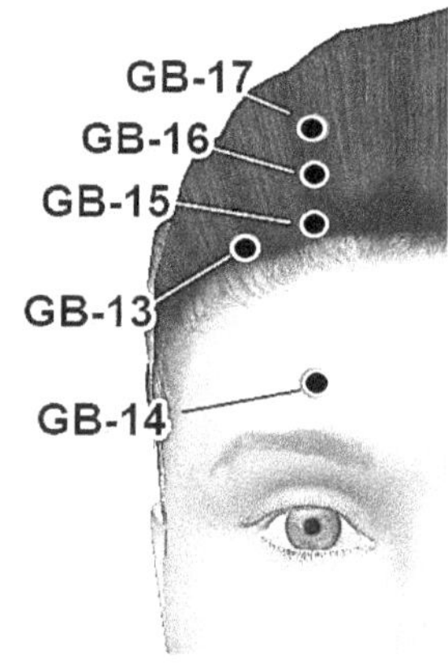

# GB-14 Yangbai

(YANG WHITE)

MEETING POINT OF THE GALL BLADDER WITH THE YANG LINKING VESSEL AND THE TRIPLE ENERGIZER, STOMACH, AND LARGE INTESTINE CHANNELS.

**Location:**
1.0 cun above the midpoint of the eyebrow, straight above the pupil.

**Dermatome:** Trigeminal nerve

**Main Action Areas:** Forehead, Eyes, Supraorbital area

**Main Functions:** Calms the mind and relaxes the body. Dispels wind and heat. Dispels stasis. Alleviates pain. Improves appearance

**Indications:**
Facial paralysis, frontal headache, frontal sinusitis, night blindness, glaucoma and other eye diseases.

**Manipulation:** Subcutaneous insertion 0.3 - 0.5 cun.

Moxibustion is applicable.

## GB-15 Toulinqi

(HEAD GOVERNOR OF TEARS)

MEETING POINT OF THE GALL BLADDER AND BLADDER CHANNELS WITH THE YANG LINKING VESSEL.

**Location:**
With the patient looking straight ahead, directly superior to the pupil and 0.5 cun superior to the anterior hairline.

**Dermatome:** Trigeminal nerve

**Main Action Areas:** Head, Forehead, Eyes

**Main Functions:** Regulates the mind, balances the emotions, clears brain, brightens eyes, frees the nose.

**Indications:**
Headache, vertigo, lacrimation, pain in outer canthus, rhinorrhea, nasal obstruction, manic depression.

**Manipulation:** Subcutaneous insertion 0.3 - 0.5 cun.

Moxibustion is applicable.

## GB-16 Muchuang

(WINDOW OF THE EYE)

MEETING POINT OF THE GALL BLADDER CHANNEL WITH THE YANG LINKING VESSEL.

**Location:**
1.5 cun superior to the anterior hairline, on the pupil line or 2.25 cun lateral to the midline (midway between DU-24 and ST-8).

**Dermatome:** Trigeminal nerve

**Main Action Areas:** Head, Brain, Eyes

**Main Functions:** Dredges the channel and dispels wind and heat. Alleviates pain.

**Indications:**
Headache, vertigo, red and painful eyes, nasal obstruction.

**Manipulation:** Subcutaneous insertion 0.3 - 0.5 cun.

Moxibustion is applicable.

**Remarks:** Treats eye disorders.

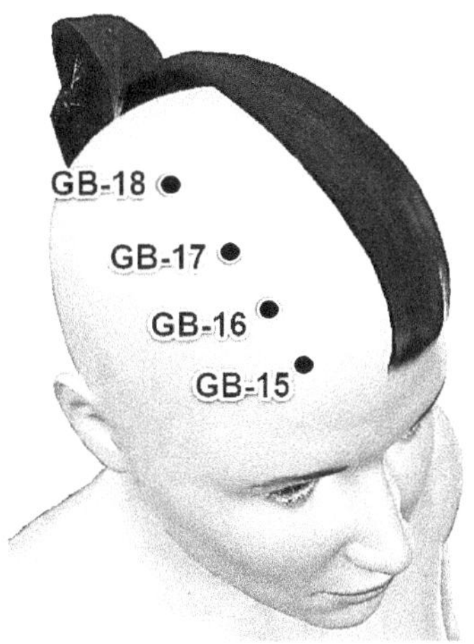


## GB-17 Zhengying

(UPRIGHT NUTRITION)

MEETING POINT OF THE GALL BLADDER AND BLADDER CHANNELS WITH THE YANG LINKING VESSEL.

**Location:**
2.5 cun superior to the anterior hairline and 2.25 cun lateral to the midline.

**Dermatome:** Trigeminal nerve

**Main Action Areas:** Head, Brain, Eyes

**Main Functions:** Alleviates pain. Calms the mind.

**Indications:**
Migraine, vertigo.

**Manipulation:** Subcutaneous insertion 0.3 - 0.5 cun.

Moxibustion is applicable.

## GB-18 Chengling

(SUPPORT SPIRIT)

MEETING POINT OF THE GALL BLADDER AND BLADDER CHANNELS WITH THE YANG LINKING VESSEL.

**Location:** 4 cun superior to the anterior hairline or 1 cun anterior to DU-20 and 2.25 cun lateral to the midline.

**Dermatome:** Trigeminal nerve, C2

**Main Action Areas:** Head, Brain, Nose, Eyes

**Main Functions:** Regulates Qi and Blood. Calms the mind and opens the orifices.

**Indications:** Headache, vertigo, epistaxis, rhinorrhea, obsessive thoughts and dementia.

**Manipulation:** Subcutaneous insertion 0.3 - 0.5 cun.

Moxibustion is applicable.

## GB-19 Naokong

(BRAIN HOLLOW)

MEETING POINT OF THE GALL BLADDER AND BLADDER CHANNELS WITH THE YANG LINKING VESSEL.

**Location:**
On the posterior aspect of the head, at the upper border of the external occipital protuberance (DU-17) and 2.25 cun lateral to the midline.

**Dermatome:** C2

**Main Action Areas:** Head, Brain, Ear

**Main Functions:** Clears the Gallbladder and drains fire, soothes the sinews and quickens the connecting vessels, rouses the brain and frees the portal.

**Indications:**
Headache, stiffness of the neck, vertigo, painful eyes, tinnitus, epilepsy.

**Manipulation:** Subcutaneous insertion 0.3 - 0.5 cun.

Moxibustion is applicable.

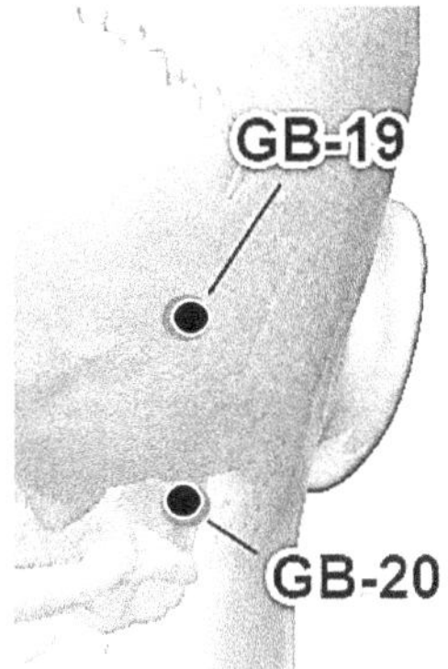


## GB-20 Fengchi

(WIND POOL)

MEETING POINT OF THE GALL BLADDER AND TRIPLE ENERGIZER CHANNELS WITH THE YANG LINKING AND YANG HEEL VESSELS.

**Location:**
In the depression lateral to the mastoid process between the origins of the trapezius and sterno-mastoid muscles.

**Dermatome:** C2/C3

**Main Action Areas:** Head, Occiput, Neck, Eyes, Ears, Brain, Mind, Muscles, Entire body

**Main Functions:** Calms the mind and relaxes the body. Descends rising Yang. Benefits the Sea of M arrow. Alleviates pain. Dispels wind and clears heat. Brightens the eyes. Benefits the ears

**Indications:**
Occipital headache, common cold, influenza, stiff neck, cervical spondylosis.

**Manipulation:** 1.0 cun with the needle directed towards the inner canthus of the opposite eye. Strong stimulation of this point is said to relieve or abort an attack of common cold.

Moxibustion is applicable.

**Cautions:** Too deep an insertion should be avoided.

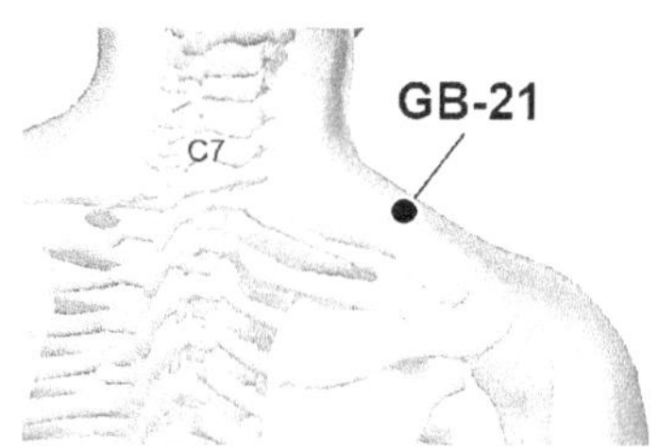


# GB-21 Jiaujing
(SHOULDER WELL)

MEETING POINT OF THE GALL BLADDER, TRIPLE ENERGIZER, AND STOMACH CHANNELS WITH THE YANG LINKING VESSEL.

**Location:**
At the highest point of the shoulder, at the midpoint of a line connecting the 7th cervical vertebra (C7) and the lateral extremity of the acromion.

**Dermatome:** C4

**Main Action Areas:** Neck, Shoulder, Upper back, Lungs, Chest, Breast, Uterus, Heat, Mind, Temple, Face, Eyes, Ears, Nose, Entire body

**Main Functions:** Strongly descends Qi. Dispels stasis. Alleviates pain. Clears the chest. Induces menstruation and labour.

**Indications:**
Pain in the shoulder region, stiffness of the neck in conditions like cervical spondylosis and ankylosing spondylitis, hyper-thyroidism, functional uterine bleeding. Headaches, trigeminal neuralgia.

**Manipulation:** 1.0 cun perpendicularly.

Moxibustion applicable.

**Cautions:** Contra-indicated in pregnancy. Deep perpendicular insertion may penetrate the Lung.

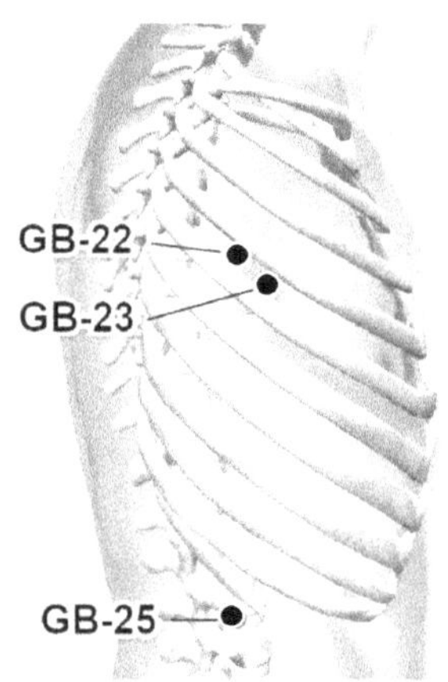


# GB-22 Yuanye
(ARMPIT ABYSS)

MUSCLE MERIDIAN MEETING POINT OF THE 3 ARM YIN.

**Location:**
On the midaxillary line, with the arm abducted approximately 3 cun inferior to the apex of the axilla, in the 4th intercostal space (according to some other text, in the 5th intercostal space).

**Dermatome:** T5

**Main Action Areas:** Axilla, Breast, Ribs

**Main Functions:** Loosens the chest and normalizes Qi, soothes the sinews and quickens the connecting vessels.

**Indications:**
Fullness of the chest, swelling of the axillary region, pain in the hypochondriac region, pain and motor impairment of the arm.

**Manipulation:** Oblique or subcutaneous insertion .3 - .5 cun.

**Cautions:** Contra-indicated for moxibustion. Deep perpendicular insertion may penetrate the Lung.

# GB-23 Zhejin
(FLANK SINEWS)

MEETING POINT OF THE GALL BLADDER AND BLADDER CHANNELS.

**Location:**
1 cun anterior to GB-22 (on the midaxillary line, 3 cun inferior to the apex of the axilla in the 4th intercostal space).

**Dermatome:** T5

**Main Functions:** Courses the Liver and rectifies Qi, calms dyspnea and downbears counterflow.

**Indications:**
Fullness of the chest, pain in the hypochondriac region, asthma.

**Manipulation:** Oblique or subcutaneous insertion .3 - .5 cun.

Moxibustion applicable.

**Cautions:** Deep perpendicular insertion may penetrate the Lung.

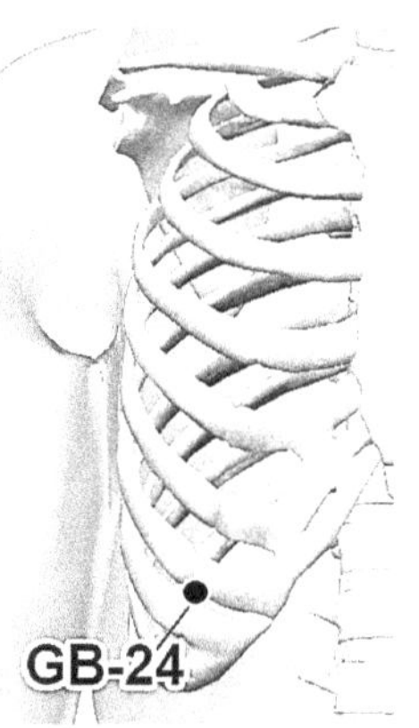


# GB-24 Riyue
(SUN AND MOON)

FRONT-MU (ALARM) POINT OF THE GB CHANNEL.

**Location:** On the nipple line in the 7th intercostal space (directly below Qimen (LIV-14) which lies in the 6th intercostal space.)

**Dermatome:** T7

**Main Action Areas:** Hypochondrium, Ribs, Gallbladder, Chest, Epigastrium, Abdomen

**Main Functions:** Regulates Gallbladder and Liver Qi. Alleviates pain. Dispels dampness and heat

**Indications:** Cholecystitis, hepatitis, hiccough, gastritis.

**Manipulation:** Oblique or subcutaneous insertion .3 - .5 cun.

Moxibustion applicable.

**Cautions:** Deep perpendicular insertion may penetrate the Lung.

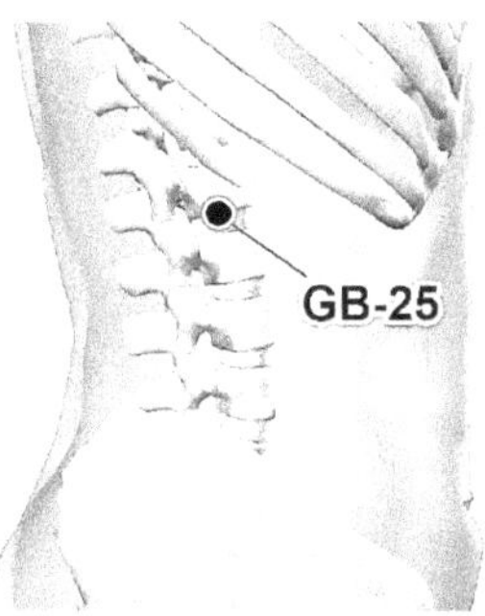


# GB-25 Jingmen

(CAPITAL GATE)

ALARM POINT (MU-FRONT) OF THE KIDNEY.

**Location:**
At the free end of the 12th rib.

**Dermatome:** T8-T10

**Main Action Areas:** Kidneys, Lumbar area, Flank

**Main Functions:** Benefits the Kidneys. Transforms dampness and heat. Regulates Qi and Blood. Alleviates pain

**Indications:**
Nephritis, costal pain, abdominal distension, flatulence.

**Manipulation:** Perpendicular insertion 0.3 - 0.5 cun.

Moxibustion applicable.

**Cautions:** Deep perpendicular insertion may penetrate the peritoneal cavity.

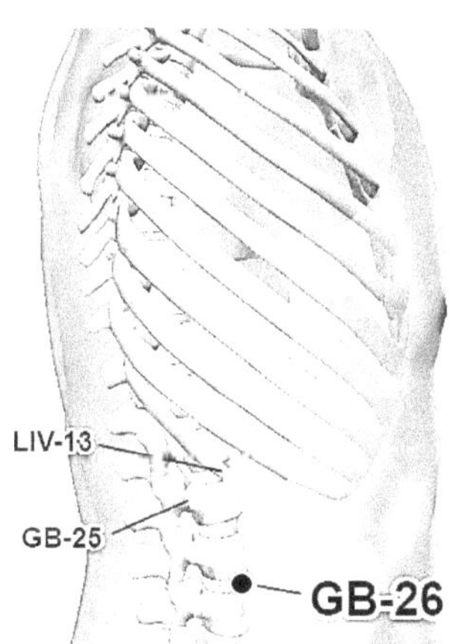


# GB-26 Daimai

(GIRDLING VESSEL)

MEETING POINT OF THE GALL BLADDER CHANNEL WITH THE GIRDLING (DIA) VESSEL.

**Location:**
At the level of the umbilicus, on the mid-point of a vertical line drawn between the free ends of the 11th and 12th ribs.

**Dermatome:** T10

**Main Action Areas:** Abdomen, Sides, Lumbar area, Uterus, Girdle Vessel

**Main Functions:** Clears dampness and heat. Benefits the lower jiao. Regulates menstruation. Aids in weight loss

**Indications:**
Pelvic disorders, costal pain, back pain.

**Manipulation:** Perpendicular insertion 0.5 - 0.8 cun.

Moxibustion applicable.

**Cautions:** Deep perpendicular insertion may penetrate the peritoneal cavity.

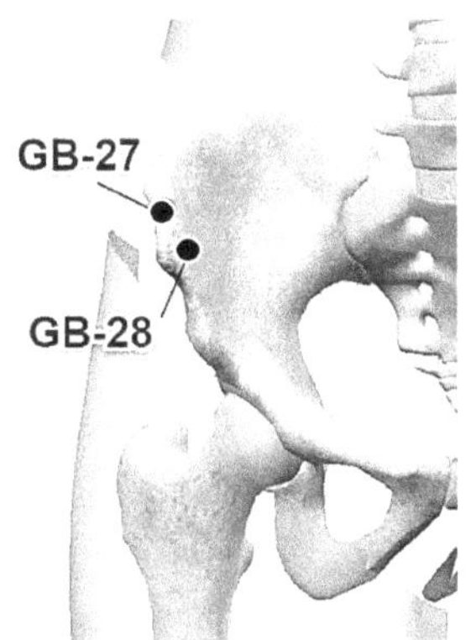


# GB-27 – Wushu

(FIFTH PIVOT)

MEETING POINT OF THE GALL BLADDER CHANNEL WITH THE GIRDLING (DIA) VESSEL.

**Location:**
In the depression medial to the anterior superior iliac spine (ASIS), approximately 3 cun inferior to the umbilicus.

**Dermatome:** T11/T12

**Main Action Areas:** Lower abdomen, Uterus, Intestines, Testicles

**Main Functions:** Regulates the lower jiao. Alleviates pain.

**Indications:**
Leukorrhea, lower abdominal pain, lumbar pain, hernia, constipation.

**Manipulation:** Perpendicular insertion 0.5 – 1.0 cun.

Moxibustion applicable.

# GB-28 Weidao

(LINKING PATH)

MEETING POINT OF THE GALL BLADDER CHANNEL WITH THE GIRDLING (DIA) VESSEL.

**Location:**
On the lateral aspect of the abdomen, anterior and inferior to the anterior superior iliac spine (ASIS), approximately 0.5 cun anterior and inferior to GB-27.

**Dermatome:** T11/T12

**Main Action Areas:** Lower abdomen, Uterus, Intestines, Testicles

**Main Functions:** Regulates the lower jiao. Alleviates pain.

**Indications:**
Leukorrhea, lower abdominal pain, hernia, prolapse of uterus

**Manipulation:** Perpendicular insertion 0.5 – 1.0 cun.

Moxibustion applicable.

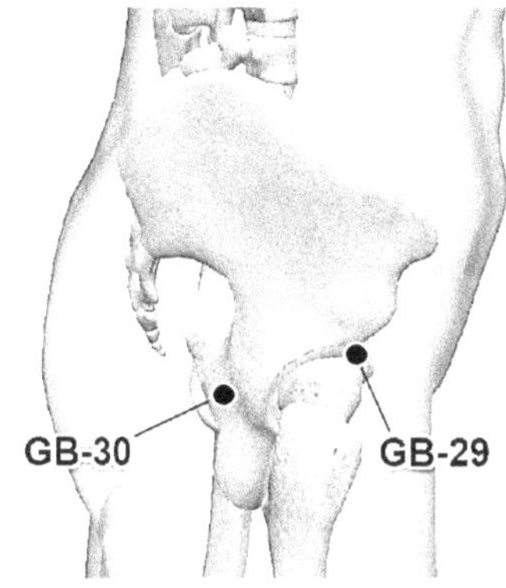


# GB-29 Juliao

(STATIONARY CREVICE)

MEETING POINT OF THE GALL BLADDER CHANNEL WITH THE YANG LINKING VESSEL.

**Location:**
At the midpoint of a line connecting the anterior superior iliac spine (ASIS) and the greater trochanter, at the anterior border of the iliac crest.

**Dermatome:** L1/L2

**Main Action Areas:** Hip, Thigh

**Main Functions:** Alleviates pain. Dispels stasis. Restores mobility to the hip.

**Indications:**
Pain and numbness in the thigh and lumbar region, paralysis, muscular atrophy of the lower limbs.

**Manipulation:** Perpendicular insertion 0.5 – 1.0 cun.

Moxibustion applicable.

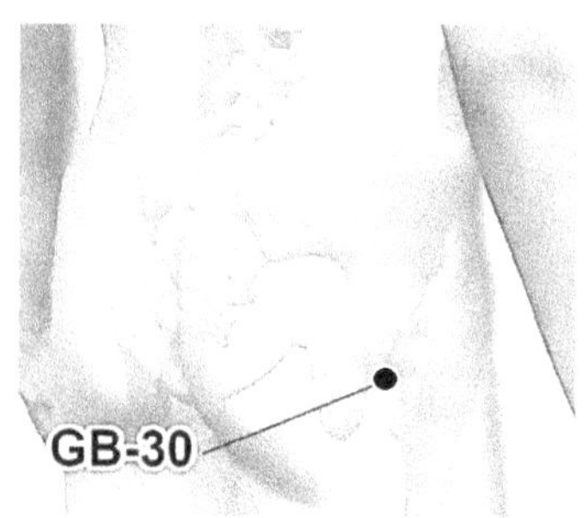


# GB-30 Huantiao

(JUMPING CIRCLE)

MEETING POINT OF THE GALL BLADDER CHANNEL AND BLADDER CHANNELS. MA DAN-YANG HEAVENLY STAR POINT.

**Location:**
Draw a line between the highest point of the greater trochanter and the sacral hiatus: the point is situated at the junction of the outer third with the medial two-thirds on this line. It is located more easily in a recumbent lateral or prone position.

**Dermatome:** L2 and S3 junction

**Main Action Areas:** Thigh. Entire lower limb, Lumbar area, Sciatic nerve

**Main Functions:** Dispels wind, cold and dampness. Regulates Qi and Blood. Alleviates pain. Strengthens the lower back

**Indications:** Sciatica, prolapsed lumbar disc, paralysis of the lower extremities, disorders of the hip joint.

**Manipulation:** Deep perpendicular insertion with a long needle (about 5 cun in length). When the needle reaches the sciatic nerve, a sensation like an electric current will be felt travelling down the leg to the ankle region. When this sensation (deqi) is elicited, good therapeutic results may be expected.

Moxibustion applicable.

**Remarks:** This is a very effective point for treating acute sciatica.

Widely used for disorders of the hip, thigh, entire lower limb, and gluteal and lower back areas.

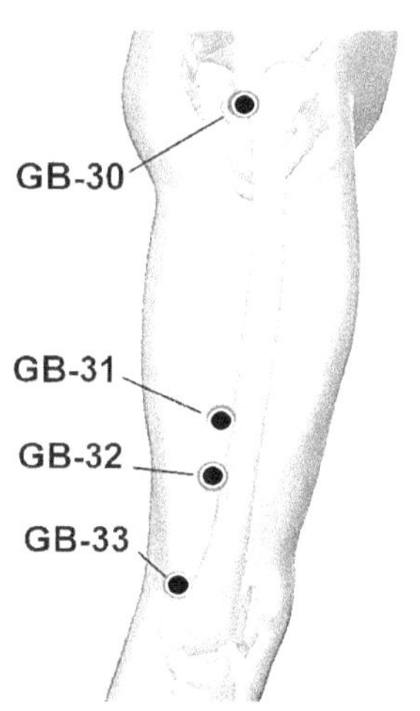


# GB-31 Fengshi

(WIND MARKET)

**Location:**
a) On the lateral aspect of the thigh, 7 cun proximal to the transverse popliteal crease, between the vastus lateralis and biceps femoris muscles.
b) with the patient standing erect or lying supine hand placed on the lateral side of the thigh, this point lies immediately distal to the tip of the middle finger.

**Shared location with Tung:** 88.25

**Dermatome:** L2

**Main Action Areas:** Thigh, Entire lower limb

**Main Functions:** Dispels wind and dampness. Regulates Qi. Alleviates pain

**Indications:**
Paralysis and pain of the lower extremities, paraesthesia in the distribution of the lateral cutaneous nerve of the thigh (meralgia paraesthetica).

**Manipulation:** 1.5 cun perpendicularly.

Moxibustion applicable.

# GB-32 Zhongdu

(MIDDLE DITCH)

**Location:**
On the lateral aspect of the thigh, 5 cun proximal to the popliteal crease, between the vastus lateralis and biceps femoris muscles.

**Shared location with Tung:** A.01

**Dermatome:** L2

**Main Action Areas:** Lateral thigh

**Main Functions:** Dissipates wind and cold. Dispels stasis of Qi and Blood. Alleviates pain.

**Indications:**
Pain and soreness of the thigh and knee, numbness and weakness of the lower limbs, hemiplegia.

**Manipulation:** Perpendicular insertion 0.7 – 1.0 cun.

Moxibustion applicable.

# GB-33 Xiyangguan

(KNEE YANG GATE)

**Location:**
On the lateral aspect of the knee. With the knee flexed, in the depression between the shaft and the lateral epicondyle and the tendon of the biceps femoris muscle, approximately 3 cun proximal to GB-34.

**Dermatome:** L2

**Main Action Areas:** Knee, Lateral thigh

**Main Functions:** Dissipates wind and cold. Dispels stasis of Qi and Blood. Alleviates pain.

**Indications:**
Swelling and pain of knee, contracture of tendons in popliteal fossa, numbness of leg.

**Manipulation:** Perpendicular insertion 0.5 – 1.0 cun.

**Cautions:** No Moxibustion.

# GB-34 Yanglingquan

(YANG MOUND SPRING)

HE-SEA, EARTH POINT OF THE GALL BLADDER CHANNEL. INFLUENTIAL POINT OF THE SINEWS. MA DAN-YANG HEAVENLY STAR POINT. LOWER HE-SEA OF THE GALL BLADDER.

**Location:**
a) In the depression anterior and inferior to the head of the fibula; or

b) at the meeting point of the two lines, one drawn vertically on the anterior margin of the head of the fibula, the other horizontally at neck of the fibula.

**Dermatome:** L5

**Main Action Areas:** Sinews (muscles, tendons, ligaments and other soft tissues), Joints, Flank,

Hypochondrium, Gallbladder, Chest, Entire body.

**Main Functions:** Regulates Qi. Smoothed the Gallbladder and Liver. Dissipates stagnation. Alleviates pain. Benefits the sinews.

**Indications:**
Hemiplegia, pain and paralysis of the leg, diseases of the gall bladder, muscle and tendon disorders, mental disorders, epilepsy.

**Manipulation:** Perpendicular insertion 0.7 – 1.0 cun.

Moxibustion applicable.

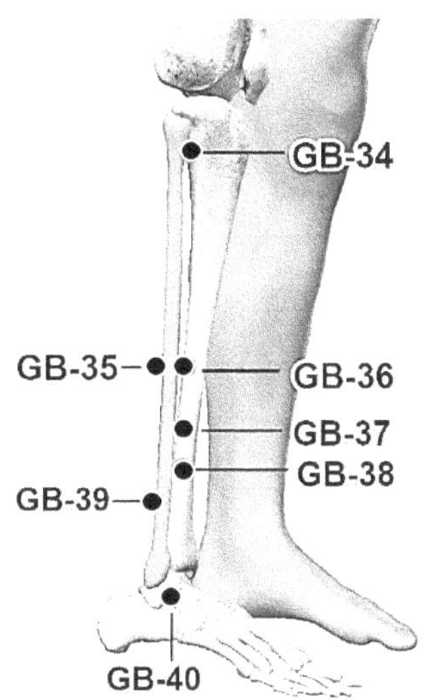


# GB-35 Yangjiao

(YANG INTERSECTION)

XI-CLEFT OF THE YANG LINKING VESSEL.

**Location:**
7 cun proximal to the highest prominence of the lateral malleolus, on the posterior border of the fibula.

**Dermatome:** L5/S1

**Main Action Areas:** Leg, Yang Wei Mai

**Main Functions:** Relaxes sinews, removes obstructions from the channel, stops pain.

**Indications:**
Fullness of chest and hypochondriac region, muscular atrophy, paralysis of leg.

**Manipulation:** Perpendicular insertion 0.5 – 0.8 cun.

Moxibustion applicable.

# GB-36 Waiqiu

(OUTER MOUND)

XI-CLEFT POINT OF THE GALL BLADDER CHANNEL.

**Location:**
7 cun proximal to the highest prominence of the lateral malleolus, on the anterior border of the fibula.

**Dermatome:** L5/S1

**Main Action Areas:** Leg, Gallbladder

**Main Functions:** Alleviates pain. Clears the Gallbladder.

**Indications:**
Pain in the neck, chest, thigh and hypochondriac region, chills and fever that accompany rabies.

**Manipulation:** Perpendicular insertion 0.5 – 0.8 cun.

Moxibustion applicable.

# GB-37 Guangming

(BRIGHT LIGHT)

LUO POINT OF THE GALL BLADDER CHANNEL

**Location:**
5 cun above the tip of the lateral malleolus, on the anterior border of the fibula.

**Dermatome:** S1

**Main Action Areas:** Eyes

**Main Functions:** Benefits eyesight and brightens the eyes. Regulates the Gallbladder

**Indications:**
Pain in the knee, muscular atrophy, motor impairment and pain of the lower extremities, blurring of vision, ophthalmalgia, night blindness, distending pain in the breast.

**Manipulation:** Perpendicular insertion 0.7 – 1.0 cun.

Moxibustion applicable.

# GB-38 Yangfu

(YANG ASSISTANCE)

JING-RIVER, SEDATION, AND FIRE POINT OF THE GALL BLADDER CHANNEL.

**Location:**
4 cun proximal to the highest prominence of the lateral malleolus, on the anterior border of the fibula.

**Dermatome:** S1

**Main Action Areas:** Gallbladder fu and channel

**Main Functions:** Subdues Liver yang, clears heat, resolves damp-heat.

**Indications:**
Migraine, pain of the outer canthus, pain in the axillary region, scrofula, lumbar pain, pain in the chest, pain in the hypochondriac region and lateral aspect of the lower extremities, malaria.

**Manipulation:** Perpendicular insertion 0.5 – 0.7 cun.

Moxibustion applicable.

# GB-39 Xuanzhong

(HANGING BELL)

INFLUENTIAL POINT FOR MARROW. GROUP LOU FOR THE 3 LEG YANG. LOWER HE-SEA OF THE TRIPLE ENERGIZER.

**Location:** 3 cun above the tip of the lateral malleolus, on the posterior border of the fibula.

**Shared location with Tung:** 77.05

**Dermatome:** S1

**Main Action Areas:** Neck, Spine, Joints, Bones, Marrow, Sinews

**Main Functions:** Benefits the Marrow, Sinews and bones. Clears heat. Regulates the Gallbladder channel

**Indications:** Paralysis of the lower limbs, stiffness of neck, disorders of the marrow.

**Manipulation:** Perpendicular insertion 0.3 – 0.5 cun.

Moxibustion applicable.

# GB-40 Qiuxu

(MOUND OF RUINS)

YUAN-SOURCE POINT OF THE GALL BLADDER CHANNEL. LOWER HE-SEA OF THE BLADDER.

**Location:**
At the meeting point of two lines, one drawn vertically on the anterior border of the lateral malleolus, the other horizontally on its inferior border.

**Dermatome:** S1

**Main Action Areas:** Ankle, Foot, Gallbladder, Mind, Emotions

**Main Functions:** Promotes the smooth flow of Liver Qi.

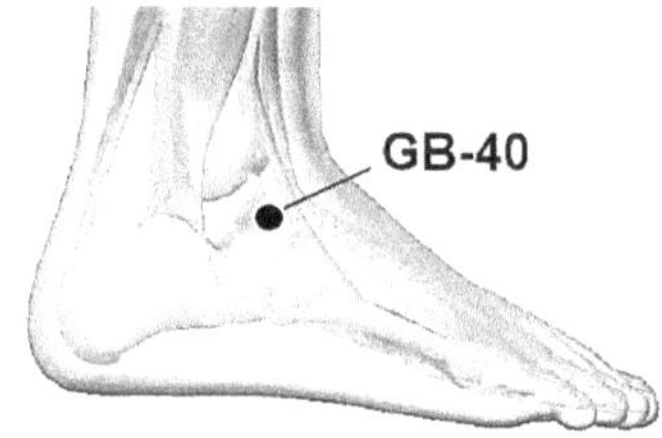


**Indications:**
Pain in the neck, swelling in the axillary region, pain in the hypochondriac region, vomiting, acid regurgitation, muscular atrophy of the lower limbs, malaria, pain and swelling of the external malleolus.

**Manipulation:** Perpendicular insertion 0.3 – 0.5 cun.

Moxibustion applicable.

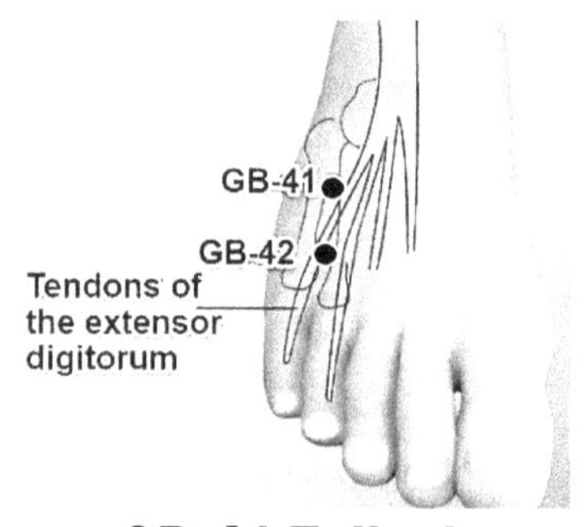


# GB-41 Zulinqi

(FOOT GOVERNOR OF TEARS)

SHU-STREAM, HORARY, AND WOOD POINT OF THE GALL BLADDER CHANNEL. MASTER POINT OF THE GIRDLING VESSEL. COMMAND POINT OF THE YANG LINKING VESSEL. EXIT POINT.

**Location:** In the depression immediately distal to the junction of the bases of the 4$^{th}$ and 5$^{th}$ metatarsals.

**Shared location with Tung:** 66.09

**Dermatome:** S1

**Main Action Areas:** Gallbladder channel, Foot, Breast, Flanks, Abdomen, Dai Mai, Gallbladder, Head, Eyes, Mind

**Main Functions:** Regulates Qi. Clears dampness and heat. Regulates the Dai Mai

**Indications:** Pain in the foot, breast disorders, ear disorders.

**Manipulation:** Perpendicular insertion 0.3 – 0.5 cun.

Moxibustion applicable.

# GB-42 Diwuhui

(EARTH FIVE MEETINGS)

**Location:**
Between the 4th and 5th metatarsal bones, proximal to the metatarso-phalangeal joints and medial to the tendon of the extensor digitorum longus muscle.

**Dermatome:** S1

**Main Action Areas:** Foot

**Main Functions:** Alleviates regional pain.

**Indications:** Pain of the canthus, tinnitus, distending pain of the breast, swelling and pain of the dorsum of foot.

**Manipulation:** Perpendicular insertion 0.3 – 0.5 cun.

**Cautions:** No Moxibustion.

# GB-43 Jiaxi/Xiaxi

(CLAMPED STREAM)

**Location:**
Between the 4th and 5th toes, proximal to the margin of the interdigital web.

**Shared location with Tung:** 66.08

**Dermatome:** S1

**Main Action Areas:** Gallbladder, Head, Eyes, Mind

**Main Functions:** Clears heat. Descends Yang. Clears the head, ears and eyes.

**Indications:**
Headache, dizziness, vertigo, pain in outer canthus, tinnitus, deafness, swelling of the cheek, pain in hypochondriac region, distending pain of the breast, febrile diseases.

**Manipulation:** Perpendicular insertion 0.3 – 0.5 cun.

Moxibustion applicable.

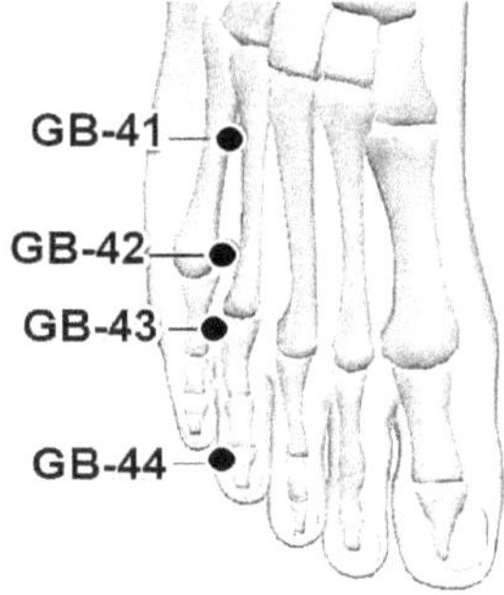


# GB-44 Zuqiaoyin

(FOOT PORTAL YIN)

JING-WELL POINT AND METAL POINT OF THE GALL BLADDER CHANNEL.

**Location:**
On the 4th toe, 0.1 cun from the lateral corner of the nail.

**Dermatome:** S1

**Main Action Areas:** Gallbladder channel, Head, Eyes, Mind

**Main Functions:** Restores consciousness. Clears the head and brain. Benefits the eyes.

**Indications:**
Migraine, deafness, tinnitus, ophthalmalgia, dream-disturbed sleep, febrile diseases.

**Manipulation:** Perpendicular insertion about 0.1 cun.

Moxibustion and prick to bleed applicable.

# LIVER MERIDIAN (Foot Jue Yin)

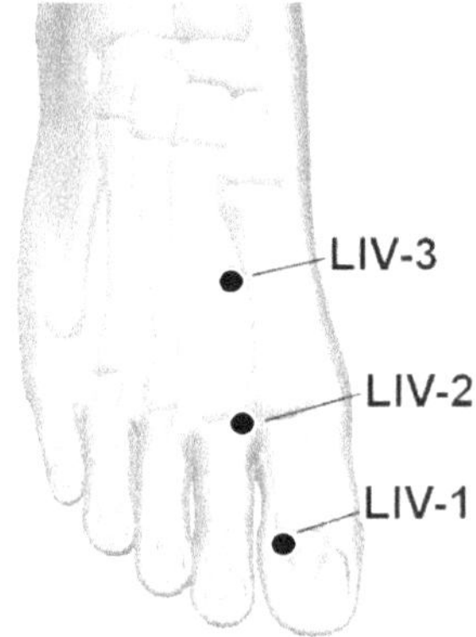


# LIV-1 Dadun

(BIG MOUND)

JING-WELL, HORARY, AND WOOD POINT OF THE LIVER CHANNEL. ENTRY POINT.

**Location:**
On the lateral aspect of the big toe, 0.1 cun proximal and lateral to the corner of the nail.

**Dermatome:** L5

**Main Action Areas:** Head, Nervous system, Uterus

**Main Functions:** Subdues interior wind. Calms the mind. Arrests bleeding.

**Indications:**
Hernia, enuresis, uterine bleeding, prolapse of the uterus, epilepsy.

**Manipulation:** Oblique insertion .1 - .2 cun, or prick to cause bleeding.

Moxibustion is applicable, except in pregnancy.

# LIV-2 Xingjian
(MOVING BETWEEN)

YING-SPRING, SEDATION, AND FIRE POINT OF THE LIVER CHANNEL.

**Location:**
Between the 1st and 2nd toes, proximal to the margin of the interdigital web.

**Shared location with Tung:** 66.03

**Dermatome:** L5

**Main Action Areas:** Head, Eyes, Nervous system, Abdomen

**Main Functions:** Clears heat and drains fire. Descends excessive Yang. Regulates Liver Qi.

**Indications:**
Incessant menorrhagia; urinary tract pain; enuresis; urinary stoppage; hernia; wryness of the mouth; red, swollen, painful eyes; pain in the lateral costal region; headache; visual dizziness; epilepsy; convulsive spasms; insomnia.

**Manipulation:** Oblique insertion 0.3 – 0.5 cun.

Moxibustion applicable.

# LIV-3 Taichung
(GREAT RUSHING)

SHU STREAM, YUAN-SOURCE AND EARTH POINT OF THE LIVER CHANNEL. MA DAN-YANG HEAVENLY STAR POINT.

**Location:**
2 cun proximal to the margin of web of the 1st and 2nd toes.

**Shared location with Tung:** 66.04

**Dermatome:** L5

**Main Action Areas:** Entire body, Abdomen, Digestive system, Reproductive systems, Chest, Head, Eyes, Nervous system, Muscles and sinews, Mind, Foot

**Main Functions:** Regulates Liver Qi. Dispels stasis. Alleviates pain. Nourishes Yin and Blood. Cools the Liver. Regulates menstruation. Calms the mind.

**Indications:**
Hypertension, headache, dizziness and vertigo, insomnia, congestion, swelling and pain of the eye, depression, infantile convulsion, deviation of mouth, pain in the hypochondriac region, uterine bleeding, hernia, enuresis, retention of urine, epilepsy, pain in the anterior aspect of the medial malleolus.

**Manipulation:** Perpendicular insertion 0.3 – 0.5 cun.

Moxibustion applicable.

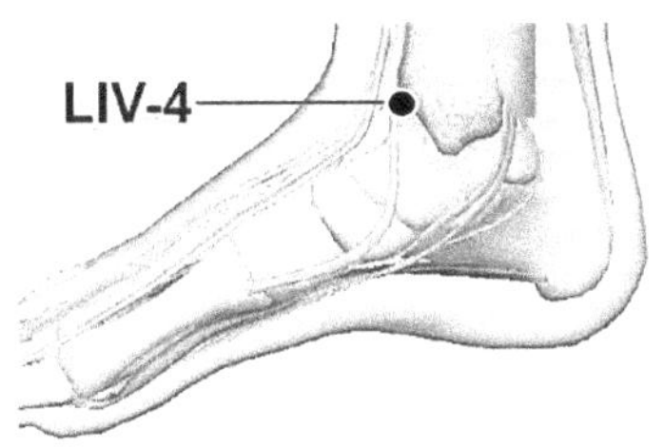


# LIV-4 Zhongfeng
(MIDDLE SEAL)

JING-RIVER AND METAL POINT OF THE LIVER CHANNEL.

**Location:**
1 cun anterior to the prominence of the medial malleolus, medial to the tendon of the tibialis anterior muscle.

**Dermatome:** L5

**Main Action Areas:** Ankle, Abdomen

**Main Functions:** Regulates Liver Qi. Harmonises the lower jiao. Alleviates swelling and pain.

**Indications:**
Hernia, pain in the external genitalia, nocturnal emission, retention of urine, distending pain in the hypochondrium.

**Manipulation:** Perpendicularly 0.3  0.5 cun.

Moxibustion applicable.

# LIV-5 Ligou
(WOODWORM CANAL)

LUO POINT OF THE LIVER CHANNEL.

**Location:**
On the medial aspect of the lower leg, 5 cun proximal to the highest

prominence of the medial malleolus, just posterior to the medial crest of the tibia, between the crest of the tibia and the gastrocnemius muscle.

**Dermatome:** L4

**Main Action Areas:** Genitourinary system, Mind, Liver

**Main Functions:** Regulates Liver Qi. Benefits the genitals and uterus. Clears damp heat

**Indications:** Retention of urine, enuresis, hernia, irregular menstruation, leukorrhea, pruritus or itchy vulvae, weakness and atrophy of the leg.

**Manipulation:**
0.5–1 cun vertically or obliquely in a posterior direction towards the fibula or transversely (subcutaneously) along the tibia towards the abdomen.

Moxibustion applicable.

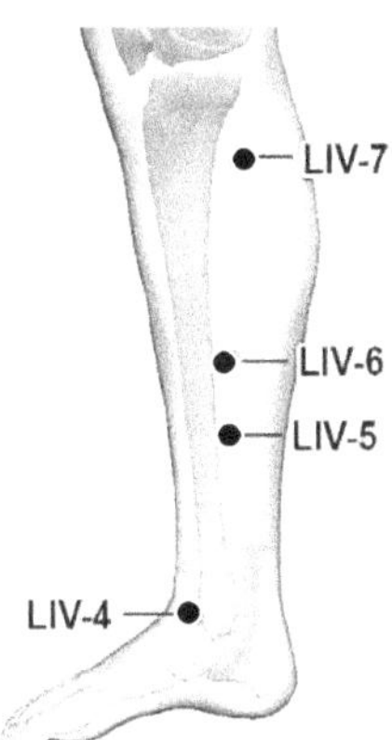


# LIV-6 Zhongdu
(CENTRAL CAPITAL)

XI-CLEFT POINT OF THE LIVER CHANNEL.

**Location:**
7 cun proximal to the highest prominence of the medial malleolus, just posterior to the medial crest of the tibia.

**Dermatome:** L4

**Main Action Areas:** Leg, Liver

**Main Functions:** Dispels Blood stasis. Alleviates pain

**Indications:**
Abdomen and hypochondriac pain, diarrhea, hernia, uterine bleeding, prolonged lochia.

**Manipulation:** 0.5–1 cun vertically or obliquely in a posterior direction towards the fibula or transversely (subcutaneously) in a proximal direction along the tibia.

Moxibustion applicable.

## LIV-7 Xiguan
### (Knee Joint)

**Location:**
At the junction of the shaft and the medial condyle of the tibia, 1 cun posterior to SP-9.

**Dermatome:** L4

**Main Action Areas:** Knees

**Main Functions:** Dispels dampness. Alleviates swelling and pain

**Indications:**
Pain of the knee, especially if pain in on the inner (medial) knee.

**Manipulation:** Perpendicular insertion 0.5 – 1.0 cun.

Moxibustion applicable.

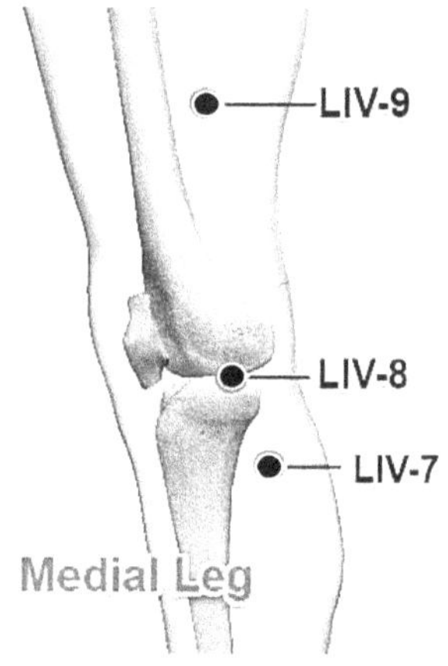


## LIV-8 Ququan
### (Spring at the Crook)

He-Sea, Tonification and Water point of the Liver channel.

**Location:** With the knee flexed, LIV-8 is located directly proximal to the medial end of the popliteal crease, in a depression anterior to the tendons of the semitendinosus and semi-membranosus muscles.

**Dermatome:** L3/L4

**Main Action Areas:** Lower jiao, Genitourinary system, Uterus, Knee

**Main Functions:** Nourishes Blood and Yin. Cools the Liver. Clears dampness and heat.

**Indications:**
Prolapse of uterus, lower abdominal pain, retention of urine, nocturnal emission, pain the external genitalia, pruritus vulvae, pain in medial aspect of the knee and thigh.

**Manipulation:** Perpendicular insertion 0.5 – 1.0 cun.

Moxibustion applicable.

## LIV-9 Yinbao
### (Yin Wrapping)

**Location:**
4 cun proximal to the medial condyle of the femur, between the sartorius and vastus medialis muscles.

**Dermatome:** L3

**Main Action Areas:** Genitals, Uterus, Thigh

**Main Functions:** Regulates Qi. Benefits the lower jiao. Alleviates pain.

**Indications:**
Pain in the lumbosacral region, lower abdominal pain, enuresis, retention of urine, irregular menstruation.

**Manipulation:** Perpendicular insertion 0.5 – 0.7 cun.

Moxibustion applicable.

## LIV-10 Zuwuli
### (Leg Five Miles)

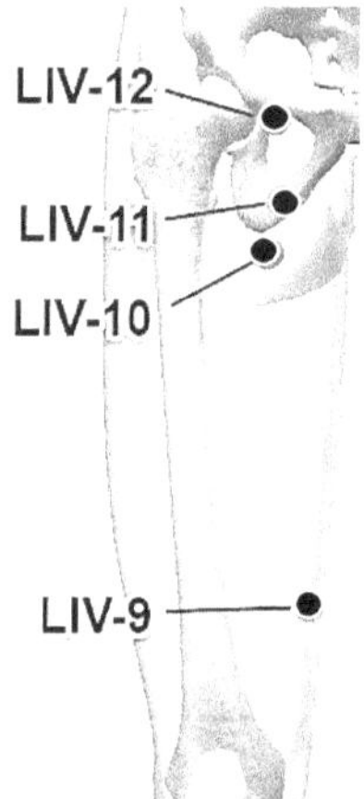


**Location:**
On the anterior aspect of the thigh, 3 cun inferior to the upper border of the symphysis, on the lateral border of the adductor longus muscle.

**Dermatome:** L1

**Main Action Areas:** Thigh, Groin, Genitals

**Main Functions:** Regulates Qi and dispels stasis. Dissipates cold from the Liver channel. Alleviates pain

**Indications:**
Lower abdominal distension and fullness, retention of urine.

**Manipulation:** Vertically 0.5–1.5 cun. Moxibustion applicable.

**Caution:** Great saphenous vein, femoral artery/nerve.

## LIV-11 Yinlian
### (Yin Corner)

**Location:**
On the anterior aspect of the thigh, 2 cun inferior to the upper border of the symphysis and on the lateral border of the adductor longus muscle.

**Dermatome:** L1

**Main Action Areas:** Thigh, Genitals, Uterus

**Main Functions:** Dispels cold and pain

**Indications:**
Irregular menstruation, leukorrhea, lower abdominal pain, pain in the thigh and leg.

**Manipulation:** Vertically 0.5–1.0 cun. Moxibustion for female sterility.

**Caution:** Great saphenous vein, femoral artery/vein/nerve.

## LIV-12 Jimai
### (Urgent Pulse)

**Location:**
In the inguinal groove, 2.5 cun lateral to the anterior midline and 1 cun inferior to the upper border of the symphysis.

**Dermatome:** L1

**Main Action Areas:** Groin, Genitals, Blood vessels, Entire lower limb

**Main Functions:** Improves Qi and Blood circulation. Dispels cold. Alleviates pain

**Indications:**
Lower abdominal pain, hernia, pain in the external genitalia.

**Manipulation:** Slightly obliquely 0.5–0.8 cun.

**Caution:** Femoral artery/vein. To avoid injury to the vein, LIV-12 should not be needled medial to the artery. Owing to its tricky location, classical texts recommend moxi-bustion only, while in modern texts moxibustion is contraindicated for the same reason.

## LIV-13 Zhangmen
### (COMPLETION GATE)

FRONT-MU (ALARM) POINT OF THE SPLEEN CHANNEL. INFLUENTIAL POINT OF THE ZANG ORGANS, MEETING POINT OF THE LIVER AND SPLEEN CHANNELS. FRONT-MU POINT OF THE SPLEEN. HUI-MEETING POINT OF THE ZANG (5 YIN ORGANS). MEETING POINT OF THE LIVER AND GALLBLADDER CHANNELS.

**Location:**
At the free end of the llth rib.

**Dermatome:** T10/T11

**Main Action Areas:** Abdomen, Hypochondrium, Chest, Digestive system

**Main Functions:** Harmonises the Liver and Spleen. Boosts Spleen Qi

**Indications:**
Liver disorders, disorders of the Spleen. Abdominal distension, borborygmus, pain in the hypochondriac region, vomiting, diarrhea, indigestion.

**Manipulation:** Perpendicular insertion .5 - .8 cun. Moxibustion is applicable.

**Cautions:** Deep needling may injure an enlarged Spleen or Liver.

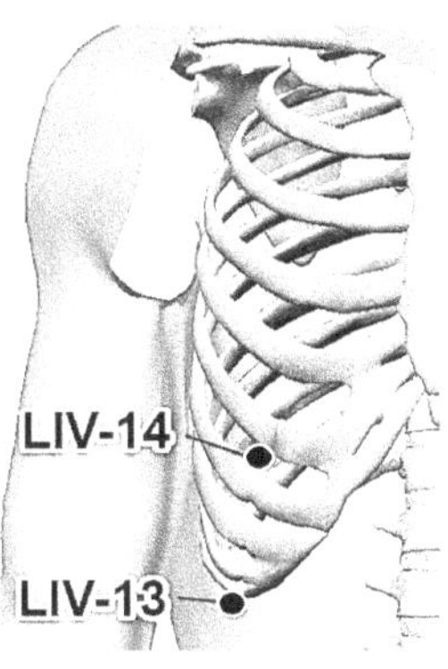


## LIV-14 Qimen
### FRONT-MU (ALARM) POINT OF THE LIVER CHANNEL

FRONT-MU (ALARM) POINT OF THE LIVER CHANNEL. MEETING POINT OF THE LIVER AND SPLEEN CHANNELS WITH THE YIN LINKING VESSEL. EXIT POINT.

**Location:** Vertically below the nipple, in the intercostal space between the 6th and 7th ribs.

**Dermatome:** T6

**Main Action Areas:** Hypochondrium, Chest, Breast, Abdomen

**Main Functions:** Regulates Liver Qi. Dispels stasis. Cools Blood.

**Indications:**
Hepatitis, chest pain. Hypochondriac pain, abdominal distension, hiccups, acid regurgitation, mastitis, depression, febrile diseases.

**Manipulation:** Oblique or sub-cutaneous insertion .3 - .5 cun.

Moxibustion is applicable.

**Cautions:**
Deep perpendicular needling has a risk of pneumothorax.

# DU (Governing Vessel, GV) MERIDIAN

## DU-1 Changqiang
### (LONG STRONG)

LUO-CONNECTING POINT OF THE GOVERNING VESSEL, MEETING POINT OF

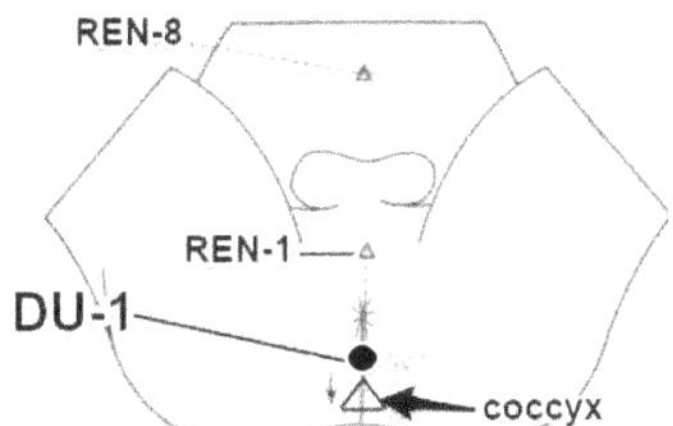


THE GOVERNING VESSEL WITH THE CONCEPTION VESSEL AND THE GALL BLADDER AND KIDNEY CHANNELS.

**Location:**
Midway between the tip of the coccyx and the anus., The point is best located with the patient in the prone or lateral position.

**Dermatome:** S4

**Main Action Areas:** Anus, Coccyx, Spine

**Main Functions:** Benefits the anus and rectum. Regulates Qi and alleviates pain. Benefits the spine

**Indications:**
Diarrhea, bloody stools, hemorrhoids, prolapse of the rectum, constipation, pain in the lower back, epilepsy.

**Manipulation:** Perpendicular or oblique insertion .5 - 1.0 cun right in front of the coccyx.

Moxibustion is applicable.

**Cautions:** Too deep insertion can injure the rectum.

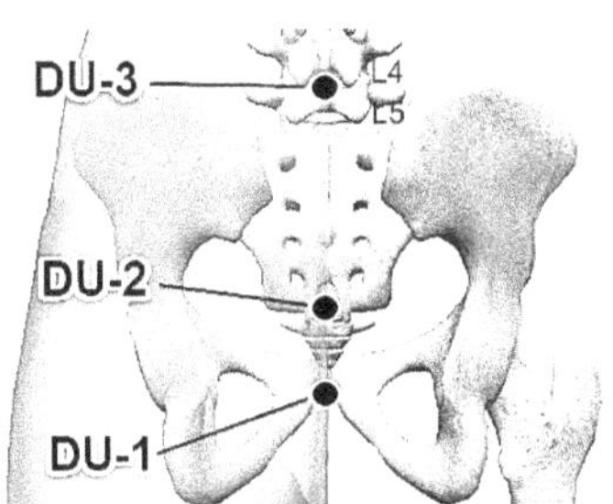


## DU-2 Yaoshu
### (LUMBAR SHU)

**Location:**
On the midline, in the sacral hiatus.

**Dermatome:** S3

**Main Action Areas:** Sacrum, Coccyx, Lumbar Spine

**Main Functions:** Regulates Qi and Blood. Alleviates pain. Benefits the spine.

**Indications:**
Irregular menstruation, pain and stiffness of the lower back, hemorrhoids, muscular atrophy of the lower extremities, epilepsy.

**Manipulation:** Oblique upward insertion 0.5 – 1.0 cun.

Moxibustion is applicable.

## DU-3 Yaoyangguan
### (LUMBAR YANG GATE)

**Location:**
On the back midline, between the dorsal spines of the 4th and 5th lumbar vertebrae (at the level of the upper border of the iliac crest).

**Dermatome:** T12/L1

**Main Action Areas:** Lumbar area, Spine, Lower limbs, Urogenital system, Uterus

**Main Functions:** Dispels dampness, heat and cold. Benefits the genitourinary system

**Indications:**
Irregular menstruation, nocturnal emission, impotence, pain in the lumbosacral region, muscular atrophy, motor impairment, numbness and pain of the lower extremities, epilepsy.

**Manipulation:** 1.0 cun perpendicularly, the needle may be tilted slightly upwards.

Moxibustion applicable.

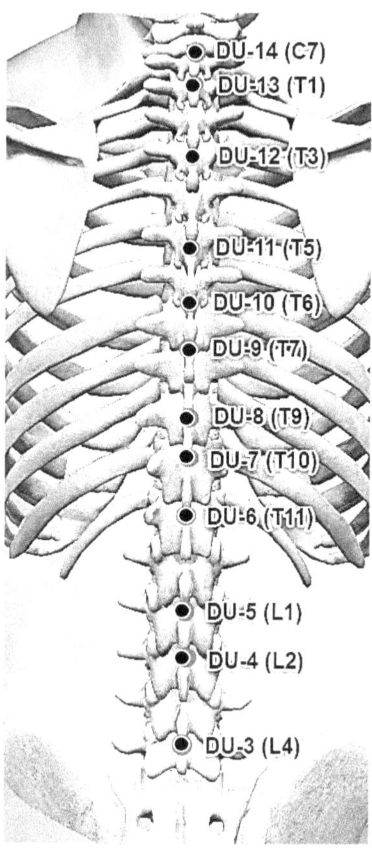



# DU-4 Mingmen
(GATE OF LIFE)

**Location:**
On the back midline, between the dorsal spines of the 2nd and 3rd lumbar vertebrae (at the level of the lower border of the rib cage).

**Dermatome:** T9-T12

**Main Action Areas:** Lumbar area, Spine, Lower limbs, Urogenital system, Uterus, Entire body

**Main Functions:** Tonifies Kidney jing and Kidney Yang. Dispels cold and dampness. Alleviates pain. Clears heat. Benefits the lower jiao and genitourinary system. Increases fertility and vitality. Treats chronic diseases.

**Indication:**
Stiffness of the back, lumbago, impotence, nocturnal emission, indigestion, irregular menstruation, diarrhea, leukorrhea.

**Manipulation:** 1.0cun perpendicularly; the needle may be tilted slightly upwards.

Moxibustion applicable only for over 20 years of age.

# DU-5 Xuanshu
(SUSPENDED PIVOT)

**Location:**
On the midline, below the spinous process of the 1st lumbar vertebra (L1).

**Dermatome:** T9-T12

**Main Action Areas:** Lumbar area, Spine

**Main Functions:** Strengthens the lumbar area. Alleviates pain. Boosts Spleen Qi and harmonises the Stomach.

**Indications:**
Pain and stiffness of the lower back, diarrhea, indigestion.

**Manipulation:** Perpendicular or oblique insertion upward .5 - 1.0 cun.

Moxibustion is applicable.

# DU-6 Jizhong
(CENTRE OF THE SPINE)

**Location:**
On the back midline, between the dorsal spines of the 11th and 12th thoracic vertebrae.

**Dermatome:** T8-T11

**Main Action Areas:** Spine, Middle jiao

**Main Functions:** Strengthens the spine and alleviates pain. Boosts Spleen Qi

**Indications:**
Haemorrhoids, epilepsy. This point causes muscular relaxation in spastic states.

**Manipulation:** 0.5 cun obliquely upwards.

**Caution:** No moxibustion

# DU-7 Zhongshu
(CENTRAL PIVOT)

**Location:**
On the midline, below the spinous process of the 10th thoracic vertebra (T10).

**Dermatome:** T8-T10

**Main Action Areas:** Spine, Stomach

**Main Functions:** Strengthens the spine. Alleviates pain.

**Indications:**
Pain in the epigastric region, lower back pain, stiffness of the back.

**Manipulation:** Perpendicular or oblique insertion .5 - 1.0 cun.

Moxibustion is applicable.

**Cautions:** Too deep insertion can injure the spinal canal.

# DU-8 Jinsuo
(SINEW CONTRACTION)

**Location:**
On the midline, below the spinous process of the 9th thoracic vertebra (T9).

**Dermatome:** T7-T9

**Main Action Areas:** Spine, Liver

**Main Functions:** Relaxes the spine and alleviates pain. Regulates Liver Qi.

**Indications:**
Epilepsy, stiffness of the back, gastric pain.

**Manipulation:** Perpendicular or oblique insertion .5 - 1.0 cun.

Moxibustion is applicable.

**Cautions:** Too deep insertion can injure the spinal canal.

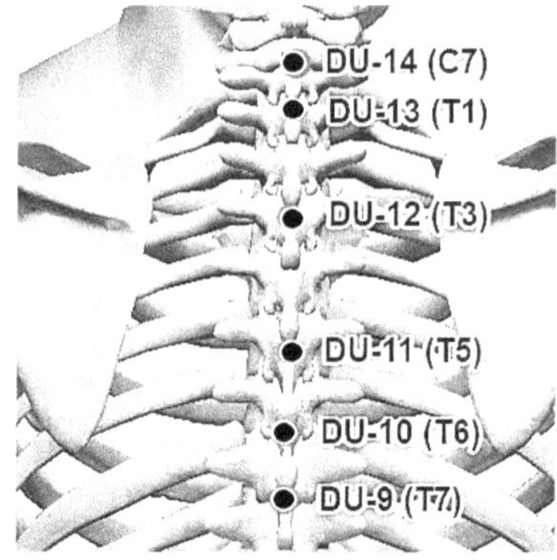



# DU-9 Zhiyang
(REACHING YANG)

**Location:**
On the midline, below the spinous process of the 7th thoracic vertebra (T7).

**Dermatome:** T6-T8

**Main Action Areas:** Spine, Diaphragm, Liver, Middle jiao

**Main Functions:** Clears dampness and heat. Regulates the Liver. Harmonises the middle jiao.

**Indications:**
Jaundice, cough, asthma, stiffness of the back, pain in the chest and back.

**Manipulation:** Perpendicular or oblique insertion upward .5 - 1.0 cun.

Moxibustion is applicable.

**Cautions:** The spinal canal lies beneath this point.

# DU-10 Lingtai
### (Spirit Tower)

**Location:**
On the midline, below the spinous process of the 6th thoracic vertebra (T6).

**Dermatome:** T6

**Main Action Areas:** Chest, Lungs, Spine, Spirit and Emotions

**Main Functions:** Treats cough. Clears heat. Alleviates pain. Calms spirit. Frees emotions.

**Indications:**
Cough, asthma, furuncles, back pain, neck rigidity.

**Manipulation:** Perpendicular or oblique insertion upward .5 - 1.0 cun.

Moxibustion is applicable.

**Cautions:** The spinal canal lies beneath this point. Several texts contra-indicate this point for needling

# DU-11 Shendao
### (Spirit Pathway)

**Location:**
On the back midline, between the dorsal spines of the 5th and 6th thoracic vertebrae.

**Dermatome:** T5

**Main Action Areas:** Chest, Heart, Spine

**Main Functions:** Regulates upper jiao Qi. Calms the mind.

**Indications:** Poor memory, anxiety, palpitation, pain and stiffness of the back, cough, cardiac pain.

**Manipulation:** 0.5 cun obliquely upwards.

Moxibustion is applicable.

**Cautions:** The spinal canal lies beneath this point. Several texts contra-indicate this point for needling

# DU-12 Shenzhu
### (Body Pillar)

**Location:**
On the midline, below the spinous process of the 3rd thoracic vertebra (T3).

**Dermatome:** T2/T3

**Main Action Areas:** Chest, Lungs, Spine

**Main Functions:** Eliminates interior wind, calms spasms, tonifies Lung Qi, strengthens the body.

**Indications:**
Cough, asthma, epilepsy, pain and stiffness of the back, furuncles.

**Manipulation:** Perpendicular or oblique insertion upward .5 - 1.0 cun.

Moxibustion is applicable.

**Cautions:** The spinal canal lies beneath this point.

# DU-13 Taodao
### (Way of Happiness)

Meeting point of the Governing vessel with the Bladder channel.

**Location:**
On the midline, below the spinous process of the 1st thoracic vertebra (T1).

**Dermatome:** T1

**Main Action Areas:** Chest, Lungs, Spine

**Main Functions:** Stiffness of the back, headache, malaria, febrile diseases.

**Indications:**
Clears heat, releases the exterior, regulates the Lesser Yang.

**Manipulation:** Perpendicular or oblique insertion upward .5 - 1.0 cun.

Moxibustion is applicable.

**Cautions:** The spinal canal lies beneath this point.

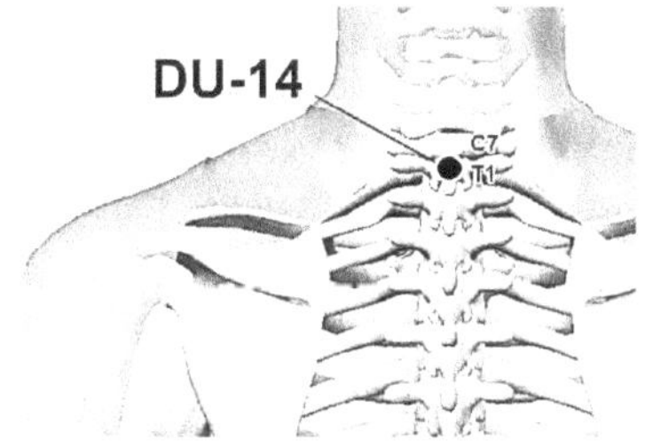


# DU-14 Dazhui
### (Large Vertebra)

Meeting point of the Governing vessel with the 6 Yang channels of the hand and foot. Point of the Sea of Qi.

**Location:**
On the back midline, between the dorsal spines of the 7th cervical (veterbra prominence) and the 1st thoracic vertebra.

**Dermatome:** C6-T1

**Main Action Areas:** Tai Yang area, Lungs, Chest, Heart, Mind, Cervical spine, Head

**Main Functions:** Regulates ascending and descending of Yang Qi. Clears heat. Subdues interior wind. Releases the exterior. Regulates Qi and Blood. Benefits the spine

**Indications:**
Neck pain and rigidity, malaria, febrile diseases, epilepsy, afternoon fever, cough, asthma, common cold, back stiffness.

**Manipulation:** Perpendicular or oblique insertion upward .5 - 1.0 cun.

Apply moxibustion for early cold and respiratory infections.

**Cautions:** The spinal canal lies beneath this point.

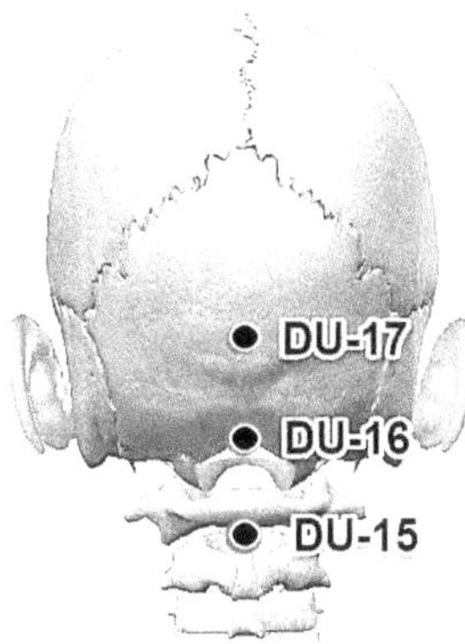


# DU-15 Yamen
### (Gate of Muteness)

Meeting point of the Governing and Yang Linking vessels. Point of the Sea of Qi and Bone.

**Location:**
a) At the nape of the neck on the midline, between the dorsal spines of the 1st and 2$^{nd}$ cervical vertebrae.
b) On the midline 0.5 cun above the posterior hairline.
c) On the midline 3.5 cun above the spinous process of the 7th cervical vetebrae when the head is erect.

**Shared location with Tung:** 1010.07

**Dermatome:** C3

**Main Action Areas:** Tongue, Head, Spine

**Main Functions:** Subdues wind. Benefits the tongue. Opens the sense organs and benefits the brain

**Indications:**
Mental disorders, epilepsy, deafness and mute, sudden hoarseness of voice, apoplexy, stiffness of the tongue and aphasia, occipital headache, neck rigidity.

**Manipulation:** This is a Dangerous point and improper needling can cause serious complications from damage to the medulla oblongata. The patient should be instructed to bend his neck slightly forwards and the needle should be inserted perpendicularly and slowly in the direction of the point of the chin. The depth of insertion should not generally exceed 1.0 cun and there should be no manipulation. If any discomfort is felt, the needle should be removed immediately.

Caution: No moxibustion.

# DU-16 Fengfu

(PALACE OF WIND)

MEETING POINT OF THE GOVERNING AND YANG LINKING VESSELS. POINT OF THE SEA OF MARROW AND BONE, WINDOW OF HEAVEN POINT, SUN SI-MIAO GHOST POINT.

**Location:**
a) At the nape of the neck, on the midline in the depression directly below the occipital protuberance.

b) On the midline 1.0 cun above the posterior hairline.

**Shared location with Tung:** 1010.07

**Dermatome:** C3

**Main Action Areas:** Head, Brain, Sense organs, Spine

**Main Functions:** Dissipates wind. Regulates Qi and Blood. Alleviates stiffness and pain. Clears the sense organs. Relaxes the body and calms the mind. Balances the nervous system

**Indications:**
Headache, neck rigidity, blurring of vision, epistaxis, sore throat, post-apoplexy, aphasia, hemiplegia, mental disorders.

**Manipulation:** This is very dangerous point. As in needling Yamen (DU-15.), care should be taken not to damage the medulla oblongata. It is

perhaps the most vulnerable acupuncture point in the body and it is best that the novice treats this as a Prohibited point. Also, unlike Yamen (DU-15). its usefulness is limited.

**Caution:** Moxibustion forbidden.

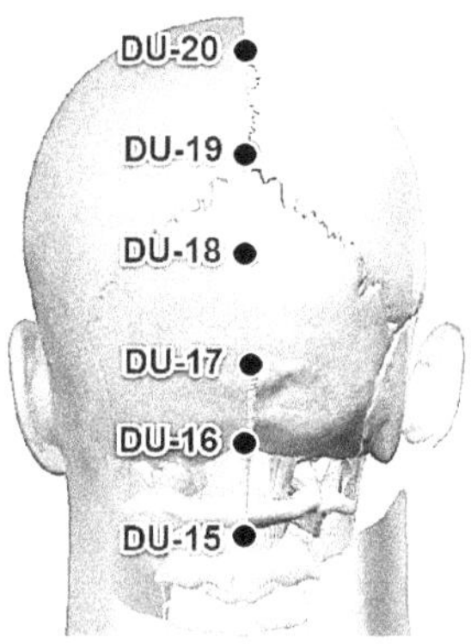


# DU-17 Naohu

(BRAIN'S DOOR)

MEETING POINT OF THE GOVERNING VESSEL AND THE BLADDER CHANNEL.

**Location:**
In a depression superior to the external occipital protuberance, approximately 2.5 cun superior to the posterior hairline or 1.5 cun superior to DU-16.

**Dermatome:** C2

**Main Action Areas:** Head, Sense organs

**Main Functions:** Dispels wind. Clears heat. Calms the mind.

**Indications:**
Epilepsy, dizziness, pain and stiffness of the neck.

**Manipulation:** Subcutaneous insertion .3 - .5 cun.

**Cautions:** According to several texts, this point is contra-indicated for needling and moxibustion.

# DU-18 Qiangjian

(UNYIELDING SPACE)

**Location:**
On the posterior midline, 1.5 cun superior to DU-17 (directly superior to the external occipital protuberance) or 3 cun inferior to DU-20 (on the vertex).

**Dermatome:** C2

**Main Action Areas:** Back of head. Brain

**Main Functions:** Sedates wind. Clears heat. Calms the mind.

**Indications:**
Headache, neck rigidity, blurring of vision, mania.

**Manipulation:** Subcutaneous insertion 0.3 - 0.5 cun.

Moxibustion is applicable.

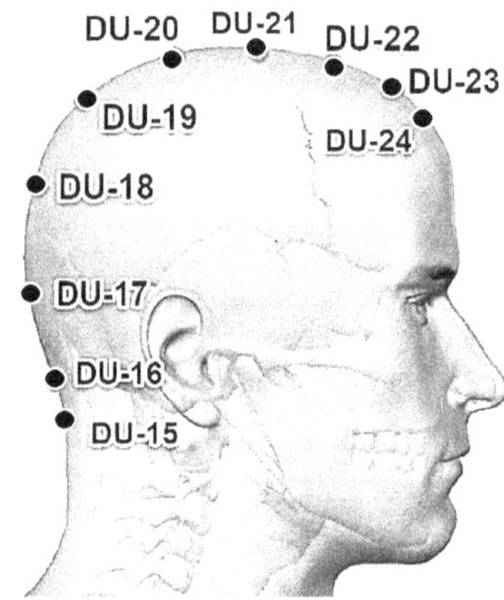


# DU-19 Houding

(BEHIND THE CROWN)

SEA POINT FOR BONE.

**Location:**
On the midline, 3 cun superior to DU-17 (directly superior to the external occipital protube-rance) or 1.5 cun posterior to DU-20.

**Shared location with Tung:** 1010.06

**Dermatome:** C2

**Main Action Areas:** Head, Brain

**Main Functions:** Dispels wind. Clears heat. Calms the mind.

**Indications:**
Headache, vertigo, epilepsy, mania.

**Manipulation:** Subcutaneous insertion 0.3 - 0.5 cun.

Moxibustion is applicable.

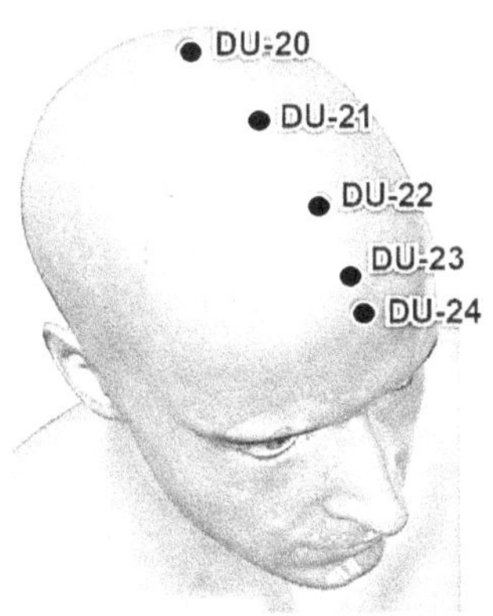

# DU-20 Baihui

(Hundred Meetings)

MEETING POINT OF THE GOVERNING VESSEL WITH THE BLADDER, GALL BLADDER, TRIPLE ENERGIZER, AND LIVER CHANNELS. POINT OF THE SEA OF MARROW AND BONE.

**Location:**
At the junction of a line connecting the apices of the ears and the midline, 5 cun from the anterior or 7 cun from the posterior hairline respectively.

**Shared location with Tung:** 1010.01

**Dermatome:** C2

**Main Action Areas:** Head, Sense organs, Rectum, Uterus, Entire body

**Main Functions:** Clears the mind, lifts the spirits, tonifies yang, strengthens the ascending function of the Spleen, eliminates interior wind, promotes resuscitation.

**Indications:**
Dizziness, headache, vertigo, tinnitus, nasal obstruction, aphasia by and the uterus. Direct moxibustion at apoplexy, coma, mental disorders, prolapse of the rectum this point is effective for hemorrhoids.

**Manipulation:** Subcutaneous insertion 0.3 - 0.5 cun.

Moxibustion is applicable.

**Remarks:**
a) This is a powerful sedative and tranquilizing point. As psychogenic factors are present in almost all diseases the use of this point on a general basis with other specific points is recommended for good therapeutic results.

b) Since this point also acts as governor, it has a coordinating effect when points are used on a number of channels.

c) This is a good point to commence the first therapy as it is a relatively painless point and the patient does not see the insertion of the needle.

# DU-21 Qianding

(In Front of the Crown)

**Location:**
On the midline, 3.5 cun superior to the anterior hairline or 1.5 cun anterior to DU-20.

**Shared location with Tung:** 1010.05

**Dermatome:** C2

**Main Action Areas:** Head, Brain

**Main Functions:** Sedates wind. Calms the mind. Alleviates pain.

**Indications:**
Epilepsy, dizziness, blurring of vision, vertical headache, rhinorrhea.

**Manipulation:** Subcutaneous insertion 0.3 - 0.5 cun.

Moxibustion is applicable.

**Caution:** Contra-indicted in infants whose fontanel has not closed.

# DU-22 Xinhui

(Fontanelle Meeting)

**Location:**
On the midline, 2 cun superior to the anterior hairline.

**Dermatome:** C2, Trigeminal nerve

**Main Action Areas:** Top of head, Nose, Brain

**Main Functions:** Benefits the nose. Alleviates pain. Sedates wind. Calms the mind.

**Indications:**
Dizziness, headache, blurring of vision, rhinorrhea, infantile convulsion.

**Manipulation:** Subcutaneous insertion 0.3 - 0.5 cun towards the nose. Do not use thick needles. Can use press needle if long retention required.

Moxibustion is applicable.

**Caution:** Contra-indicted in infants whose fontanel has not closed. Excessive stimulation is to be avoided.

# DU-23 Shangxing

(Upper Star)

SUN SI-MIAO GHOST POINT

**Location:**
1.0 cun above the midpoint of the anterior hairline.

**Dermatome:** Trigeminal nerve

**Main Action Areas:** Nose, Eyes, Face, Forehead

**Main Functions:** Dispels wind. Clears heat. Opens the nose. Clears the face and eyes. Calms the mind

**Indications:**
Headache, ophthalmalgia, epistaxis, nasal discharge (effective if moxibustion applied), mental disorders.

**Manipulation:** 0.5 cun obliquely downwards.

**Manipulation:** Subcutaneous insertion 0.3 - 0.5 cun or prick to bleed.

Moxibustion is applicable.

**Caution:** Contra-indicted in infants whose fontanel has not closed.

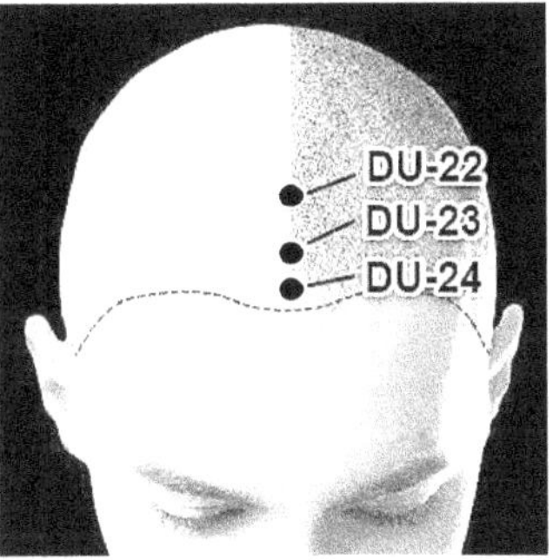


# DU-24 Shenting

(Courtyard of the Spirit)

MEETING POINT OF THE GOVERNING VESSEL WITH THE BLADDER AND STOMACH CHANNELS.

**Location:**
On the midline, 0.5 cun superior to the anterior hairline or 4.5 cun anterior DU-20.

**Dermatome:** Trigeminal nerve

**Main Action Areas:** Head, Mind, Nose, Eyes

**Main Functions:** Descends rising Yang and subdues wind. Calms the mind. Clears the face and eyes.

**Indications:**
Epilepsy, anxiety, vertigo, palpitation, insomnia, headache, rhinorrhoea.

**Manipulation:** Subcutaneous insertion 0.3 - 0.5 cun or prick to bleed.

Moxibustion is applicable.

# DU-25 Suliao
(WHITE CREVICE)

**Location:** At the tip of the nose.

**Shared location with Tung:** 1010.12

**Dermatome:** Trigeminal nerve

**Main Action Areas:** Nose, Lungs, Eyes, Mind

**Main Functions:** Benefits the nose. Clears the face and eyes. Revives Yang, stimulates the mind and restores consciousness

**Indications:** Loss of consciousness, nasal obstruction, epistaxis, rhinorrhea, rosacea..

**Manipulation:** Perpendicular or oblique insertion 0.2 - 0.3 cun or prick to bleed.

**Cautions:** No moxibustion.

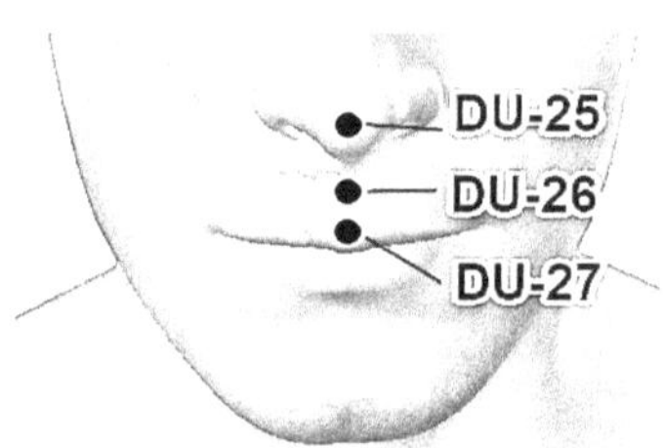


# DU-26 Renzhong
(MAN'S MIDDLE)

MEETING POINT OF THE GOVERNING VESSELS WITH THE LARGE INTESTINE AND STOMACH CHANNELS. SUN SI-MIAO GHOST POINT.

**Location:**
At the junction of the upper third and lower two thirds of the philtrum of the upper lip, in the midline.

**Dermatome:** Trigeminal nerve

**Main Action Areas:** Mind, Nose, Face, Lumbar Spine

**Main Functions:** Benefits the nose. Clears the face and eyes. Restores consciousness and stimulates the mind. Regulates Qi and Blood. Alleviates lumbar pain.

**Indications:**
Mental disorders, epilepsy, hysteria, infantile convulsion, coma, deviation of the mouth, apoplexy-faint, trismus, puffiness of the face, pain and stiffness of the lower back.

**Manipulation:** Oblique insertion upwards .3 - .5 cun.

**Cautions:** Contraindicated for moxibustion.

**Remarks:**
a) In traditional Chinese medicine this point is known as the point of re-animation as it is used as emergency treatment for sudden fainting.

b) In the treatment of emergency conditions, the needle may be manipulated and removed as soon as pain is felt by the patient. It is not necessary to keep the needle longer. c) Acupressure applied with the nail of the index finger (and applied obliquely backwards and upwards) is often found to be equally effective. Firm pressure should be maintained till the patient recovers.

# DU-27 Duiduan
(EXTREMITY OF THE MOUTH)

**Location:**
On the midline, on the margin of the upper lip and the philtrum.

**Dermatome:** Trigeminal nerve

**Main Action Areas:** Upper Lip, Supralabial area, Mouth, Mind

**Main Functions:** Clears heat. Regulates Qi and alleviates pain. Calms the mind.

**Indications:**
Mental disorders, lip twitching, lip stiffness, pain and swelling of the gums.

**Manipulation:** Oblique insertion upwards .2 - .3 cun.

**Cautions:** Contraindicated for moxibustion.

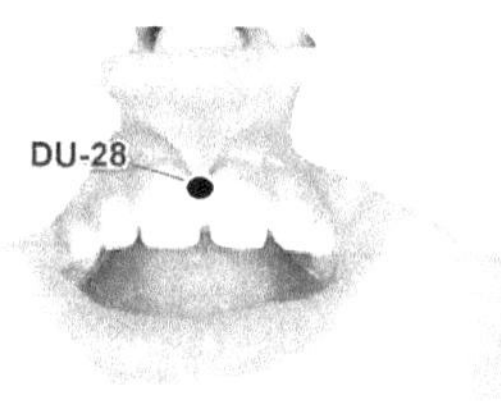


# DU-28 Yinjiao
(GUM INTERSECTION)

MEETING POINT OF THE GOVERNING VESSEL WITH THE STOMACH CHANNEL.

**Location:**
Between the gum and upper lip in the frenulum of the upper lip.

**Dermatome:** Trigeminal nerve

**Main Action Areas:** Gums, Mouth, Nose

**Main Functions:** Benefits the gums. Clears heat

**Indications:**
a) Pain and swelling of the gums and other oral diseases. b) Haemorrhoids, as a distal point.

**Manipulation:** 0.1-0.2 cun obliquely upwards or prick to bleed with the three-edged needle.

**Caution:** No moxibustion

# REN (Conception Vessel, CV) MERIDIAN

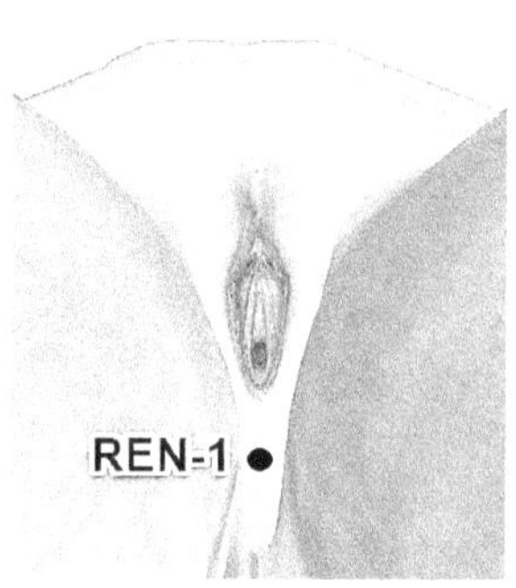


# REN-1 Huiyin
(MEETING OF THE YIN)

MEETING POINT OF THE CONCEPTION, PENETRATING, AND GOVERNING VESSELS. SI-MIAO GHOST POINT

**Location:**
In the center of the perineum, Males: between the anus and the scrotum, Females: between the anus and the posterior labial commissure.

**Dermatome:** S4

**Main Action Areas:** Genitals, Mind, Entire body

**Main Functions:** Boosts the lower jiao. Lifts sinking Qi. Increases libido.

**Indications:**
Vaginitis, retention of urine, hemorrhoids, nocturnal emission, enuresis, irregular menstruation, mental disorders.

**Manipulation:** Perpendicular insertion 0.5 - 1.0 cun.

Moxibustion is applicable.

**Cautions:** Contraindicated in pregnancy

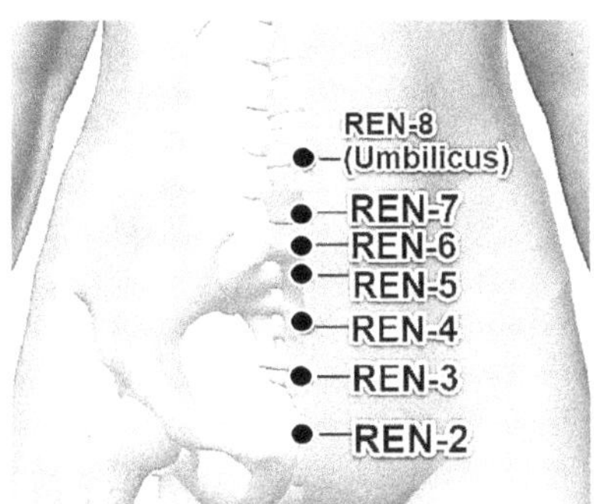


# REN-2 Qugu
(CURVED BONE)

MEETING POINT OF THE CONCEPTION VESSEL AND THE LIVER CHANNEL.

**Location:**
Immediately above the midpoint of the superior border of the symphysis pubis.

**Dermatome:** T5-T12

**Main Action Areas:** Bladder, Genitals, Uterus

**Main Functions:** Benefits the genitourinary system and lower jiao

**Indications:**
Retention and dribbling of urine, enuresis, nocturnal emission, impotence, morbid leukorrhea, irregular menstruation, dysmenorrhea, hernia.

**Manipulation:** Perpendicular insertion 0.5 - 1.0 cun.

Moxibustion is applicable.

**Cautions:** Deep insertion may penetrate a full bladder.

# REN-3 Zhongji
(MIDDLE POLE)

FRONT MU (ALARM) POINT OF THE BLADDER CHANNEL. MEETING POINT OF THE CONCEPTION VESSEL WITH THE SPLEEN, LIVER, AND KIDNEY CHANNELS. MUSCLE MERIDIAN MEETING POINT OF THE 3 LEG YIN

**Location:**
In the front midline 4 cun below the umbilicus, 1 cun above REN-2.

**Dermatome:** T5-T12

**Main Action Areas:** Bladder, Uterus, Lower jiao

**Main Functions:** Dispels dampness, heat and cold. Strengthens the genitourinary system

**Indications:** Enuresis, nocturnal emission, impotence, hernia, uterine bleeding, irregular menstruation, dysmenorrhea, morbid leukorrhea, frequency of urination, retention of urine, pain in the lower abdominal, prolapse of the uterus, vaginitis.

**Manipulation:** Perpendicular insertion 0.5 - 1.0 cun.

Moxibustion is applicable.

**Cautions:** Deep insertion may penetrate a full bladder. No deep needling in pregnancy.

# REN-4 Guanyuan
(GATE OF THE SOURCE)

FRONT-MU (ALARM) POINT OF THE SMALL INTESTINE CHANNEL. MEETING POINT OF THE CONCEPTION VESSEL WITH THE SPLEEN, LIVER, AND KIDNEY CHANNELS.

**Location:**
In the front midline, 3 cun below the umbilicus. 2 cun above Qugu (REN-2)

**Dermatome:** T12

**Main Action Areas:** Entire body, Abdomen, Small Intestine, Bladder, Uterus

**Main Functions:** Augments yuan Qi. Nourishes Yin and Blood. Calms the mind. Reinforces the Kidneys. Regulates Qi and Blood. Strengthens the lower jiao. Benefits the Small Intestine.

**Indications**
Enuresis, nocturnal emission, frequency of urination, retention of urine, hernia, dysmenorrhea, uterine bleeding, irregular menstruation, morbid leukorrhea, lower abdominal pain, prolapse of the rectum, post-partum hemorrhage, indigestion, diarrhea, flaccid type apoplexy.

**Manipulation:** Perpendicular insertion 0.8 - 1.2 cun.

Moxibustion is applicable.

**Cautions:** Deep insertion may penetrate a full bladder. No deep needling in pregnancy.

# REN-5 Shimen
(STONE GATE)

FRONT-MU (ALARM) POINT OF THE TRIPLE ENERGIZER CHANNEL.

**Location:**
In the front midline, 2 cun below the umbilicus.

**Dermatome:** T10

**Main Action Areas:** Abdomen, Uterus

**Main Functions:** Mobilises yuan Qi. Warms and strengthens the lower jiao

**Indications:**
Oedema and ascites. Abdominal pain, diarrhea, hernia, anuria, enuresis, uterine bleeding, amenorrhea, morbid leukorrhea, postpartum haemorrhage.

**Manipulation:** Perpendicular insertion 0.5 - 1.0 cun.

Moxibustion is applicable.

**Cautions:** Deep insertion may penetrate the peritoneal cavity.

# REN-6 Qihai
(SEA OF QI)

**Location:**
In the front midline, 1.5 cun below the umbilicus.

**Dermatome:** T10

**Main Action Areas:** Entire body, Lower jiao, Abdomen

**Main Functions:** Tonifies and warms Yang. Lifts sinking Qi. Warms the abdomen. Regulates Qi in the lower jiao

**Indications:**
Neurasthenia. This is a good Tonification point and used in conjunction with Zusanli [ST-36] and Sanyinjiao [SP-6] for chronic fatigue and hypotension. Abdominal pain, enuresis, nocturnal emission, impotence, hernia, edema, asthma, diarrhea, dysentery, uterine bleeding, irregular menstruation, dysmenorr-hea, morbid leukorrhea, amenorrhea, postpartum hemorrhage, constipation, flaccid type apoplexy.

**Manipulation:** Perpendicular insertion 0.8 - 1.2 cun.

Moxibustion is applicable.

**Cautions:** Deep insertion may penetrate the peritoneal cavity. No deep needling in pregnancy.

# REN-7 Yinjiao

### (YIN INTERSECTION)

MEETING POINT OF THE CONCEPTION AND PENETRATING VESSELS WITH THE KIDNEY CHANNEL. UPPER ENERGIZER POINT.

**Location:**
On the anterior midline, 1 cun inferior to the umbilicus.

**Dermatome:** T9/T10

**Main Action Areas:** Abdomen, Umbilicus, Uterus

**Main Functions:** Regulates Qi in the lower jiao. Alleviates pain.

**Indications:**
Abdominal distension, edema, hernia, irregular menstrua-tion, uterine bleeding, morbid leukorrhea, pruritus vulvae, post-partum hemorrhage, abdominal pain around the umbilicus.

**Manipulation:** Perpendicular insertion 0.8 - 1.2 cun.

Moxibustion is applicable.

**Cautions:** Deep insertion may penetrate the peritoneal cavity. No deep needling in pregnancy.

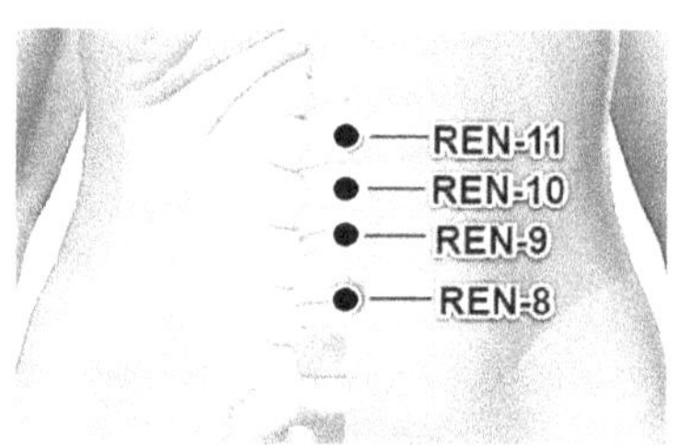


# REN-8 Shenque

### (SPIRIT GATEWAY)

CONSIDERED TO BE THE POINT WHERE QI ENTERS AT BIRTH AND LEAVES AT DEATH.

**Location:**
In the centre of the umbilicus.

**Dermatome:** T9

**Main Action Areas:** Navel, Abdomen, Entire body

**Main Functions:** Tonifies, warms, lifts and revives Yang. Regulates Qi in the abdomen.

**Indications:**
Abdominal pain, borborygmus, flaccid type of apoplexy, prolapse of the rectum, unchecked diarrhea.

**Manipulation:** While it is forbidden for acupuncture, it is an important moxibustion point. The umbilicus is also used as an anatomical landmark to locate other points.

# REN-9 Shuifen

### (WATER SEPARATION)

**Location:**
In the front midline, 1.0 cun above the umbilicus.

**Dermatome:** T8

**Main Action Areas:** Abdomen, Entire body

**Main Functions:** Reduces oedema

**Indications:**
Specific point for oedema and ascites.

**Manipulation:** Perpendicular insertion 0.5 - 1.0 cun.

Moxibustion is applicable.

**Cautions:** Deep insertion may penetrate the peritoneal cavity. Contraindicated in pregnancy.

# REN-10 Xiawan

### (LOWER CAVITY)

MEETING POINT OF THE CONCEPTION VESSEL AND THE SPLEEN CHANNEL.

**Location:**
On the anterior midline, 2 cun superior to the centre of the umbilicus.

**Dermatome:** T8

**Main Action Areas:** Stomach, Abdomen

**Main Functions:** Descends rebellious Qi. Relieves food stagnation

**Indications:**
Epigastric pain, abdominal pain, borborygmus, indigestion, vomiting, diarrhea.

**Manipulation:** Perpendicular insertion 0.5 - 1.0 cun.

Moxibustion is applicable.

**Cautions:** Deep insertion may penetrate the peritoneal cavity. Contraindicated in pregnancy.

# REN-11 Jianli

### (INTERIOR STRENGTHENING)

**Location:**
On the anterior midline, 3 cun superior to the umbilicus. **Dermatome:** T7/T8

**Main Action Areas:** Stomach, Middle jiao

**Main Functions:** Harmonises the middle jiao

**Indications:**
Stomach ache, vomiting, edema, abdominal distension, borborygmus, anorexia.

**Manipulation:** Perpendicular insertion 0.5 - 1.2 cun.

Moxibustion is applicable.

**Cautions:** Deep insertion may penetrate the peritoneal cavity. No deep needling in pregnancy.

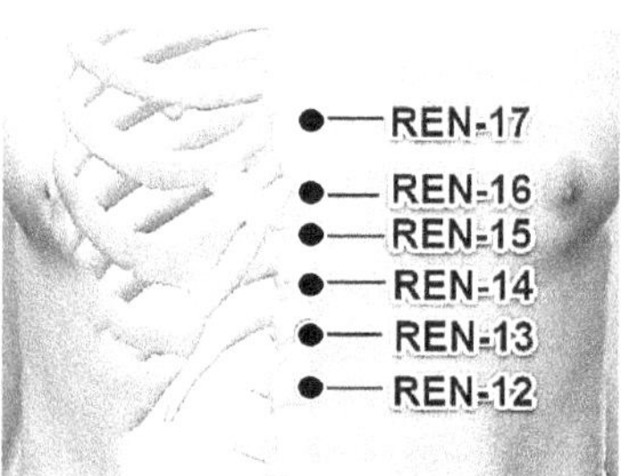


# REN-12 Zhongwan

### (MIDDLE CAVITY)

FRONT-MU (ALARM) POINT OF THE STOMACH. INFLUENTIAL POINT OF THE FU ORGANS, MEETING POINT OF THE CONCEPTION VESSEL AND THE SMALL INTESTINE, TRIPLE ENERGIZER, AND STOMACH CHANNELS. MIDDLE ENERGIZER POINT.

**Location:**
In the front midline, midway between the xyphoid process and the umbilicus [or 4 cun directly above the umbilicus].

**Dermatome:** T7

**Main Action Areas:** Middle jiao, Epigastrium, Stomach, Abdomen, Entire body

**Main Functions:** Tonifies the Stomach and Spleen. Transforms dampness. Dispels cold. Harmonises the middle jiao and descends rebellious Qi. Nourishes fluids and Yin. Soothes the Heart and calms the mind.

**Indications:**
Stomach ache, abdominal distension, borborygmus, nausea, vomiting, acid regurgitation, diarrhea, dysentery, jaundice, indigestion, insomnia.

**Manipulation:** Perpendicular insertion 0.5 - 1.2 cun.

Moxibustion is applicable.

**Cautions:** Deep insertion may penetrate the peritoneal cavity. No deep needling in pregnancy.

# REN-13 Shangwan

(UPPER CAVITY)

MEETING POINT OF THE CONCEPTION VESSEL AND THE STOMACH AND SMALL INTESTINE CHANNELS.

**Location:**
On the anterior midline, 3 cun inferior to the sternocostal angle.

**Dermatome:** T7

**Main Action Areas:** Stomach

**Main Functions:** Harmonises the Stomach.

**Indications:**
Stomach ache, abdominal distension, nausea, vomiting, epilepsy, insomnia.

**Manipulation:** Perpendicular insertion 0.5 - 1.2 cun.

Moxibustion is applicable.

**Cautions:** Deep insertion may penetrate the peritoneal cavity. No deep needling in pregnancy.

# REN-14 Juque

(GREAT GATEWAY)

FRONT-MU (ALARM) POINT OF THE HEART CHANNEL.

**Location:**
On the anterior midline, 2 cun inferior to the sternocostal angle or 6 cun superior to the umbilicus.

**Dermatome:** T6/T7

**Main Action Areas:** Heart, Chest, Epigastrium

**Main Functions:** Soothes the Heart and calms the mind. Harmonises the Heart and Stomach.

**Indications:**
Pain in cardiac region and chest, nausea, acid regurgitation, difficulty in swallowing, vomiting, mental disorders, epilepsy, palpitations.

**Manipulation:** Perpendicular or oblique insertion 0.3 – 0.8 cun.

Moxibustion is applicable.

**Cautions:** Deep insertion may penetrate an enlarged Liver and Heart. No deep needling in pregnancy.

# REN-15 Jiuwei

(TURTLEDOVE TAIL)

LUO POINT OF THE CONCEPTION VESSEL.

**Location:**
On the anterior midline, 1 cun inferior to the sternocostal angle or 7 cun superior to the umbilicus.

**Dermatome:** T6

**Main Action Areas:** Chest, Abdomen

**Main Functions:** Regulates Qi and dispels stasis. Calms and balances the mind.

**Indications:**
Pain in the cardiac region and the chest, nausea, mental disorders, epilepsy, palpitations, difficulty swallowing, itchy skin on abdomen.

**Manipulation:** Oblique insertion downwards .4 - .6 cun.

Moxibustion is applicable.

**Cautions:** Deep insertion may penetrate an enlarged Liver and Heart. No deep needling in pregnancy.

# REN-16 Zhongting

(CENTRAL COURTYARD)

**Location:**
On the anterior midline, on the level of the sternocostal angle.

**Dermatome:** T5

**Main Action Areas:** Chest, Abdomen

**Main Functions:** Regulates Qi and dispels stasis. Calms and balances the mind.

**Indications:**
Distension and fullness in the chest and intercostal region, hiccups, nausea, anorexia.

**Manipulation:** Subcutaneous insertion .3 - .5 cun.

Moxibustion is applicable

# REN-17 Danzhong

(CHEST CENTRE)

FRONT-MU (ALARM) POINT OF THE PERICARDIUM. INFLUENTIAL POINT OF THE QI. POINT OF THE SEA OF QI, MEETING POINTING OF THE CONCEPTION VESSEL WITH THE SPLEEN, KIDNEY, SMALL INTESTINE, AND TRIPLE ENERGIZER CHANNELS. UPPER ENERGIZER POINT

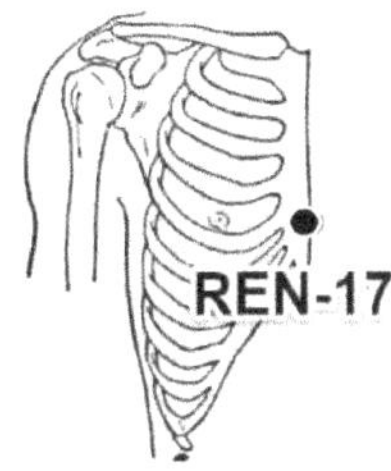


**Location:**
On the sternum, midway between the two nipples [at the the level of the 4th intercostal space].

**Dermatome:** T4

**Main Action Areas:** Heart, Lungs, Chest, Breast, Entire body

**Main Functions:** Regulates Qi and dispels stasis. Tonifies Qi. Calms and balances the mind. Benefits the chest.

**Indications:**
Heart disease, bronchial asthma, and other lung disorders, breast disorders.

**Manipulation:** 1.0 cun horizontally downwards; in breast disease the needle may be directed laterally towards the diseased breast.

Moxibustion is applicable.

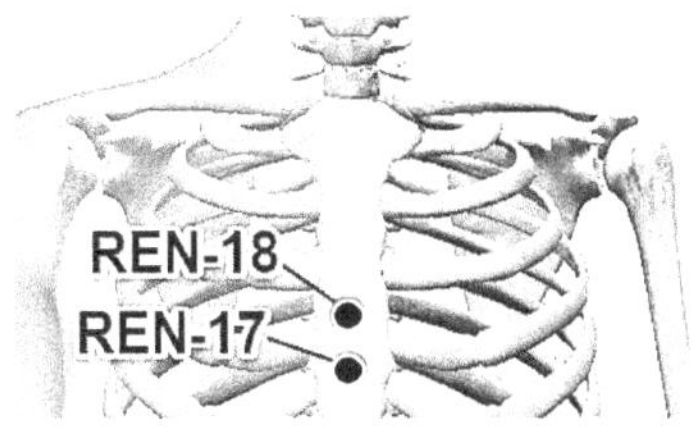


# REN-18 Yutang

(JADE HALL)

**Location:**
On the anterior midline, on the level of the 3rd intercostal space.

**Dermatome:** T3

**Main Action Areas:** Sternum, Chest, Lungs, Heart, Breast

**Main Functions:** Regulates Qi, dissipates stasis and alleviates pain. Calms and balances the mind. Benefits the chest.

**Indications:**
Pain in the chest, cough, asthma, vomiting.

**Manipulation:** Subcutaneous insertion 0.3 - 0.5 cun.

Moxibustion is applicable.

## REN-19 Zigong

(PURPLE PALACE)

**Location:**
On the anterior midline, on the level of the 2nd intercostal space.

**Dermatome:** T2

**Main Action Areas:** Sternum, Chest, Lungs, Heart, Breast

**Main Functions:** Regulates Qi, dissipates stasis and alleviates pain. Calms and balances the mind. Benefits the chest

**Indications:**
Pain in the chest, cough, asthma.

**Manipulation:** Subcutaneous insertion 0.3 - 0.5 cun.

Moxibustion is applicable.

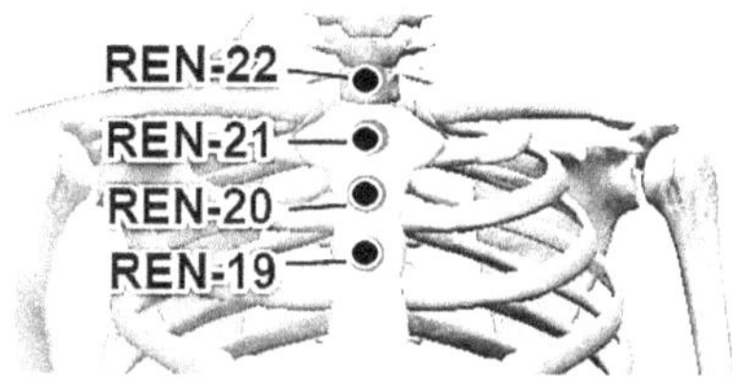


## REN-20 Hua gai

(MAGNIFICENT CANAPY)

**Location:**
On the anterior midline, on the lower part of the manubrium sterni, on the level of the 1st inter-costal space.

**Dermatome:** C4-T2

**Main Action Areas:** Heart, Lungs, Chest

**Main Functions:** Regulates Qi. Relaxes the chest.

**Indications:**
Fullness and pain in the chest and intercostal region, cough, asthma.

**Manipulation:** Subcutaneous insertion 0.3 - 0.5 cun.

Moxibustion is applicable.

## REN-21 Xuanji

(JADE PIVOT)

**Location:**
On the anterior midline, below the upper border of the manubrium sterni.

**Dermatome:** C4

**Main Action Areas:** Chest, Throat

**Main Functions:** Relaxes the chest. Descends rebellious Qi

**Indications:**
Pain in the chest, cough, asthma.

**Manipulation:** Subcutaneous insertion 0.3 - 0.5 cun.

Moxibustion is applicable.

## REN-22 Tiantu

(HEAVENLY PROMINENCE)

MEETING POINT OF THE CONCEPTION AND YIN LINKING VESSELS. WINDOW OF HEAVEN POINT.

**Location:**
At the centre of the suprasternal fossa, 0.5 cun above the sternal notch.

**Dermatome:** C3

**Main Action Areas:** Throat, Chest

**Main Functions:** Descends rebellious Qi. Alleviates dyspnoea and cough. Treats asthma.

**Indications:**
Asthma, cough, sore throat, dry throat, hiccups, sudden hoarseness of the voice, difficulty in swallowing, goiter.

**Manipulation:** For insertion, the following procedures should be observed in sequence:

a) Have the patient comfortably seated.

b) Locate the point.

c) Insert the needle about 0.3 cun perpendicularly.

d) Extend the patient's neck.

e) Change the direction of the needle and then insert further 1.0 - 1.5 cun downwards along the posterior border of the sternum.

f) Ensure that the patient can swallow without pain and is otherwise comfortable.

All manoeuvres must be carried out gently and precisely.

Moxibustion apploicable.

**Remarks:** Caution required.

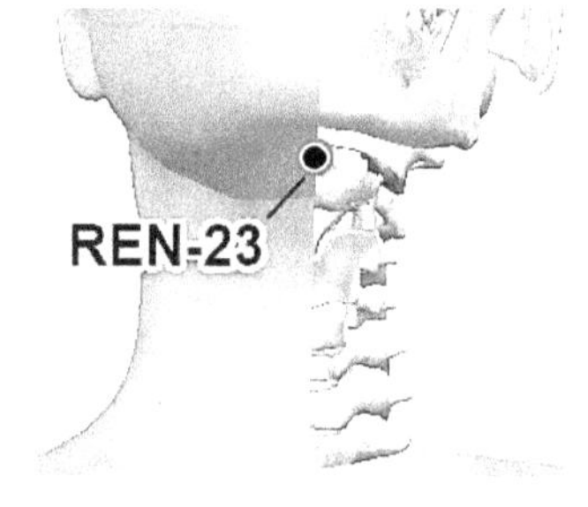


## REN-23 Lianquan

(CORNER SPRING)

MEETING POINT OF THE CONCEPTION AND YIN LINKING VESSELS.

**Location:**
On the middle of the neck, midway between the upper border of the cartoid cartilage and the lower border of the mandible.

**Dermatome:** C3

**Main Action Areas:** Tongue, Submandibular area, Throat

**Main Functions:** Resolves phlegm and clears heat. Descends rebellious Qi.

**Indications:**
Aphasia, mutism, dysarthria, sndden loss of speech, dysphagia., speech difficulties following paralytic strokes, stammering, excessive salivation, pharyngitis, pseudobulbar palsy, speech disorders due to Parkinsonism.

**Manipulation:** 1.0-1.5 cun obliquely towards the root of the tongue, or towards Baihui [DU-20].

Moxibustion applicable.

**Remarks:** Care should be taken to insert in the midline and in the correct direction.

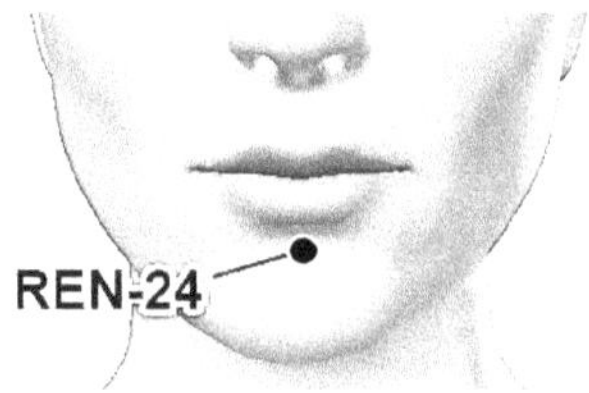


## REN-24 Chengjiang

(CONTAINER OF FLUIDS)

MEETING POINT OF THE CONCEPTION VESSEL WITH THE GOVERNING VESSEL AND THE LARGE INTESTINE AND STOMACH CHANNELS.

**Location:**
In the middle of the mento labial groove, in the depression between the point of the chin and midpoint of the lower lip.

**Dermatome:** Trigeminal nerve

**Main Action Areas:** Chin, Face

**Main Functions:** Dispels wind and clears heat. Treats paralysis. Alleviates pain. Improves appearance.

**Indications:**
Facial paralysis, trigeminal neuralgia, toothache of the lower incissors, swelling of the gums, excessive salivation, anaesthetic point for tooth extraction.

**Manipulation:** Oblique upward insertion 0.2 - 0.3 cun.

Moxibustion is applicable.

# EXTRA POINTS: Head and Neck (EX-HN)

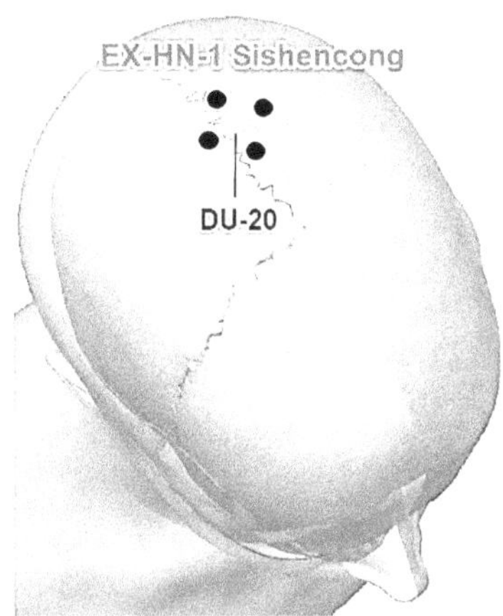


# EX-HN-1 Sishencong
(FOUR ALERT SPIRIT)

**Location:**
These are four points situated on the vertex, 1.0 cun anterior, posterior and lateral to the point Baihui (DU-20).

**Dermatome:** C2

**Main Action Areas:** Head, Mind

**Main Functions:** Clears the head and calms the mind. Subdues wind

**Indications:**
Wind strike hemiplegia; headache; dizziness; epilepsy; mental disorders.

**Manipulation:** 0.5 cun horizontally towards Baihui (DU-20.).

Moxibustion applicable.

**Remarks:** Usually used with Baihui (DU-20).

# EX-HN-2
DANGYANG
(ABOVE THE YANG)

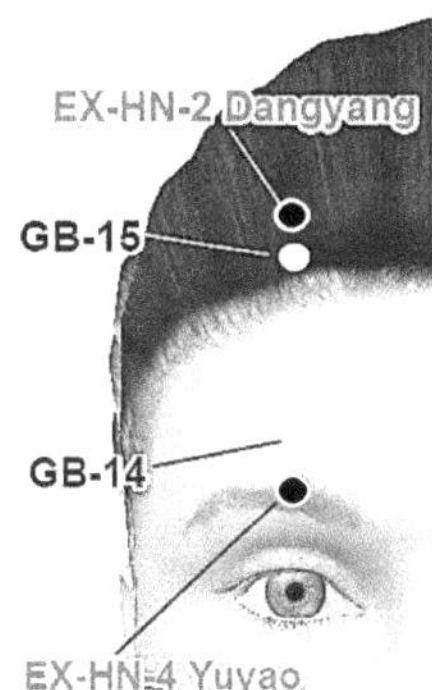


**Location:**
With the patient looking straight ahead, vertically above the pupil, 1 cun above the anterior hairline.

**Actions/Indications:**
Dispels Wind and Heat, alleviates pain

**Manipulation:** 0.5 cun transversely (subcutaneously) towards the site of the disorder/pain.

Moxibustion applicable.

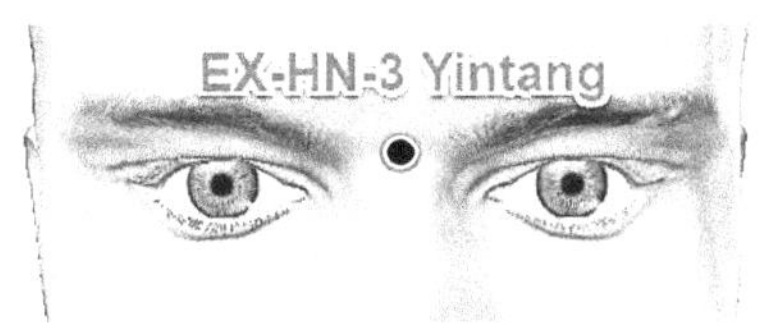


# EX-HN-3 Yintang
(HALL OF IMPRESSION)

**Location:**
On the bridge of the nose, midway between the medial ends of the two eyebrows.

**Shared location with Tung:** 1010.08

**Dermatome:** Trigeminal nerve

**Main Action Areas:** Mind, Forehead, Eyes, Nose, Lumbar spine, Entire body

**Main Functions:** Calms the mind and relaxes the body. Clears wind and heat from the face. Benefits the eyes and nose. Subdues wind. Complements the treatment.

**Indications:**
Rhinitis, sinus, nasal diseases, headache, eye disease.

**Manipulation:** 0.5 cun horizontally downwards. Blood-letting applicable.

# EX-HN-4 Yuyao
(FISH WAIST)

**Location:**
At the midpoint of the eyebrow, vertically above the midpoint of the pupil.

**Shared location with Tung:** 1010.10

**Dermatome:** Trigeminal nerve

**Main Action Areas:** Eyes, Forehead

**Main Functions:** Regulates Qi and Blood. Alleviates pain and swelling. Benefits the eyes

**Indications:**
Frontal sinusitis, eye disorders, facial paralysis. Neuralgia of the supraorbital nerve, eye strain and eye fatigue.

**Manipulation:** 0.5 cun horizontally along the skin: i) directed medially for frontal sinusitis; ii) directed downwards for eye disorders; iii) directed laterally for facial paralysis.

**Caution:** No moxibustion.

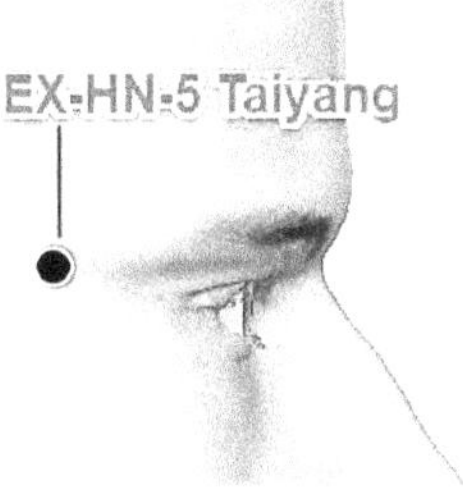


# EX-HN-5 Taiyang
(SUPREME YANG)

**Location:**
At the temple, in the depression approximately 1 cun posterior to the midpoint between the lateral extremity of the eyebrow and the outer canthus of the eye.

**Dermatome:** Trigeminal nerve

**Main Action Areas:** Temples, Eyes, Head

**Main Functions:** Regulates Qi and Blood. Alleviates pain and swelling. Benefits the eyes

**Indications:**
Headache, migraine, eye diseases, facial paralysis, trigeminal neuralgia, toothache, sinusitis.

**Manipulation:** Perpendicular insertion .3 - .5 cun., or prick to cause bleeding.

**Caution:** No Moxibustion

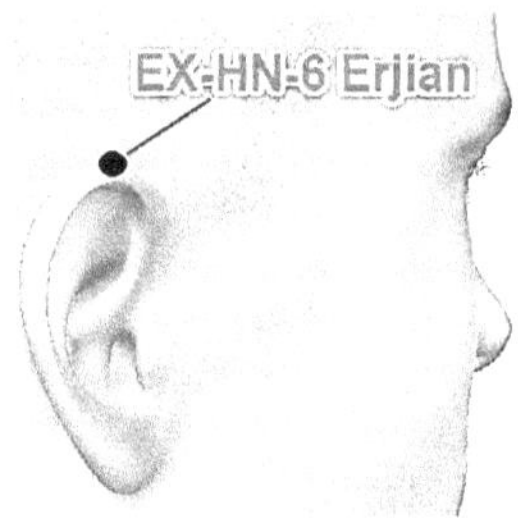


# EX-HN-6 Erjian
(TIP OF THE EAR)

**Location:**
On the apex of the ear, on the helix.

**Dermatome:** C2, Trigeminal nerve

**Main Action Areas:** Eyes, Head, Liver, Entire body

**Main Functions:** Descends Yang and clears heat. Alleviates pain

**Indications:**
Eye screens; redness, swelling and pain of the eyes; high fever

**Manipulation:** Perpendicular insertion .1 - .2 cun., or prick to cause bleeding. Indirect moxibustion for eye disorders.

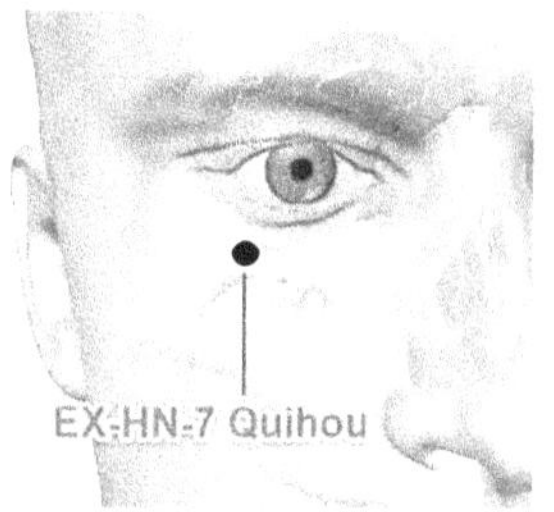


# EX-HN-7 Quihou
(BEHIND THE BALL)

Dangerous point.

**Location:**
At the junction of the lateral fourth and the medial three-fourths of the infra-orbital border.

**Dermatome:** Trigeminal nerve

**Main Action Areas:** Eyes and area below

**Main Functions:** Benefits the eyes and improves vision

**Indications:**
Myopia, optic nerve disorders, glaucoma and other eye disorders.

**Manipulation:** 1.0 cun perpendicularly with the patient looking upwards. The needle should be directed along the floor of the orbit in the direction of the optic foramen [i.e., slightly medially and superiorly].

**Caution:** No moxibustion.

**Remarks:** This is a Dangerous point as it is located in the orbit.

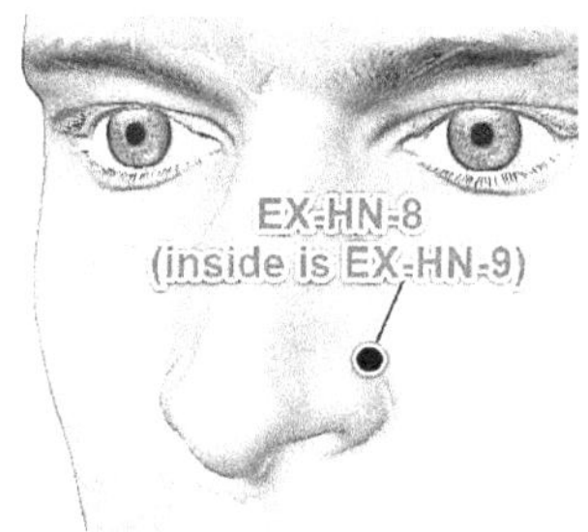


# EX-HN-8 Shangyingxiang/ Bitong
(UPPER YINGXIANG/ CLEAR NOSE)

**Location:**
At the upper end of the nasiolabial groove, at the junction of the maxilla and the nasal cavity.

**Dermatome:** Trigeminal nerve

**Main Action Areas:** Nose

**Main Functions:** Clears wind and heat. Opens the nose

**Indications:**
Nasal obstruction, rhinitis.

**Manipulation:** 0.3–0.5 cun vertically towards the centre of the nasal cavity.

**Caution:** No moxibustion.

# EX-HN-9 Neiyingxiang
(INNER YINGXIANG)

**Location:**
Inside the nasal cavity, at the junction of the nasal bone and the nasal cartilage. First find Shangyingxiang EX-HN-8 which is at the upper end of the nasolabial groove. Neiyingxiang EX-HN-9 is inside the nasal cavity, opposite of the external point of EX-HN-8

**Actions/Indications:**
Clears Heat, drains Fire

**Manipulation:** Prick to bleed with a needle, lancet or three-edged needle. Caution: Contraindicated in patients with bleeding disorders (or taking anticoagulants). Needling may be painful!

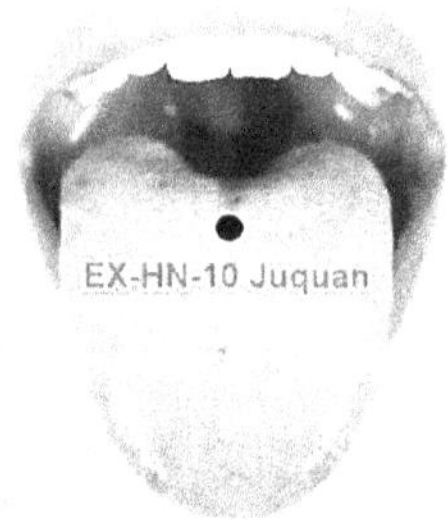


# EX-HN-10 Juquan
(GATHERING SPRING)

**Location:**
With maximal extension of the tongue, in the centre of the tongue body.

**Actions/Indications:**
Deviation of the tongue, impaired mobility or atrophy of the musculature of the tongue: for example, after a stroke or with loss of sense of taste

**Manipulation:** Vertically 0.2 cun. Needling may be painful!

# EX-HN-11 Haiquan
(SEA SPRING)

**Location:**
Below the tongue, in the centre of the frenulum, between the points EX-HN-12 (jinjin) and EX-HN-13 (yuye).

**Actions/Indications:**
Mouth and tongue ulcers, hiccups

**Manipulation:** Vertically 0.2 cun. Remove needle immediately after short stimulation. Needling may be painful!

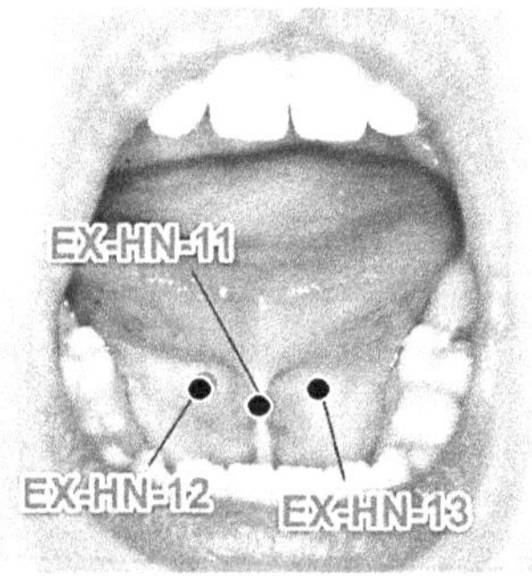


# EX-HN-12/EX-HN-13 Jinjin/Yuye
(GOLDEN LIQUID/JADE FLUID)

**Location:**
On the sublingual veins on either side of the root of the tongue.

**Indications:**
Swelling of the tongue, ulceration of the mucous membrane of the mouth, thrush, aphasia, nausea, vomiting.

**Manipulation:** With the tongue rolled upwards, 0.5 cun perpendicularly, or prick to bleed with the three-edged needle. Contraindicated with bleeding disorders or in patients taking anticoagulant medication.

**Caution:** No moxibustion.

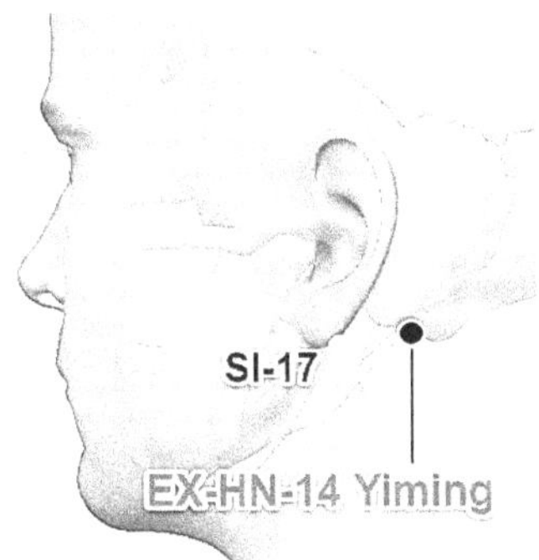


# EX-HN-14 Yiming
(EYE BRIGHTENING)

**Location:**
1.0 cun posterior to Yifeng (SI-17), This point lies on a straight line between Yifeng (SI-17), and Fengchi (GB-20.).

**Dermatome:** C3

**Main Action Areas:** Sub-occipital headaches, Eye conditions.

**Main Functions:** Clears and sharpens vision

**Indications:**
Ear and eye disorders. Tinnitus, insomnia, mouth disorders.

**Manipulation:** 0.5cun perpendicularly.

**Caution:** No moxibustion.

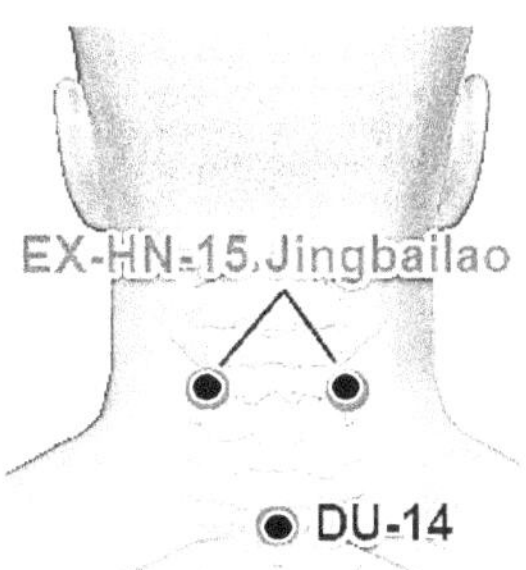


# EX-HN-15
# Jingbailao/Bailao
(HUNDRED TAXATIONS)

**Location:**
2 cun superior to DU-14 and 1 cun lateral to the midline

**Dermatome:** C3/C5

**Main Action Areas:** Mid to lower cervical spine, cervicogenic headaches

**Main Functions:** Reduces tension in lower cervical musculature

**Indications:**
Postpartum body pain; cough; scrofula; whooping cough; sprain or spasms of the neck muscles; lung diseases

**Manipulation:** Vertically 0.5–0.8 cun.

Moxibustion applicable.

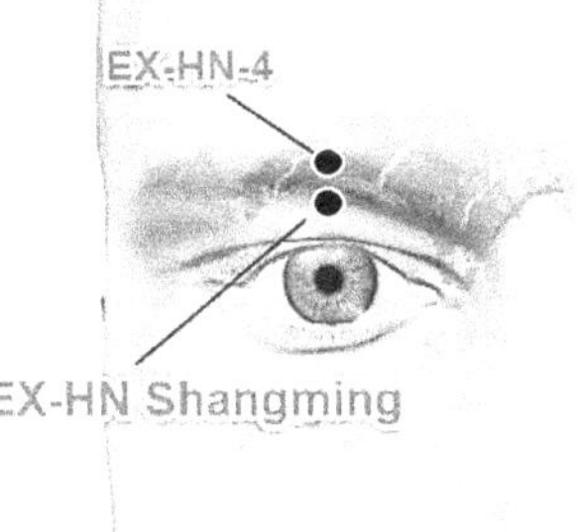


# EX-HN Shangming
(UPPER BRIGHTNESS)

**Location:**
Directly superior to the pupil, below the margin of the orbit.

**Actions/Indications:**
Disorders of the eyes

**Manipulation:** Gently push the eyeball downward. Slowly insert the needle 0.5–1 cun vertically into the fatty tissue immediately below the bone (orbit).

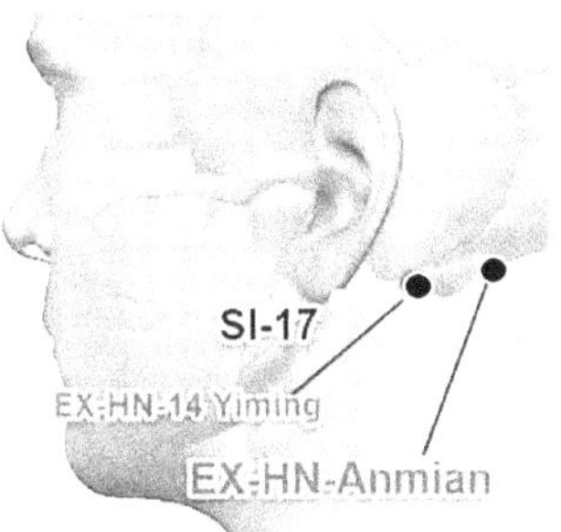


**Caution:** Pay attention to any pain from needling. No stimulation. After removal of the needle, compress the site for 10 minutes.

# EX-HN-Anmian
(PEACEFUL SLEEP)

**Location:**
Posterior to the ear, bet-ween SJ-17 and GB-20, posterior to the mastoid process.

**Dermatome:** C2/C3

**Main Action Areas:** Mind, Head, Eyes

**Main Functions:** Promotes relaxation and sleep. Regulates Liver Qi. Benefits the eyes

**Indications:**
Insom

nia; dizziness; headache; high blood pressure; mental disorders; hysteria.

**Manipulation:** 0.5–1 cun vertically or obliquely towards SJ-17 (yifeng) or GB-20 (fengchi).

**Caution:** No moxibustion.

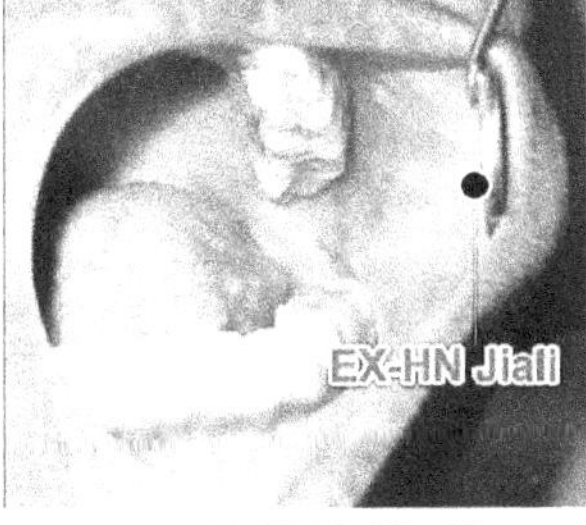


# EX-HN Jiali
(CHEEK CENTRE)

**Location:**
Inside the mouth, on the mucosa of the cheek, 1 cun posterior to the corner of the mouth.

**Actions/Indications:**
Clears Heat, for inflammations of the mouth and throat, for gastritis

**Manipulation:** 0.3–0.5 cun obliquely in a posterior direction, prick to bleed.

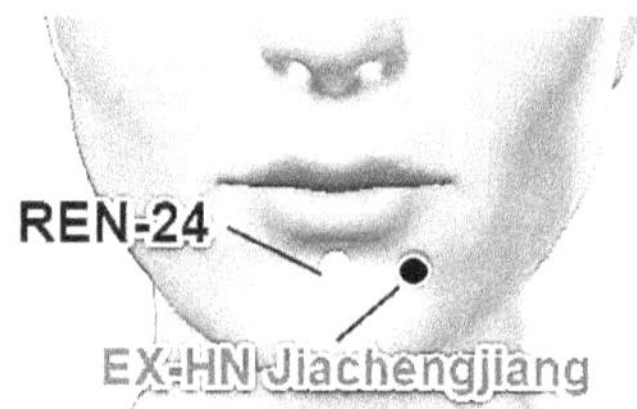


## EX-HN Jiachengjiang
(ADJACENT TO CONTAINER OF FLUIDS)

**Location:**
In the depression on the mental foramen, 1.0 cun lateral Chengjiang [REN-24].

**Dermatome:** Trigeminal nerve

**Main Action Areas:** Mouth, Chin

**Main Functions:** Regulates Qi and Blood. Dispels wind. Alleviates pain

**Indications:**
Facial paralysis, trigeminal neuralgia, lower toothache.

**Manipulation:** 0.2 cun perpendicularly.

**Caution:** No moxibustion.

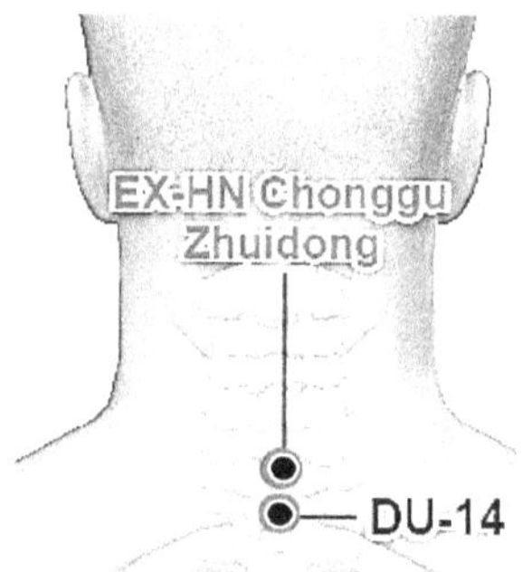


## EX-HN Chonggu Zhuidong
(PROMINENT BONE)

**Location:**
Below the spinous process of the 6th cervical vertebra (C6).

**Actions/Indications:**
Dispels external pathogenic factors. Harmonises the shen

**Manipulation:** 0.5–1 cun obliquely in a superior direction.

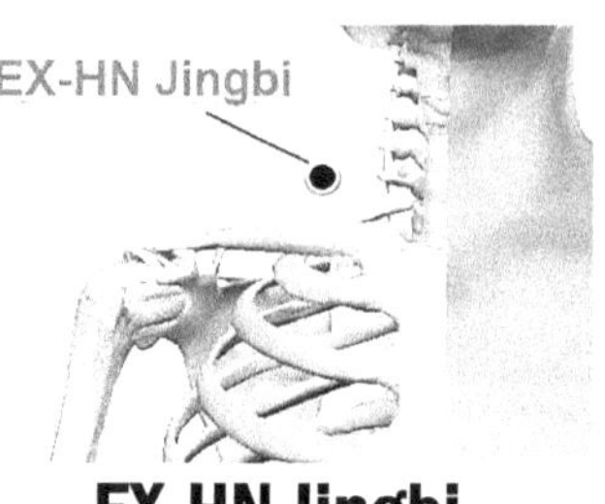


## EX-HN Jingbi
(UPPER ARM)

**Location:**
1 cun superior to the junction of the proximal and middle third of the clavicle.

**Actions/Indications:**
Paraesthesia and paralysis of the upper extremity

**Manipulation:** Vertically 0.3–0.5 cun. During insertion or stimulation, a tingling or warm sensation should be felt radiating to the fingers.

**Caution:** Pneumothorax.

# EXTRA POINTS: Chest and Abdomen (EX-CA)

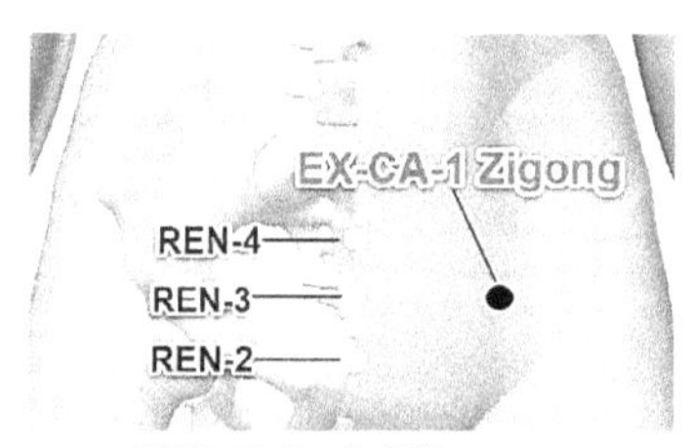


## EX-CA-1 Zigong
(PALACE OF THE CHILD)

**Location:**
3 cun lateral to the anterior midline and 1 cun superior to the upper border of the pubic symphysis.

**Dermatome:** T11/T12

**Main Action Areas:** Uterus, Ovaries, Abdomen

**Main Functions:** Increases fertility. Regulates menstruation. Benefits the uterus.

**Indications:**
Prolapse of the uterus; irregular menstruation; infertility; eclampsia; pain due to hernia; orchitis.

**Manipulation:** 0.5–1 cun vertically or 1–2 cun obliquely towards the upper border of the pubic symphysis.

Moxibustion applicable.

**Caution:** Peritoneum, pregnancy, full bladder.

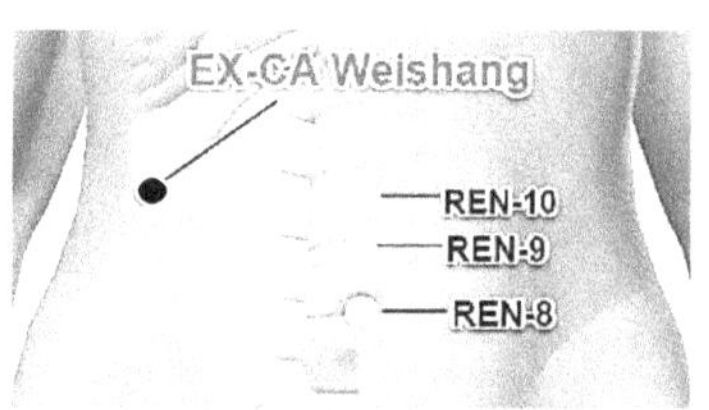


## EX-CA Weishang
(LIFTING THE STOMACH)

**Location:**
On the Spleen channel, 4 cun lateral and 2 cun superior to the umbilicus. Same level as REN-10.

**Actions/Indications:**
Gastroptosis, abdominal pain

**Manipulation:** 2–3 cun obliquely in the direction of the umbilicus.

**Caution:** Peritoneum, pregnancy.

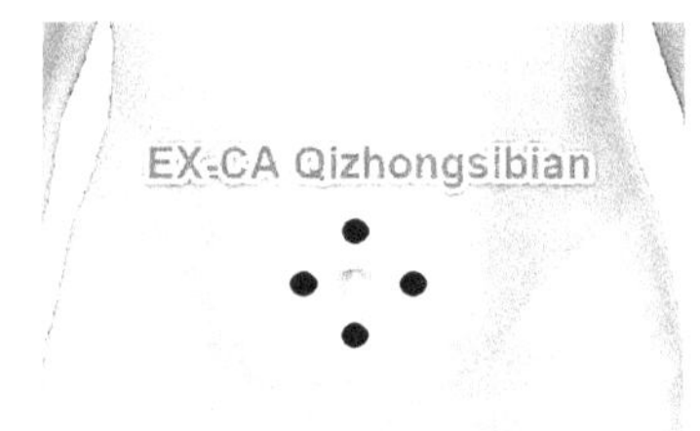


## EX-CA Qizhongsibian
(FOUR POINTS AROUND THE UMBILICUS)

**Location:**
Four points, 1 cun lateral, superior and inferior to the umbilicus.

**Indications:**
Distension, diarrhoea, dyspepsia, dysmenorrhoea

**Manipulation:** Vertically 0.5–1 cun.

**Caution:** Peritoneum, pregnancy.

## EX-CA Yijing
### (Loss of Semen)

**Location:**
1 cun lateral to the anterior midline and 2 cun superior to the upper border of the pubic symphysis. Same level as REN-4.

**Indications:**
Ejaculation disorders, impotence, scrotal eczema.

**Manipulation:** 0.5–1 cun. Caution: Peritoneum, full bladder, pregnancy.

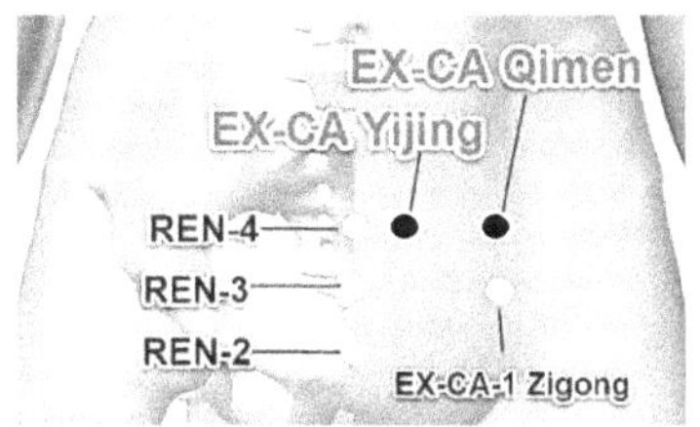


## EX-CA Qimen
### (Qi Gate)

**Location:**
3 cun lateral to the anterior midline and 2 cun superior to the upper border of the pubic symphysis. Same level as REN-4.

**Indications:**
Metrorrhagia, female infertility, orchitis, urinary tract infections, persistent lochial discharge

**Manipulation:** Vertically 0.5–1 cun.

**Caution:** Peritoneum, pregnancy.

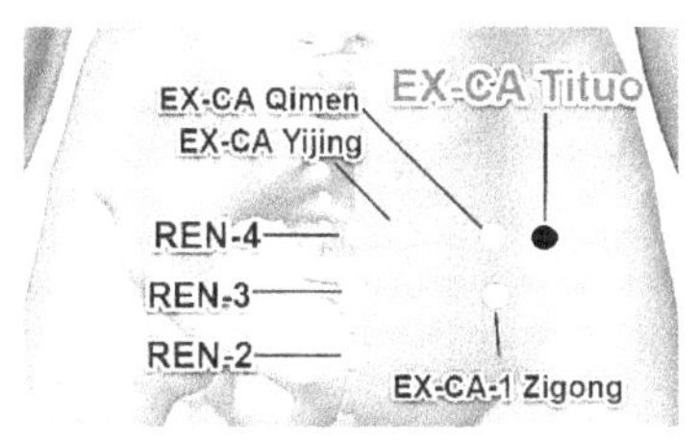


## EX-CA Tituo
### (Lift and Support)

**Location:**
4 cun lateral to the anterior midline and 2 cun superior to the upper border of the pubic symphysis. Same level as REN-4.

**Indications:**
Strengthens the rising Qi and alleviates organ prolapse. Important point for prolapse of the uterus.

**Manipulation:** Vertically 0.5–1 cun.
**Caution:** Peritoneum, pregnancy.

## EX-CA Zhixie
### (End Diarrhea)

**Location:**
On the anterior midline, 2.5 cun inferior to the umbilicus.

**Indications:**

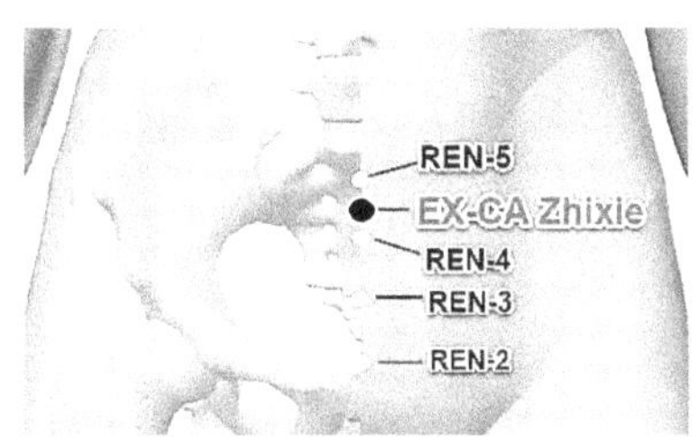


Stops diarrhea

**Manipulation:** Vertically 0.5–1 cun.

**Caution:** Peritoneum, full bladder, pregnancy.

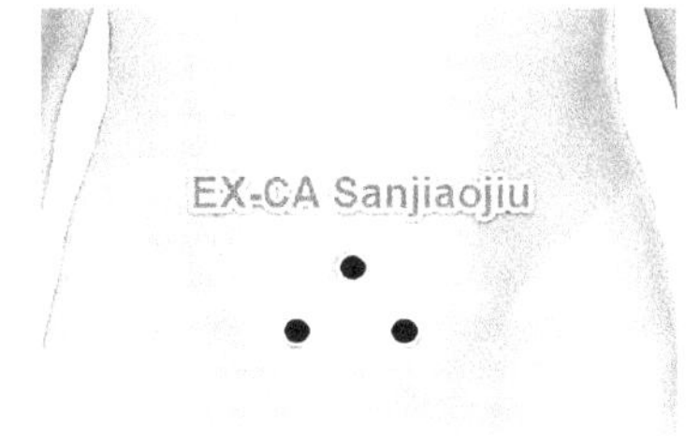


## EX-CA Sanjiaojiu
### (Triangle Moxibustion)

**Location:**
These three points are located on the corners of an equilateral triangle, the apex of which is formed by the umbilicus, while the base forms a horizontal line on the abdomen. The sides are equal to the patient's smile.

**Dermatome:** T10-T12

**Main Action Areas:** Abdomen, Intestines

**Main Functions:** Regulates Qi. Alleviates pain. Stops diarrhoea

**Indications:**
Regulate Qi and stop diarrhea.

**Manipulation:** Moxibustion only, no needling.

# EXTRA POINTS: Back (EX-B)

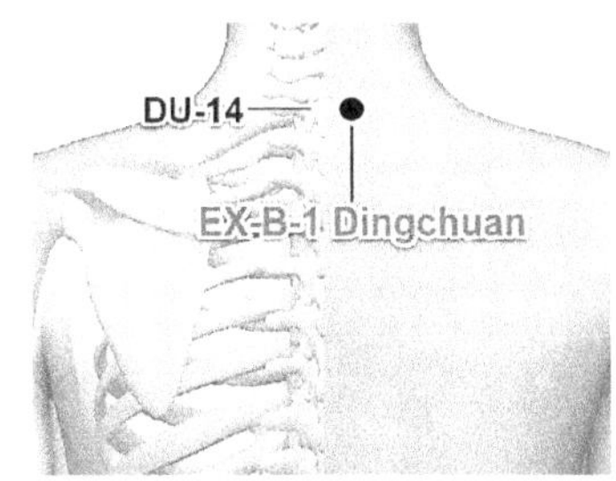


## EX-B-1 Dingchuan
### (Calm Dyspnea)

**Location:**
0.5 cun lateral to Dazhui (DU-14.). (This is also one of the Huatuojiaji points.)

**Dermatome:** C5-T1

**Main Action Areas:** Chest, Lungs, Neck, Upper back

**Main Functions:** Benefits the breathing and alleviates coughing

**Indications:**
Bronchial asthma, local point for the neck and shoulders, effective for dyspnea.

**Manipulation:** 0.5 cun with the needle directed slightly medially.

Moxibustion applicable.

## EX-B-2 Huatuojiaji
### (Hua Tuo's Paravertebral Points)

**Location:**
17 point pairs, 0.5 cun lateral to the lower borders of the spinous processes, close to the spinal facet joints:

- 12 thoracic point pairs (xiongjiaji): between T1 and T12
- 5 lumbar point pairs (yaojiaji): between L1 and L5, Depending on the school of thought, corresponding points lateral to the cervical spine are described as 'additional huatuojiaji'.

**Dermatome:** C3-L5

**Main Action Areas:** Entire body, Spine, Nervous system, Internal organs

**Main Functions:** Alleviates pain. Regulates the pertaining internal

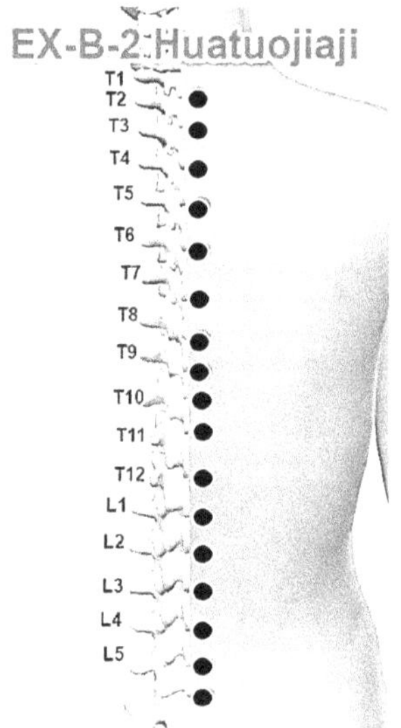



organs and the nervous system. Relaxes the body and mind

**Indications**:

Similar to those of the associated-shu points. The para-vertebral points on the upper back are indicated in disorders of the chest, heart and upper abdomen, liver, gallbladder, spleen and stomach; those in the lumbar region are used in disorders of the lower abdomen, kidney, intestines, bladder and lower extremities.

**Manipulation:** 0.5 - 1.0 cun in the cervical and thoracic regions. 1.0 - 1.5 cun in the lumbar and sacral regions. The needle should be directed slightly obliquely towards the median plane.

Moxibustion applicable.

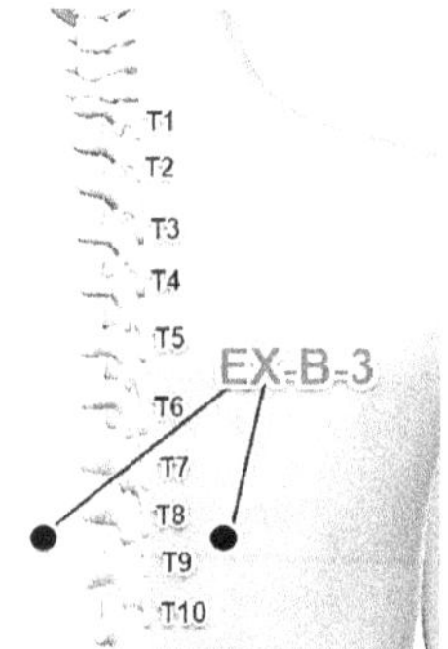



# EX-B-3 Weiwanxiashu

(STOMACH CONTROLLER LOWER SHU)

**Location:**

1.5 cun lateral to the lower border of the spinous process of the 8th thoracic vertebra (T8).

**Indications:**

Diabetes; pain in the stomach, chest and hypochondriac regions.

**Manipulation:** 0.5–1 cun vertically or up to 1.5 cun obliquely in a medial direction. Do not needle in a lateral direction. Moxibustion applicable.

**Caution:** Pneumothorax.

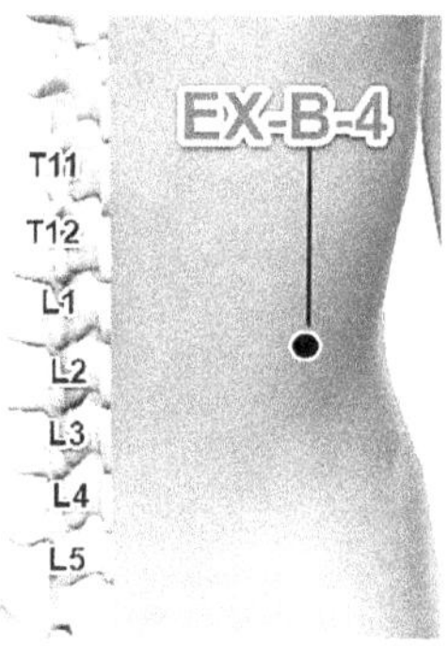



# EX-B-4 Pigen

(FULLNESS ROOT)

**Location:**

3.5 cun lateral to the posterior midline, on the level of the lower border of the spinous process of the 1st lumbar vertebra (L1).

**Indications:**

Lump glomus (specifically hepatosplenomegaly); diarrhea; hernia; lumbar pain; stomach pain.

**Manipulation:** 0.8–1 cun obliquely in a medial direction.

Moxibustion applicable.

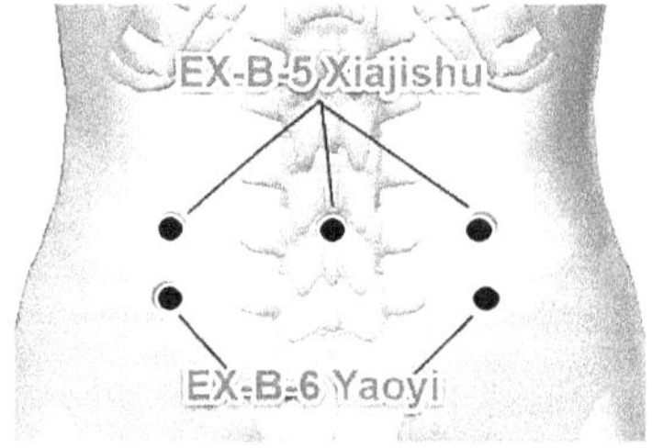



# EX-B-5 Xiajishu

(LOWER SHU POINT)

**Location:**

Three points: one point on the midline below the spinous process of the 3rd lumbar vertebra (L3) (this is the more common and single location of this extra point), complemented by two lateral points 3 cun lateral to the centre point on the midline.

**Manipulation**: 0.5–0.8 cun vertically to the skin or obliquely in an inferior direction. The patient's back should be straight or overextended to avoid a spinal puncture. Oblique insertions in a superior direction should only be carried out by experienced practitioners, as in small persons (regardless of their weight), the spinal canal can be reached after only 1.25 cun.

**Caution:** In pregnant women about to go into labour, this point might have a labour-promoting effect.

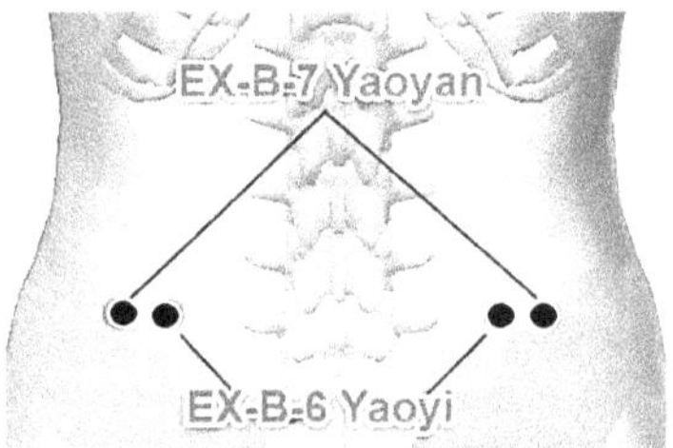



# EX-B-6 Yaoyi

(BACK PAIN POINT)

**Location:**

3 cun lateral to the midline, on the level of the lower border of the spinous process of the 4th lumbar vertebra (L4).

**Dermatome:** T12/L1

**Indications:**

Chronic back pain

**Manipulation:** Vertically 0.5–0.8 cun

# EX-B-7 Yaoyan

(LUMBAR EYES)

**Location:**

3.5 cun lateral to the midline, on the level of the lower border of the spinous process of the 4th lumbar vertebra (L4).

**Dermatome:** T10/T11

**Main Action Areas:** Lower back, Uterus, Urinary system

**Main Functions:** Alleviates pain. Regulates Qi in the lower jiao

**Indications:**

Pulmonary tuberculosis; frequent urination; irregular menstruation; backache.

**Manipulation:** Vertically 0.5-0.8 cun.

Moxibustion applicable.

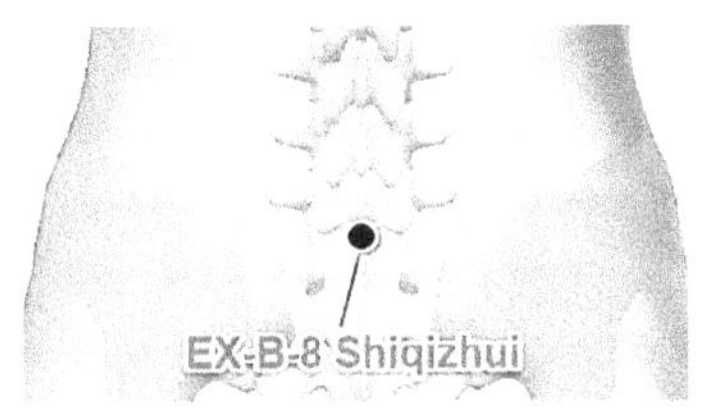

# EX-B-8 Shiqizhui/
### SHIQIZHUIXIA
### (BELOW THE 17TH VERTEBRA)

**Location:**
On the midline, below the spinous process of the 5th lumbar vertebra (L5).

**Dermatome:** T12/L1

**Main Action Areas:** Lower back, Uterus, Urinary system

**Main Functions:** Alleviates pain. Regulates Qi in the lower jiao

**Indications:**
Lumbar pain

**Manipulation:** 0.5–1 cun vertically to the skin or obliquely in an inferior direction.

Moxibustion applicable.

**Caution:** In pregnant women about to go into labour, this point might have a labour-promoting effect.

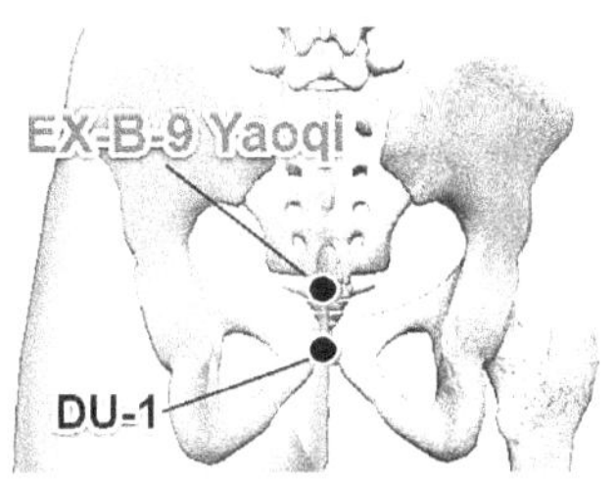

# EX-B-9 Yaoqi
### (MIRACULOUS LUMBAR POINT)

**Location:**
2 cun superior to the tip (inferior end) of the coccyx.

**Indications:**
Insomnia, constipation, epilepsy, headache.

**Manipulation:** Subcutaneous insertion upwards 1.0 - 2.0 cun.

Moxibustion is applicable.

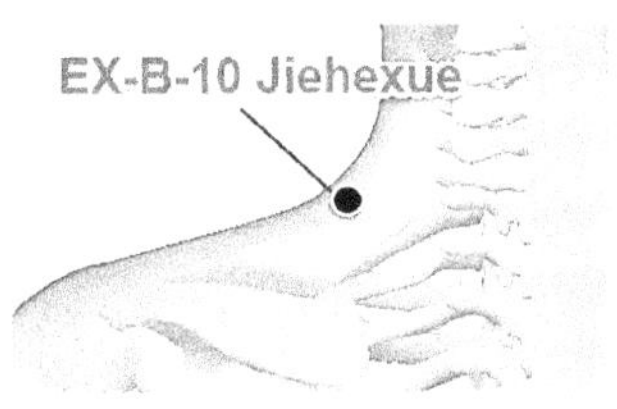

# EX-B-10 Jiehexue
### (TUBERCULOSIS POINT)

**Location:**
3.5 cun lateral to the lower border of the spinous process of the 7th cervical vertebra (C7).

**Actions/Indications:**
Tonifies the Lung, Opens the channel locally.

**Manipulation:** Vertically 0.5–0.8 cun.
**Caution:** Pneumothorax.

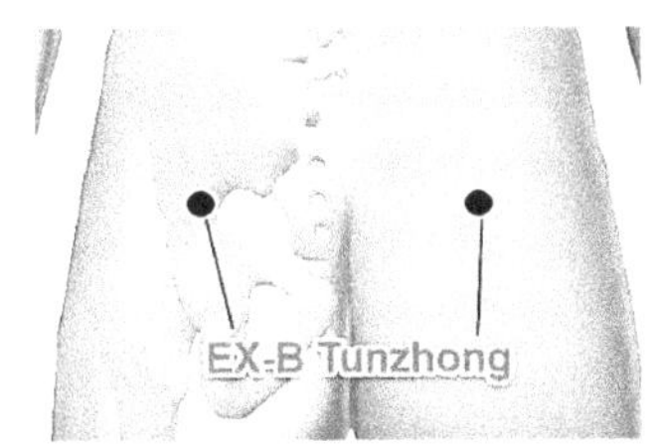

# EX-B Tunzhong
### (BUTTOCK CENTRE)

**Location:**
At the centre of the buttock, 3.5 cun lateral to the posterior midline, on the level of the 4th sacral foramen.

**Actions/Indications:**
Opens the channel and luo vessels locally

**Manipulation:** Vertically 2–3 cun

# EXTRA POINTS: Upper Extremities (EX-UE)

# EX-UE-1 Zhoujian
### (ELBOW TIP)

**Location:**
On the tip of the olecranon. Best located with elbow flexed.

**Indications:**
Scrofula; yong and clove sores.

**Manipulation:** Moxibustion only!

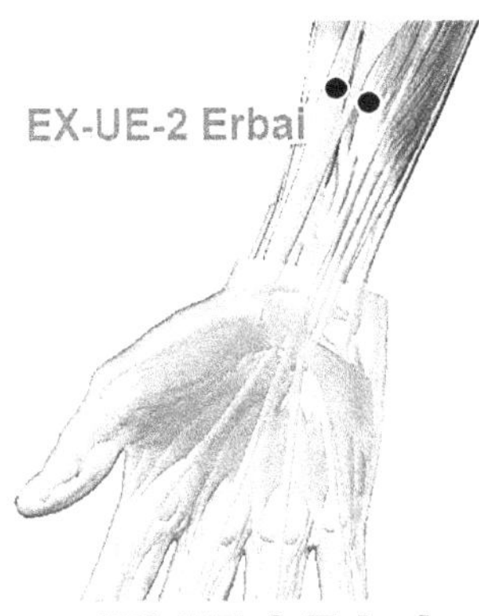

# EX-UE-2 Erbai
### (TWO WHITES)

**Location:**
A pair of points on the palmar aspect of the forearm, 4 cun proximal to the wrist joint space (most distal wrist crease), on either side of the tendon of the flexor carpi radialis muscle.

**Indications:**
Raises Qi to treat prolapse of the rectum and haemorrhoids

**Manipulation:** Up to 1 cun vertically or up to 1.5 cun obliquely towards proximal.

Moxibustion applicable.

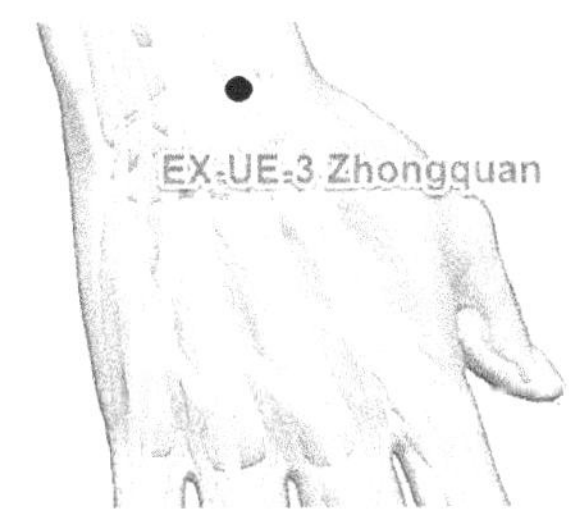

# EX-UE-3 Zhongquan
### (POSTERIOR SPRING)

**Location:**
On the dorsal aspect of the wrist joint space (dorsal wrist crease), radial to the tendon of the extensor digitorum communis muscle.

**Indications:**
Fullness in the chest and spitting of blood.

**Manipulation:** Vertically 0.3–0.5 cun. Moxibustion applicable.

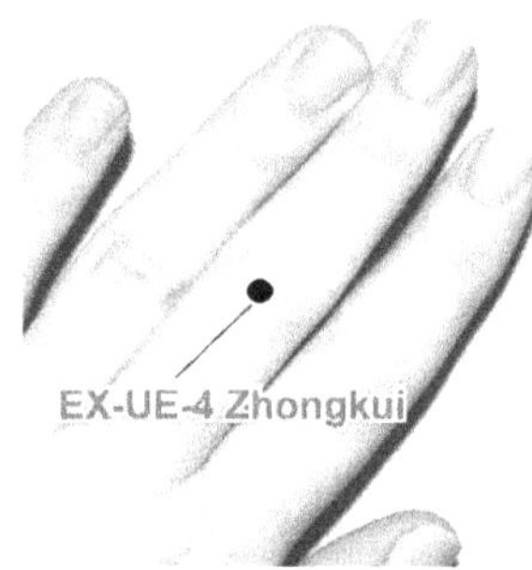


## EX-UE-4 Zhongkui
### (BACK OF THE MIDDLE FINGER)

**Location:**
As the name implies, on the dorsal aspect of the middle finger,

in the centre of the transverse creases of the proximal interphalangeal joint (PIP).

**Indications:**
Hiccup, nausea and vomiting.

**Manipulation:** Prick to bleed or moxibustion.

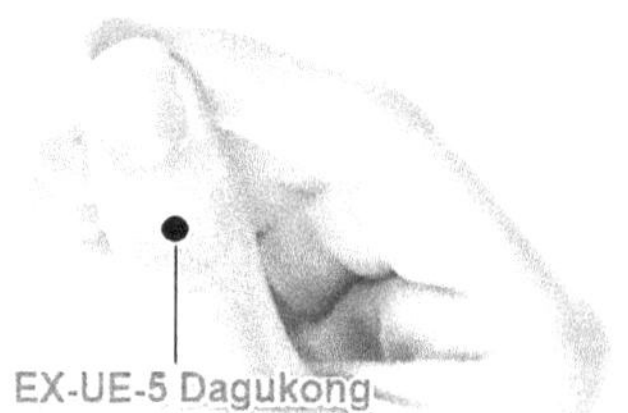


## EX-UE-5 Dagukong
### (THUMB JOINT)

**Location:**
As the name implies, on the dorsal aspect of the thumb, in the centre of the transverse creases of the interphalangeal joint.

**Actions/Indications:**
Clears Heat, Harmonises the Middle Burner

**Manipulation:** Prick to bleed or moxibustion.

## EX-UE-6 Xiaogukong
### (LITTLE FINGER JOINT)

**Location:**
As the name implies, on the dorsal aspect of the little finger, in the centre of the transverse creases of the

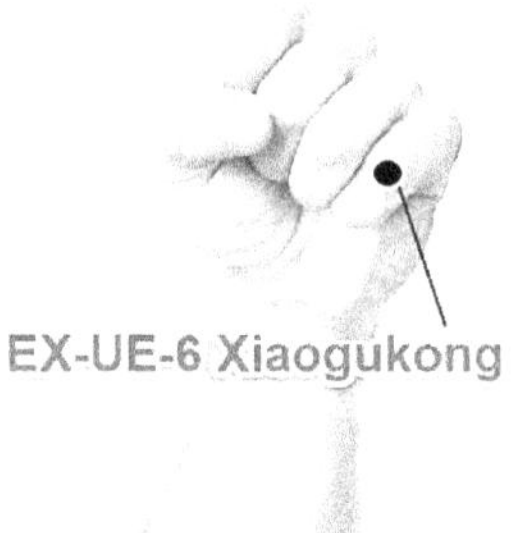


proximal interphalangeal joint (PIP).

**Actions/Indications:**
Clears Heat

**Manipulation:** Prick to bleed

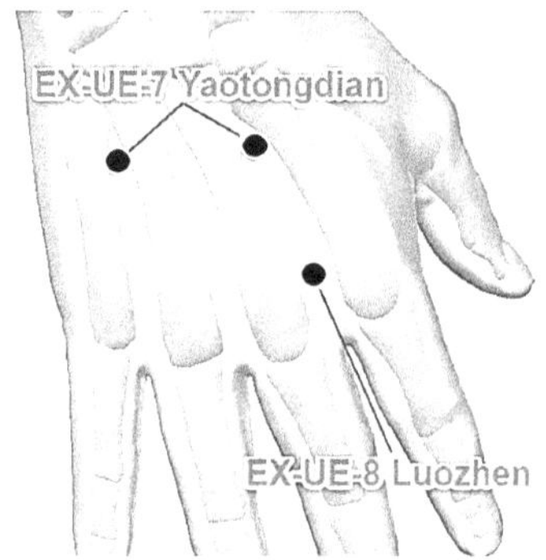


## EX-UE-7 Yaotongdian
### (LUMBAR PAIR POINT)

**Dermatome:** C7/C8

**Main Action Areas:** Lower back

**Main Functions:** Regulates Qi and Blood. Alleviates stiffness and pain

**Indications:**
Lumbar pain; acute lumbar sprain; diabetes; gyneco- logical disorders; orchitis.

**Manipulation:** 0.5–0.8 cun vertically or slightly obliquely towards the centre of a loose fist.

**Caution:** No moxibustion.

## EX-UE-8 Luozhen/ Xianqiang/ Wailaogong
### (STIFF NECK)

**Location:**
On the dorsal aspect of the hand, between the 2nd and 3$^{rd}$ metacarpal bones, proximal to the metacarpophalangeal joints, at the junction of the heads and the shafts of the metacarpal bones.

**Dermatome:** C7

**Main Action Areas:** Neck, Upper limbs

**Main Functions:** Regulates Qi and Blood. Alleviates pain and stiffness

**Indications:**
Inability to turn the head; crick in the neck; pain in the shoulder and arm; stomach pain.

**Manipulation:** 0.5–1 cun vertically or slightly obliquely.

**Caution:** No moxibustion.

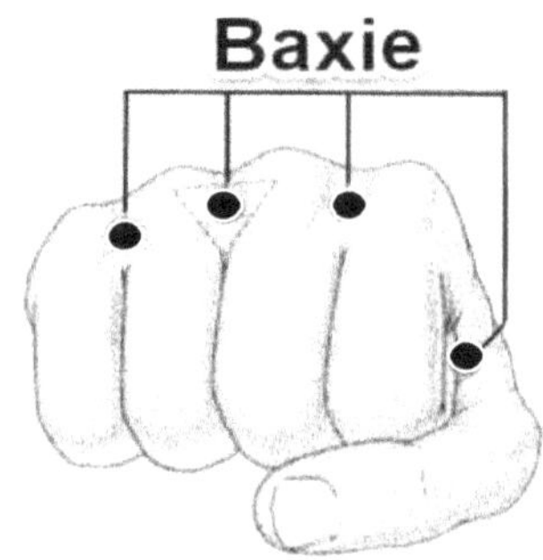


## EX-UE-9 Baxie
### (EIGHT PATHOGENS)

**Location:**
On the dorsum of the hand, on the webs between the 5 fingers; 4 points in each hand, totalling 8 points. (Ba means eight in Chinese.) These points are best located having the patient form a fist.

**Dermatome:** C7/C8

**Main Action Areas:** Head, Redness of throat, Hand and Finger conditions

**Main Functions:** Alleviates pain and stiffness of the hands and fingers

**Indications:**
Disorders of the fingers, rheumatoid arthritis, numbness of fingers.

**Manipulation:** 1.0 cun obliquely proximally.

Moxibustion applicable.

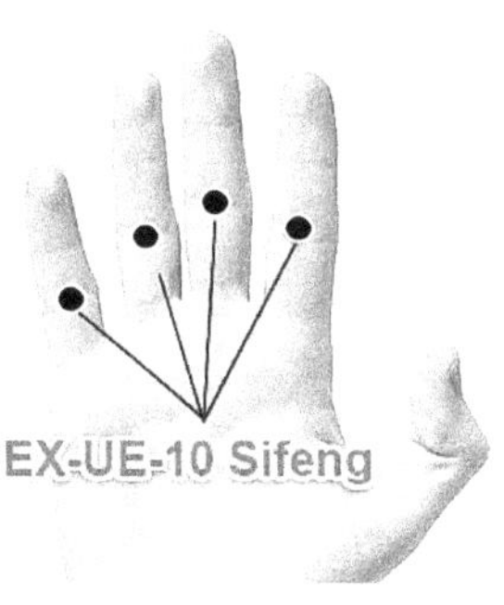



## EX-UE-10 Sifeng
(FOUR SEAMS)

**Location:**
On the palmar aspect of the 2nd to 5th fingers, at the midpoint of the transverse creases of the proximal interphalangeal joints (PIP).

**Dermatome:** C7/C8

**Main Action Areas:** Abdomen, Chest, Fingers

**Main Functions:** Boosts the middle jiao and tonifies the Spleen. Relieves accumulation

**Indications:**
Eating disorders in children; infantile indigestion; whooping cough; roundworm. Pain and stiffness of the fingers.

**Manipulation:** Prick to cause bleeding, or squeeze out a small amount of yellowish viscous fluid locally.

**Caution:** No Moxibustion

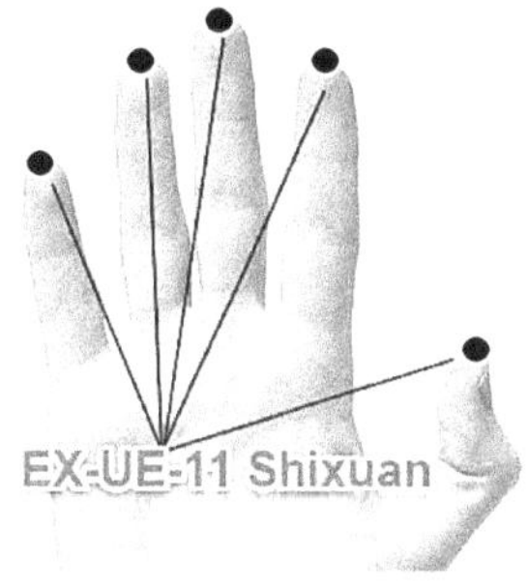



## EX-UE-11 Shixuan
(TEN DIFFUSIONS)

**Location:**
On the tips of the 10 fingers.

**Dermatome:** C7/C8

**Main Action Areas:** Brain, Senses, Abdomen

**Main Functions:** Restores consciousness. Subdues wind and stops seizures.

---

Clears the brain and sense organs. Clears heat and dispels exterior wind.

**Indications:**
Acute tonsillitis; child fright wind; hypertension; wind strike; syncope due to high fever; mania and withdrawal; fright wind; vomiting; diarrhea; numbness of the fingers.

**Manipulation:** Pucture .1 - .2 cun. superficially, or prick to cause bleeding.

**Caution:** No Moxibustion

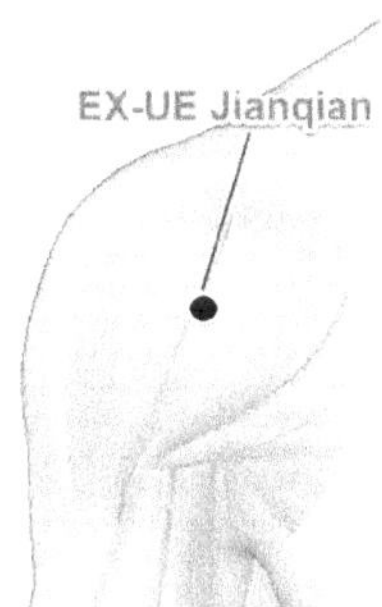



## EX-UE Jianqian/Jianneiling
(FRONT OF THE SHOULDER)

**Location:**
On the midpoint of a line connecting the end of the anterior axillary fold and LI-15.

**Dermatome:** C3/C4

**Main Action Areas:** Shoulder, Upper arm

**Main Functions:** Regulates Qi and Blood. Alleviates stiffness and pain

**Indications:**
Pain in the shoulder and arm; paralysis of the upper extremities.

**Manipulation:**
Vertically up to 1.5 cun.

Moxibustion applicable.

## EX-UE Bizhong
(ARM CENTRE)

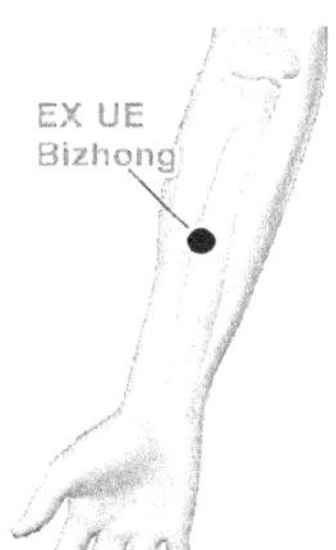



**Location:**
On the palmar aspect of the forearm, midway between the cubital crease and the wrist joint space ('most distal wrist crease').

---

**Indications:**
Pain, spasm or paralysis of the forearm.

**Manipulation:** Vertically 1–1.5 cun. Moxibustion applicable.

# EXTRA POINTS: Lower Extremities (EX-LE)

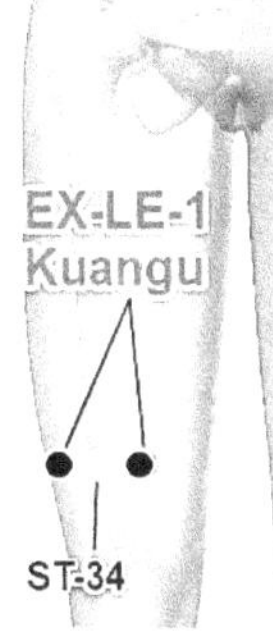



## EX-LE-1 Kuangu
(HIP BONE)

**Location:**
A pair of points 2 cun superior to the patella and 1.5 cun lateral and medial to ST-34 (liangqiu).

**Actions:**
Alleviate pain

**Manipulation:** Vertically 1–1.5 cun

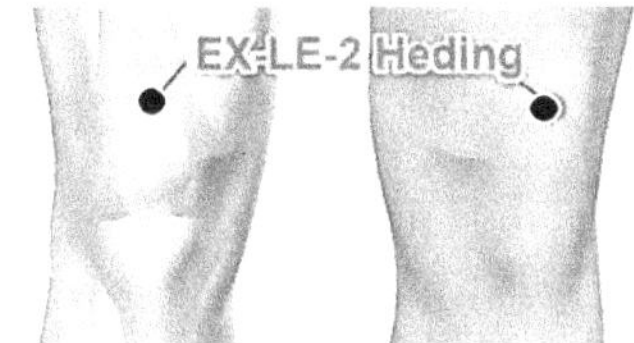



## EX-LE-2 Heding/Xiding
(CRANE'S SUMMIT)

**Location:**
On the midpoint of the upper border of the patella.

**Dermatome:** L3

**Main Action Areas:** Knees, Patella

**Main Functions:** Alleviates stiffness and pain

**Indications:**
Disorders of the knee joint.

**Manipulation:** 0.5 cun perpendicularly.

Moxibustion applicable.

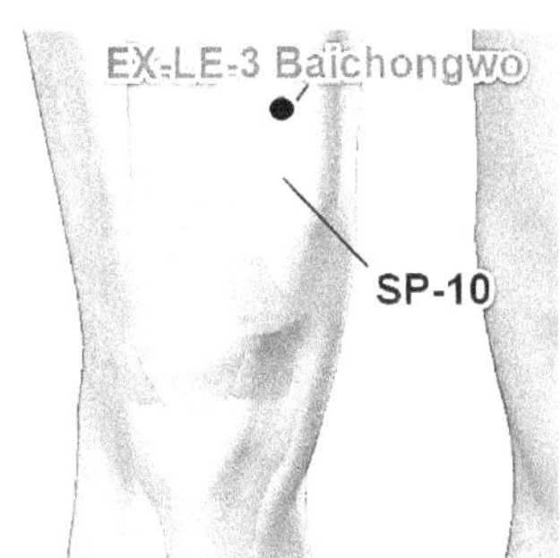

## EX-LE-3 Baichongwo
### (Hundred Insect Burrow)

**Location:**
3 cun superior and 1 cun medial to the upper medial border of the patella, in a small depression on the vastus medialis muscle or 1 cun superior to SP-10.

**Indications:** Parasitic diseases, rubella, eczema.

**Manipulation:** Vertically 1–2 cun.
Moxibustion applicable.

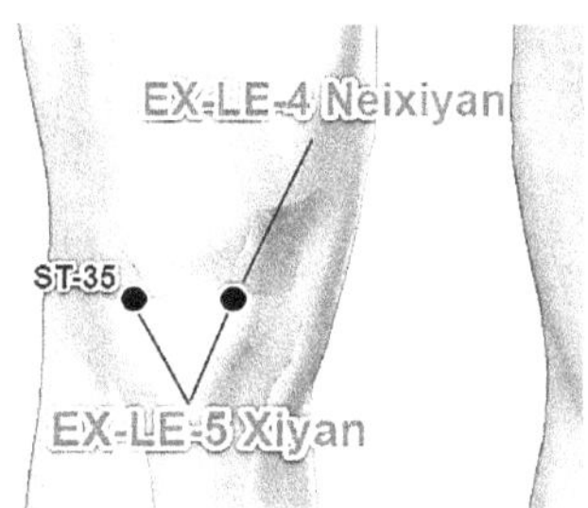


## EX-LE-4 Neixiyan
### (Inner Eye of the Knee)

**Location:**
With the knee flexed, inferior to the patella, in a depression medial to the patellar ligament.

**Indications:**
Disorders of the knee joint

**Manipulation:** 0.5–1 cun vertically or obliquely towards the lateral eye of the knee.

**Caution:** Too deep insertion may injure Knee joint.

## EX-LE-5 Xiyan
### (Eyes of the Knee)

**Location:**
With the knee flexed, this pair of points is located inferior to the patella, medial and lateral to the patellar ligament. EX-LE-5 includes two points: the medial eye of the knee corresponds to EX-LE-4 and the lateral eye of the knee to ST-35.

**Dermatome:** L3-L5 junction at knee

**Main Action Areas:** Knees, Lower limbs

**Main Functions:** Regulates Qi and Blood. Alleviates stiffness, swelling and pain

**Indications:**
Numbness, pain, or swelling of the knee; limpness of the lower extremities.

**Manipulatrion:** Medial eye of the knee: 0.5–1 cun vertically or obliquely towards the lateral eye of the knee; lateral eye of the knee: 0.5–1 cun vertically or obliquely towards the medial eye of the knee.

Moxibustion applicable.

**Caution:** Do not needle too deeply to avoid intra-articular puncture.

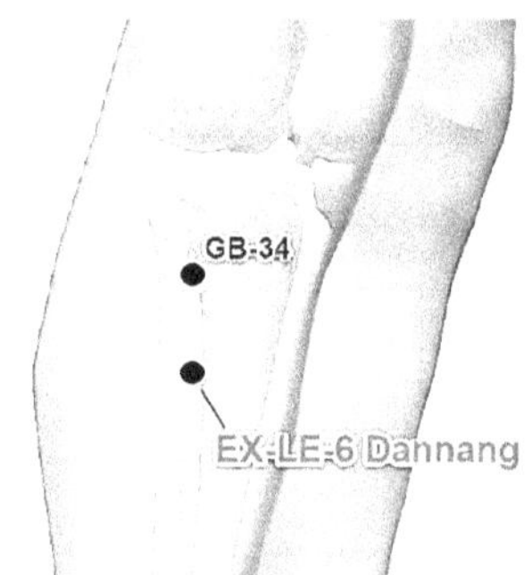


## EX-LE-6 Dannang/
### Dannangxue
### (Gall Bladder Point)

Alarm point of the Gall Bladder Channel.

**Location:**
1.0 to 2.0 cun below Yanglingquan (GB-34.), on the Gall Bladder Channel. Check for tenderness.

**Dermatome:** L5

**Main Action Areas:** Gallbladder, Digestive system

**Main Functions:** Regulates Qi, dispels stasis and alleviates pain. Benefits the gallbladder

**Indications:**
Diseases of the gall bladder such as such as cholecystitis and cholelithiasis and the liver.

**Manipulation:** 1.0 cun perpendicularly. (Tenderness on this point is diagnostically significant).

**Caution:** No moxibustion.

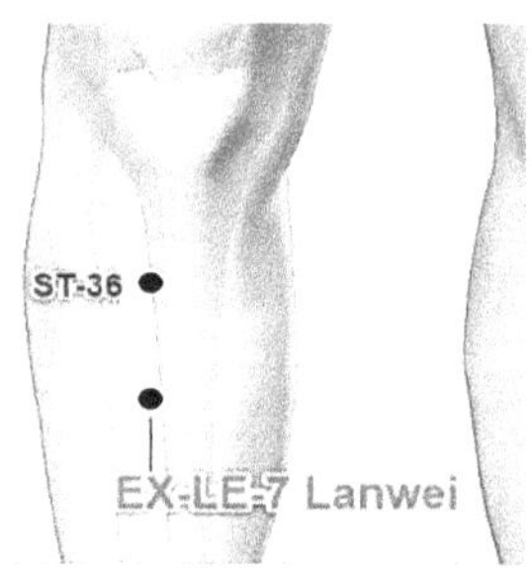


## EX-LE-7
## Lanwei/Lanweixue
### (Appendix Point)

Alarm point of the vermiform appendix.

**Location:**
Approximately 2 cun below ST-36, on the Stomach Channel. Check for tenderness.

**Dermatome:** L5

**Main Action Areas:** Appendix, Large Intestine, Shin

**Main Functions:** Clears heat, dampness and fire poisons from the Large Intestine. Alleviates pain

**Indications:**
Appendicitis, post-operative pain after appendicectomy. Muscular atrophy; loss of locomotive ability of the lower extremities.

**Manipulation:** 1.0 cun perpendicularly.

**Caution:** No moxibustion.

**Remarks:** This point becomes tender in acute appendicitis and is therefore particularly useful in confirming the diagnosis.

## EX-LE-8 Neihuaijian
### (Medial Malleolus Tip)

**Location:**

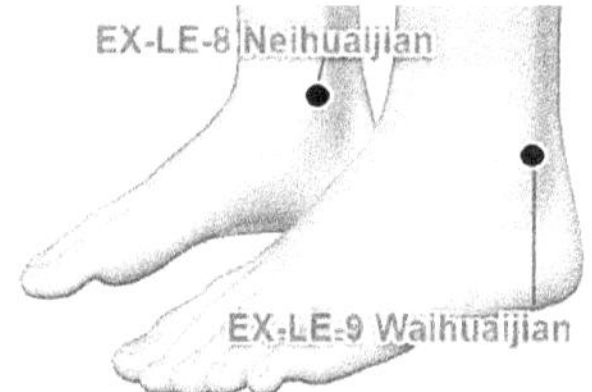


On the highest point of the medial malleolus.

**Indications:**
Pain in the medial ankle region

**Manipulation:** 0.1 cun transversely (subcutaneously) or prick to bleed.

## EX-LE-9 Waihuaijian
(OUTER MALLEOLUS TIP)

**Location:**
On the highest point of the lateral malleolus.

**Indications:**
Pain in the lateral ankle region

**Manipulation:** 0.1 cun transversely (subcutaneously) or prick to bleed.

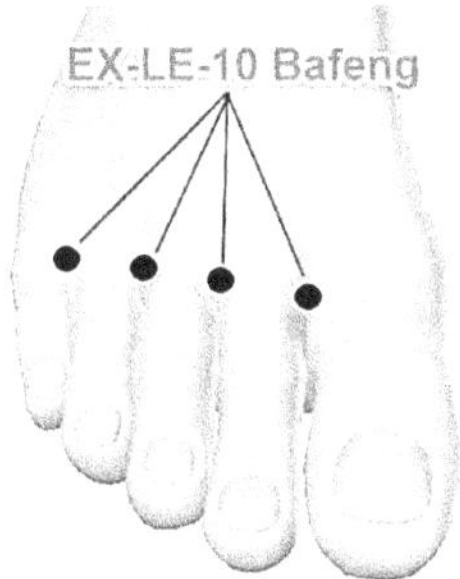


## EX-LE-10 Bafeng
(EIGHT WINDS)

**Location:**
On the dorsum of the foot, 0.5 cun proximal to the borders of the webs between the 5 toes; 4 points on each foot totalling 8 points.

**Dermatome:** L5/S1

**Main Action Areas:** MTP joints

**Main Functions:** Alleviates stiffness and pain. Regulates Qi and Blood. Clears heat

**Indications:**
Arthritis of toes, numbness of foot and toes.

**Manipulation:** 0.5 cun obliquely and proximally.

Moxibustion applicable.

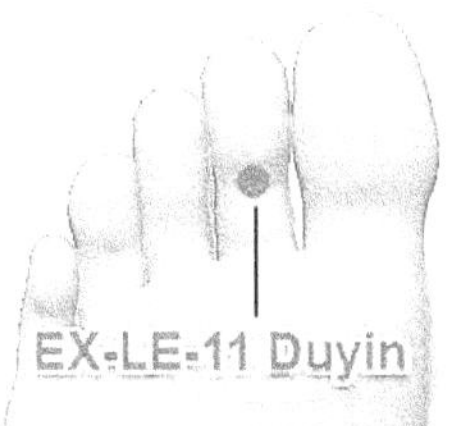


## EX-LE-11 Duyin
(SOLITARY YIN)

**Location:**
On the plantar aspect of the 2nd toe, at the midpoint of the transverse crease of the distal interphalangeal joint.

**Shared location with Tung:** 55.01

**Indications:**
Acute angina, thoracic and hypochondriac pain, nausea, vomiting, retention of the lochia, irregular menstruation, inguinal hernia

**Manipulation:** 0.2–0.3 cun vertically or transversely (subcutaneously) or prick to bleed or moxibustion.

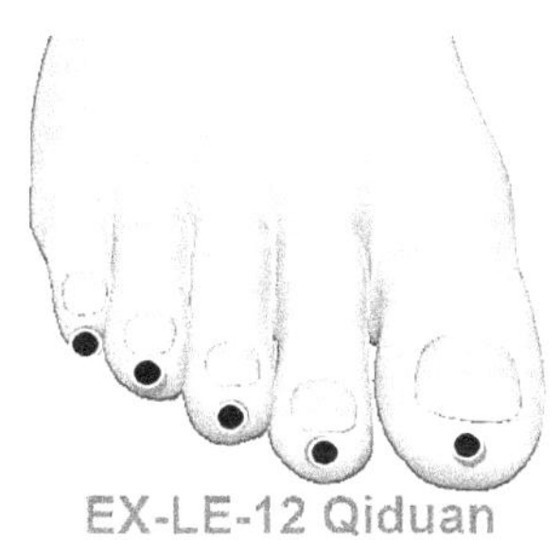


## EX-LE-12 Qiduan
(END OF QI)

**Location:**
On the tips of the 10 toes.

**Indications:**
Syncope, edema of the feet, acute abdominal pain

**Manipulation:** Prick to bleed

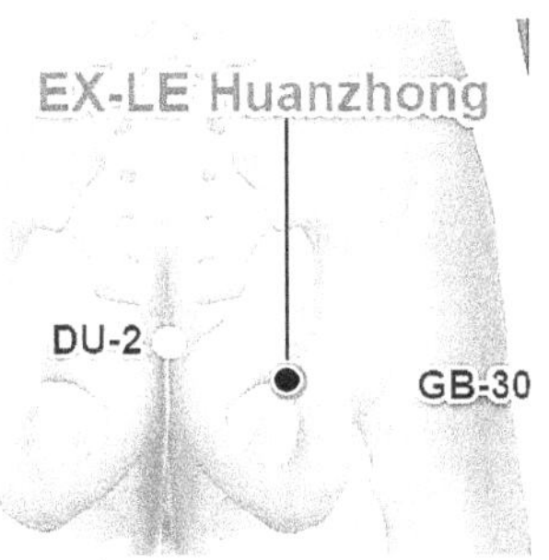


## EX-LE Huanzhong
(CIRCLE CENTRE)

**Location:**
Midway between GB-30 (huantiao) and DU-2 (yaoshu).

**Indications:**
Sciatica, urinary tract infection, haemorrhoids, paralysis of the lower extremities

**Manipulation:** Vertically 2–2.5 cun.

Moxibustion applicable.

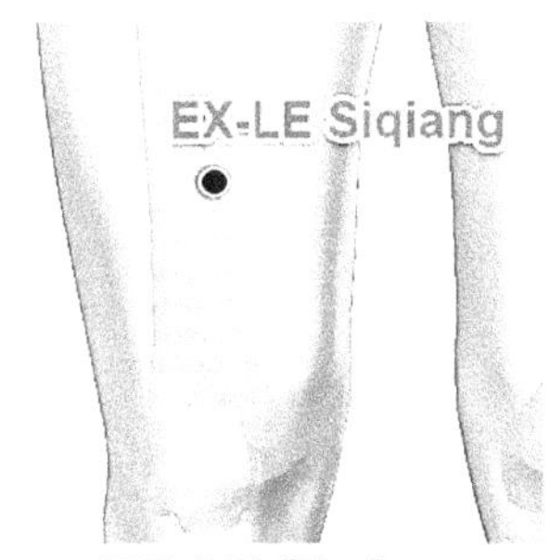


## EX-LE Siqiang
(FOUR MUSCLES STRENGTHENING POINT)

**Location:**
4.5 cun superior to the centre of the upper patellar border.

**Indications:**
Paralysis and atrophy of the muscles of the lower extremities,

especially of the quadriceps femoris muscle

**Manipulation:** Vertically 1–2 cun

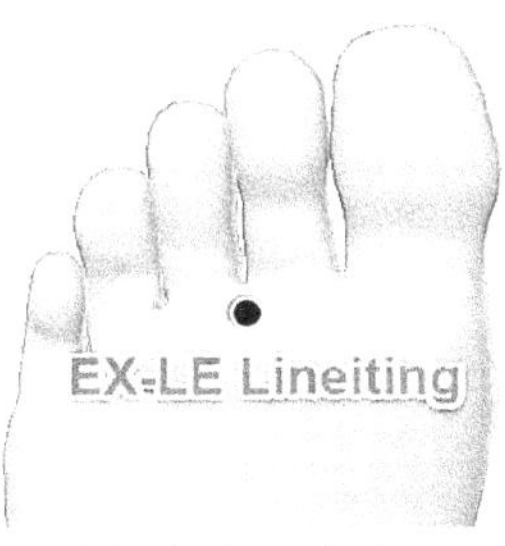


## EX-LE Lineiting
(PLANTAR INNER SPACE)

**Location:**
On the plantar aspect of the foot, between the 2nd and 3rd metatarsal bones, opposite ST-44 (neiting).

**Indications:**
Acute epigastric pain, local pain, epilepsy, restlessness

**Manipulation:** 0.2–0.3 cun vertically towards ST-44.

Moxibustion applicable.

# DISEASES TREATED BY MASTER TUNG AND TCM ACUPUNCTURE

# HOW TO SELECT TREATMENT POINTS

When it comes to choosing acupuncture points for treatment, acupuncturists follow general guidelines that are applicable to both the 14 Channels Acupuncture System and the Master Tung System. The guidelines used in this book include:

1. **Acupuncture Points can treat pathology in their local area**

   For example, to treat knee pain, points on the knee can be chosen. This is sometimes referred to as local or Ashi treatment although the point used need not necessarily be tender.

2. **Disorder can be treated on points of the meridians which pass the affected area.**

   For example, all the points along the Stomach meridian can treat digestive disorders and also headache because the meridian transverses the affected (sick) areas. This explains the effective use of ST-44 to treat headaches.

3. **Treating in response to pathological changes**

   Where there is tenderness, swelling, pain, injury or change of skin color/texture, treatments like guasha, moxibustion or blood-letting can be used, in addition to needling. The treatment area does not necessarily have to be on established acupuncture points or pathways. Example is cupping the shoulder and scapula to treat shoulder issues.

4. **Highly effective points on every meridian**

   Every meridian has points which are more effective than others. In particular, the Transport or Five Shu Points on each meridian. Other special points used in this book include front-mu, back-shu, xi-cleft, influential and luo-connecting points. Examples are: LIV-3 (Shu-Stream), LI-4 (Yuan Source), P-6 (Luo-connecting) – some of the most commonly used acupuncture points.

5. **Creating Balance in a Treatment through Channel or Holographic Correspondence**

   Needling points from another meridian can be used to balance the "sick" meridian. This is the underlining principle of the Dr. Tan Balance method. Example, the Hand Tai Yin (Lung meridian) treats the Foot Tai Yin (Spleen meridian)

6. **Each point has Reaction Areas which influences particular organs**

   Master Tung's points are categorized based on their corresponding reaction areas, which reflect the functions of both TCM and Western organs. This means that if a point's reaction area is associated with the Kidney, example 77.18 Shen Guan, it has the potential to address both the physical dysfunction of the kidney diagnosed through clinical tests and diarrhea caused by Kidney deficiency (a TCM diagnosis).

7. **Choosing treatment points through Imaging Correspondence**

   Every part of the body has various corresponding parts which can be used for treatment. Example, the point on the elbow, LI-11, corresponds to the knee and can be used to treat knee pain. Similarly, the pain on the sole of the foot can be treated with points on the palm of the hand.

8. **Choosing Points through Tissue Correspondence**

   Each tissue resonates with its specific tissue. Example needling the Achilles tendon, 77.01+77.02, on the ankle will treat neck issues related to tendons, "tendon treats tendon". Similarly, "muscle treats muscle", "bone treats bone", "skin treats skin" etc.

# MASTER TUNG ACUPUNCTURE SYSTEM

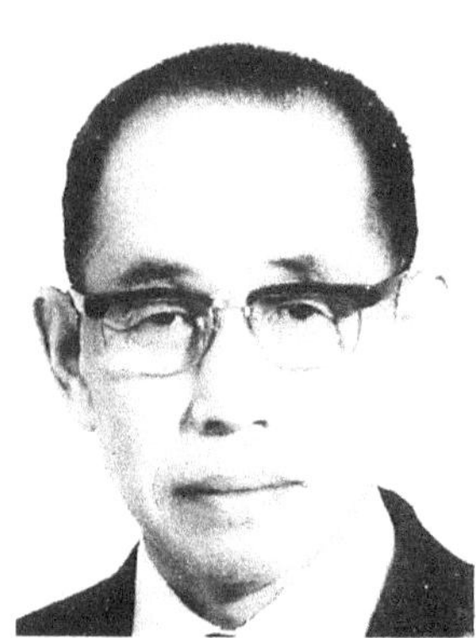

Master Tung, also known as Tung Ching-Chang, was born in 1916 in Ping Du County, Shan Dong Province, China, into a family of acupuncturists. He began providing acupuncture treatment to his fellow soldiers when he joined the Nationalist army at a young age. Following the end of the China-Japan war, he returned to Qing Dao City and opened an acupuncture clinic. In 1949, he relocated to Taiwan and established his acupuncture clinic in Taipei City, where he began accepting students in 1962. A total of 73 students studied with him.

Master Tung's acupuncture points are organized into 10 areas, as well as the dorsal and ventral trunk, which is similar to the Systematic Classic of Acupuncture and Moxibustion from 256-260 AD. This suggests that his family's acupuncture tradition has a long history. However, Tung's acupuncture points differ from the traditional 14-channel acupuncture points in terms of their location and system of channels, and has distinct treatment principles and diagnostic methods.

Here are some underlying principles of the Master Tung style acupuncture:

- Local pain/injured areas are seldom needled.
- Distal treatment – the more distal (below knees and elbows) the more effective.
- Contralateral needling for pain or structural problems.
- For chronic conditions and treating organ issues, needle bilaterally.
- When carrying out blood-letting, treat affected side.
- Blood-letting techniques are effective in chronic and difficult cases.

Master Tung Acupuncture has several needling techniques peculiar to the system:

## Dao Ma Technique

One of the most unique features of Master Tung's Acupuncture is the use of synergistic needling, which he called Dao Ma. The Dao Ma technique uses two or three points combined, most commonly arranged in a vertical line or along a channel, to increase needle stimulation. These points are located relatively close to each other, usually no more than two or three cun apart. Dao Ma groups are usually needled in combination rather than as single points. The goal is to achieve more effective and immediate results.

## Active Qi Moving technique

When inserting a needle to treat an injured area, the patient will be asked to move that area, example the wrist for wrist pain, or to assist him to move the affected area if he is unable to do so. This helps to direct or focus Qi/Blood to the affected area. The patient will be asked to report any relieve of symptoms. Thus, assisting the practitioner to instantly assess the effectiveness of his treatment approach.

## Guide Point

Another method to bring focus to the affected area is the use of guide points. Guide points are always located on the same side as the affected area but distally. Shu-stream point of the affected meridian are usually chosen.

# DR. TAN BALANCE METHOD

The Balance Method is a form of acupuncture that was developed by a Taiwanese-American acupuncturist, Dr. Richard Teh-Fu Tan. Dr. Tan developed a logical system to determine the body's energetic points. By providing a strategical method to the ancient practice of acupuncture, the Balance Method ensures the efficacy of each acupuncture session, often bringing about immediate relief from pain.

The three important steps when using the Dr. Tan Balance Method are:

Step 1: Diagnose the sick meridian

Step 2: Determine the Treating Meridian based on the chart below

Step 3: Point selection based on Step 2 with correspondence to mirroring and imaging.

| SYSTEM | 1 | 2 | 3 | 4 | 5 | 6 |
|---|---|---|---|---|---|---|
| **SICK MERIDIAN** | HAND/ FOOT | YIN/YANG HAND/FOOT | INTERNAL/ EXTERNAL | CLOCK OPPOSITE | CLOCK NEIGHBOR | SAME MERIDIAN |
| **Needle** | Opposite Side | Either Side | Opposite Side | Either Side | Opposite Side | Same Side |
| **LU** Hand Taiyin | **SP** Foot Taiyin | **BL** Foot Taiyang | **LI** Hand Yangming | **BL** Foot Taiyang | **LIV** Foot Jueyin | **LU** Hand Taiyin |
| **LI** Hand Yangming | **ST** Foot Yangming | **LIV** Foot Jueyin | **LU** Hand Taiyin | **KI** Foot Shaoyin | **ST** Foot Yangming | **LI** Hand Yangming |
| **ST** Foot Yangming | **LI** Hand Yangming | **P** Hand Jueyin | **SP** Foot Taiyin | **P** Hand Jueyin | **LI** Hand Yangming | **ST** Foot Yangming |
| **SP** Foot Taiyin | **LU** Hand Taiyin | **SI** Hand Taiyang | **ST** Foot Yangming | **SJ** Hand Shaoyang | **HT** Hand Shaoyin | **SP** Foot Taiyin |
| **HT** Hand Shaoyin | **KI** Foot Shaoyin | **GB** Foot Shaoyang | **SI** Hand Taiyang | **GB** Foot Shaoyang | **SP** Foot Taiyin | **HT** Hand Shaoyin |
| **SI** Hand Taiyang | **BL** Foot Taiyang | **SP** Foot Taiyin | **HT** Hand Shaoyin | **LIV** Foot Jueyin | **BL** Foot Taiyang | **SI** Hand Taiyang |
| **BL** Foot Taiyang | **SI** Hand Taiyang | **LU** Hand Taiyin | **KI** Foot Shaoyin | **LU** Hand Taiyin | **SI** Hand Taiyang | **BL** Foot Taiyang |
| **KI** Foot Shaoyin | **HT** Hand Shaoyin | **SJ** Hand Shaoyang | **BL** Foot Taiyang | **LI** Hand Yangming | **P** Hand Jueyin | **KI** Foot Shaoyin |
| **P** Hand Jueyin | **LIV** Foot Jueyin | **ST** Foot Yangming | **SJ** Hand Shaoyang | **ST** Foot Yangming | **KI** Foot Shaoyin | **P** Hand Jueyin |
| **SJ** Hand Shaoyang | **GB** Foot Shaoyang | **KI** Foot Shaoyin | **P** Hand Jueyin | **SP** Foot Taiyin | **GB** Foot Shaoyang | **SJ** Hand Shaoyang |
| **GB** Foot Shaoyang | **SJ** Hand Shaoyang | **HT** Hand Shaoyin | **LIV** Foot Jueyin | **HT** Hand Shaoyin | **SJ** Hand Shaoyang | **GB** Foot Shaoyang |
| **LIV** Foot Jueyin | **P** Hand Jueyin | **LI** Hand Yangming | **GB** Foot Shaoyang | **SI** Hand Taiyang | **LU** Hand Taiyin | **LIV** Foot Jueyin |

# IMAGING CORRESPONDENCE

The mirror/imaging theory suggests that each point on the body has a corresponding point on the opposite side of the body. For example, a point on the left hand may correspond to a point on the right foot. By treating these corresponding points, acupuncturists aim to balance the flow of Qi in the body. The most commonly used image correspondences are shown in this chapter. *Pics on this page is credited to Alex Costa.*

"**Man corresponds with nature**: In heaven, there are Yin and Yang;
in man, there are 12 large joints of the limbs,"
"When one **understands the principles of the 12 joints,**
a sage will never surpass him."
"Diverse pricking to the right side or to the left,
contralateral insertion of pricking
the **upper part to cure the lower disease,**
and pricking the **left side to cure the right.**"

"Nei Jing"

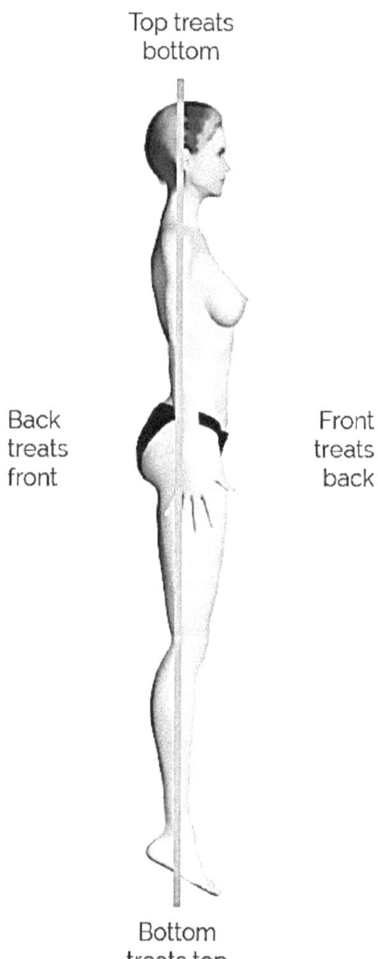


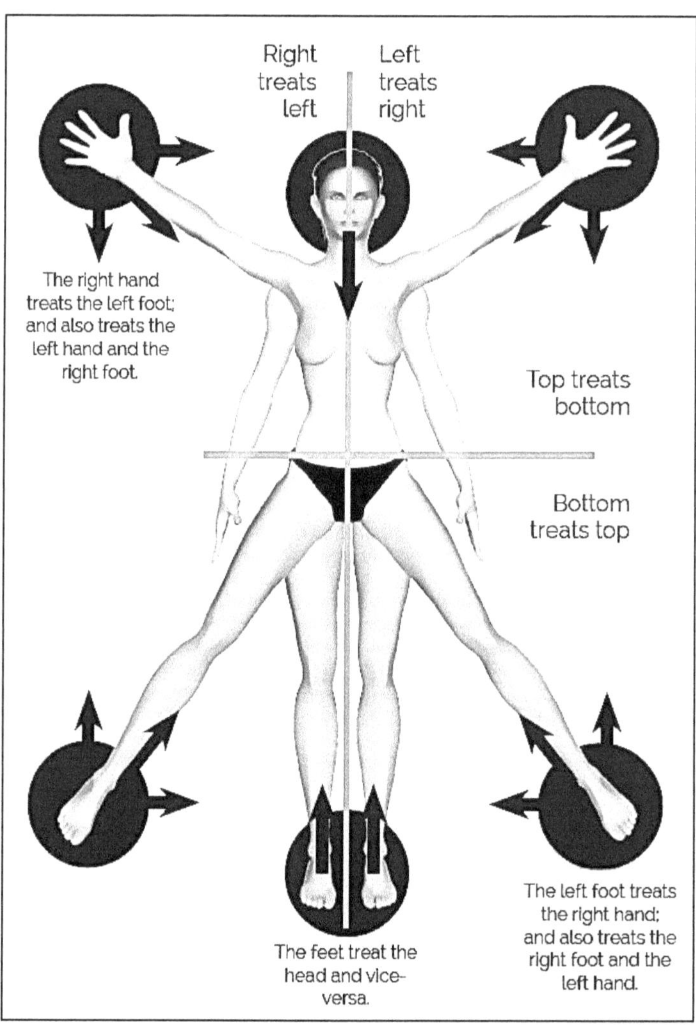

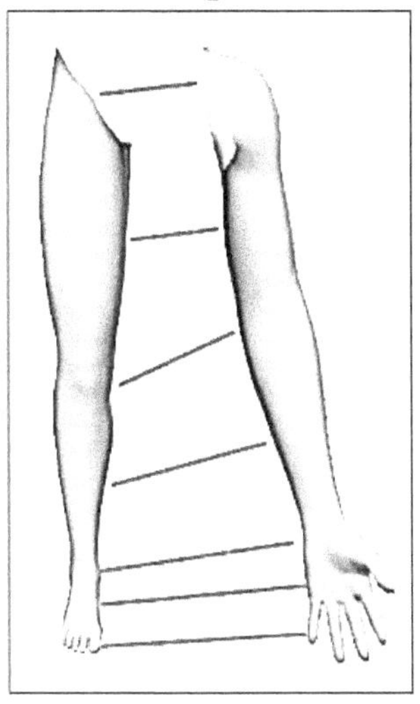

Mirroring Format

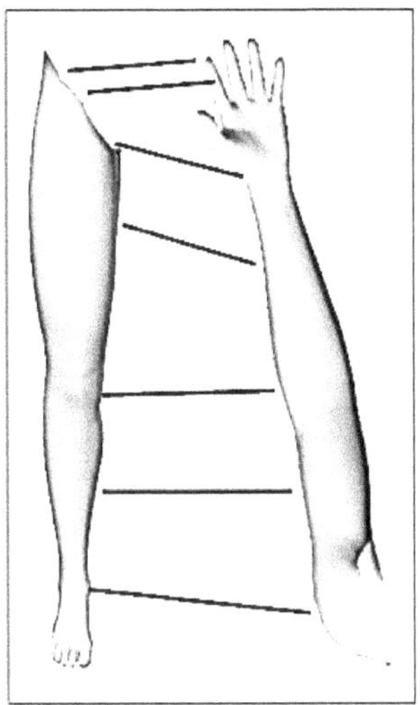

Reverse Mirroring Format

| Mirror Format | Reverse Mirror Format |
|---|---|
| Finger - Toe | Finger – Top of Hip |
| Hand - Foot | Hand - Hip |
| Wrist - Ankle | Wrist – Hip Joint |
| Forearm – Lower Leg | Forearm - Thigh |
| Elbow - Knee | Elbow - Knee |
| Upper Arm - Thigh | Upper Arm – Lower Leg |
| Shoulder - Hip | Shoulder - Ankle |

## IMAGE OF LOWER LIMB TO HEAD AND TRUNK

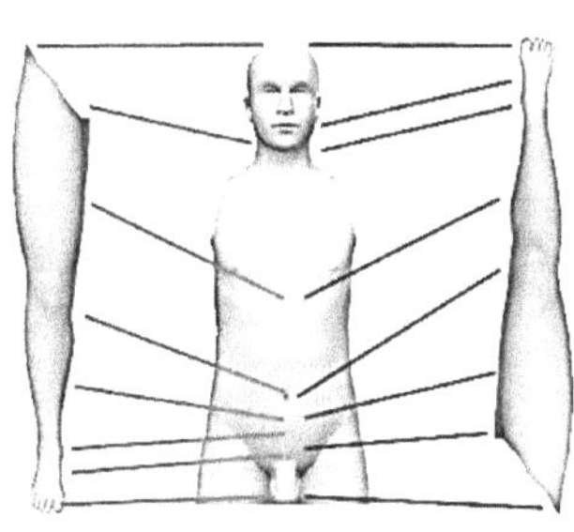

| Needled Area | Image | Reverse Image |
|---|---|---|
| Toe | Testicles and anus | Top of head |
| Foot | Genitals, coccyx, lower sacrum | Head and base of skull |
| Ankle | Genitals, bladder, sacrum | Neck and neck joint |
| Lower Leg | Lower abdomen, lower back | Upper abdomen, rib cage, chest, mid-upper back |
| Knee | Umbilicus level, Lumbar 2, waist | Umbilicus level, Lumbar 2, waist |
| Upper leg | Upper abdomen, rib cage, chest, mid-upper back | Lower back, lower abdomen |
| Hip Joint | Neck, jaw, base of skull | Sacrum, genitals, coccyx |
| Top of hip | Top of head | Testicles and anus |

## IMAGE OF UPPER LIMB TO HEAD AND TRUNK

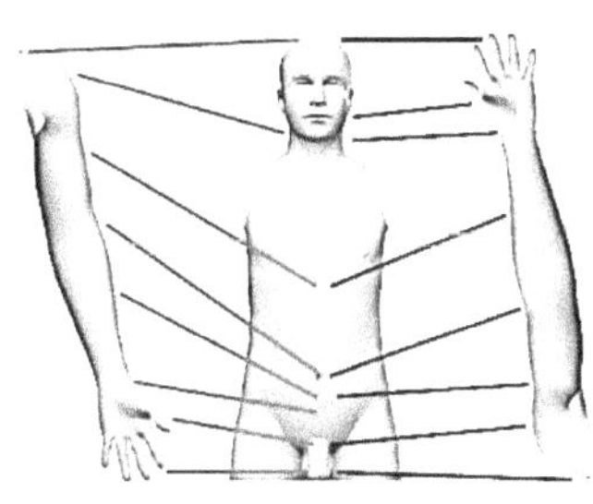

| Needled Area | Image | Reverse Image |
|---|---|---|
| Finger | Testicles and anus | Top of head |
| Hand | Genitals, coccyx, lower sacrum | Head and base of skull |
| Wrist | Genitals, bladder, sacrum | Neck and neck joint |
| Forearm | Lower abdomen, lower back | Upper abdomen, rib cage, chest, mid-upper back |
| Elbow | Umbilicus level, Lumbar 2, waist | Umbilicus level, Lumbar 2, waist |
| Upper arm | Upper abdomen, rib cage, chest, mid-upper back | Lower back, lower abdomen |
| Shoulder | Neck, jaw, base of skull | Sacrum, genitals, coccyx |
| Top of shoulder | Top of head | Testicles and anus |

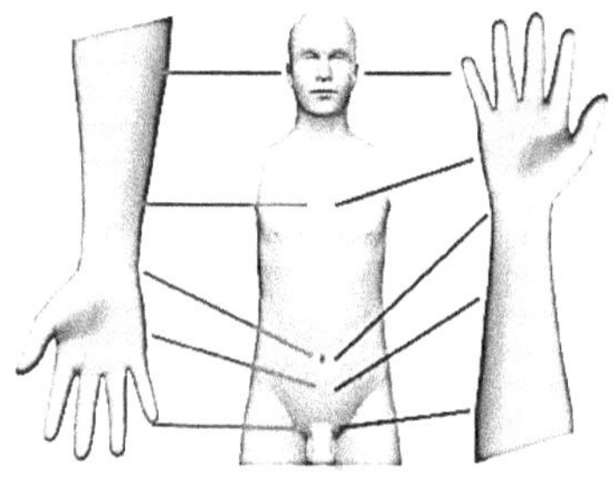

### IMAGE OF BELOW ELBOW TO HEAD AND TRUNK

| Needled Area | Image | Reverse Image |
| --- | --- | --- |
| Forearm (A) | Head, Face | Fingers |
| Forearm (B) | Thorax, Upper Back | Hand |
| Wrist | Navel, Waist | Wrist |
| Hand | Abdomen, Low Back | Forearm (B) |
| Fingers | Genitalia, Tailbone | Forearm (A) |

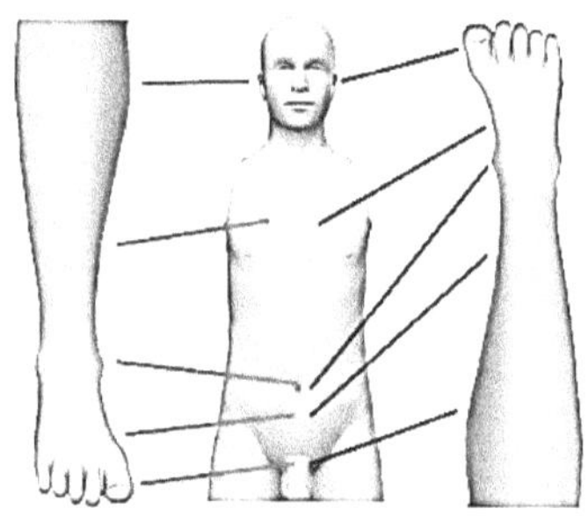

### IMAGE OF BELOW KNEE TO HEAD AND TRUNK

| Needled Area | Image | Reverse Image |
| --- | --- | --- |
| Lower Leg (A) | Head, Face | Toes |
| Lower Leg (B) | Thorax, Upper Back | Foot |
| Ankle | Navel, Waist | Ankle |
| Foot | Abdomen, Low Back | Lower Leg (B) |
| Toes | Genitalia, Tailbone | Lower Leg (A) |

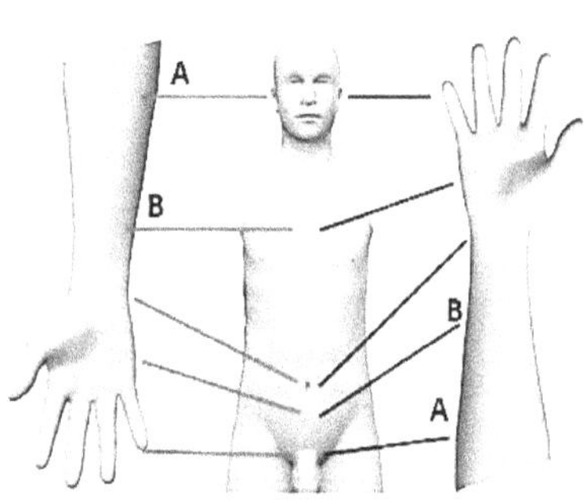

### IMAGE OF BELOW ELBOW TO HEAD AND TRUNK

| Needled Area | Image | Reverse Image |
| --- | --- | --- |
| Forearm (A) | Head, Face | Fingers |
| Forearm (B) | Thorax, Upper Back | Hand |
| Wrist | Navel, Waist | Wrist |
| Hand | Abdomen, Low Back | Forearm (B) |
| Fingers | Genitalia, Tailbone | Forearm (A) |

## IMAGE OF BELOW KNEE TO HEAD AND TRUNK

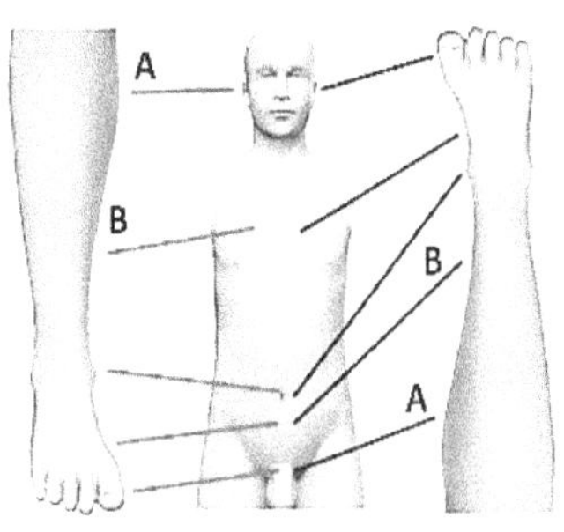

| Needled Area | Image | Reverse Image |
| --- | --- | --- |
| Lower Leg (A) | Head, Face | Toes |
| Lower Leg (B) | Thorax, Upper Back | Foot |
| Ankle | Navel, Waist | Ankle |
| Foot | Abdomen, Low Back | Lower Leg (B) |
| Toes | Genitalia, Tailbone | Lower Leg (A) |

## REVERSE IMAGE OF HEAD TO UPPER AND LOWER LIMBS

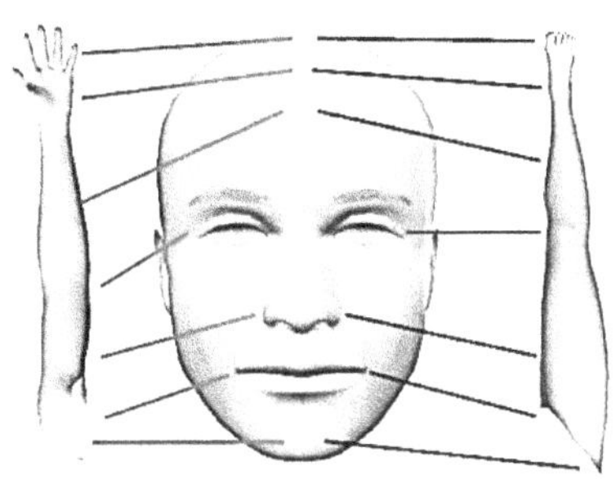

| Needled Area | Upper Limb | Lower Limb |
| --- | --- | --- |
| Top of Head | Fingers | Toes |
| Between Forehead and Top of Head | Wrist and hand | Ankle and foot |
| Forehead Level | Forearm | Lower leg |
| Eye, Ear, Occiput | Elbow | Knee |
| Nose Level | Upper arm | Upper leg |
| Mouth Level | Shoulder | Hip |
| Chin Level | Shoulder joint | Hip joint |

## Image of Scalp to the Spine

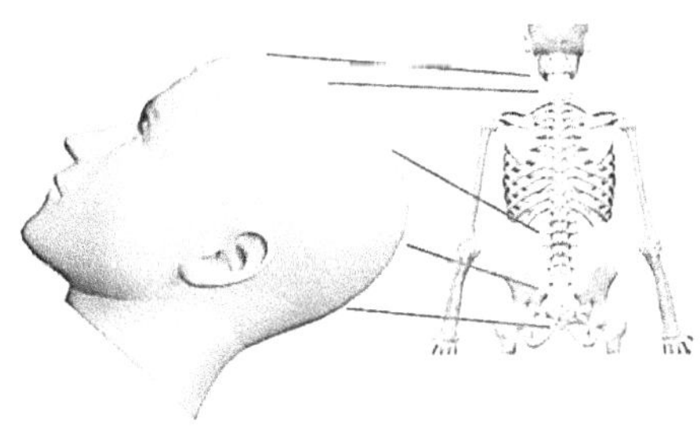

| Hairline | C-1, C-2 |
| --- | --- |
| Du 24-22 | C3-C5 |
| Du 22-20 | Thoracic vertebra |
| Du 20 | Lumbar 2 (waist level) |
| Du 19 | L2-L5 |
| Du 18-16 | Sacral area |
| Du 16 | Tailbone |

# HEAD AND FACE

## Frontal Headache

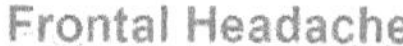
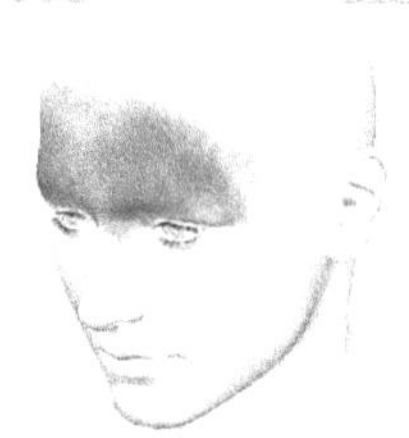
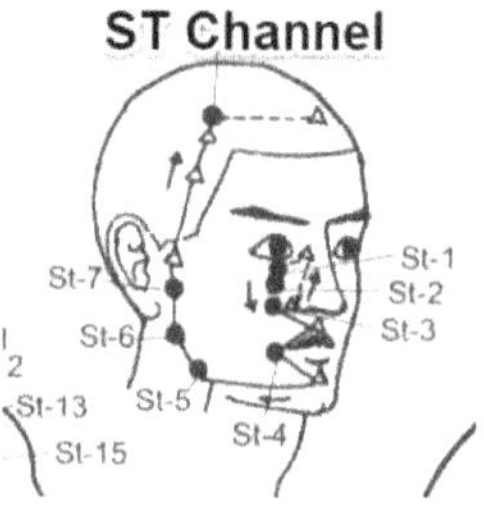
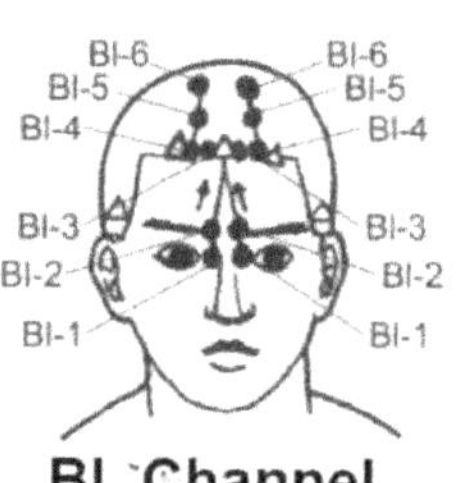
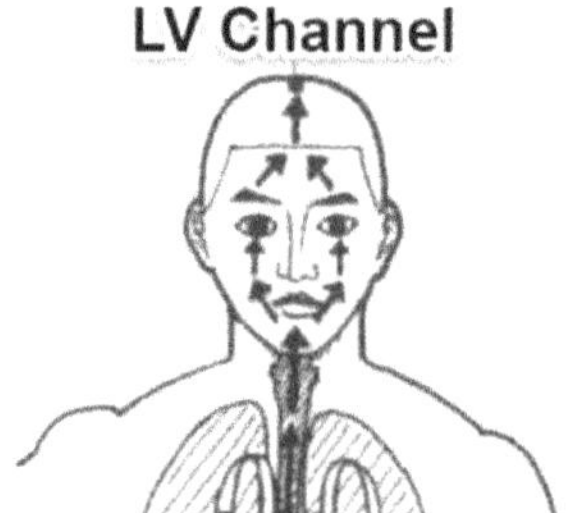



**Affected (Sick) Meridians: Stomach, Bladder, Liver**

**Effective points:**
- LI-3 (22.04) - Large Intestine treats Stomach (System 1 Balance Method)
- ST-8 (bilateral) – Treats own meridian
- BL-60, BL-65- Bladder Channel treats its own channel (System 6 Balance Method)
- Yintang [Ex. 1.] or Ex-HN-3, BL-2 - guide points (needle same side as pain)
- REN-12, Front-mu point of the ST Meridian.

**Headache which aggravates with heat/pressure (Excess-type)**
- Needle 77.08 Si Hua Shang (ST-36), 77.09 Si Hua Zhong or/and bleed 77.14 Si Hua Wai (ST-40)
- 66.04 Huo Zhu (LIV-3)

**Headache which feels better with warmth/pressure (Deficient-type)**
- Bilaterally needle 77.18 Shen Guan or 77.17 Tian Huang (SP-9)
- 66.10 Huo Lian+66.11 Huo Ju (SP-3 + SP-4)

---

### Cupping/Blood-letting

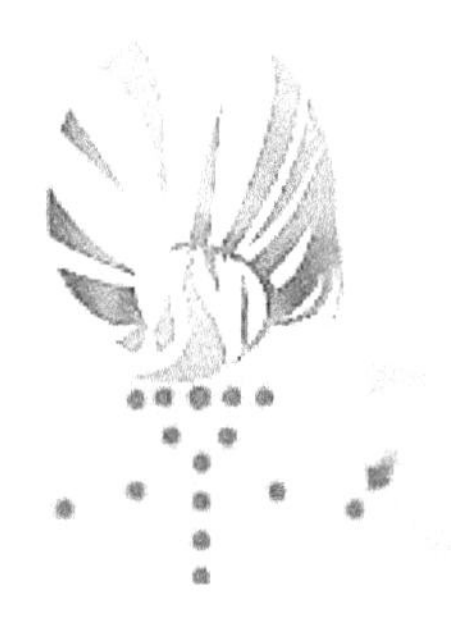

- Dry cup (1 or 2 minutes) or mild gua sha upper back on the side with symptoms, or both sides if the symptoms are on both sides
- Bleed the patient's EX-HN-6 ERJIAN ear apex on the same side as the headache, or both ears if necessary.
- Bleed BL-40 area – relates to the occipital region in Master Tung's Correspondence
- Also look for bleed-able veins elsewhere on the legs, especially lateral lower legs and around 77.09, 77.14
- Prick-bleed 1010.09 Shang Li, 1010.10 Si Fu Er, 1010.11 Si Fu Yi. Avoid arteries.

*Points Illustrations for treatment of Frontal Headache*

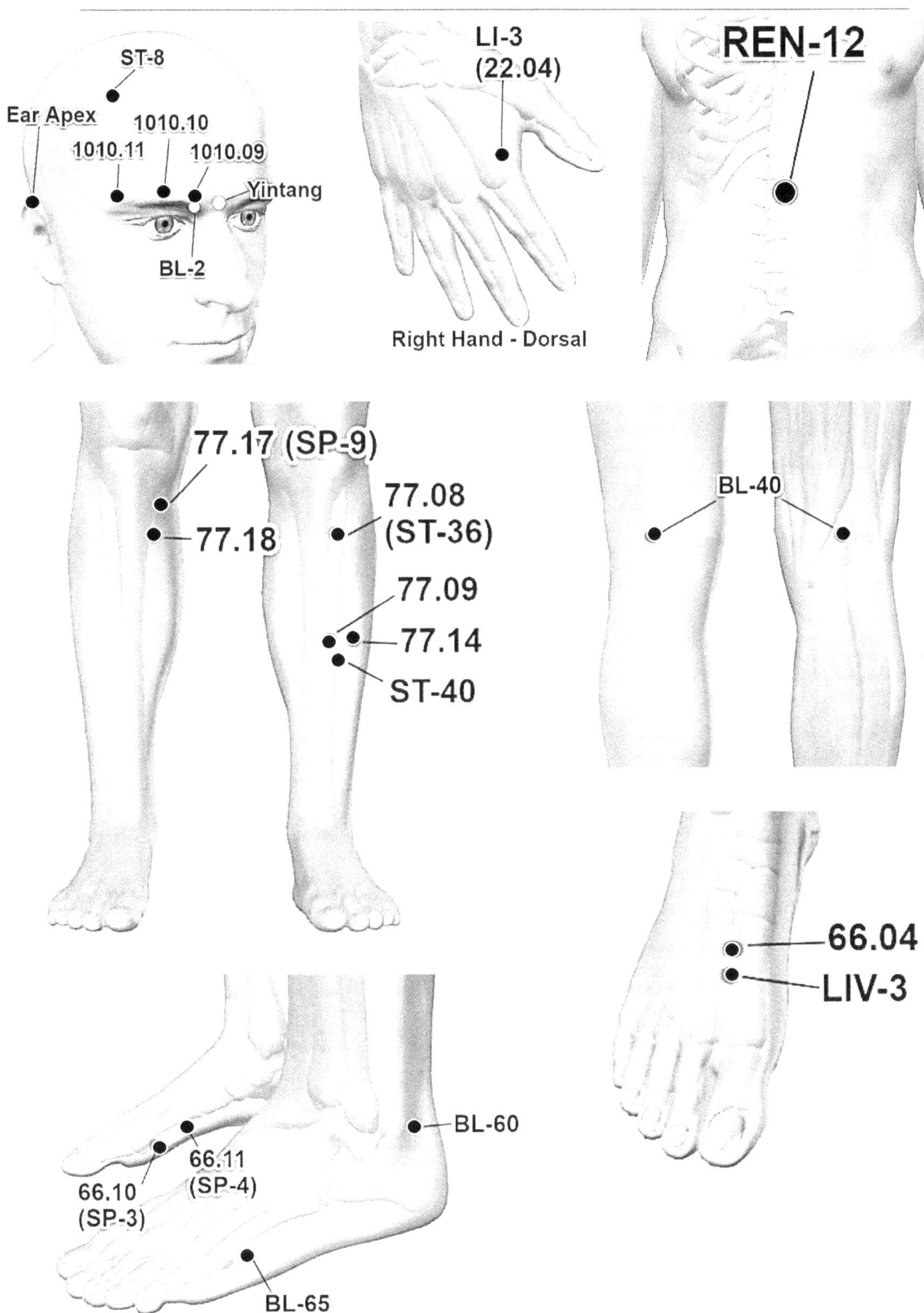

# Migraine Headache

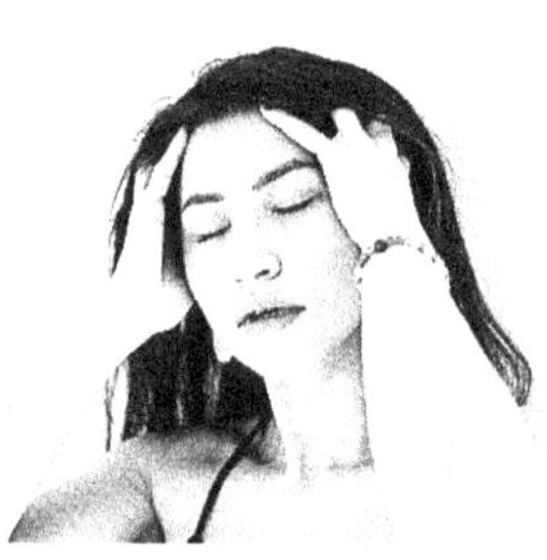

*According to TCM theory, there are several meridians, or energy pathways, in the body that are involved in the onset and progression of migraines.*

*The **Liver Meridian**: The Liver Meridian runs through the head, and any blockages or imbalances in this meridian can cause headaches and migraines.*

*The **Gallbladder Meridian**: The Gallbladder Meridian is closely related to the liver and is responsible for the decision-making process in the body. When the gallbladder is imbalanced or blocked, it can result in migraines.*

*The **Bladder Meridian**: The Bladder Meridian runs along the back of the head and neck, and any blockages or imbalances in this meridian can cause tension headaches and migraines.*

*The **Stomach Meridian**: The Stomach Meridian runs through the forehead, temples, and eyes, and any blockages or imbalances in this meridian can cause migraines.*

*The **Triple Warmer Meridian (Sanjiao)**: The Triple Warmer Meridian is responsible for regulating the body's temperature and energy flow. When there is an excess of heat in the head, it can result in migraines. The Triple Warmer Meridian runs along the sides of the head and neck.*

**Affected (Sick) Meridians: Sanjiao, Gall Bladder, Stomach, Liver, Bladder**

**Migraine treatment options (generally needle on contralateral side)**

- 88.25 Zhong Jiu Li (GB-31) and GB-32 treat all kinds of pain.
- Add 22.04 Da Bai+22.05 Ling Gu or LI-4
- ST-36, 77.22 Ce San Li+77.23 Ce Xia San Li (near GB-34) help ST and GB Meridians headache.
- 66.05 Men Jin (ST-43) and 66.09. Help ST and GB Meridians/premenstrual headache.
- 66.12 Huo San (KI-2) to treat migraines due to hypertension.
- P-6. Pericardium treats Liver, Stomach and Sanjiao
- BL-60, treats Bladder Meridian
- Guide Points - GB-4 and GB-5, GB-20, DU-20 (needle on same side)

## Cupping and Blood-letting

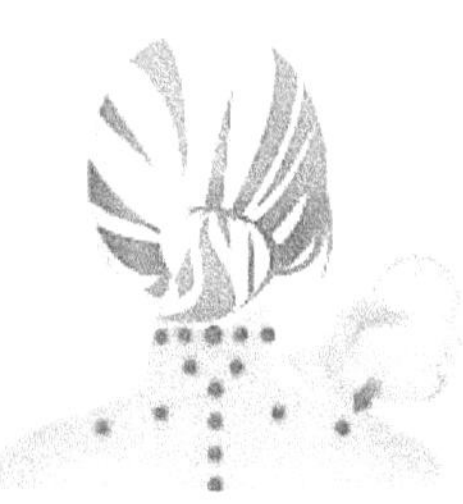

- Cup the neck and shoulders to improve blood circulation to the head. Include the area directly behind the ear (SJ-17).
- Bleeding 99.07 Er Bei Ear Back or 99.08 Er San Ear Apex or Taiyang [Ex.2.] clears excesses from the head.
- Bleed SJ-23
- For nausea and vomiting, bleed 1010.07 Zong Shu.
- Prick 77.07 San Zhong/77.14 Si Hua Wai (near to each other).

*Points Illustrations for treatment of Migraine Headache*

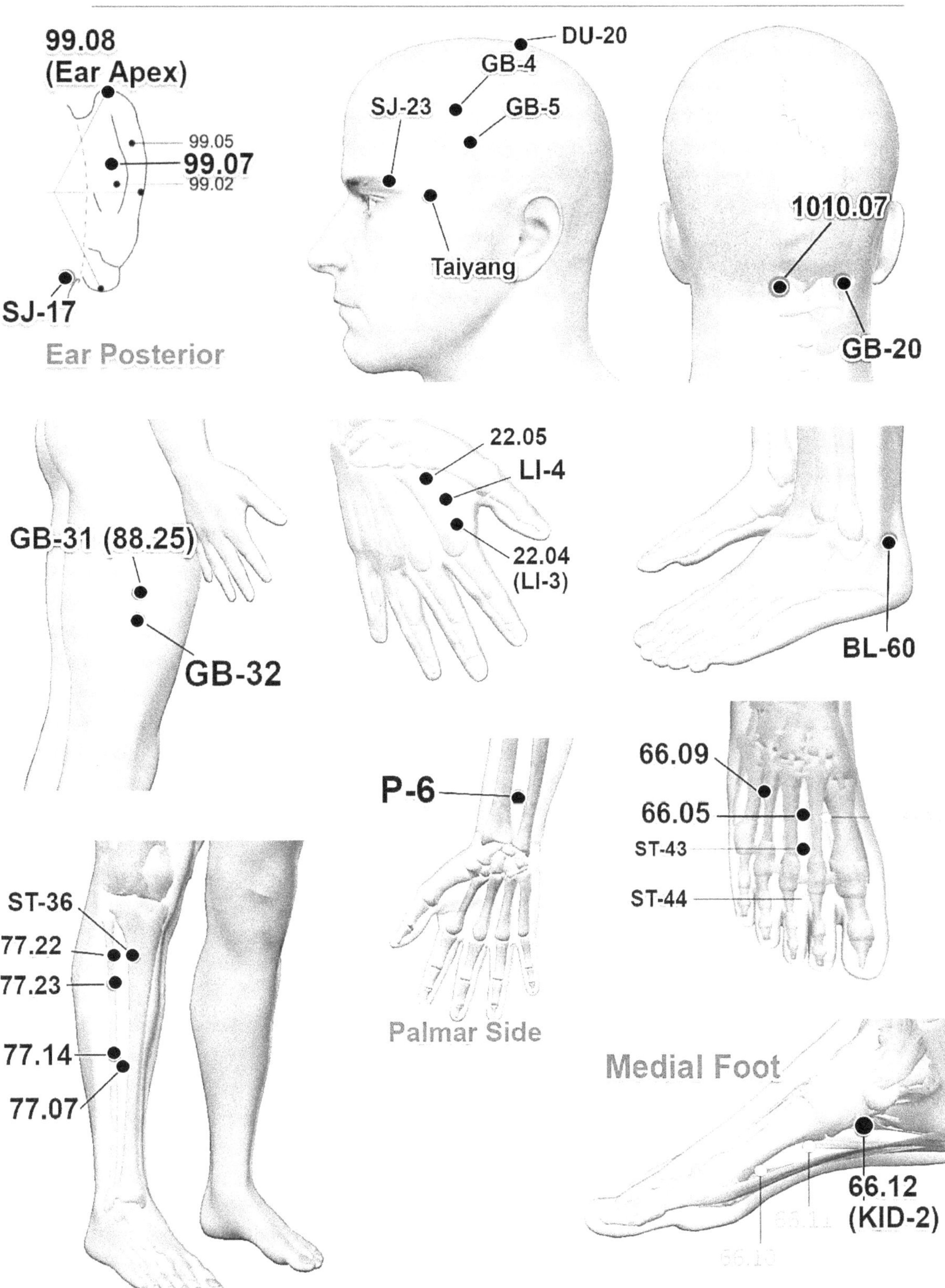

# Vertex Headache

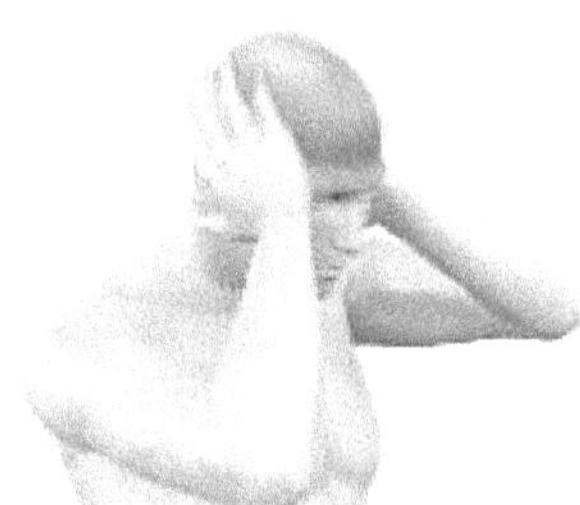

**Highly effective points:**
- 66.04 Huo Zhu (LIV-3)
- BL-65 toward KI-1.
- LI-4 (22.04)

| AFFECTED (SICK) MERIDIANS | TREATMENT POINTS |
|---|---|
| **DU (GV)** | • 55.06, KID-1 - Sole treats vertex |
| **BLADDER** (FOOT TAIYANG) | • BL-60, BL-65, BL-67 (Bilateral) - treats same channel, foot treats head (Jing-well, Shu-stream, Jing-River points)<br>• SI-3 - SI treats BL (System 1)<br>• 77.01, 77.02 – near Bladder meridian, "bottom treats top"<br>• LU-7 - Lung treats Bladder (System 2), Luo-connecting point. |
| **LIVER** (FOOT JUEYIN) | • LIV-3 - Treats same channel. Yuan source point.<br>• SI-3 - SI treats Liver (System 4), Shu-stream point<br>• LU-7 - Lung treats Liver (System 5)<br>• P-6 - Pericardium treats Liver (System 1), Luo-connecting point. |
| **SAN JIAO** (HAND SHAOYANG) | • KID-1 - Kidney treats Sanjiao (System 2), Jing-well point. |
| **GALL** BLADDER (FOOT SHAO YANG) | • LIV-3 - Liver treats Gall bladder (System 3), Shu-stream point |

**Guide Point** - 1010.01 (DU-20) - Meeting Point on the Governing Vessel with the six yang channels.

---

### Blood-letting for Vertex Headache
- Dry cup (1 or 2 minutes) or mild gua sha upper back/neck on the side(s) with symptoms.
- Bleed the patient's EX-HN-6 ERJIAN ear apex on the same side(s) as the headache.
- Prick bleed-able veins on lateral lower legs.
- Yintang [Ex. 1.] or Ex-HN-3 (Using a bleed lancet to obtain a few drops of blood is effective. Bleed-cupping can be used but can cause undesirable cupping marks.)
- Bleed Jing Well Points (hand and foot)
- Bleed around BL-40

*Points Illustrations for treatment of Vertex Headache*

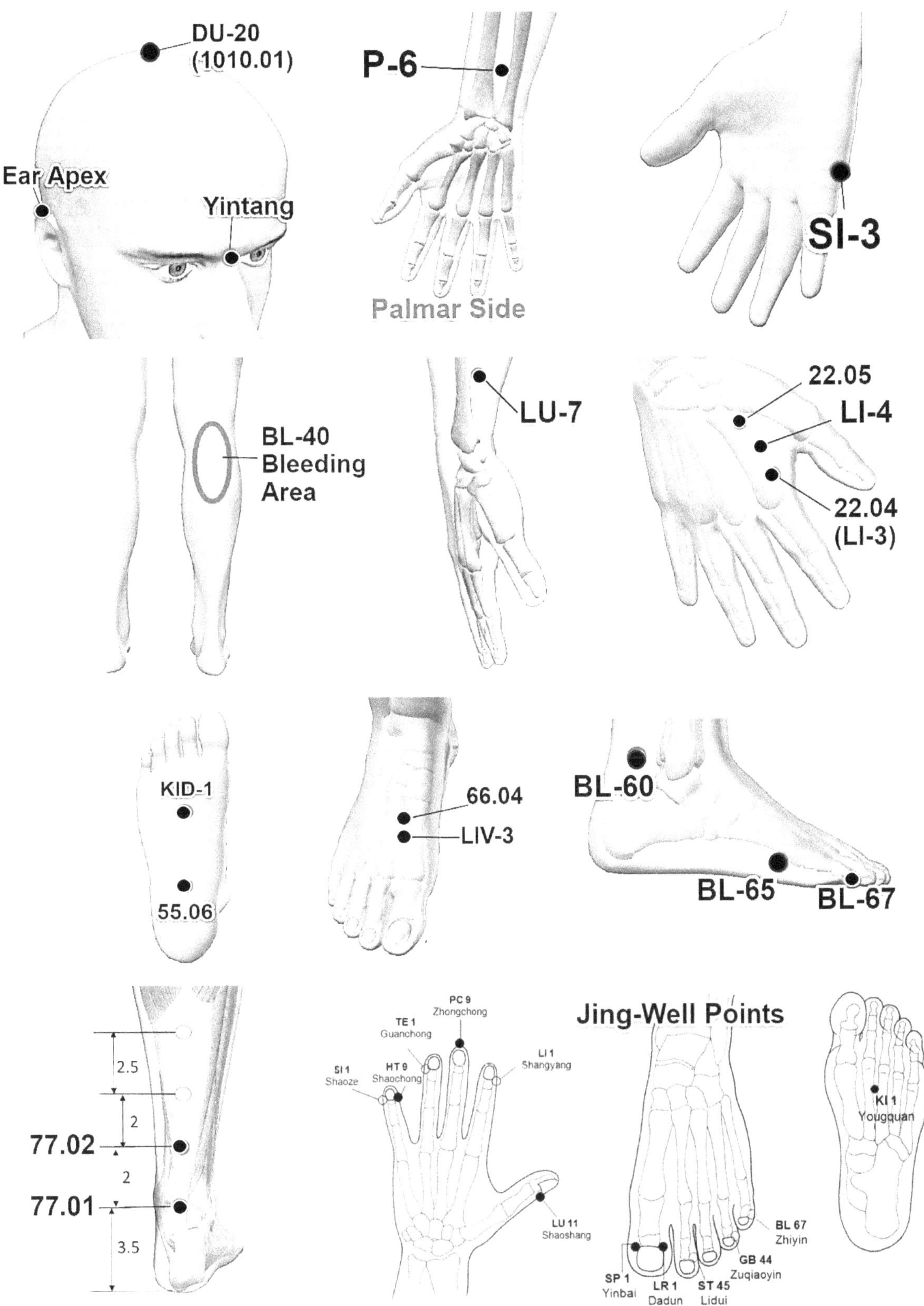

# Occipital Headache

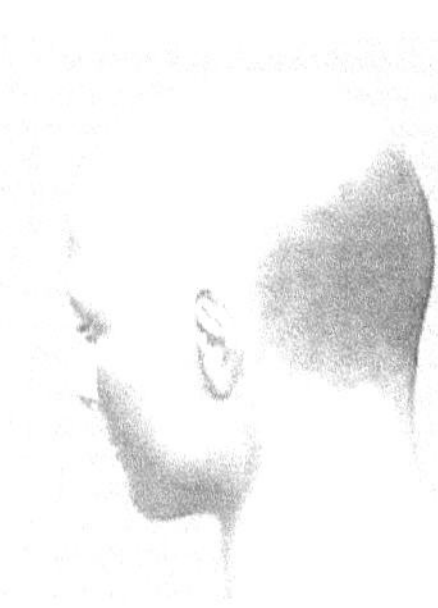

**Highly effective treatment points:**
- 22.04 (LI-3), 22.05, LI-4
- 66.04 Huo Zhu (LIV-3)
- BL-65 toward KI-1.

**Brain tumor, meningitis or severe occipital headache:**
- 55.06 Shang Liu, KID-1
- 77.01 Zheng Jin+77.02 Zheng Zong

| AFFECTED (SICK) MERIDIANS | TREATMENT POINTS |
|---|---|
| **BLADDER -**<br><br>FOOT TAIYANG | • BL-65 - treats same channel, foot treats head, Shu-stream point<br>• BL-60 - treats same channel, foot treats head, Jing-river point<br>• SI-3 - SI treats Bladder, Shu-stream point<br>• BL-67 - treats same channel, foot treats head, Jing-well point |
| **GALL BLADDER**<br><br>FOOT SHAO YANG | • GB-20, GB-34 - Treats the same meridian. Meeting point of SJ and GB meridians |

**Guide points-** BL-10

---

### Blood-letting Treatment
- EX-HN-6 ERJIAN ear apex
- Visible veins on the leg, especially BL-40 general area
- Bleed-cup any tender spots lateral to the spine at the lumbar/sacrum region, around DU-4 and DT.17 Chong Xiao (around DU-2).
- Bleed jing-wells BL-67 and GB-44 followed by needling BL-65

*Points Illustrations for treatment of Occipital Headache*

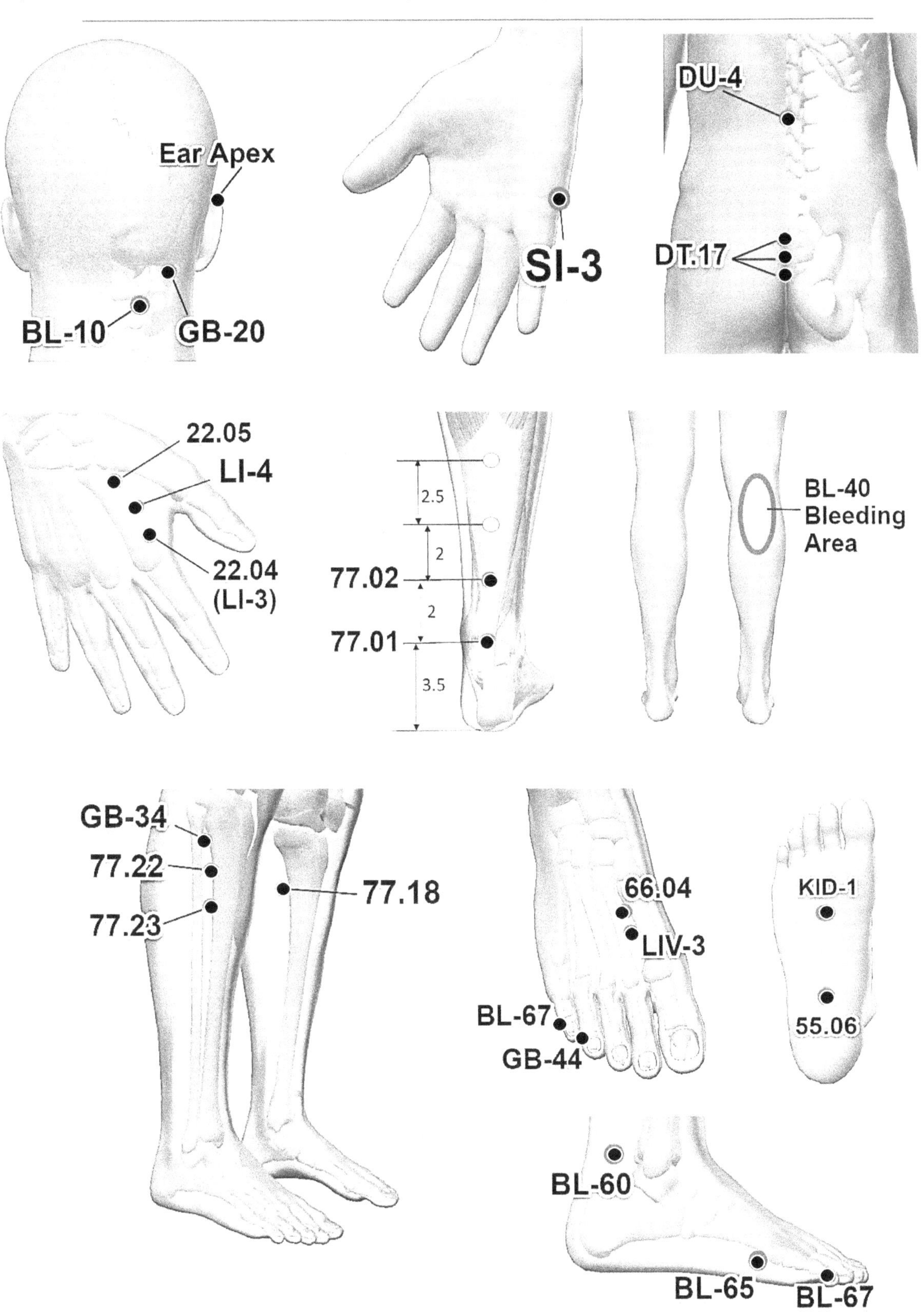

# Whole Head Pain

**Affected (Sick) Meridians**: Sanjiao, Gall Bladder, Urinary Bladder, Stomach, Large Intestine

| SICK MERIDIAN | TREATMENT POINTS |
|---|---|
| **SANJIAO MERIDIAN** | • SJ-2 (Ying-spring point), A.04 San Cha San (SJ-2) 22.06 Zhong Bai (SJ-3) |
| **GALLBLADDER MERIDIAN** | • GB-20, 77.22 Ce San Li, 77.23 Ce Xia San Li |
| **BLADDER MERIDIAN** | • LU-7, LU-9 (Lung treats BL). BL-65, 77.01+77.02 |
| **STOMACH MERIDIAN** | • 77.18 Shen Guan (Spleen treats Stomach Channel) |
| **LARGE INTESTINE MERIDIAN** | • LU-7, LU-9 (Lung treats LI)<br>• LI-3 (22.04 Da Bai) + 22.05 Ling Gu |

**Meningitis**
- 77.05+77.06+77.07
- Bleed 77.14, needle 77.01

**Brain Tumor**
- 1010.03 (BL-8)+1010.04 (BL-6) – Treats BL Meridian
- 77.05 (GB-39) +77.06+77.07
- 55.06
- 77.01 + 77.02

**Hydrocephalus**
- 77.01, 55.06
- Bleed around 77.07

> ### Cupping/Blood-letting Treatment
> - Dry cup (1 or 2 minutes) or mild gua sha upper back/neck on the side(s) with symptoms.
> - Bleed the patient's EX-HN-6 ERJIAN ear apex on the same side as the headache, or both ears if the pain is bilateral.
> - Bleed BL-40- it is the Master Tung occipital region.
> - Bleed bleed-able veins elsewhere on the legs, especially lateral lower legs around 77.07.
> - Bleed Taiyang [Ex.2.] or Ex-HN-5
> - Bleed around ST-40 or 77.14 (eliminates phlegm)

*Points Illustrations for treatment of Whole Head Pain*

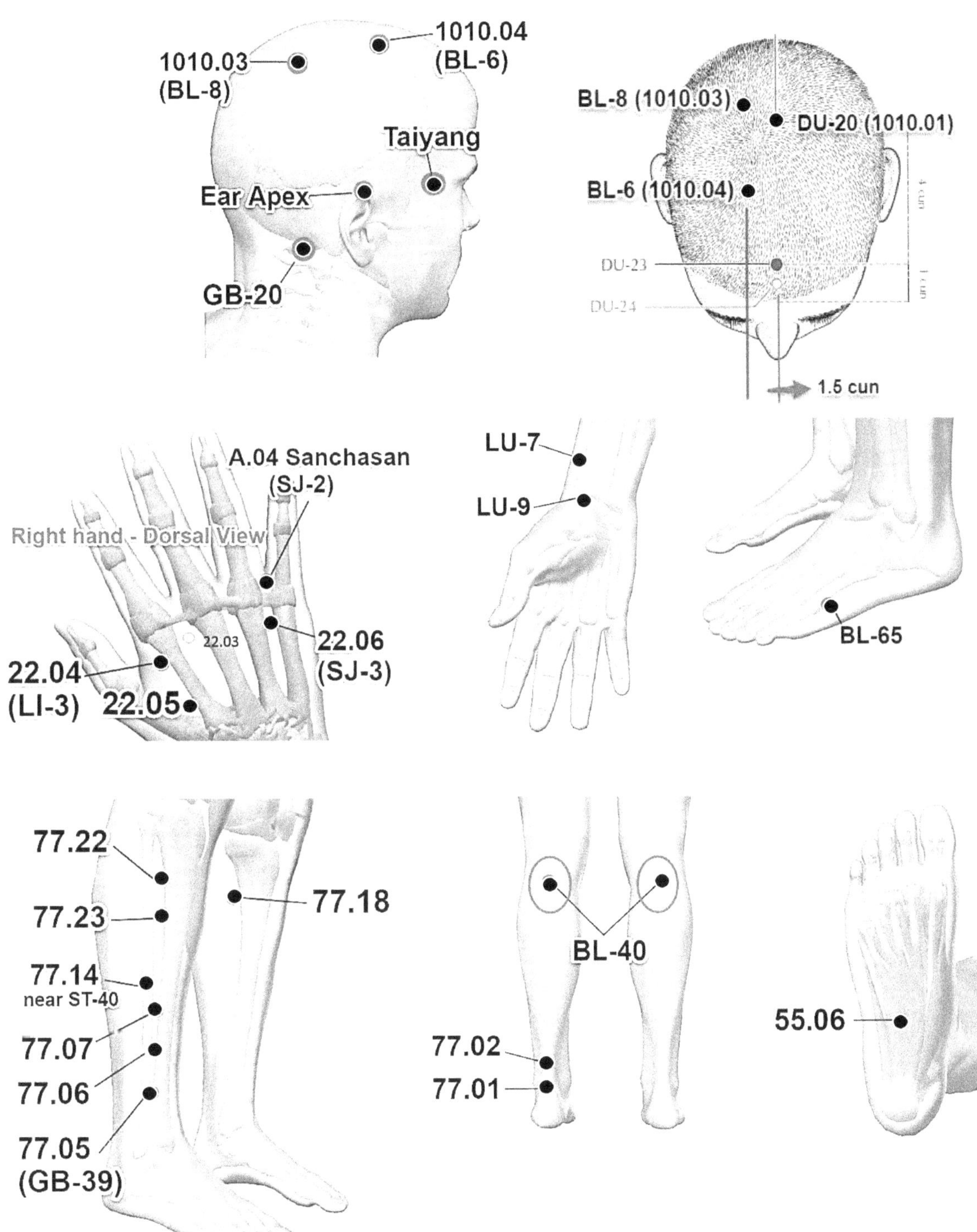

# Eye Pain

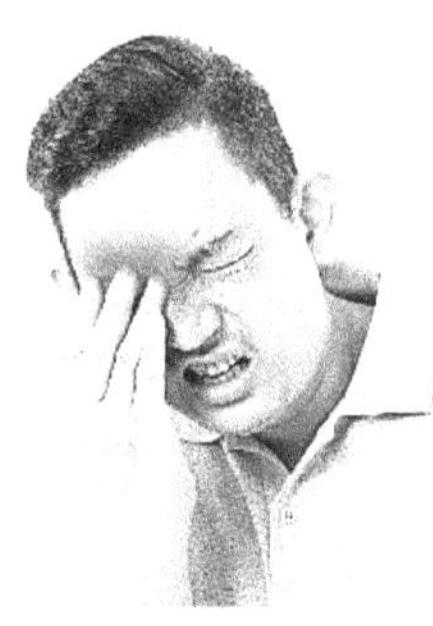

*Discussion on glaucoma, red eye (acute catarrhal conjunctivitis), conjunctiva and corneal pain caused by foreign objects.*

**Liver**    governs eye ball
**Kidney**    governs the power of vision
**Spleen**    governs the eye lid
**Lung**    governs the sclera

| AFFECTED (SICK) CHANNELS | TREATMENT POINTS |
| --- | --- |
| **LIVER**<br>Foot Jue Yin | • LIV-2 - Ying-spring point. Treats own meridian pathway.<br>• LI-11 - He-sea point. LI treats LIV (System 2)<br>• LI-3 (22.04 Da Bai) - Shu-stream point of LI Meridian. LI treats LIV (System 2)<br>• GB-41 + GB-43 + GB-37 - GB treats Liver (System 3)<br>• 55.02<br>• 88.12 + 88.13 + 88.14 |
| **SMALL INTESTINE**<br>Hand Taiyang | • Taiyang [Ex.2.]. or Ex-HN-5. Meeting point of GB, ST, SI and SJ meridians.<br>• SI-4 |
| **GALL BLADDER**<br>Foot Shao Yang | • GB-41 (66.09 Shui Qu) - Shu-stream of GB Meridian. Treats own meridian.<br>• GB-43 - Ying-Spring point.  Treats own meridian. |
| **STOMACH**<br>FOOT YANGMING | • ST-43. Shu-stream point |

---

### Blood-letting Treatment

- Bleed EX-HN-6 ERJIAN (Ear Apex) -Traverses BL, GB, SI and SJ Channels. Treats all head issues.
- Bleed Taiyang [Ex.2.]. or Ex-HN-5.
- Bleed blue veins at 66.03, 66.04
- Gua sha Eye Area on the 3rd Cervical Vertebrae

*Points Illustrations to treat Eye Pain*

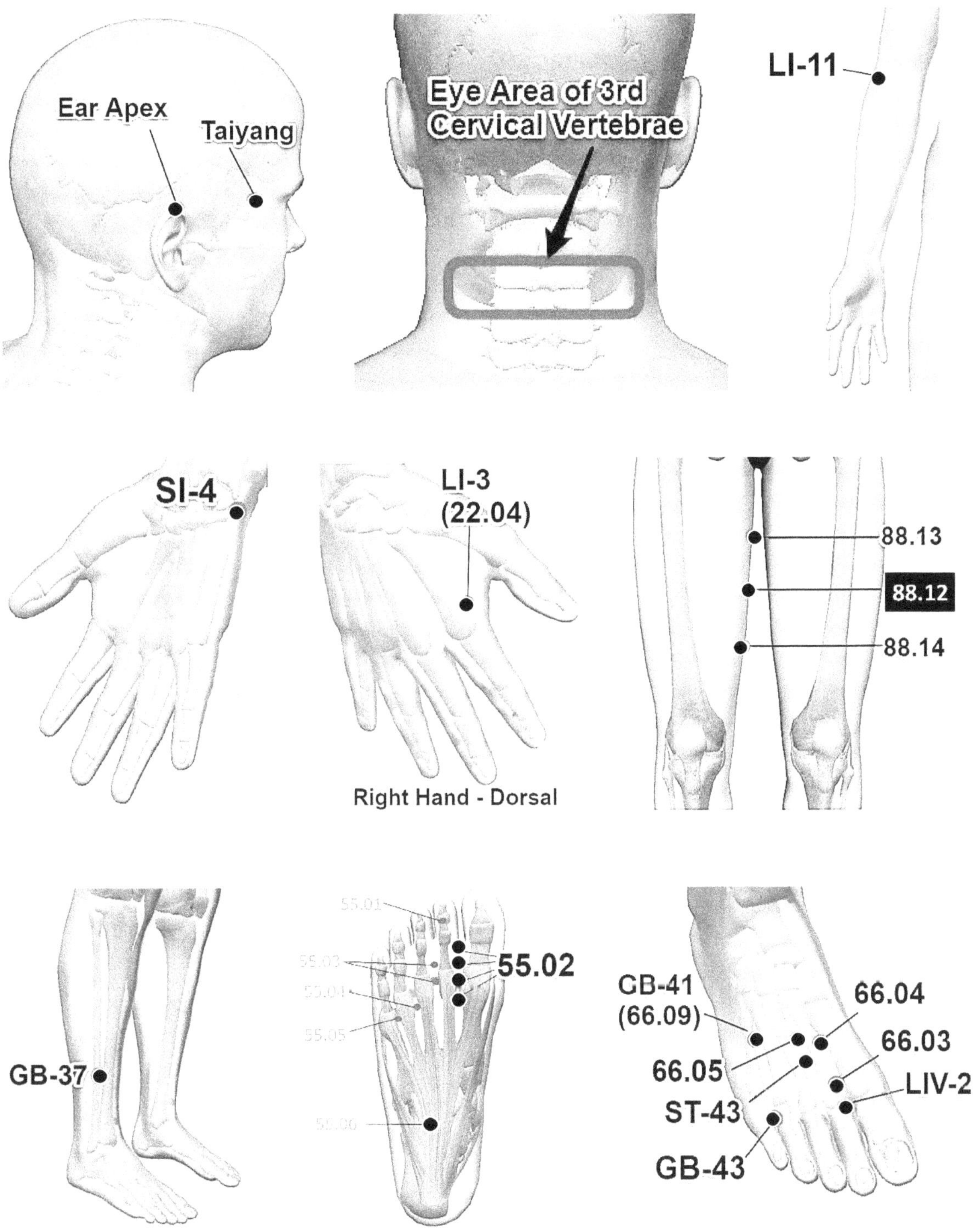

# Eye Issues

*While the anatomy of the eye is governed by the **Liver** (wood), the power of vision comes from the **Kidneys.***

**Miscellaneous eye diseases (near-sightedness, farsightedness, astigmatism, night blindness, eye inflammation, photophobia, trachoma macular degeneration and eyelid infection), failing vision**
- 55.02 Hua Gu Yi
- 77.18 Shen Guan+77.19 Di Huang+77.21 Ren Huang with 77.28 Guang Ming (KI-7)
- 88.12 + 88.13 + 88.14
- LI-3 (22.04), 22.03
- GB-20, GB-37, LIV-3
- Cup the neck and shoulders

**Conjunctivitis**
- 88.17+88.18+88.19 (both sides)
- LIV-3

**Cataract**
- 77.18+77.19+77.21
- 77.28 (KID-7)
- LIV-3

**Glaucoma**
- LIV-2, LIV-3, 66.03 and 66.04 (Liver to eyes relationship)
- 55.02 Hua Gu Yi with 77.18 Shen Guan+77.19 Di Huang+77.21 Ren Huang, 77.28 (KID-7)
- GB-20 and GB-37
- If pressure on the eyes aggravates, use 77.08 Si Hua Shang+77.09 Si Hua Zhong.

**Floaters**
- 77.18 Shen Guan with 77.28 Guang Ming (KI-7) with A.04 San Cha San and 66.05 Men Jin (ST-43) - for treating floaters in the field of vision

**Optic nerve atrophy**
- 55.02 Hua Gu Yi, LIV-3
- GB-20 that helps to nourish the optic nerves
- 77.18 and 77.28 (KID-7)

**Dry or tearing eyes**
- Bilaterally: 11.17 Mu (Anger), 55.02 Hua Gu Yi, 77.18 Shen Guan with 77.21 Ren Huang (SP-6 or 77.28 Guang Ming (KI-7)
- 77.07 for chronic cases

**Eyes twitching**
- 22.08 + 22.09, Shu-stream point SI-3
- 77.22+77.23, and 77.18
- GB-31 and KID-7
- 88.20+88.21+88.22

**Difficult to open the eyes**
- A.04 Sanchasan, 66.05 and 66.11
- 77.28+77.21

---

### Blood-letting for Eye Issues
- Bleed Taiyang [Ex.2.]. or Ex-HN-5 area or EX-HN-6 ERJIAN Ear Apex
- Gua sha Eye Area on the 3rd Cervical Vertebrae

*Points Illustrations for treatment of Eye Issues*

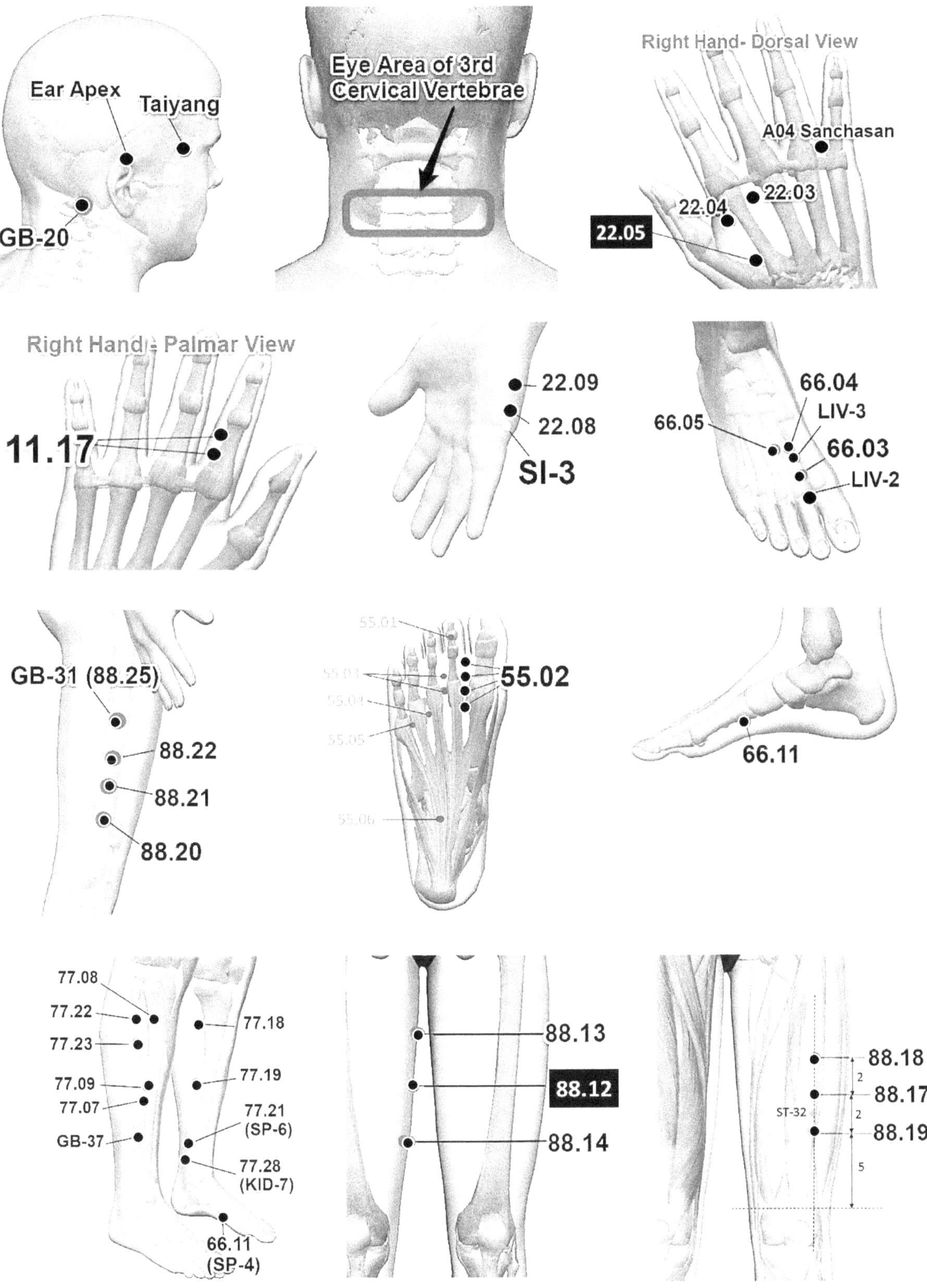

# Trigeminal Neuralgia

*Characterized by sudden attacks of spasmodic electric shock-like severe pain in the facial areas, supplied by the trigeminal nerve, ophthalmic (1), maxillary (2) and mandibular (3) divisions (most commonly along the maxillary division). Attacks may recur several times daily, generally when the patient is washing the face, brushing the teeth, eating or walking.*

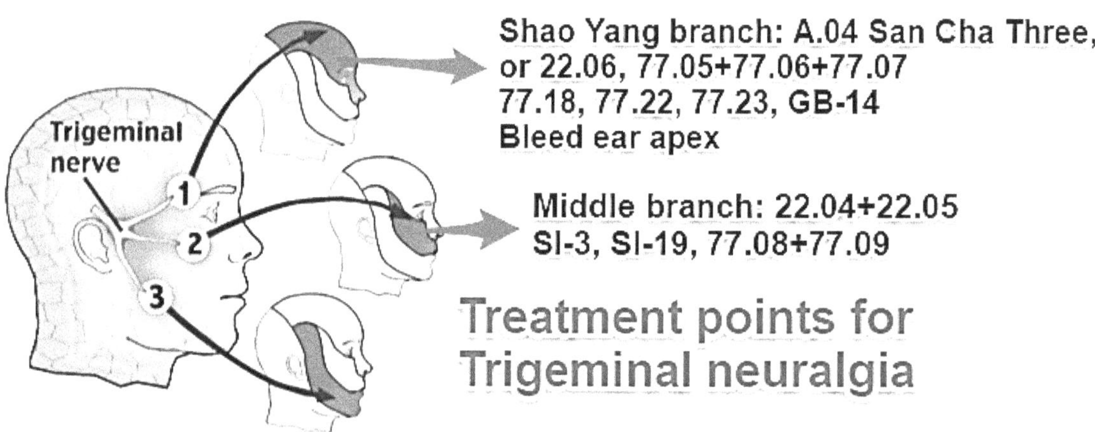


| AFFECTED (SICK) CHANNEL | TREATMENT POINTS |
|---|---|
| **Branch 1:**<br><br>**Sanjiao,**<br><br>**Gall Bladder** | • A.04 San Cha San or 22.06 Zhong Bai<br>• 77.05 Yi Zhong+77.06 Er Zhong+77.07 San Zhong,<br>• 77.22 Ce San Li+77.23 Ce Xia San Li (Reaction area of the teeth)<br>• or 66.06 Mu Liu+66.07 Mu Dou<br>• 77.18 Shen Guan (System 2 and 4) for chronic cases.<br>• GB-14, Taiyang |
| **Branch 2 (Middle):**<br><br>**Small Intestine,**<br><br>**Large Intestine,**<br><br>**Stomach** | • SI-3, SI-18, SI-19<br>• 22.04 Da Bai (LI-3) +22.05, LI-4<br>• ST-7, LI-20 (Local area)<br>• 77.08 Si Hua Shang+77.09 Si Hua Zhong<br>• SP-3 - Shu-stream point. Spleen treats SI channel.<br>• SP-6 - Spleen treats SI channel (System 2)<br>• ST-43 (Shu-stream point) |
| **Branch 3:**<br><br>**Large Intestine** | • 22.04 Da Bai (LI-3) +22.05<br>• ST-7, LI-20 (local area) |

## Cupping/Blood-letting Treatment
- Bleed ear-apex (EX-HN-6 ERJIAN). Bleed a few points along the helix.
- Bleed Taiyang [Ex.2.]. or Ex-HN-5 for serious conditions, avoid the artery.
- Bleed around 77.14 Si Hua Wai and ST-40
- Dry cupping can help but start gently and check for results to decide continuance. Cupping has been known to cause aggravation.

*Points Illustrations for treatment of Trigeminal Neuralgia*

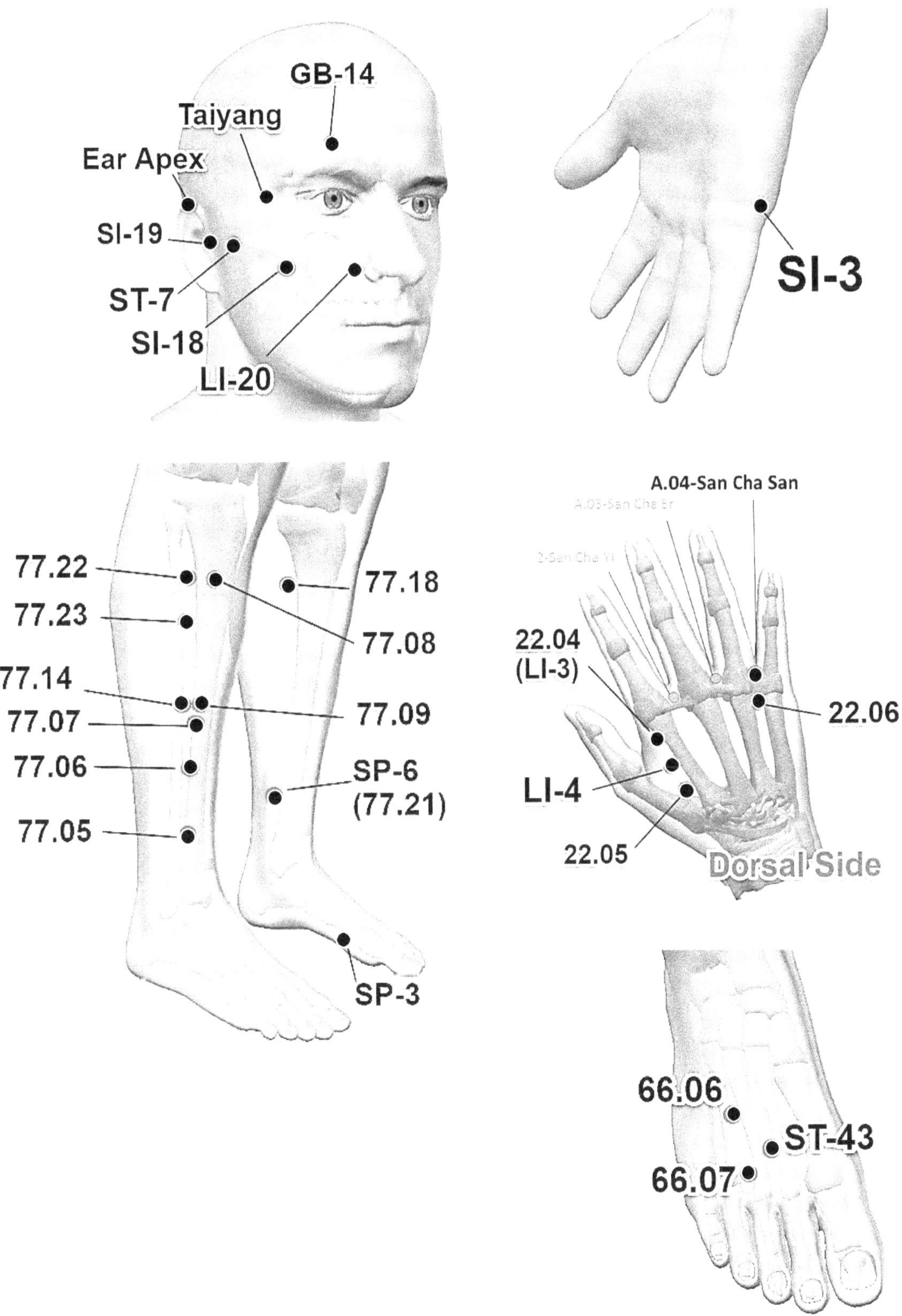

# Bell's palsy, Facial paralysis, Jaw pain

***Bell's palsy*** *is a condition that causes temporary weakness or paralysis of the muscles in one side of the face.*

***Temporomandibular Joint (TMJ)*** *disorders are conditions affecting the jaw joints and surrounding muscles and ligaments. It can be caused by trauma, an improper bite, arthritis or wear and tear. Common symptoms include jaw tenderness, headaches, earaches and facial pain.*

*Facial paralysis is commonly associated with dysfunction of the facial nerve (cranial nerve VII), which controls the muscles of the face. In TCM, the meridians involved in facial paralysis are the Yangming meridian of the hand and foot (**Large Intestine and Stomach**), the Taiyang meridian of the hand and foot (**Small Intestine and Urinary Bladder**), and the Shaoyang meridian of the hand (**Sanjiao**).*

### Treatment for Bell's palsy, facial paralysis
- 66.04 Huo Zhu with strong stimulation
- 77.05 Yi Zhong+77.06 Er Zhong+77.07 San Zhong
- 77.22 Ce San Li+77.23 Ce Xia San Li (treat both ST and GB Meridians). Alternatively, use ST-36 and ST-37.
- 88.25 Zhong Jiu Li (GB-31) and/or 88.17 +88.18 +88.19
- 11.14 Zhi San Zhong -difficulty smiling; LI-4 – difficulty whistling
- REN-24 acts as a Guiding Point.
- Treat frequently with long needle retention.  Be prepared for possible "healing crisis".

### Facial twitch
- 88.25 Zhong Jiu Li (GB-31) and/or 88.17 +88.18 +88.19
- 77.22 Ce San Li+77.23 Ce Xia San Li
- 22.04
- SI-3

### Deviation of the mouth
- Bleed 77.07
- Bleed ear apex
- 88.17 +88.18 +88.19

### Treatment for TMJ Disorder/Jaw pain
- Bilaterally 66.03 Huo Ying or 66.04 Huo Zhu helps to open the jaw.
- KI-1, 55.06 Shang Liu and the extra point 1.0 cun distal for clenching jaw.
- If the pain is arthritic, ST-41 is useful.
- Other point options include: SJ-5 or SJ-6, GB-34, P-5.
- When the TMJ is chronic and severe, cupping is useful.

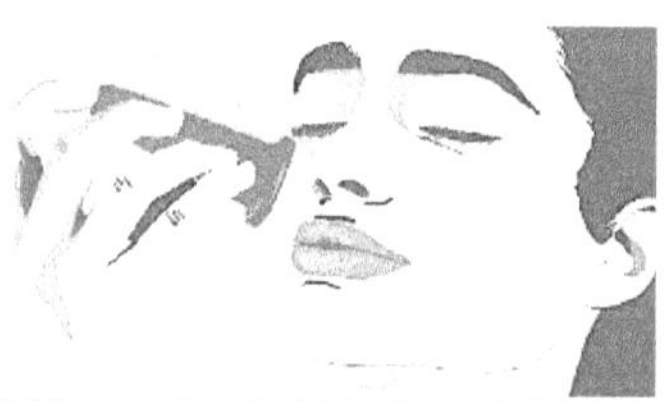

**Cupping The Face and Jaw**
- Cup the face and/or jaw to improve blood circulation.
Go gradually because aggravation might occur.
- Gua sha applicable.
- 

## Blood-letting for Facial Paralysis/Jaw Pain
- Yang jing well points on ipsilateral hand
- Weekly or twice weekly, bleed inside of cheek on diseased side.
- Bleed or bilaterally deeply needle (2.0-3.0 cun) 77.08 Si Hua Shang (ST-36) + 77.09 Si Hua Zhong
- Bleeding options include 99.08 Er San Ear Apex, veins around Taiyang [Ex.2.] and 33.16 Qu Ling (LU-5).

*Points Illustrations for treatment of Bell's Palsy*

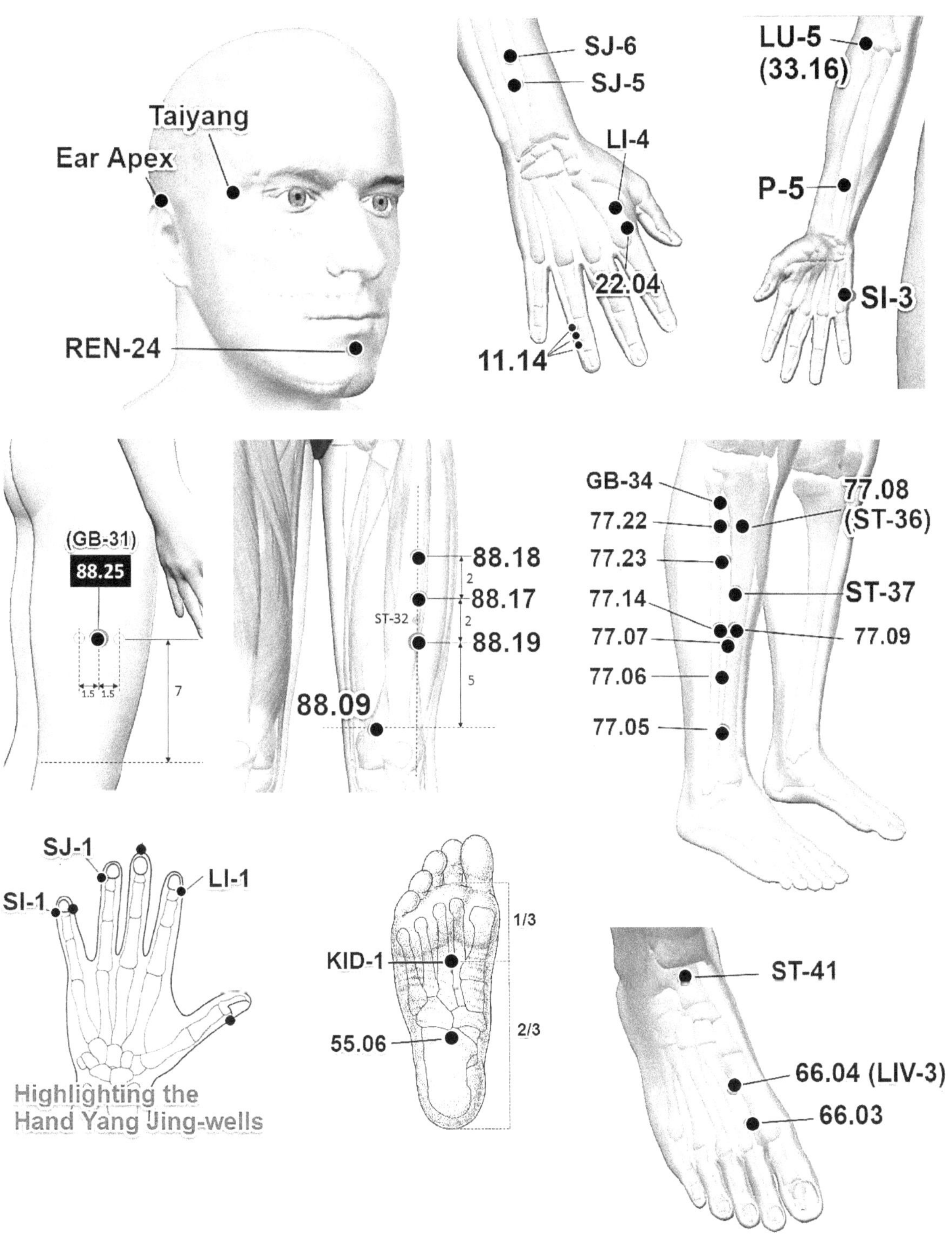

# Earache

*Inflammation of the ear, usually distinguished as otitis externa (of the passage of the outer ear), otitis media (of the middle ear), and otitis interna (of the inner ear; labyrinthitis)*

*The meridians that are commonly involved in earache include:*

***GB meridian**: Ear pain along this meridian may be associated with issues such as headaches, dizziness, and tinnitus.*
***SJ meridian**: Ear pain along this meridian may causes issues such as throat inflammation, fevers, and sinusitis.*
***SI meridian**: Ear pain along this meridian may causes toothaches, sore throats, and neck pain.*
***BL meridian**: Ear pain along this meridian may causes issues such as back pain, urinary problems, and constipation.*

**Points for Otitis media and ear pain**
- 77.22 Ce San Li+77.23 Ce Xia San Li- the Gallbladder meridian goes around the ear. Needle the side opposite the pain or bleed the same side.
- Needle opposite-side 22.06 Zhong Bai (SJ-3) or A.04 San Cha San - opposite side for treatment and same side for guide.
- 88.17 +88.18 +88.19 - bilateral

**Other Needling Treatment Protocols**

| AFFECTED (SICK) MERIDIANS | TREATMENT POINTS |
|---|---|
| **SANJIAO** Hand Shaoyang encircles the ear. | <ul><li>KI-3 - Kidney opens to the ears. Shu Stream Point on the Kidney Channel. Yuan Source on the Kidney Channel. KID treats SJ (System 2)</li><li>SJ-2 - Ying-spring point. Treats own meridian.</li><li>SJ-3 - Shu-stream point of SJ meridian. Treats own meridian.</li><li>A.04 San Cha San - Treats own meridian.</li><li>KI-1 - Kidney opens to the ears. Jing-well point of Kidney Meridian.</li><li>LI-10 - LI treats Kidney (System 4)</li></ul> |
| **GALL BLADDER** Foot Shao Yang traverses the ear. | <ul><li>GB-31 -Treats own meridian.</li></ul> |
| **URINARY BLADDER** Foot Taiyang | <ul><li>Bleed 11.26 Zhi Wu - Traverses Lung Meridian. Lung treats Bladder (System 2)</li></ul> |

## Blood-letting Treatment
- Apex of the ear EX-HN-6 ERJIAN
- Bleed visible veins on the leg especially around the ankle
- Bleed 11.26 Zhi Wu, if a vein is visible (for otitis media) – heals wounds.
- Bleed 77.22 Ce San Li+77.23 Ce Xia San Li
- Bleed 77.07 San Zhong and 77.14 Si Hua Wai simultaneously – for severe case
- Bleed 77.05 Yi Zhong+77.06 Er Zhong+77.07 San Zhong

*Points Illustrations for treatment of Earache*

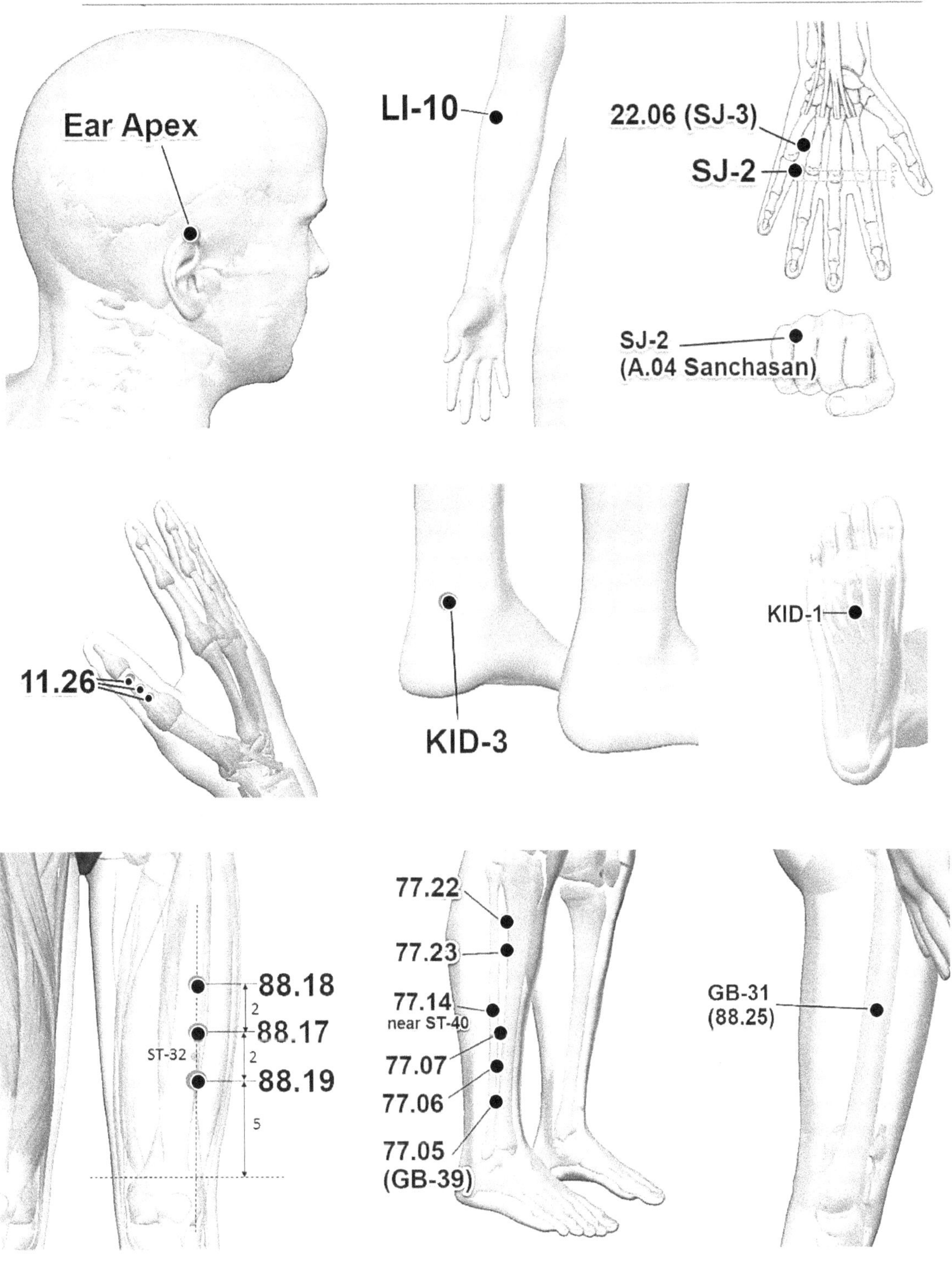

# Deafness and Tinnitus

*The meridians that are commonly involved in deafness and tinnitus include:*

***Kidney meridian:*** *Deafness and tinnitus along this meridian may be associated with issues such as aging, weakness, and poor circulation.*

***Gallbladder meridian:*** *Deafness and tinnitus along this meridian may be associated with issues such as liver problems, headaches, and stress.*

***Bladder meridian:*** *Deafness and tinnitus along this meridian may be associated with issues such as back pain, urinary problems, and fatigue.*

***Triple Burner (Sanjiao)meridian:*** *Deafness and tinnitus along this meridian may be associated with issues such as throat inflammation, fevers, and sinusitis.*

**Sudden hearing loss (opposite side treatment points)**
- 77.22 Ce San Li+77.23 Ce Xia San Li
- SI-19+GB-2+SI-4
- SJ-21
- GB-20

**Tinnitus or deafness**
- Combine SI-3 with 88.17 Si Ma Zhong+88.18 Si Ma Shang+88.19 Si Ma Xia, because the Small Intestine channel ends at SI-19, just in front of the ear opening.
- Guiding Point for Deafness and tinnitus (other than otitis media) - SJ-17
- Cup the area of SJ-17 to clear stagnation
- 88.32 Shi Yin
- 88.25 (GB-31)
- GB-20

**Tinnitus**
- Chronic hearing loss due to Kidney-deficient - 77.18 Shen Guan (Kidney Gate) 22.06, 22.07, 22.08, 22.09
- 88.17 Si Ma Zhong+88.18 Si Ma Shang+88.19 Si Ma Xia with A.04 San Cha San and 22.05 Ling Gu
- 66.08 Liu Wan- dizziness, GB migraine, tinnitus
- SI-3
- Scalp acupuncture: For difficult tinnitus, thread needles horizontally for 4cm, starting 1.5cm above ear apex, 2cm to the right and 2 cm to the left (see illustration) This area is known in scalp acupuncture as the "vertigo and hearing area".
- Guiding Points: SI-19 with SJ-21 or SJ-22 or GB-20 (same side).

---

### Blood-letting for Deaf-Mutism
- Bleed 77.07 San Zhong then needle 88.17 Si Ma Zhong+88.18 Si Ma Shang+88.19 Si Ma Xia (bilateral)
- Prick point 1010.07 Zong Shu (DU-15-DU16) to cause bleeding – sudden hearing loss
- Bleed 33.16 (LU-5)
- Bleed the Ashi points around the external malleolus.

---

*Points Illustrations for treatment of Deafness and Tinnitus*

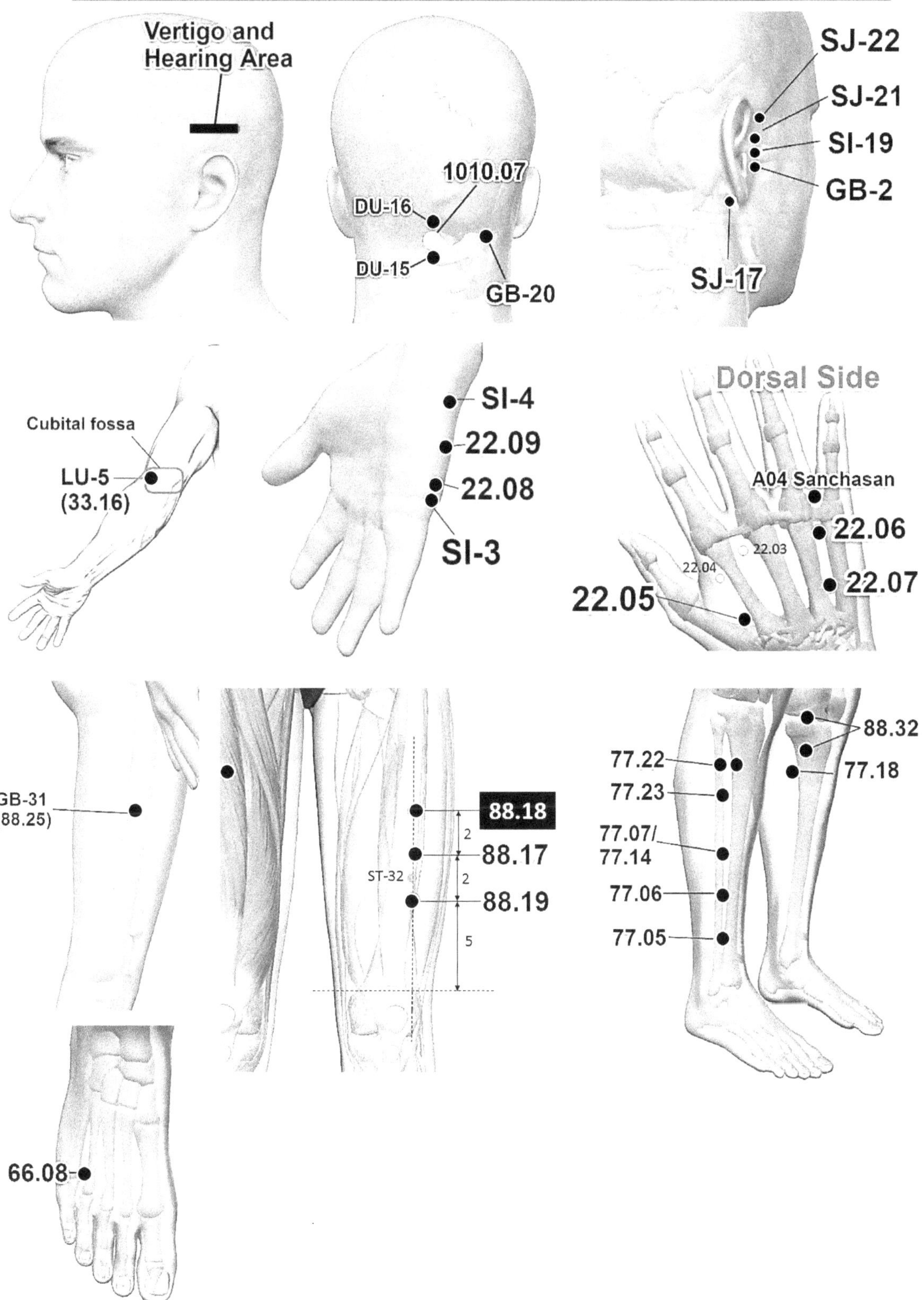

# <u>NECK</u>

## Neck Pain and Injury

*Head and neck injuries like whiplash, concussion, neck pain or stiffness (including protruding or herniated discs and stenosis), occipital headaches, as well as intracranial injury or disease.*

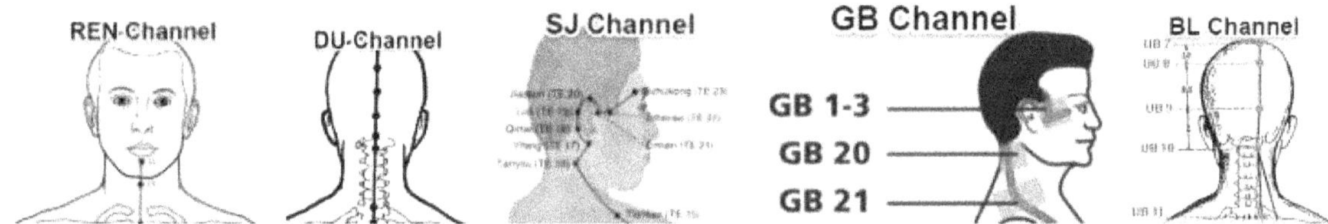


**Affected (Sick) Meridians: REN, DU, Sanjiao, Gallbladder, Urinary Bladder**

### Needling

- 77.01 Zheng Jin+77.02 Zheng Zong+77.03 Zheng Shi, 77.04 Bo Qiu (same side), situated on the back of the Achilles tendon, between the Urinary Bladder and Kidney meridians. They correspond to the Reaction Areas of Brain and Spine,
- For an acute neck sprain, needle 22.01 Chong Zi and 22.02 Chong Xian on the opposite side with REN-24 and /or DU-26. To improve outcome, rotate the neck every 10 minutes while needling.

### Neck and back pain

- BL-60, BL-65 with SI-3 (Guide point) treats the back and stiff neck
- 77.05 Yi Zhong (GB-39) +77.06 Er Zhong+77.07 San Zhong treats the neck
- 22.01 Chong Zi+22.02 Chong Xian covers neck and back.
- 77.26 Qi Hu and/or  77.27 Wai San Guan covers neck to shoulder pain

### Other Points:

- DU-26 - Treats same channel. Holographic front to back.
- SJ-3 - Treats the same meridian, SJ Shu-stream point
- P-6 - Luo connecting point, PC treats SJ Channel.
- 22.03 Shang Bai - Pericardium treats SJ channel

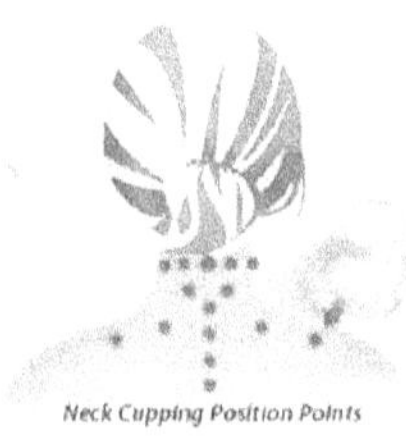
Neck Cupping Position Points

### Cupping/Blood-letting Treatment

- Cup the entire upper back and neck before needling
- Apex of the ear
- Visible veins in the leg, especially ST-36/GB-34 area and BL-40 area
- Visible veins in the cubital fossa (around LU-5)
- Bleed or gua sha local pain area

## Holographic Correspondence Treatment for Cervical Scapula Pain

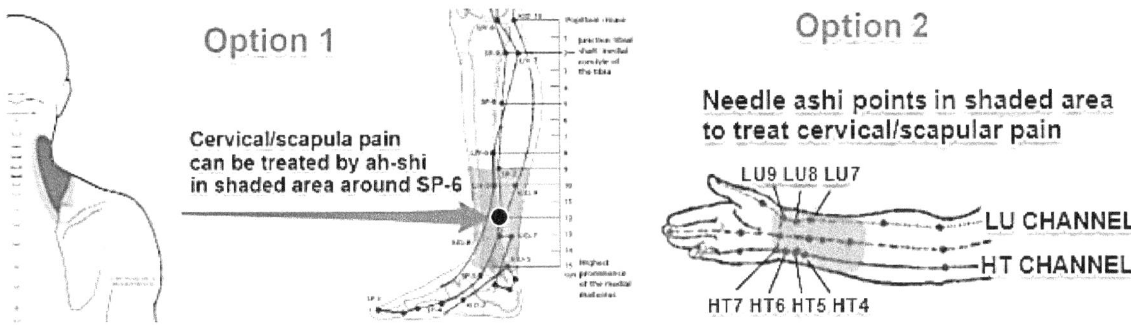


- Palpate for tender (ashi) points around SP-9, LU-7, LU-8, LU-9 and HT-4, HT-5, HT-6, HT-7

---

*Points Illustrations for treatment of Neck Pain and Injury*

---

# UPPER LIMBS

# Periarthritis of the Shoulder

*Shoulder Periarthritis **(frozen shoulder)** is a condition that leads to pain and stiffness in and around the shoulder joint. With a frozen shoulder, the capsule of the humerus – which is a loose joint capsule over the shoulder – becomes thick, tight, and difficult to move.*

**Affected (Sick) Meridians**: **Small Intestine, Large Intestine, Sanjiao, Gallbladder, Stomach, Lung**

**Treatment sequence**: Cupping, blood-letting then needling with Active Qi Moving.  Exercise at home.

**Needling Opposite-side**
- 77.18 Shen Guan - cannot raise arm
- Fan Hou Jue/San Jian
- 77.24 Zu Qian Jin+77.25 Zu Wu Jin - arm cannot go behind
- 88.25 Zhong Jiu Li (GB-31)
- 44.06 Jian Zhong (add extra needles to form Shoulder Triangle)
- 11.16 Huo Xi or left-side 1010.22 Bi Yi – for serious pain

**Needle same-side**
- ST-38 towards BL-57 (or chose side which is more tender), with stimulation
- 77.08 Si Hua Shang, 77.09 Si Hua Zhong (or chose side which is more tender)
- Choose from:  SI-3, A.04 San Cha San, or 22.06 or 22.04 (for anterior shoulder pain)

**For Pain along Large Intestine Meridian**: LI-15(44.07), LI-16, LI-14, LI-11 LI-4, ST-38
**For Pain along Sanjiao Meridian**: SJ-14, SJ-13, SJ-5, LI-4, ST-38
**For Pain along Small Intestine Meridian**: SI-9, SI-10, SI-11, DU-14, SI-6, SI-3, GB-34, ST-38

**Cupping**
Apply cupping around the shoulder girdle, including the scapula's outer edge and the LU-1 and LU-2 area. The skin may turn black. Cup over several sessions until the skin stops coloring. Encourage exercise to maintain the improvement in range of motion.

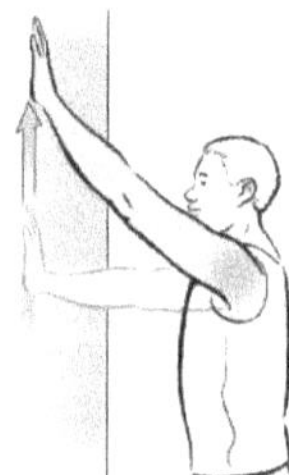

**Daily Exercise**
Daily performing the finger walking exercise is of utmost importance for the patient. The objective is to gradually move their armpit closer to the wall by walking their fingers up, which can be especially difficult and uncomfortable if the shoulder joint is significantly restricted in motion.

<table>
<tr><td>

### Blood-letting for Frozen Shoulder
- EX-HN-6 ERJIAN Apex of the ear
- Bleed-cup any tender spots around the shoulder and scapular
- Visible veins in the cubital fossa, around LU-5
- Visible veins on the leg, especially lower part of lateral leg
- Upper limb area of the back, general area of SI-10
- DT.16 Shuang He
- Shoulder pain (anterior) - bleed LU-11, LI-1 followed by needling 44.06 Jian Zhong, 77.18 Shen Guan
- Shoulder pain (posterior) - bleed SI-1, SJ-1 followed by needling 44.06 Jian Zhong, 77.18 Shen Guan
- Shoulder pain (at apex) - bleed LI-1 followed by needling 44.06 Jian Zhong, 77.18 Shen Guan

</td></tr>
</table>

*Points Illustrations for treatment of Shoulder Pain*

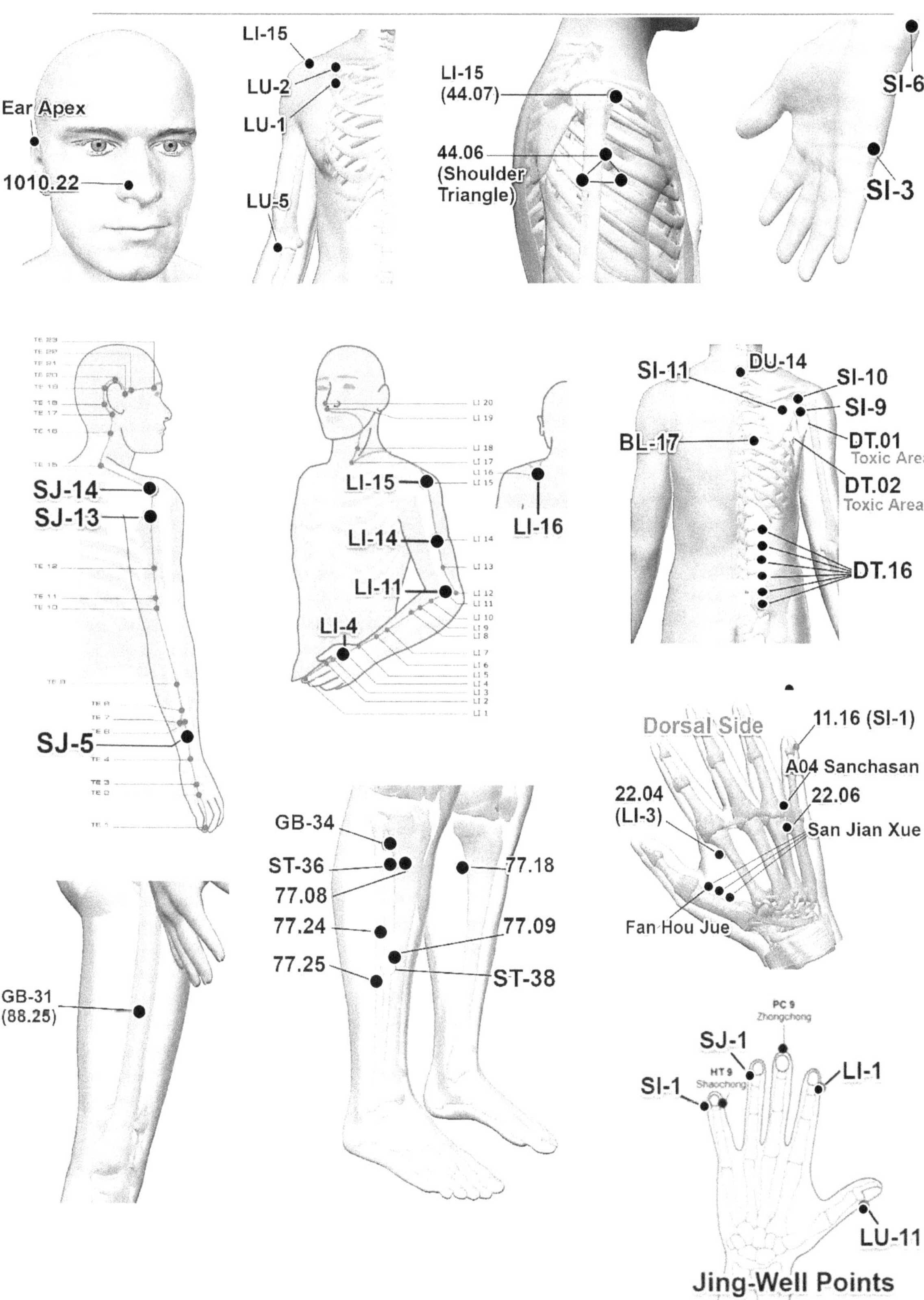

# Carpal Tunnel Syndrome/Wrist pain

*The meridians that are commonly involved in wrist pain include:*
***Heart meridian, Pericardium meridian, Large Intestine meridian, Lung meridian***

**Treatment for Wrist pain or carpal tunnel:**
- For carpal tunnel pain, use 77.22 Ce San Li + 77.23 Ce Xia San Li   and SJ-5 on the opposite side, with SI-3 on the same side.
- Alternately, you can use SI-3 with 22.04 Da Bai, threading each through to the other.
- If the pain is on the ulnar side, use opposite side SI-4 with same side SI-3 as a Guiding Point.
- Select and needle the relative ashi on the ankle area.

**Hand pain:** If the patient has difficulty opening and closing the hands, sedate or bleed same side 33.16 Qu Ling (LU-5), and then needle 22.01 Chong Zi+22.02 Chong Xian on the opposite side. For joint pain in the fingers, needle SJ-5.

**Thenar eminence pain**: Needle opposite side:  22.01 Chong Zi+22.02 Chong Xian, 22.04 Da Bai+22.05 Ling Gu, SJ-5 and 33.04 Huo Chuan (SJ-6), or 22.11 Tu Shui. These points are all effective for hand pain.

**Alternate treatment approach**

| AFFECTED(SICK) MERIDIANS | TREATMENT POINTS |
| --- | --- |
| **PERICARDIUM** Hand Jueyin | • P-6<br>• 77.22 Ce San Li + 77.23 Ce Xia San Li - ST treats PC (System 2 and 4)<br>• LIV-4, LIV-5, LIV-6 - for carpal tunnel syndrome (Balance Method, Liver treats PC) |
| **SANJIAO** Hand Shao Yang | • SJ-5, SJ-3, SJ-4<br>• 77.22 Ce San Li + 77.23 Ce Xia San Li - GB treats SJ (System 1) |
| **Large Intestine** - Hand Yang Ming | • 77.22 Ce San Li + 77.23 Ce Xia San Li - ST treats LI (System 1) |
| **LUNG** Hand Taiyin | • 11.27 Wu Hu #1, healthy side |

**Blood-letting for Wrist pain**
- Apex of the ear
- Visible veins in the cubital fossa and/or affected area
- Visible veins on the leg, especially lower part of lateral leg
- General area of SI-10
- Bleed jing-well of affected meridian followed by needling 77.22

*Points Illustrations for treatment of Wrist Pain*

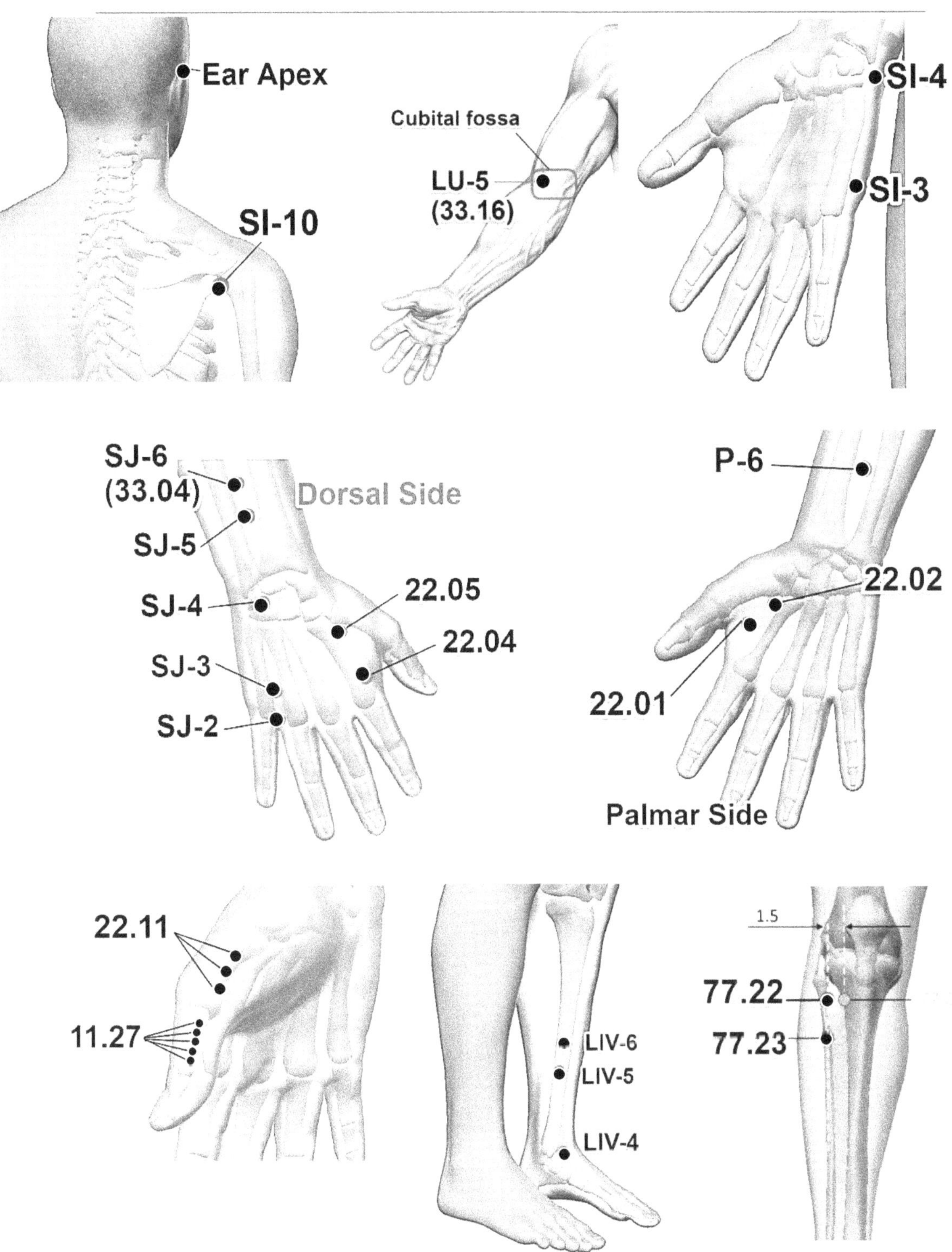

# Finger Pain/Trigger Finger

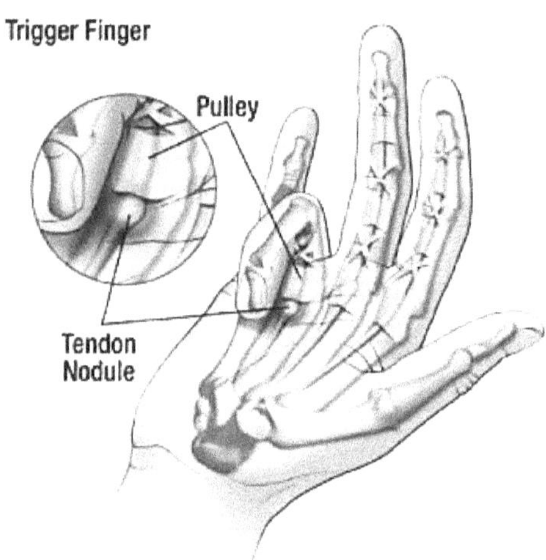


*Trigger finger is a condition in which one of your fingers gets stuck in a bent position. Your finger may bend or straighten with a snap — like a trigger being pulled and released. Trigger finger is also known as stenosing tenosynovitis. It occurs when inflammation narrows the space within the sheath that surrounds the tendon in the affected finger. If trigger finger is severe, your finger may become locked in a bent position.*

**Affected meridians: LI, Sanjio, LU, SI**

**Needling Treatment - Trigger finger/Finger pain**
- Needle opposite side 11.27 Wu Hu #1, #2 (can use same side if used as guide points)
- SJ-5 – effective for pain of all fingers (needle same side)
- Mu Guan and Gu Guan
- 33.08 Shou Wu Jin+33.09 Shou Qian
- Middle or Ring Finger locking: 66.06 Mu Liu+66.07 Mu Dou (opposite-side)
- 88.01 Tong Guan+88.02 Tong Shan+88.03 Tong Tian - bilateral for rheumatic arthritis
- Ashi points (can use press needles)
- Needle to the nodule
- Fingers mirror the toes and vice versa.  Locate and needle ashi points on mirror and opposite side.
- Moxibustion is suitable for injured finger joints

**Thumb pain:**
- Needle opposite-side:  11.27 Wu Hu #1, #2 and 66.01 Hai Bao, while the patient rotates the affected thumb until the pain is gone (approximately two minutes); then add 11.27 Wu Hu #1 on the same side as a Guiding Point. Can add 22.11 Tu Shui.

**Hand pain**
- Opposite side:  22.01 Chong Zi+22.02 Chong Xian, 22.11 Tu Shui.

---

### Blood-letting for Hand and finger pain and numbness
- Apex of the ear
- Visible veins on the leg, especially lower part of lateral leg
- General area of SI-10
- Bleed jing-well point of affected meridian
- Bleed same side 33.16 Qu Ling (LU-5).
- Prick hardening of the ganglion

*Points Illustrations for treatment of Finger Pain/Trigger Finger*

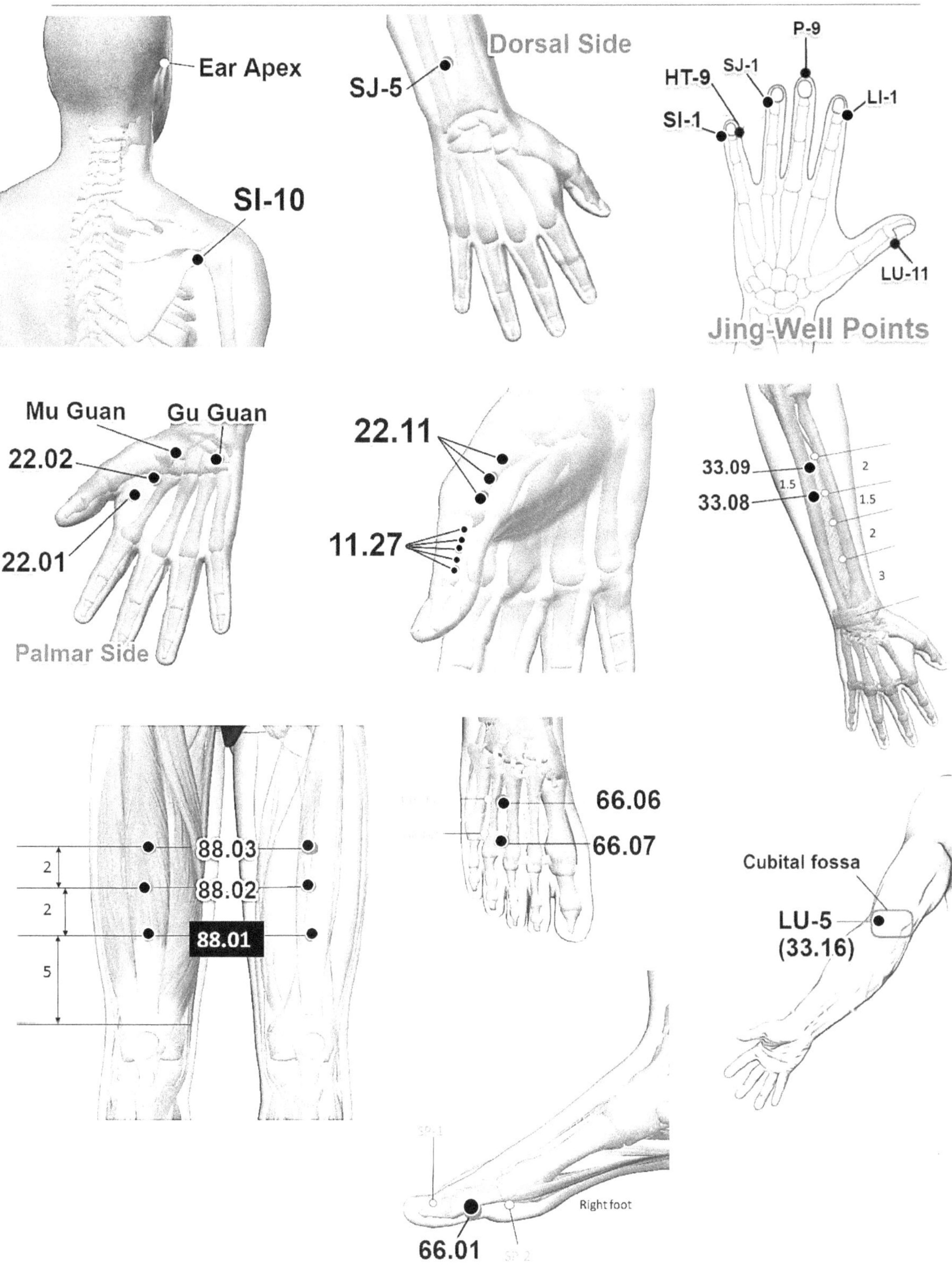

# "Tennis" Elbow Pain

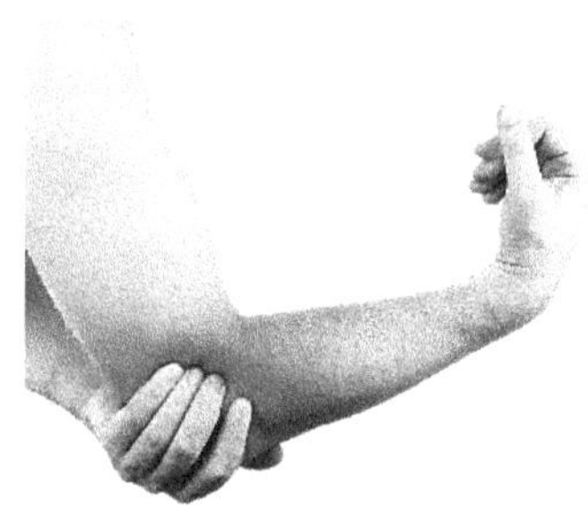

*Tennis elbow (lateral epicondylitis) is a painful condition that occurs when tendons in your elbow are overloaded, usually by repetitive motions of the wrist and arm.*

**Tennis elbow (Affected Channel: San Jiao meridian)**
- Needle opposite-side 77.22 Ce San Li + 77.23 Ce Xia San Li
- Or 88.25 Zhong Jiu Li (GB-31) with A.01 Qi Li (GB-32)
- Needle same side A.04 San Cha San or 22.06 Zhong Bai (SJ-3) – acting as Guiding Points.
- Treat ashi points on healthy elbow (mirror correspondence)

**Tennis Elbow (Affected Channel: Large Intestine meridian)**
- Needle opposite-side 33.07 Huo Fu Hai (LI-10), LI-11
  (needle both LI-10 and LI-11 just above the radius, sliding the needle along the bone)
- Needle same-side 22.04 Da Bai or 22.05 Ling Gu – acting as a Guiding Points.
- Treat ashi points on healthy elbow (mirror correspondence)

**Medial Elbow (Golfer's Elbow) pain (Affected Meridian), pain on Small Intestine meridian**

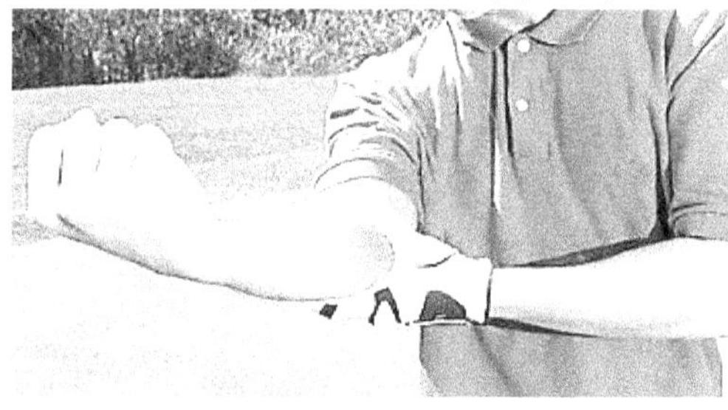

- Needle opposite-side 33.12 Xin Men with same-side SI-3 as guide point.
- Opposite side HT-3, LU-5
- Treat ashi points on healthy elbow (mirror correspondence)

---

### Blood-letting Treatment
- Moxibustion on local pain spots.
- Bleed Ashi
- Bleed LU-5
- Bleed 77.14
- Bleed DT.16 or around BL-25 and BL-27

*Points Illustrations for treatment of Elbow Pain*

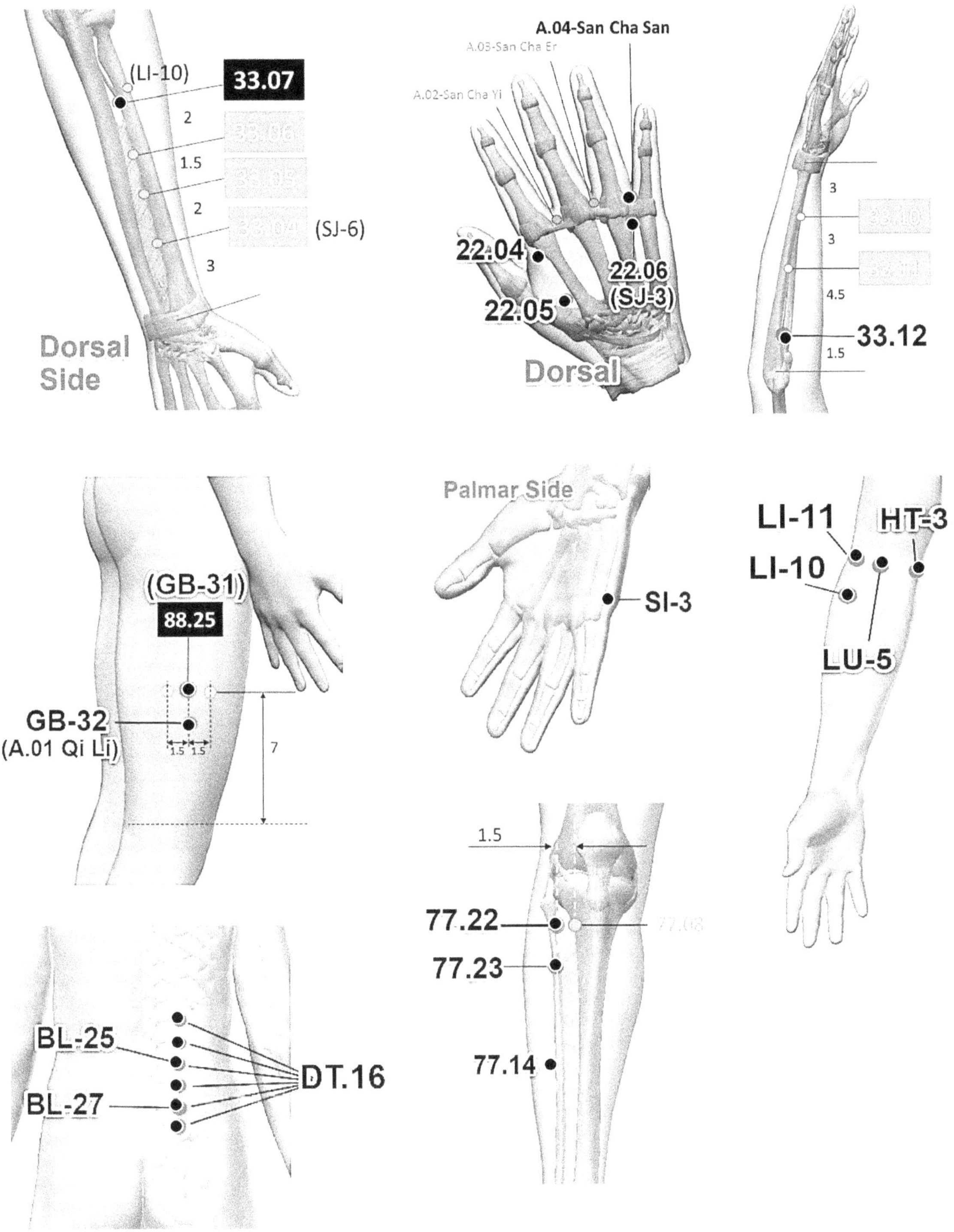

# LOWER LIMBS

## Groin pain

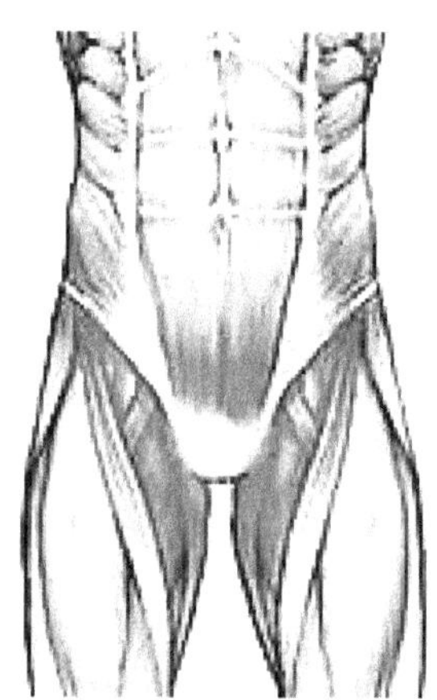

*According to TCM, groin pain is commonly associated with imbalances in the **kidney, bladder, and liver meridians**.*

*The **kidney meridian** governs the lower back, knees, and feet, and its imbalance can result in groin pain.*

*The **bladder meridian** runs along the back of the body and governs the lower back, buttocks, and legs. Imbalance in this meridian can lead to pain in the groin area.*

*The **liver meridian** governs the tendons, ligaments, and muscles, and its imbalance can result in groin pain due to tension or stiffness in the muscles and tendons.*

*Additionally, groin pain can also be associated with an imbalance in the qi and blood flow in the affected area, which can lead to stagnation and pain.*

**Treatment Points**

**Groin pain**

- 33.12 Xin Men on the opposite side
- KI-2(66.12), SP-4 (66.11) - groin injury


**Groin pain with sciatica**:

- Cup both GB-29 and GB-30.
  Recommend to cup BL-36 while the patient is lying on their side,
  as the skin color after cupping here is often extremely dark
  (indicating toxin buildup).
- 33.12 Xin Men can be used in conjunction with
  SI-3, 22.04 Da Bai+22.05 Ling Gu, and/or 22.06 Zhong Bai, 22.07 Xia Bai.


---

**Blood-letting**
- Bleed Ashi areas

*Points Illustrations for treatment of Groin Pain*

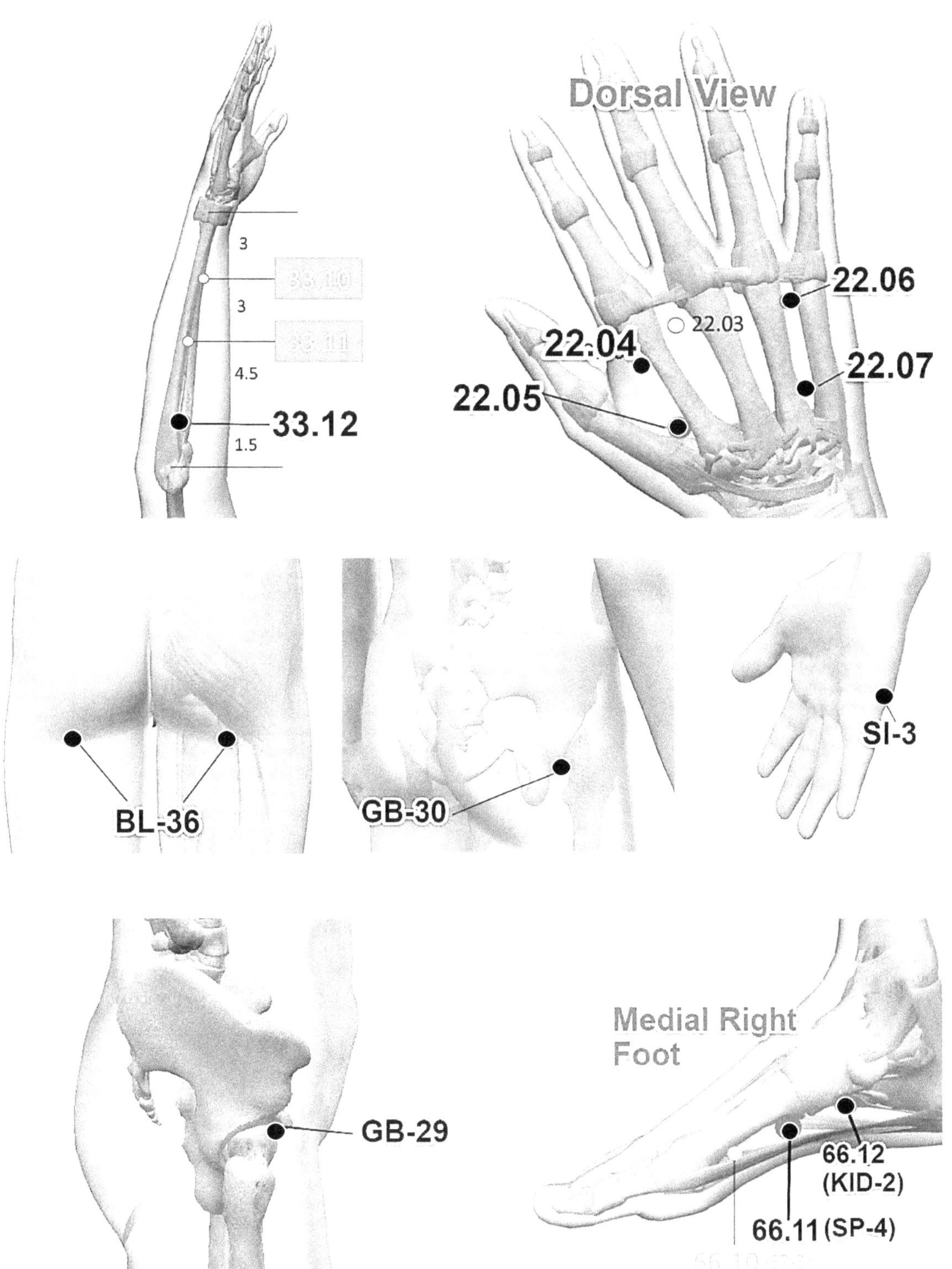

# Hip Pain

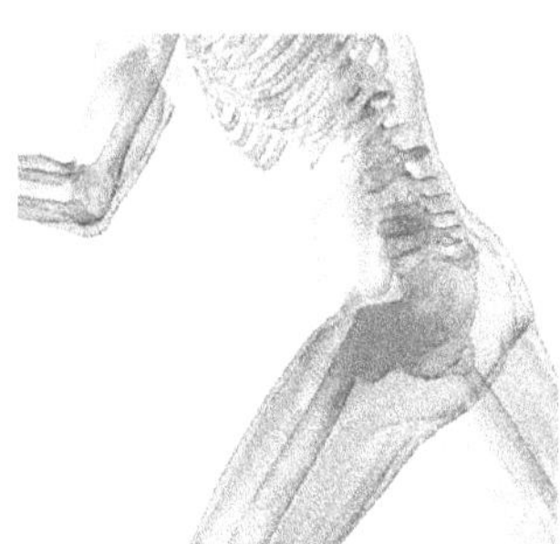

*The meridians that are commonly involved in hip pain include:*

***Gallbladder meridian:*** *Hip pain along this meridian may be associated with issues such as indecisiveness, anger, and resentment.*

***Bladder meridian:*** *Hip pain along this meridian may be associated with issues such as fear, stress, and low back pain.*

***Liver meridian:*** *Hip pain along this meridian may be associated with issues such as anger, frustration, and menstrual problems.*

***Kidney meridian:*** *Hip pain along this meridian may be associated with issues such as fear, stress, and low back pain.*

**Needle**

- Opposite-side 22.04 Da Bai+22.05 Ling Gu or 22.06 Zhong Bai, 22.07 Xia Bai
- 77.05 Yi Zhong+77.06 Er Zhong+77.07 San Zhong; effective for greater trochanter hip pain.
- 33.12 Xin Men – hip and groin pain
- 66.09 Shui Qu (GB-41) helps as a same-side Guiding Point.
- 88.17 + 88.18 + 88.19 – thigh numbness
- TCM points: GB-30, BL-54, BL-32, ST-31, BL-40, BL-60 (treat affected GB, BL and ST meridians)

---

### Cupping/Blood-letting

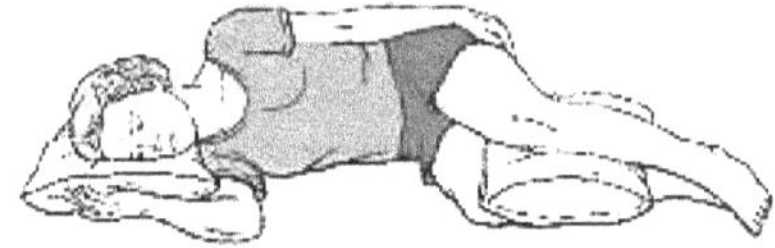

- Position the patient on their side and use a pillow to support their upper leg and knee. Next, thoroughly cup the sacrum and hip joint area, especially around GB-29, GB-30, BL-36, and BL-34.

- Wet-cup tender local areas
- Bleed BL-40

*Points Illustrations for treatment of Hip Pain*

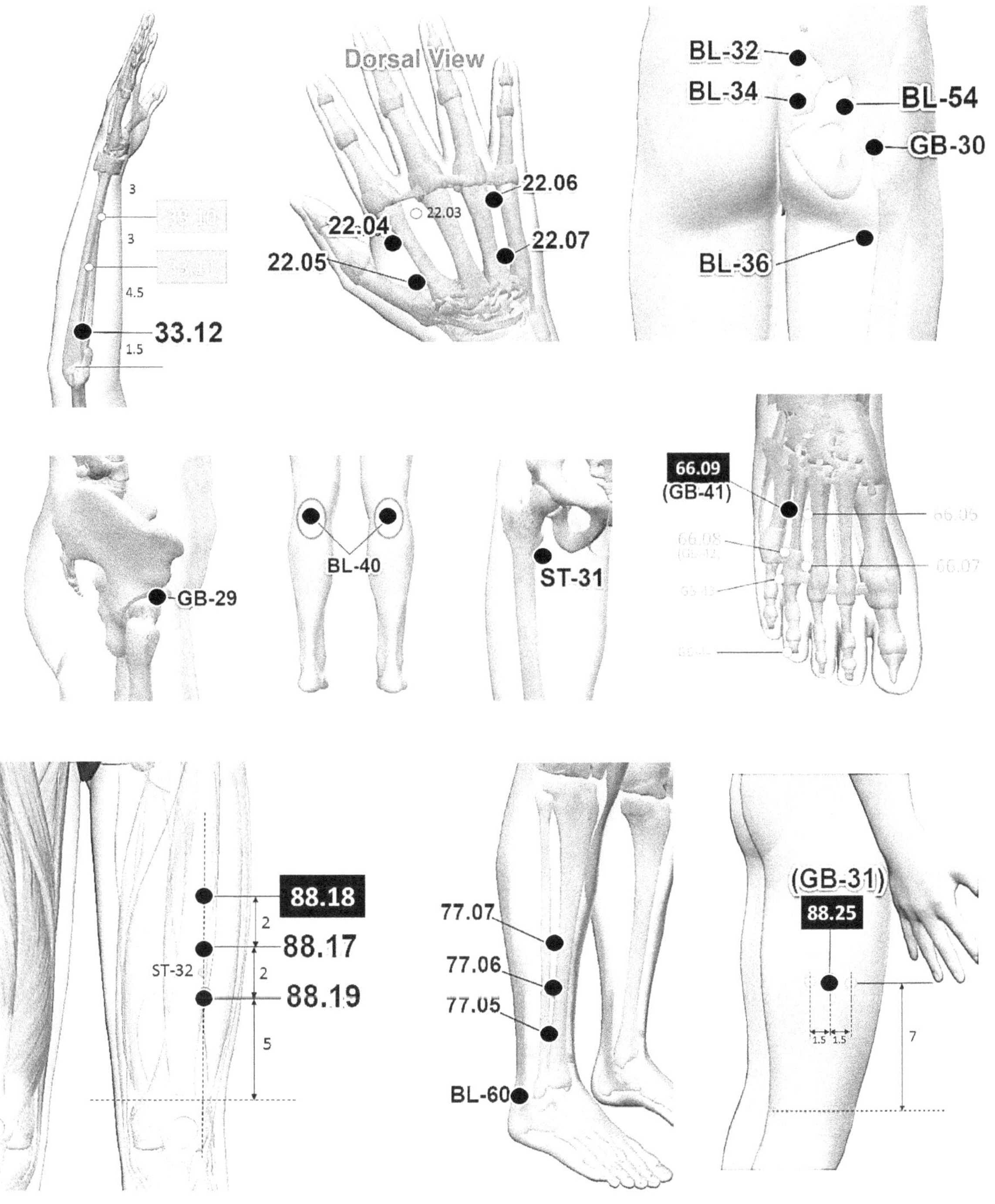

# Sciatica

*Sciatica refers to pain that radiates along the path of the sciatic nerve, which branches from your lower back through your hips and buttocks and down each leg. Typically, sciatica affects only one side of your body. Sciatica most commonly occurs when a herniated disk, bone spur on the spine or narrowing of the spine (spinal stenosis) compresses part of the nerve. This causes inflammation, pain and often some numbness in the affected leg.*

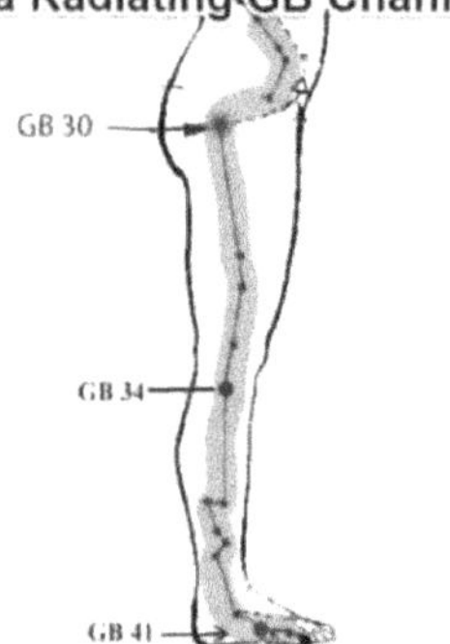


**Treatment for Pain Radiating along GB Channel (Lateral)**

- 22.05, 22.04, 22.06 Zhong Bai+ 22.07 Xia Bai - opposite side
- 33.08 Shou Wu Jin+33.09 Shou Qian Jin - opposite side
- GB-30, GB-31, GB-32 (A.01 Qi Li) - Treats own meridian.
- SJ-2 + SJ-3 - SJ treats GB (System 1)
- BL-65 or GB-41 (66.09 Shui Qu) as Guiding Points on the same side
- GB-30 + BL-60 – with electrical stimulation

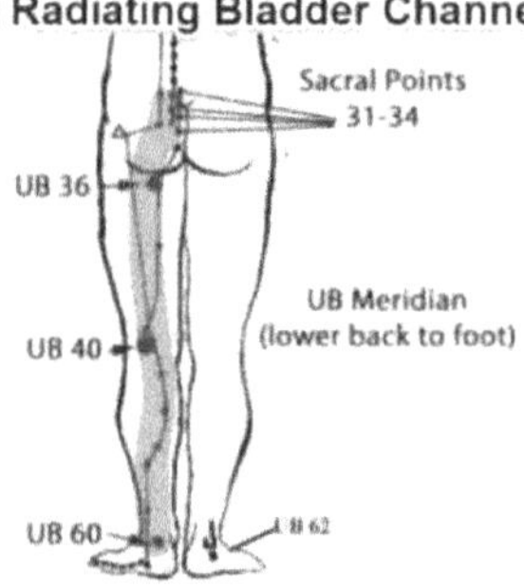


**Treatment for Pain Radiating along BL Channel (Posterior)**

- SI-3 and then add 22.04 +22.05 on opposite side, finishing with BL-65 on the affected side, acting as guide point.
- For both BL and GB channel sciatica add 22.06 Zhong Bai, 22.07 Xia Bai on the opposite side, and GB-41 (66.09 Shui Qu) on the same side.
- SI-3 +SI-4 - SI treats BL (System 1)
- 33.12 Xin Men - SI treats Bladder (System 1). Elbow images sacrum.
- BL-54 (same side) - Treats own meridian.
- 1010.25 – if pain also in sacrum
-

**Groin pain with sciatica**

- 33.12 Xin Men can be used in conjunction with SI-3, 22.04 Da Bai+22.05 Ling Gu, and/or 22.06 Zhong Bai, 22.07 Xia Bai.

---

## Cupping/Blood-letting Treatment

- Cup both GB-29 and GB-30. Recommend to cup BL-36 while the patient is lying on their side, as the skin color after cupping here is often extremely dark (indicating toxin buildup).
- Cup the entire lower back, sacral area and hip area but avoid traumatized spine/vertebrae.
- Moxibustion tender spots on lower back and sacral area
- Bleed BL-40 - Treats own meridian.  BL-40 is Xi-cleft of blood. BL treats kidney (bones)
- Bleed-cup around BL-31 if tender
- Visible veins anywhere else on the leg and thigh.
- For difficult cases, palpate the most sensitive point in the area of DT.08 Jing Zhi or DT.09 Jin Lin (or area around SI-9, SI-10), and bleed -cup tender areas.
- Bleed-cup tender point on the ipsilateral buttock.
- Sciatica (lateral) - bleed GB-44 followed by needling SJ-5, SJ-6
- Sciatica (posterior) - bleed BL-67 followed by needling SI-3, SI-4

*Points Illustrations for treatment of Sciatica*

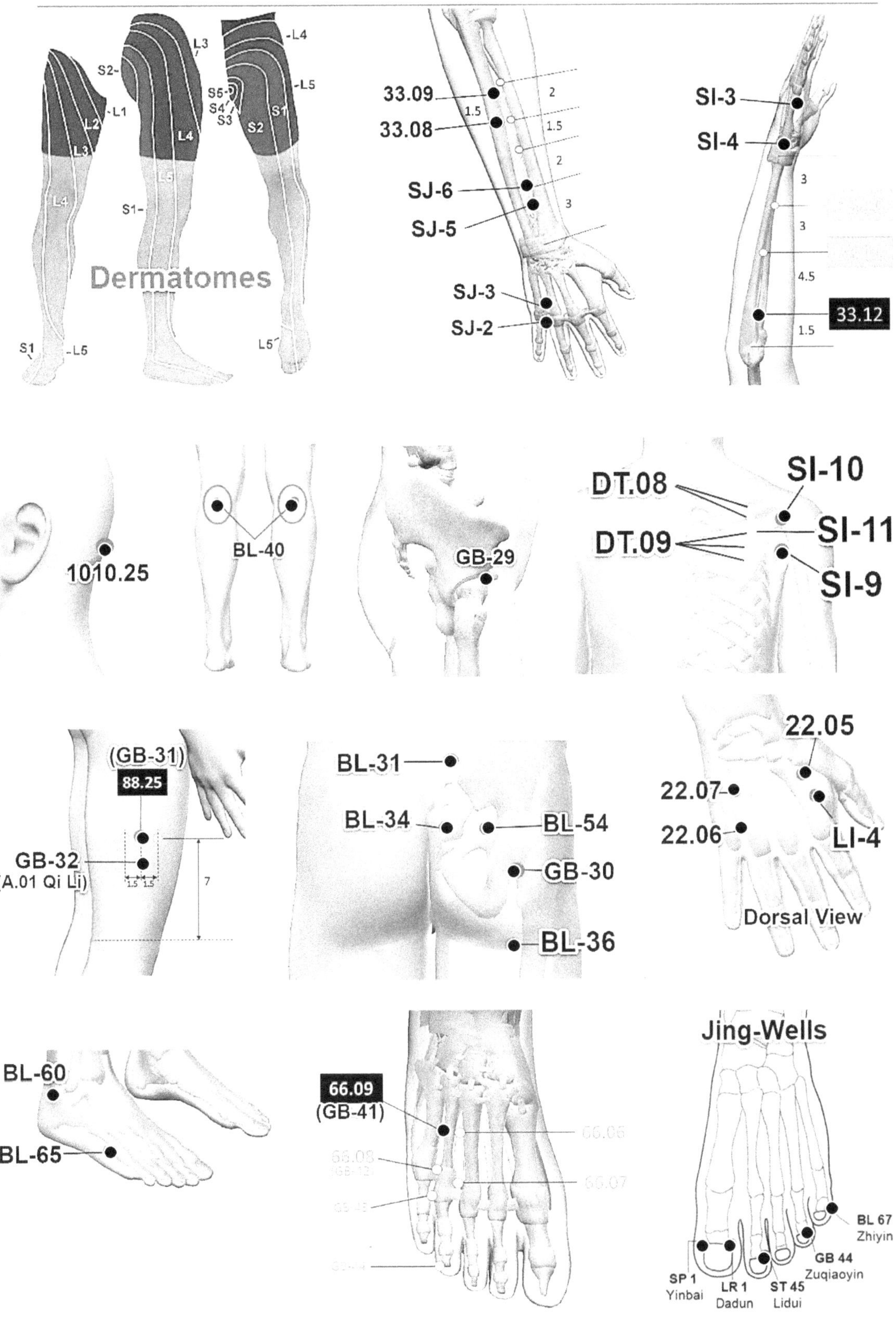

# Knee Pain

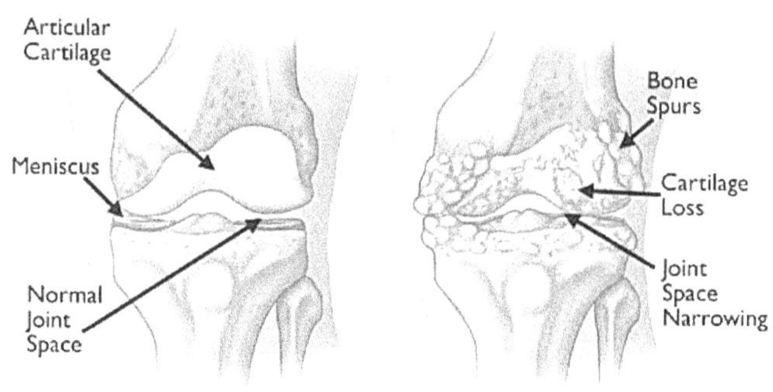


*Knee pain may be the result of an injury, such as a ruptured ligament or torn cartilage. Medical conditions — including arthritis, gout and infections — also can cause knee pain.*

*The meridians that are commonly involved in knee pain include:*

***Liver meridian***: *Knee pain along this meridian may be associated with issues such as menstrual problems, anger, and frustration.*

***Stomach meridian***: *Knee pain along this meridian may be associated with issues such as digestive problems and worry.*

***Kidney meridian***: *Knee pain along this meridian may be associated with issues such as fear, stress, and low back pain.*

***Bladder meridian***: *Knee pain along this meridian may be associated with issues such as low back pain, fear, and stress.*

**Needling Treatment (generally on opposite side)**

- Bilaterally needle 11.09 Xin Xi + 11.13 Dan - Degenerative knee pain (Osteoarthritis) causes pain when climbing and descending stairs
- 44.06 Jian Zhong - LI treats Stomach (System 1). Reaction area: Heart.  In the Master Tung System, all points relating to the Heart can be useful to treatment of knee pain
- P-6
- 33.12 Xin Men on the opposite side – when there is more pain descending stairs than ascending. Possibly bone spurs present.
- 66.03 Huo Ying or 66.04 Huo Zhu as Guiding Points on affected side.
- Can add opposite-side or same side ST-36, SP-9 and GB-34
- LI-11 on opposite side- LI treats Stomach (System 1). Elbow images the knee.
- Heding, Xiyan (Ex. 32.) or Ex-LE-5, Dubi (ST-35) – same side with electrical stimulation
- SP-10, ST-34 (same side, local needling)
- Moxibustion of local area is useful.
- Active Qi Moving technique when there are no local needles inserted.

---

**Blood-letting Treatment**

- Bleed-cup DT.07 San Jin (same side or both sides and only if tender to palpation) - For pain underneath the knee cap (inside the joint), degenerative knee pain (osteoarthritis).
- 77.08 Si Hua Shang, 77.09 Si Hua Zhong, 77.13 Si Hua Li can be needled on the opposite side or bled on the same side (if a good vein is found).
- Bleed-cup around ashi areas of the knee.
- Knee pain (medial) - bleed  LIV-1, SP-1 followed by needling  44.06 Jian Zhong,  11.09 Xin Xi
- Knee pain (lateral) - bleed  ST-45,  GB-44 followed by needling 44.06 Jian Zhong,  11.09 Xin Xi

*Points Illustrations for treatment of Knee Pain*

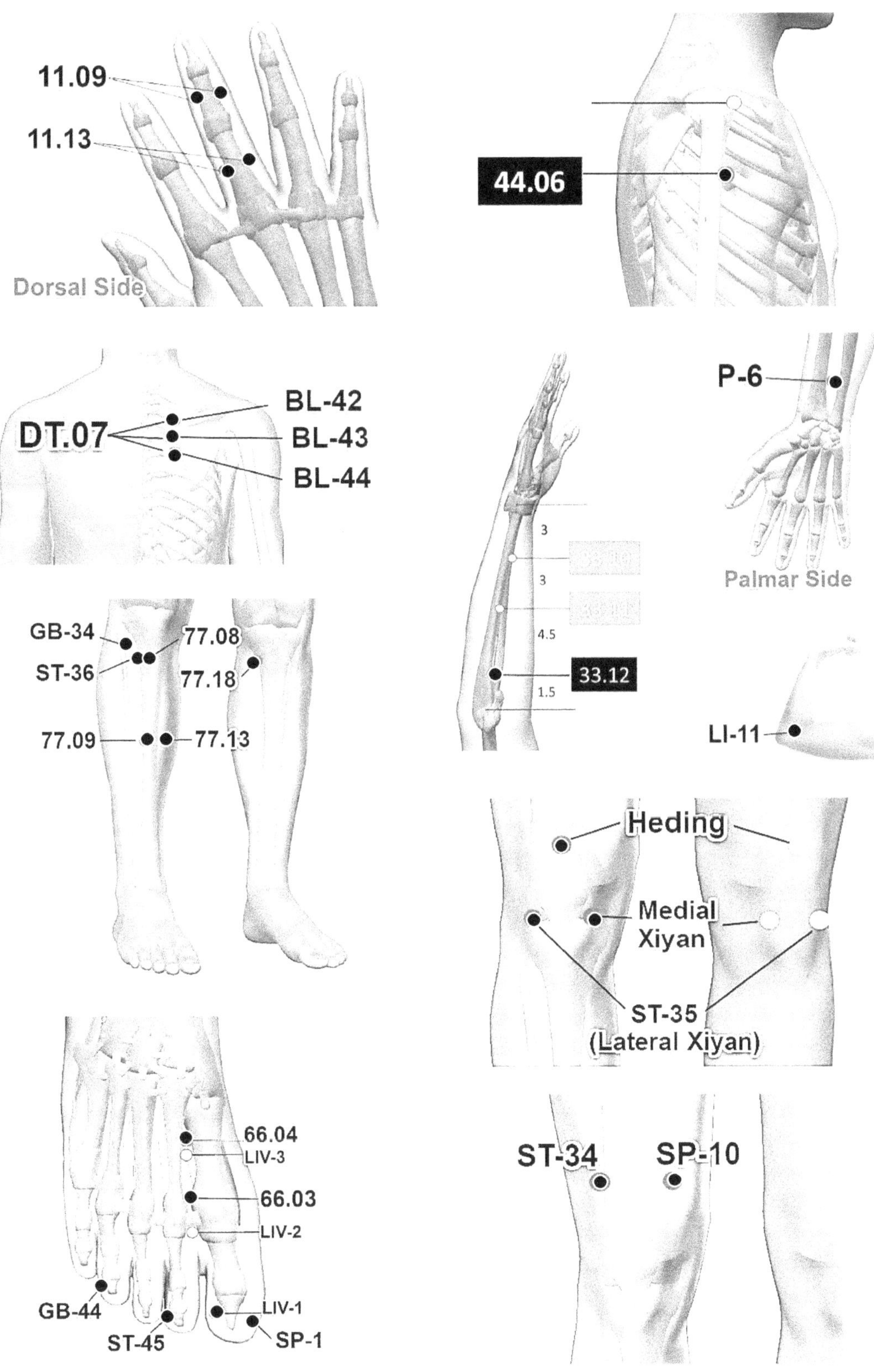

# Leg Pain

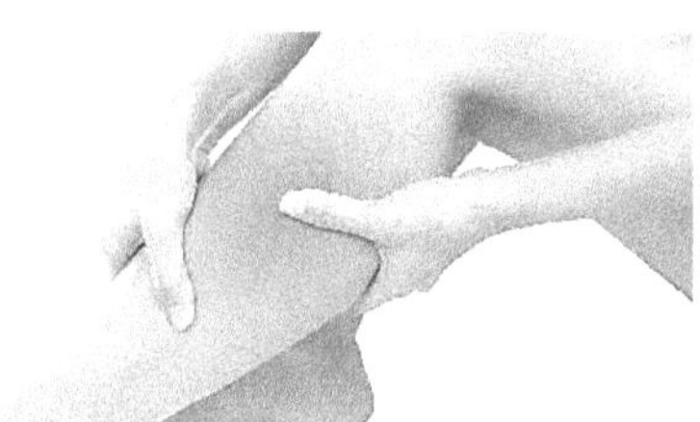

**Needling Treatment**

**Leg pain and weakness**

- 88.01 Tong Guan, 88.02 Tong Shan, 88.03 Tong Tian -for cases of poor blood circulation due to weak heart resulting in weakness, cold, pain or numbness in the lower body.
- A.06 Ci Bai on healthy side。
- 44.06 Jian Zhong on diseased side (improve heart function)
- SI-3, SI-4 + 22.04 Da Bai+22.05 Ling Gu+22.06 Zhong Bai+22.07 Xia Bai or A.04 San Cha San
- 44.08 Ren Zong+44.09 Di Zong+44.10 Tian Zong - reaction area of the legs, leg pain
- 33.07 Huo Fu Hai (due to heart and spleen), 33.08 +33.09, 44.17 Shui Yu - legs sore
- 1010.08 Zhen Jing - both legs sore
- 66.11 Huo Ju, 88.25 Zhong Jiu Li (GB-31), GB-32, 88.27 Xia Jiu Li
- 77.27 Wai San Guan for local treatment

**Leg and foot numbness**

- 55.04 Hua Gu San+55.05 Hua Gu Si on opposite side treat the entire leg as well as numbness of the legs and feet. Carry-out Active Qi Moving during treatment.

**Numbness of the hands and feet**

- Bilaterally needle 77.18 Shen Guan+77.19 Di Huang+77.21 Ren Huang or 66.11 Huo Ju (SP-4).

**Diabetic neuropathy**

- 77.18 Shen Guan+77.19 Di Huang+77.21 Ren Huang treats diabetes and diabetic neuropathy by tonifying Spleen qi and Kidney yin.
- Treat the feet with gentle Gua Sha (oil and rubbing with a finger).

**Swelling in legs and weakness**

- 77.18 Shen Guan+77.19 Di Huang+77.21 Ren Huang
- 88.01 Tong Guan, 88.02 Tong Shan, 88.03 Tong Tian

---

### Blood-letting for Lower limb conditions

- For any pain or symptom of the lower limbs, first bleed any visible veins in the BL-40 area.
- Also examine the legs and thighs for any veins that look particularly "bleed-able,"
  i.e. dark, prominent veins, and bleed those.
- DT.08 Jing Zhi/DT.09 Jin Lin area
- 44.07 Bei Mian (LI-15) - aching and soreness of both lower legs
- Avoid bleeding foot and/or areas of poor circulation

*Points Illustrations for treatment of Leg Pain*

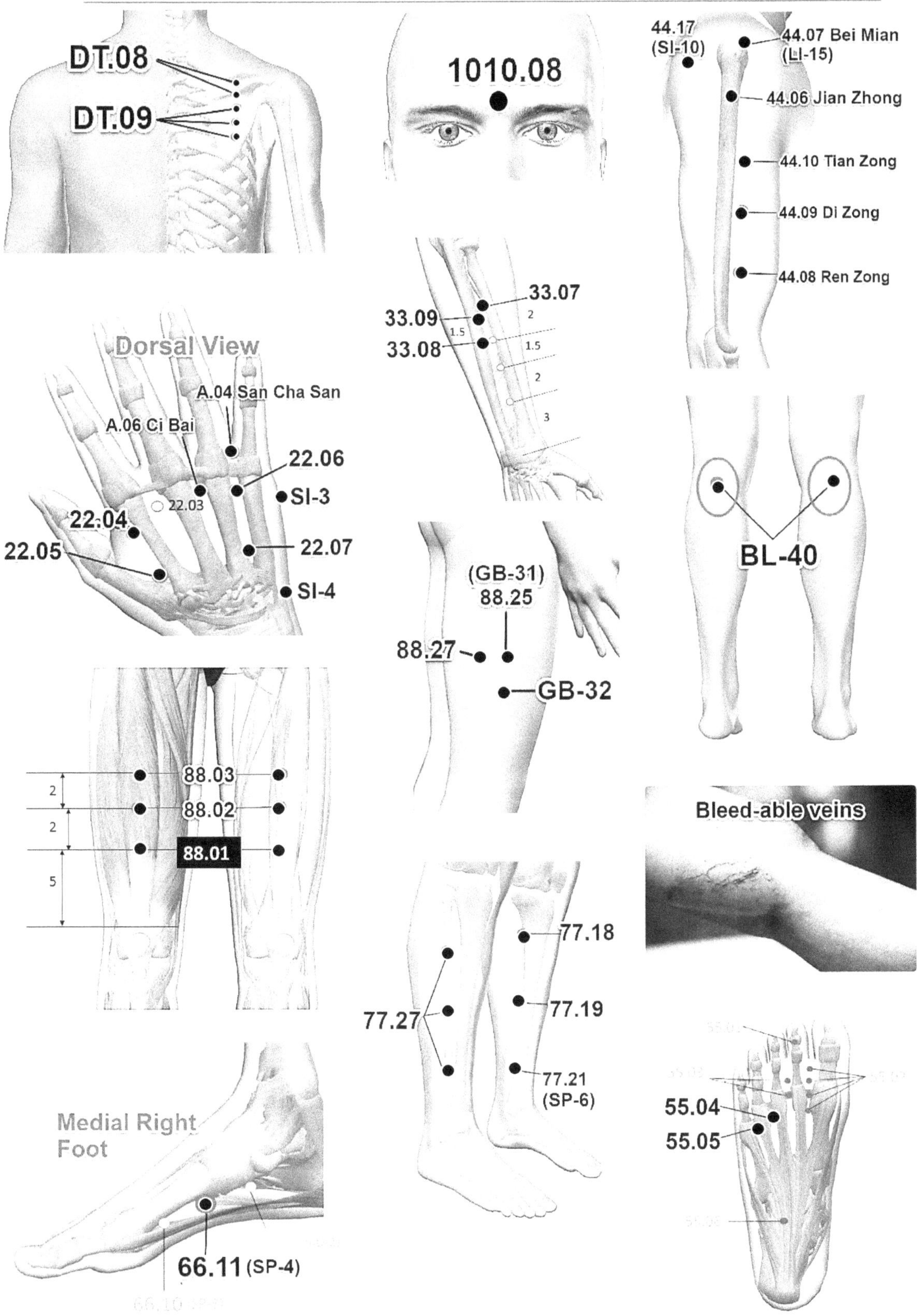

# Ankle Sprain and Pain

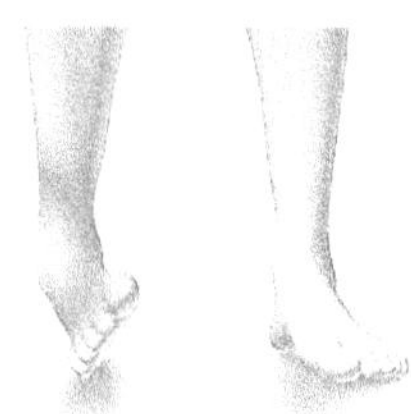

*A sprained ankle is an injury that occurs when you roll, twist or turn your ankle in an awkward way. This can stretch or tear the tough bands of tissue (ligaments) that help hold your ankle bones together. Ligaments help stabilize joints, preventing excessive movement. A sprained ankle occurs when the ligaments are forced beyond their normal range of motion. Most sprained ankles involve injuries to the ligaments on the outer side of the ankle.*

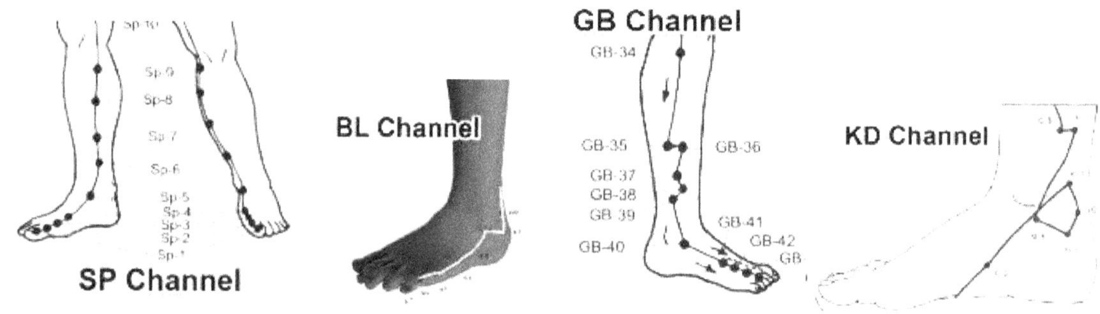


**Affected Meridians: Spleen, Urinary Bladder, Gall Bladder, Kidney**

**Needling Points for ankle pain**

- A.05 Xiao Jie (needle obliquely towards P-7) on opposite side – highly effective for acute or chronic ankle pain.  LU treats Spleen (System 1). Wrist images the ankle.
- Toe, ankle, foot or heel pain: 11.27 #3, #4, #5 Wu Hu
- Ashi around 22.10 Shou Jie opposite side (hand images foot)
- SI-6 - Xi-cleft point of SI. SI treats Spleen Channel (System 2). Wrist images the ankle.
- SJ-4, SJ-5 or 22.06 Zhong Bai+22.07 Xia Bai- lateral ankle pain, SJ treats GB Channel (System 1). Needle any other ashi points around the wrist to treat pain ankle.
- GB-41 (66.09 Shui Qu) - Shu-stream of GB Meridian
- 77.27 Wai San Guan - local treatment
- BL-60, KID-3, ST-41 – needle/moxa local area

**Dorsum of Foot Pain**

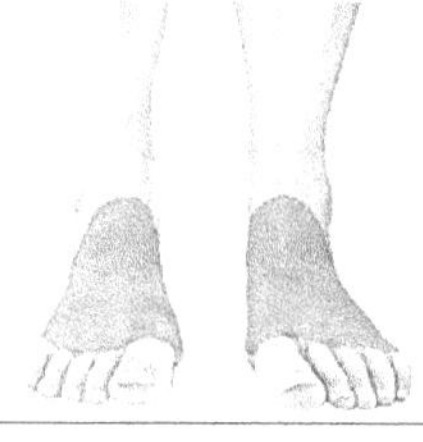

- Gently oil and rub (Gua Sha) around the painful area
- 66.03 Huo Ying, 66.04 Huo Zhu can be needled on the opposite foot

---

**Blood-letting Treatment**

- Visible veins on the leg, especially the BL-40 region, ST-36 /GB-34 region, and around the ankle
- Bleed locally, not necessarily in the bruised area but in the most painful spots.
- Bleed affected Jing Well Points
- Bleed 77.14 Si Hua Wai- to reduce swelling then needle A.05 Xiao Jie
- Bleed BL-40
- Ankle pain (medial) - bleed LIV-1, SP-1, followed by needling 11.27 #3, #4, #5
- Ankle pain (lateral) - bleed ST-45, GB-44, followed by needling 11.27 #3, #4, #5

*Points Illustrations for treatment of Ankle Sprain and Pain*

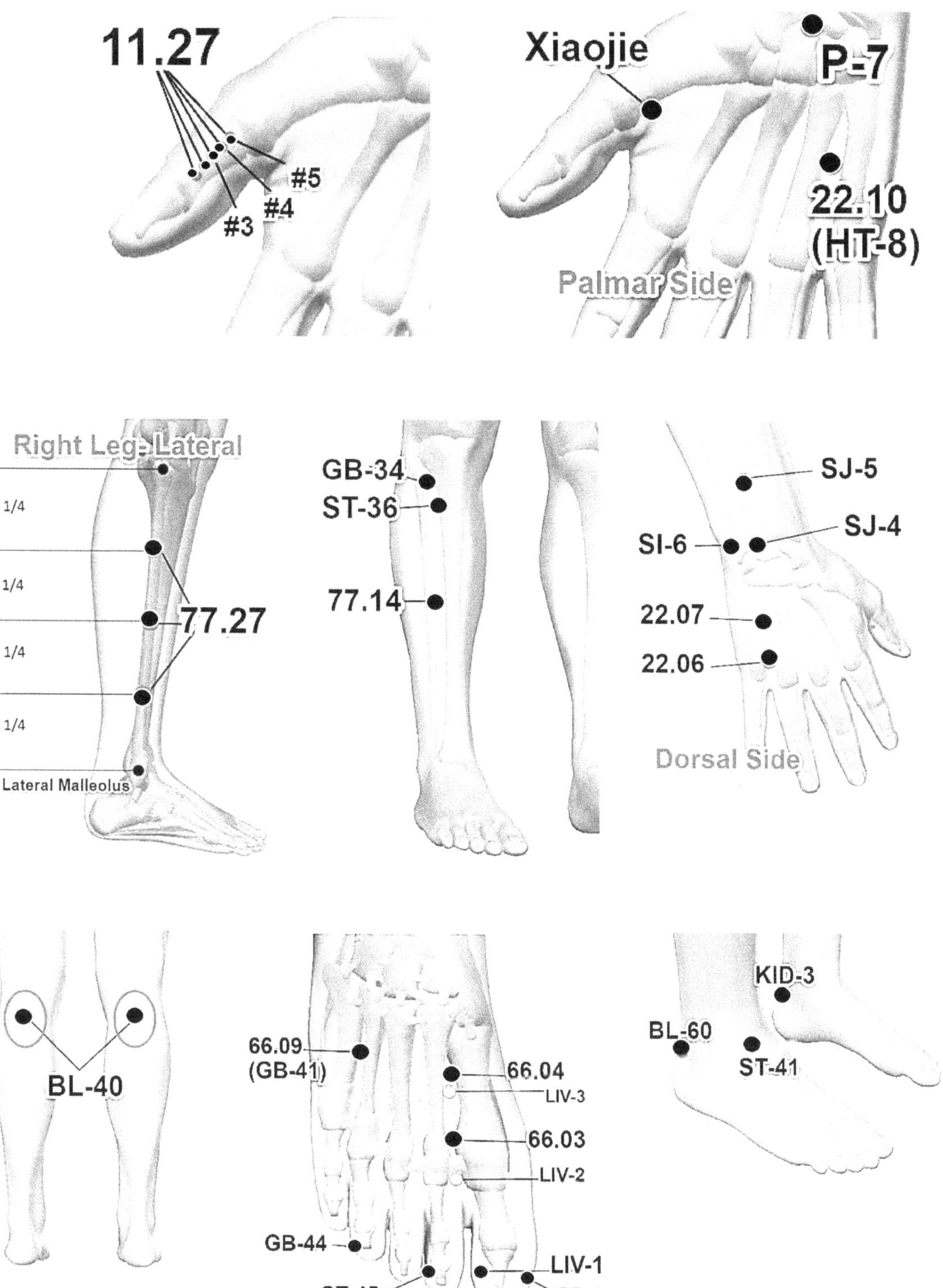

# Heel and Sole Pain

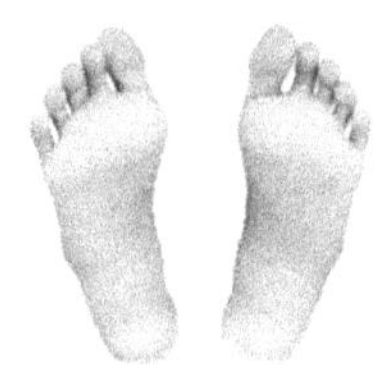

**Treatment for Ball of the foot pain**
- Moxa on 1010.01 Zheng Hui (DU-20). Top treats bottom.

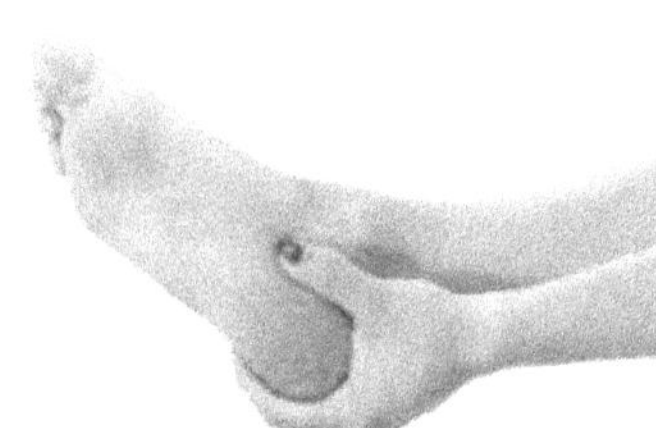

**Treatment for Heel pain**
- Mu Guan & Gu Guan, Heel Zone
- Needle bilateral or opposite-side 88.17 +88.18 +88.19
- Points P-7 and one additional point 1.0 cun distal
- Zugendian - 0.5 cm inferior to P-7. Empirical point for heel pain.
- 22.05 Ling Gu. Treating bone with bone. Wrist treats heel.
- KID-3, BL-60, BL-65- either side
- Zhu Wu Hu #5

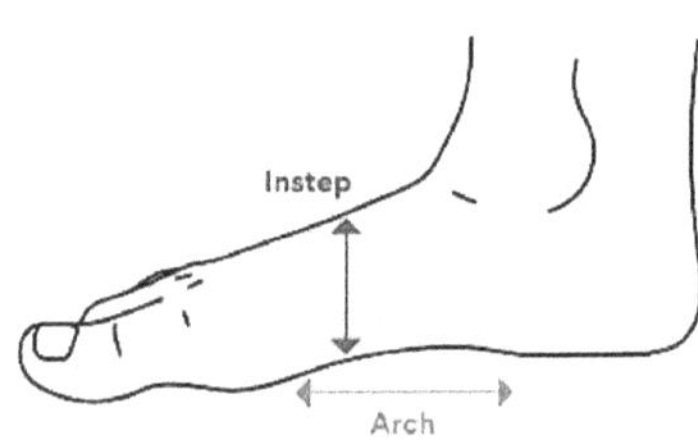


**Treatment for Sole pain (instep)**
- Needle opposite-side 11.27 Wu Hu. #3-#4
- Opposite side 44.06 Jian Zhong

**Treatment by Direct Mirror Imaging for pain at bottom of foot**
- Locate point on hand relative to pain point on foot. If ashi, needle.

Plantar Fasciitis

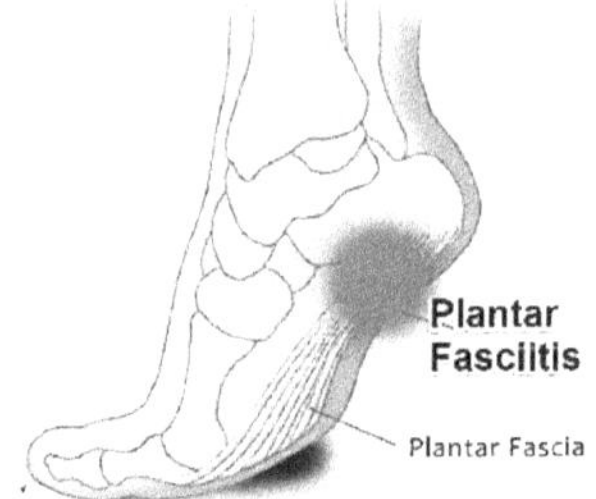


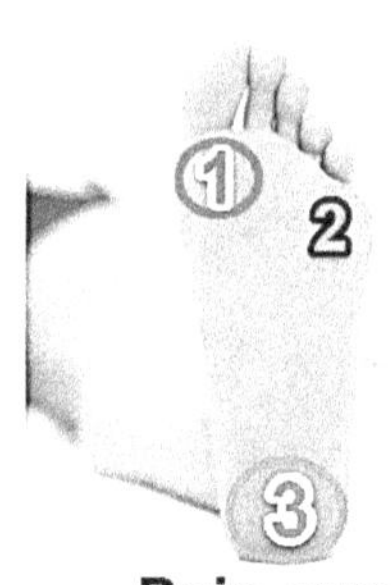


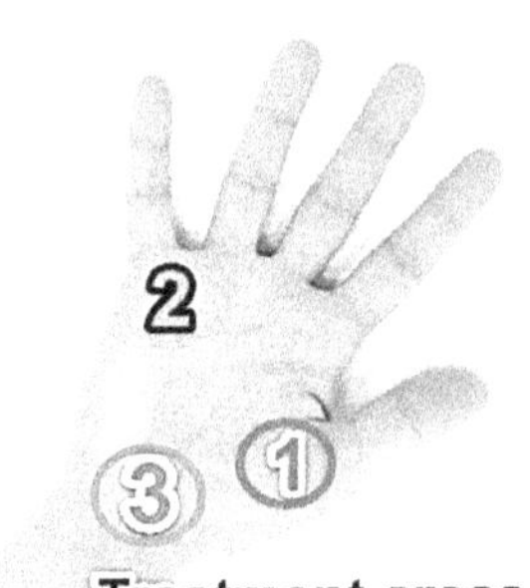


---

**Blood-letting for Heel pain/plantar fasciitis**
- Visible veins in the BL-40 region
- Visible veins around the ankle
- Visible veins anywhere else on the leg and thigh
- Bleed same-side DT.08 Jing Zhi
- Bleed 11.26 Zhi Wu for fractures which are slow to heal.
- Massage/acupressure and moxa ashi spots

*Points Illustrations for treatment of Heel and Sole Pain*

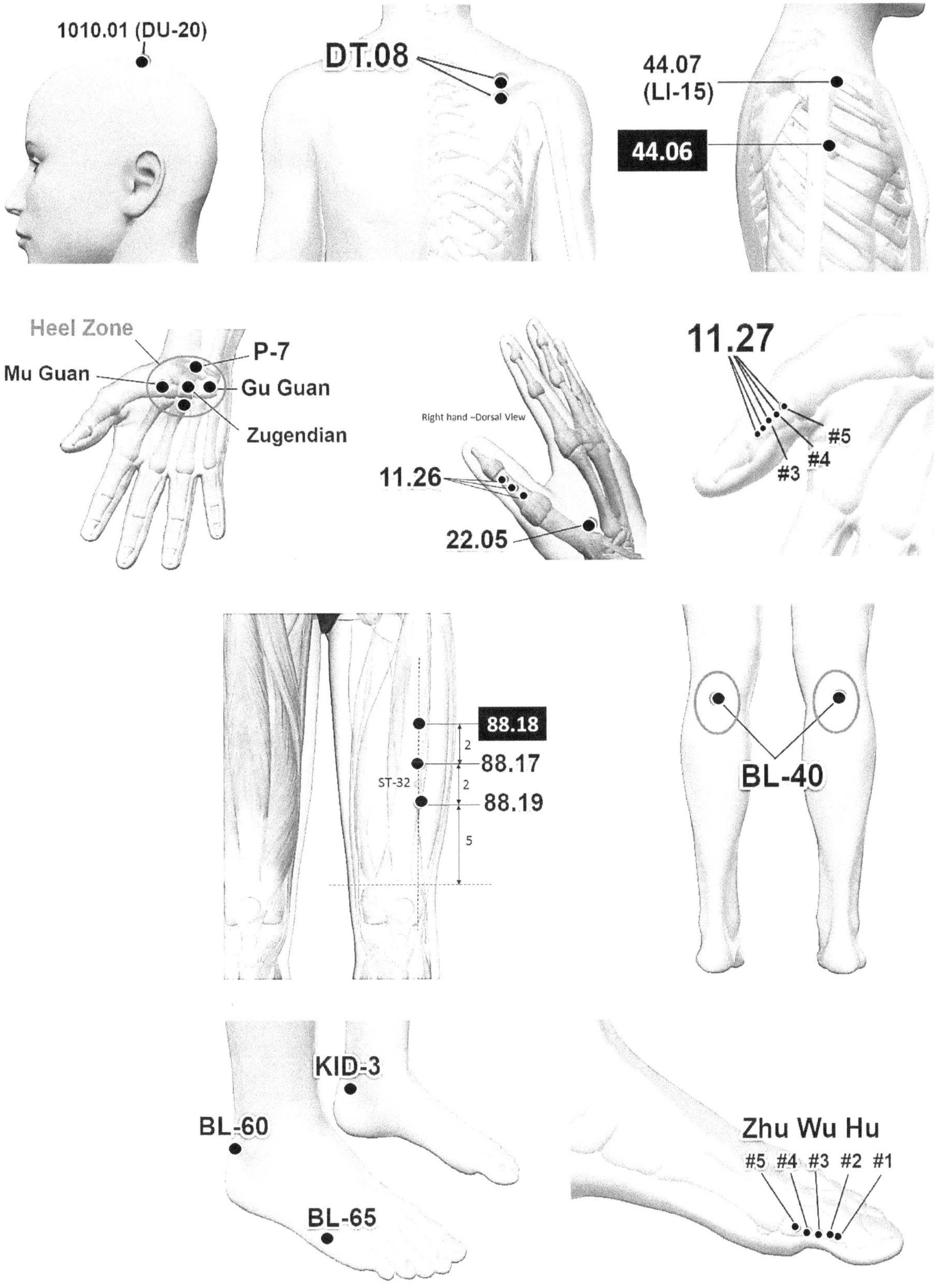

# <u>BACK AND SPINE</u>

## Back Pain

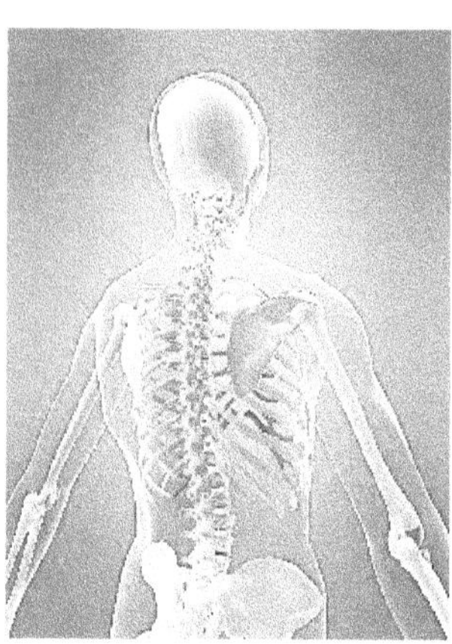

*According to TCM theory, back pain can be caused by a variety of factors, including:*

*Qi and blood stagnation - If there is stagnation of Qi and blood in the back, it can result in pain.*

*Kidney deficiency - In TCM, the kidneys are considered the root of vitality and are responsible for nourishing the muscles and bones. If there is a deficiency in kidney energy, it can lead to weakness and pain in the back.*

*Cold and dampness - Cold and dampness can obstruct the flow of Qi and blood in the back, leading to pain.*

*External factors - External factors such as wind, cold, and dampness can invade the body and cause pain in the back.*

**Affected meridians: Liver, Kidney, Bladder, Gallbladder**

**Needling Treatment**

- 22.04 Da Bai+22.05 Ling Gu on one hand and 22.06 Zhong Bai+22.07 Xia Bai on other hand
- 22.01 Chong Zi+22.02 Chong Xian + SI-3 on one hand with 22.04 Da Bai+22.05 Ling Gu on the other hand. Lung treats bladder (System 2)
- 22.03 Shang Bai with 001 Hand Golden Gate - acute twisted back, middle back and waist pain.
- Needle opposite-side or bilateral SI-3, BL-65, BL-60 on the same side acting as Guiding Points. For spine or muscle pain on both sides of the spine, use points bilaterally with strong stimulation.
- 1010.19 Shui Tong+1010.20 Shui Jin (Kidney related pain)
- 66.14 Shui Xiang (KI-3)
- 77.01 Zheng Jin+77.02 Zheng Zong - Treats own BL meridian, tendon treats tendon
- 1010.22, 1010.25

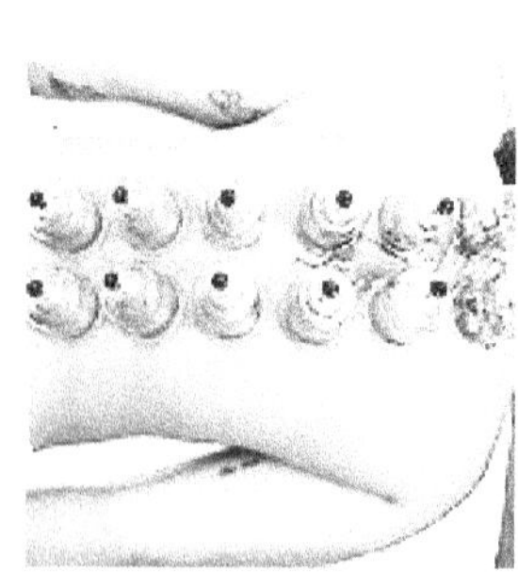

### Cupping/Blood-letting for Upper back pain

- Cup the entire back
- Apex of the ear
- Palpate for the most tender point on the back and wet-cup it directly
- Visible veins in the leg
- Bleed cup BL-40 and BL-57 regions
- Gua sha Huatuojiaji points. Start gently and assess effectiveness. Continue with more pressure if positive outcome.

*Points Illustrations for treatment of Back Pain*

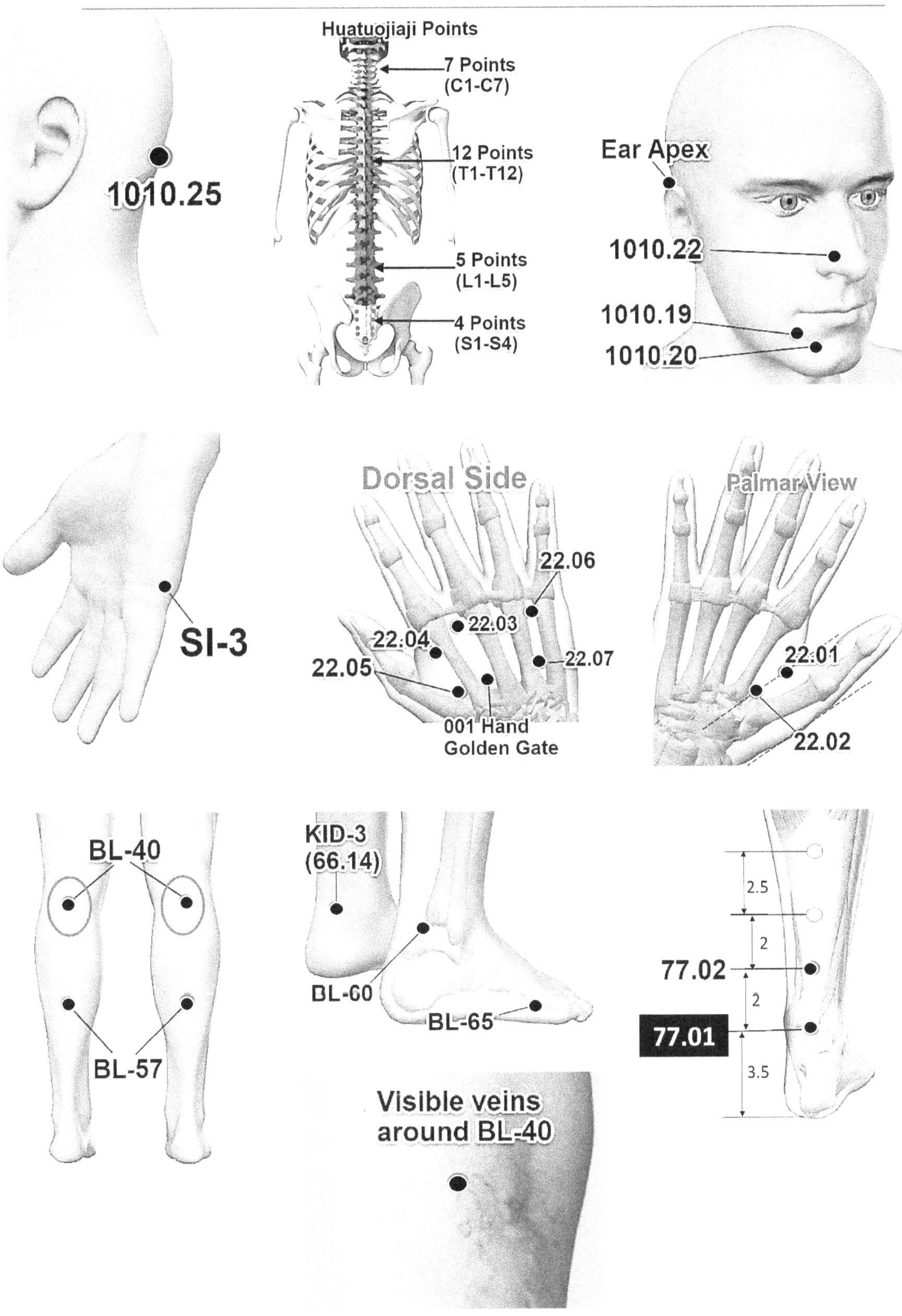

# Acute Lumbar Sprain/Low Back Pain

**Treatment for Acute lumbar sprain**
- Bleed-cup BL-40 area
- BL-60 + SI-3 + DU-26
- 1010.19 Shui Tong+1010.20 Shui Jin - opposite side
- 1010.13 Ma Jin Shui+1010.14 Ma Kuai Shui - opposite side
- Needle 11.12 Er Jiao Ming, 22.05

| AFFECTED MERIDIANS | TREATMENT POINTS |
|---|---|
| **DU (GV)** | • DU-26 - Treats own meridian.<br>• 11.12 Er Jiao Ming - Holographic the spine and DU meridian |
| **BLADDER -**<br>FOOT TAIYANG | • SI-3 - SI treats Bladder, Shu-stream point<br>• KID-7 (77.28) - Kidney treats Bladder (System 3)<br>• 22.04 Da Bai+22.05 Ling Gu - LI treats Kid (System 4).<br>• BL-58 - Luo-connecting point. Treats own meridian.<br>• BL-23, BL-25 (local treatment)<br>• SI-6 - SI treats Bladder, Xi-cleft point<br>• 77.03+77.04 - Treats own meridian. Tendon treats tendon<br>• 33.12 Xin Men - SI treats Bladder, Holographic correspondence.<br>• 1010.13 Ma Jin Shui - Along SI channel which treats BL channel. |
| **Large intestine sinew channel**<br>Hand Yangming | • 22.04 Da Bai+22.05 Ling Gu - Treats own sinew meridian<br>• LI-10 - Treats own sinew meridian.<br>• Gu YI Er San – along the LI meridian |
| **Kidney Internal Pathway (along the spine)**<br>Foot Shao Yin | • 22.04 Da Bai+22.05 Ling Gu - LI treats Kidney (System 4)<br>• KI-7 -Treats own pathway.<br>• SJ-6, SJ-3  - SJ treats Kidney (System 2)<br>• A.02 San Cha Yi - LI treats Kidney (System 4)<br>• EX-UE-7 YAOTONGDIAN - SJ treats Kid (System 2). Empirical point. |
| **Gall Bladder Sinew Channel**<br>Foot Shaoyang | • EX-UE-7 YAOTONGDIAN - SJ treats GB (System 1).  Empirical point.<br>• GB-41 (66.09 Shui Qu) - Treats own meridian<br>• 66.04 Huo Zhu - Liver governs the sinews. LV treats GB (Sys 3) |

## Cupping/Blood-letting Treatment for Low Back Pain
- Visible veins on the legs, especially the BL-40 region
- Cup the lumbar/sacral area.
- Palpate the low back and wet-cup any points that are very tender to palpation
- Prick to bleed any versicle around DU-28
- Bleed EX-HN-6 ERJIAN (Ear Apex) – Along Bladder meridian

# Treatment by Holographic Correspondence for Low Back Pain

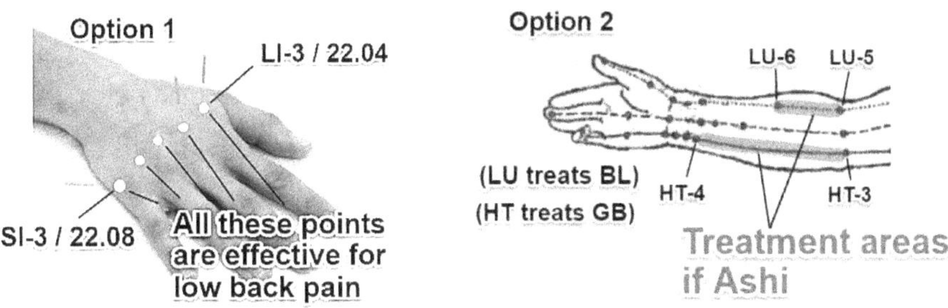


*Points Illustrations for treatment of Low Back Pain*

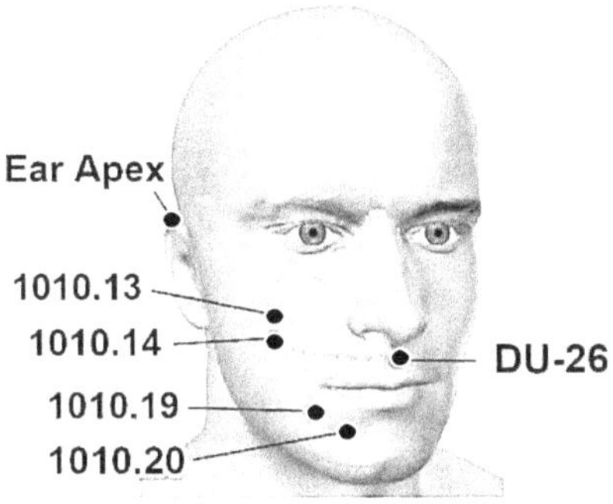

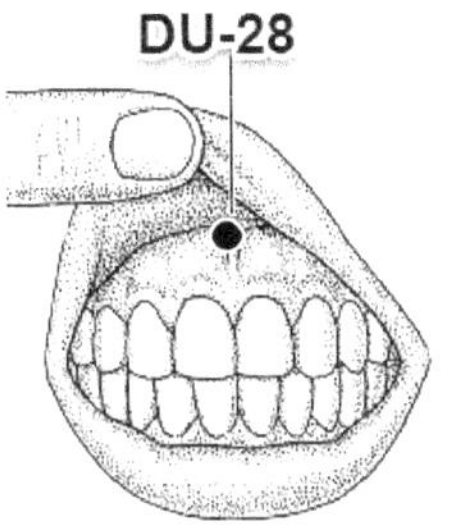

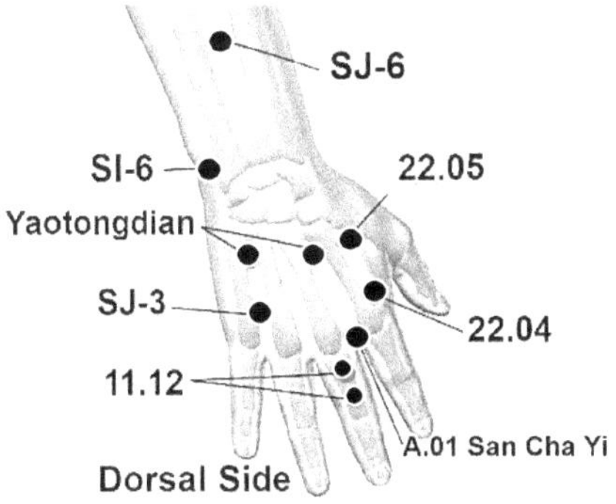

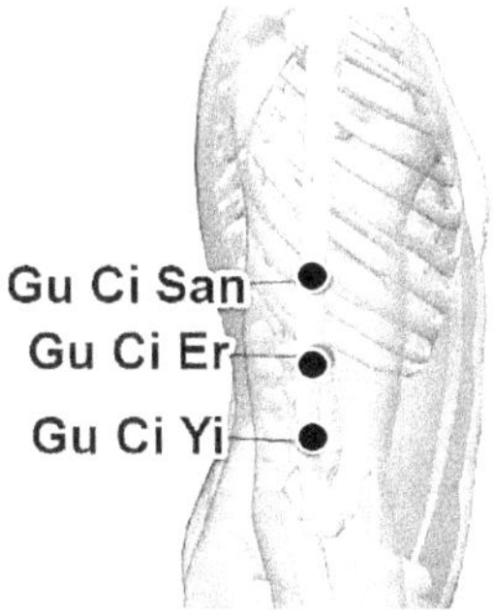

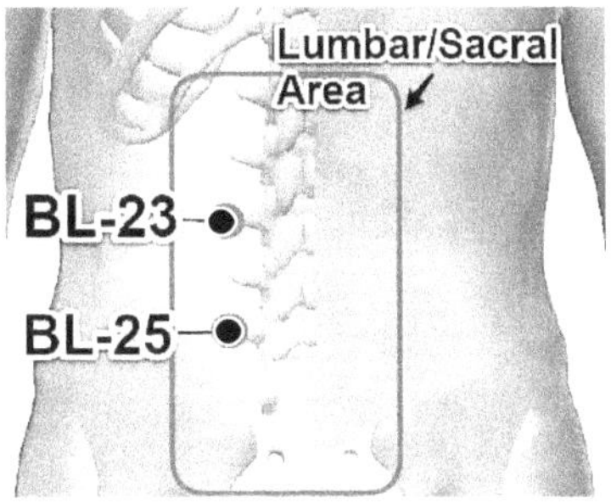

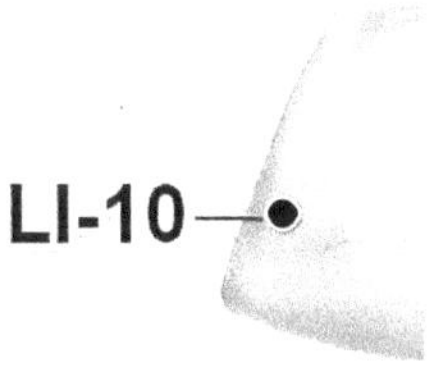

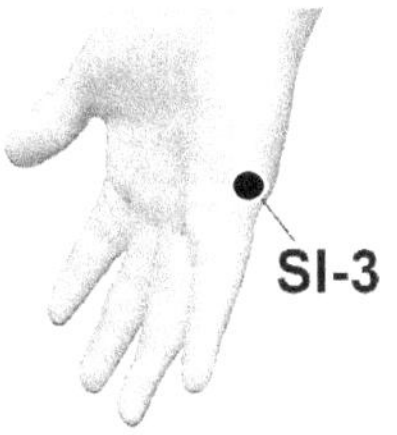

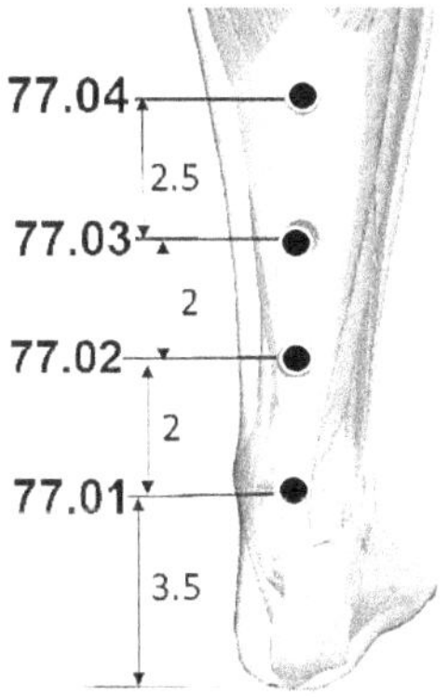

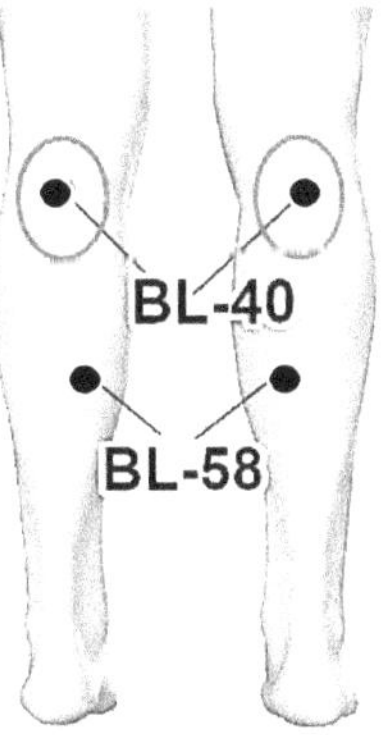

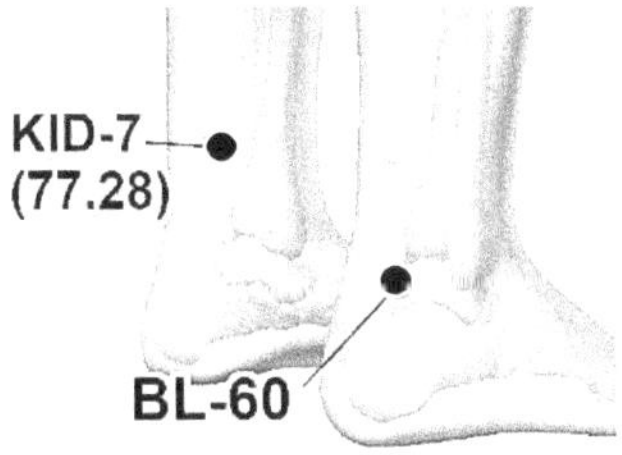

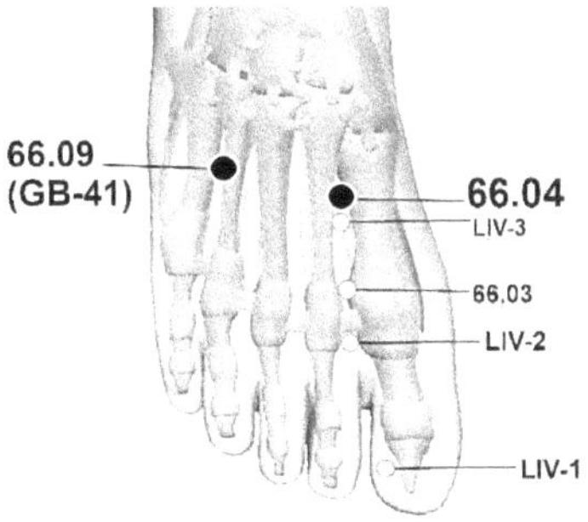

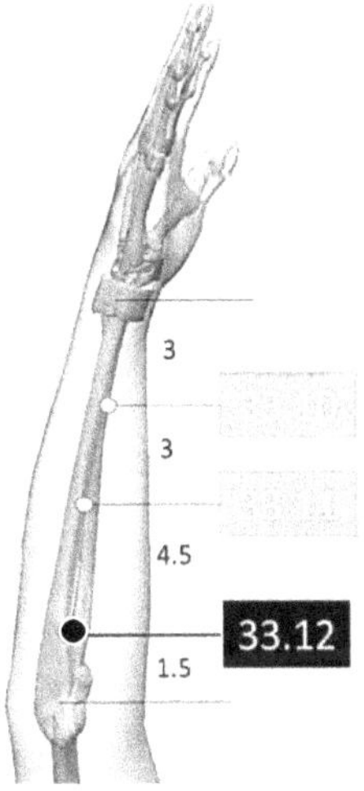

# Sacral/Coccyx Pain

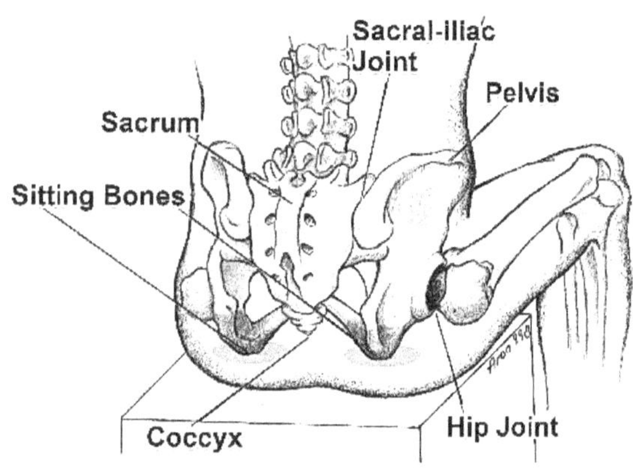



*Your coccyx is made up of three to five fused vertebrae (bones). It lies beneath the sacrum, a bone structure at the base of your spine. Several tendons, muscles and ligaments connect to it. Both the coccyx and the ischial tuberosities (two bones that make up the bottom of your pelvis) bear your weight when you sit down.*

*Pain in the coccyx area may be attributed to a blockage or imbalance of energy along the **Du Meridian**, which can be caused by various factors such as trauma, prolonged sitting, and emotional stress.*

*Other related meridians that may be involved in coccyx pain include the **Bladder Meridian** and the **Kidney Meridian**.*

*Tailbone pain ranges from a dull ache to a fierce stab. It can last for weeks, months or sometimes longer.*

## Image of Scalp to the Spine

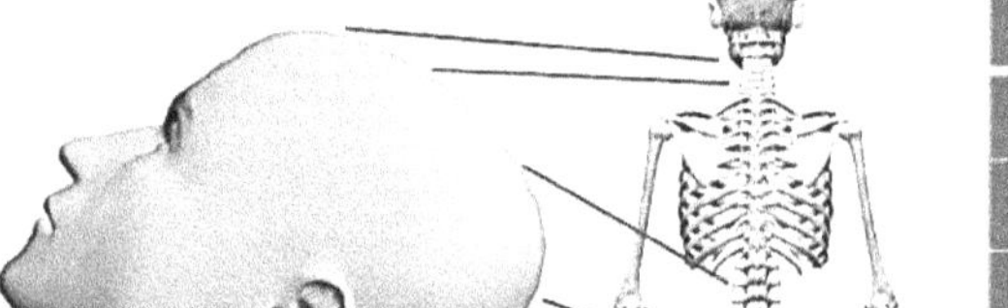

| Hairline | C-1, C-2 |
| --- | --- |
| Du 24-22 | C3-C5 |
| Du 22-20 | Thoracic vertebra |
| Du 20 | Lumbar 2 (waist level) |
| Du 19 | L2-L5 |
| Du 18-16 | Sacral area |
| Du 16 | Tailbone |

**Treatment for Tailbone pain**

- Unilaterally or bilaterally needle 33.12 Xin Men (SI treats Bladder (System 1))
- Needle 1010.01 Zheng Hui (DU-20) - images around Lumbar 2 area, see above chart.
- 1010.06 Hou Hui (DU-19 • Hou Ding) to 1010.25 – images sacral to coccyx, see above.
- Bilaterally needle 66.01 Hai Bao and SP-2 (Toe images the coccyx and genital area.)
- 11.11 + 11.12 (dorsal middle finger images the spine)
- 77.01 Zheng Jin+77.02 Zheng Zong, 77.03 Zheng Shi, 77.04 Bo Qiu
- Bilaterally needle 55.04 Hua Gu San+55.05 Hua Gu Si (see below for image correspondence)
- A.02 San Cha Yi, A.03 San Cha Er, A.04 San Cha San, 22.05 Ling Gu, SI-4 – pain at piriformis, sacrum, coccyx, ischial tuberority pain (sit bone pain)
- DU-26 - Treats own meridian. Head treats tail.
- Bilateral BL-60. Treats Bladder meridian
- If the sacral pain is related to prolapse of urinary bladder, uterine, hemorrhoid, etc., needle DU-19 and DU-21 combined, through DU-20. Can moxa DU-20. Can cup over pain area but not over a fresh trauma.
- GB-30

## Blood-letting for Coccyx pain

- Visible veins in the leg esp. around BL-40

*Points Illustrations for treatment of Sacral/Coccyx pain*

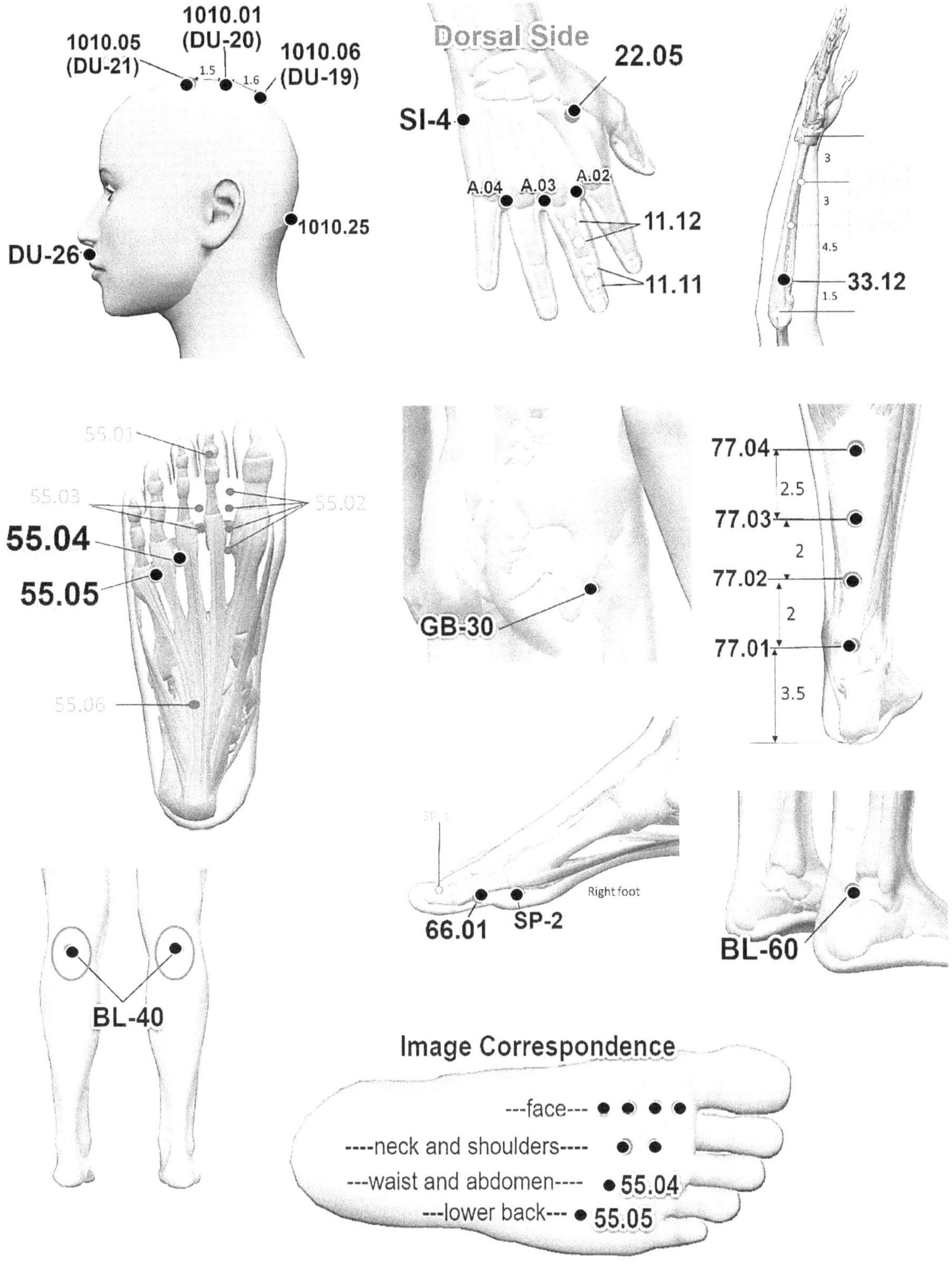

# Spine Pain

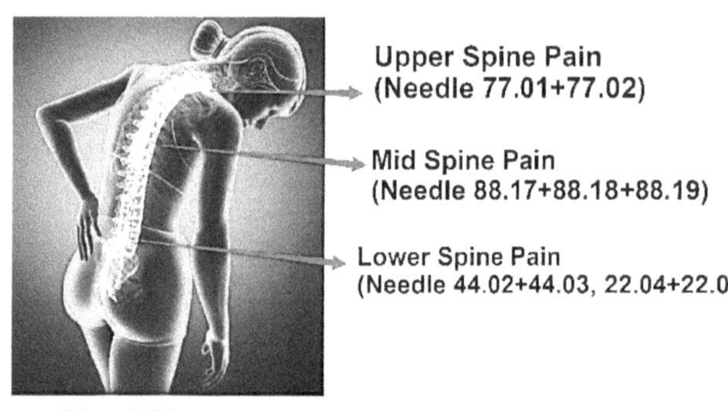


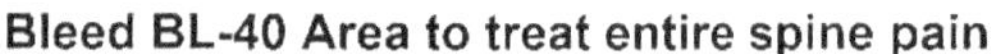

Bleed BL-40 Area to treat entire spine pain

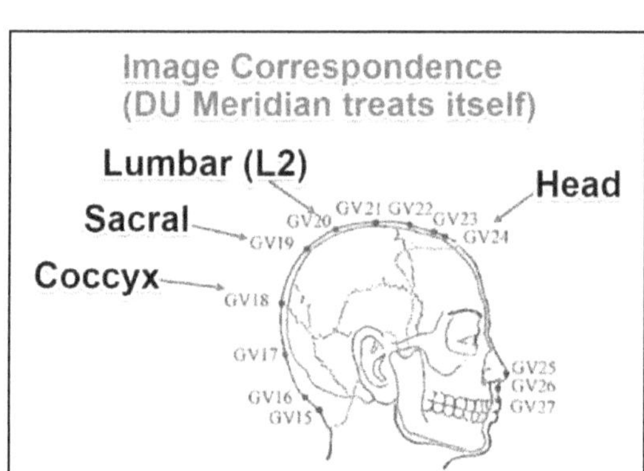


**Affected Meridians: Bladder, Gallbladder, Kidney, Governing (DU)**

**Treatment for Spine Pain:**
- 44.02 Hou Zhui + 44.03 Shou Ying. SJ treats KD (System 2)
- 77.01 Zheng Jin+77.02 Zheng Zong (every vertebra in pain)
- SI-3 opens the DU Channel. Add DU-26
- BL-60 and BL-65. Treat Bladder Meridian.
- 1010.01 Zheng Hui (DU-20), 1010.06 Hou Hui (DU-19), 1010.25 (see above for image correspondence)
- 11.11 Fei Xin, 11.12 Er Jiao Ming - back of the middle finger corresponds to the spine
- 88.25 Zhong Jiu Li ( GB-31) , 88.26 Shang Jiu Li+88.27 Xia Jiu Li

**Spinal cord injury**
- Huatuojiaji (Ex.21.) or Ex-B-2 points, the pair of points for stimulation should be one above and one below the site of injury
- Treat for affected area paralysis.

**Combine with**
- 22.04 Da Bai+22.05 Ling Gu for lumbar spine
- 88.17 Si Ma Zhong+88.18 Si Ma Shang+88.19 Si Ma Xia for thoracic spine
- 77.01 Zheng Jin+77.02 Zheng Zong for cervical spine

## Cupping/Blood-letting Treatment
- For back spasms due to problematic discs, cupping therapy can provide relief. Avoid cupping directly over a protruding or herniated disc.
- Palpate gently all along the paraspinals and wet-cup (bleed cup) wherever tender.
- Bleed around BL-40 to treat the entire spine.
- Spinal pain (thoracic) - bleed SP-1 followed by needling 22.05 Ling Gu, SP-3, DU-26

*Points Illustrations for treatment of Spine Pain*

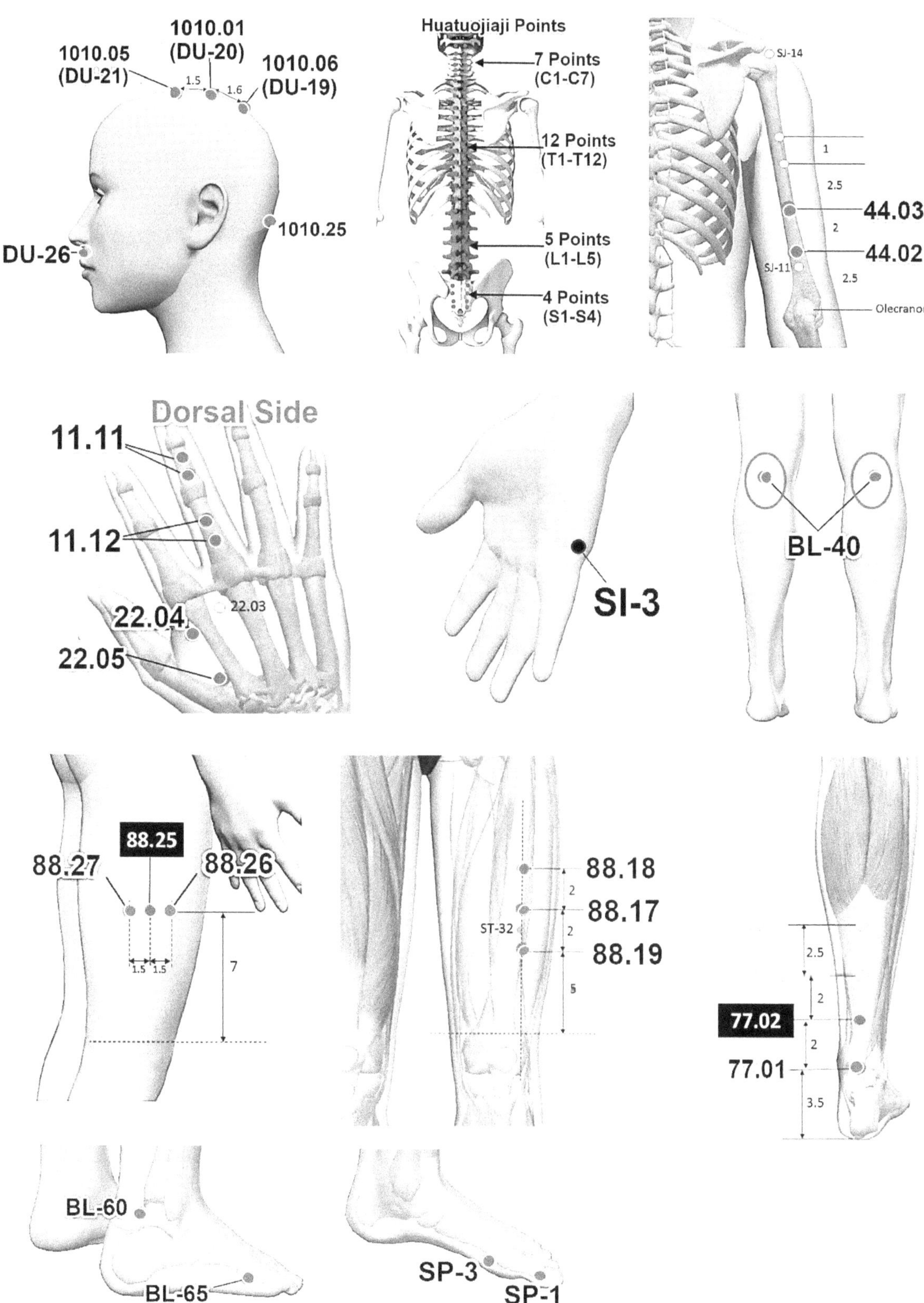

# Ankylosing Spondylitis

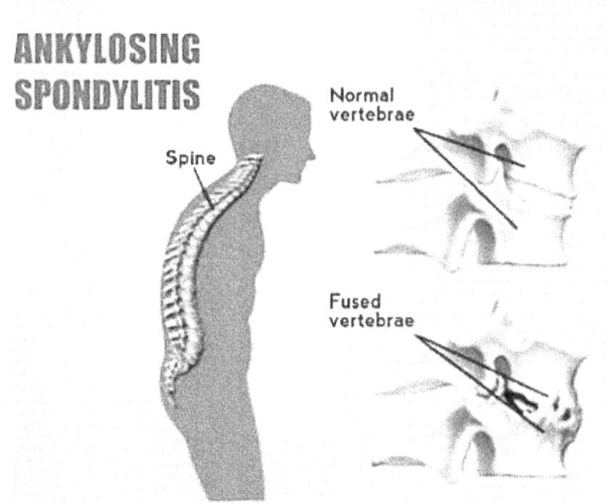


*Ankylosing spondylitis: Ankylosing spondylitis is a condition that causes the fusion of the entire spinal column.*

*The slow calcification of the spine gradually causes a bending forward*
*which results in the patient looking only at the ground when walking.*

**Affected Meridians: Bladder, Gallbladder, Kidney, Governing (DU), Liver**

**Treatment options**
- 77.01 Zheng Jin+77.02 Zheng Zong
- Bilaterally needle 88.12 Ming Huang.
- Bilaterally needle 77.08 Si Hua Shang+77.09 Si Hua Zhong, 22.06 Zhong Bai, SI-3
- 1010.13 Ma Jin Shui + 1010.14
- Bilaterally needle 88.25 Zhong Jiu Li+88.26 Shang Jiu Li+88.27 Xia Jiu Li, SI-3.
- Bilaterally 77.09 Si Hua Zhong, 77.10 Si Hua Fu.
- Bilaterally needle 77.18 Shen Guan, 77.28 Guang Ming (KI-7) and BL-65 or BL-60 (if there is Kidney deficiency).
- Needle DU-26; bilaterally needle LI-11
- Moxa BL-18, BL-19, BL-20
- Bilaterally needle 11.11 Fei Xin, 11.12 Er Jiao Ming
- Needle Huatuojiaji points of corresponding area

---

### Blood-letting Treatment
- A recommended method to promote better blood flow and prevent calcification is to perform bleed cupping between vertebrae on the spine.
- Bleed BL-40
- Gua sha Huatuojiaji points. Start gently and assess effectiveness. Continue with more pressure if positive outcome.

*Points Illustrations for treatment of Ankylosing Spondylitis*

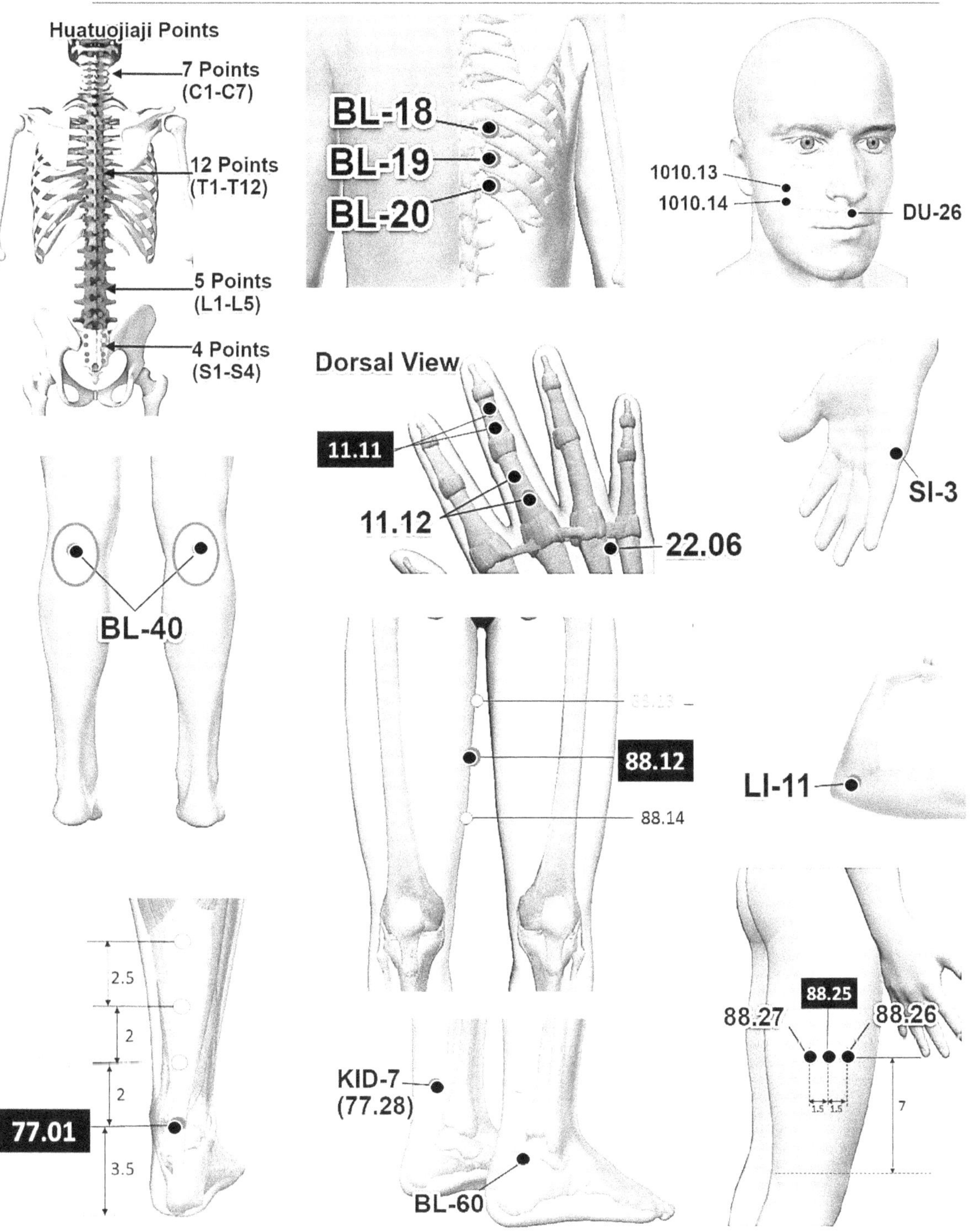

# Scoliosis

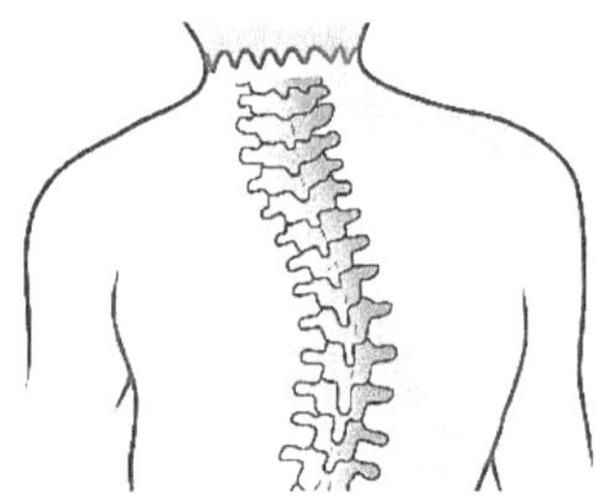

*According to TCM theory, scoliosis can be caused by a variety of factors, including:*

***Kidney deficiency*** *- In TCM, the kidneys are considered the root of vitality and are responsible for nourishing the bones. If there is a deficiency in kidney energy, it can lead to weakness and deformities in the bones, including scoliosis.*

***Liver Qi stagnation*** *- If there is stagnation of liver Qi, it can lead to tension and imbalance in the muscles of the back, which can contribute to scoliosis.*

*Blood stasis - If there is stagnation of blood in the back, it can contribute to the development of scoliosis.*

**Needle/Moxa**

- Bilaterally needle 88.12 Ming Huang+88.13 Tian Huang+88.14 Qi Huang
- Add DU-26, LI-11
- BL-60 + BL-65 bilateral
- Needle/moxa, gua sha Huatuojiaji points of corresponding area
- Refer to Spine Pain on Page 100 for additional treatment points.

Alternatively
- Needle SI-3, BL-65, 88.25 Zhong Jiu Li (GB-31) and DU-26 (Dr. Young's bone spur treatment).

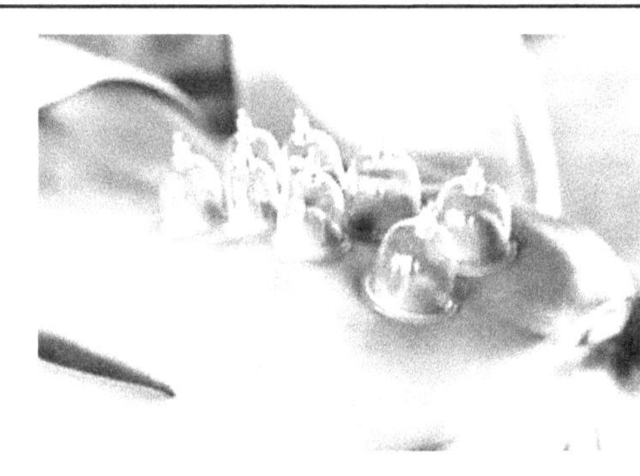

## Cupping/Blood-letting Treatment

- First relax all the muscles and movable joints along the spine with cupping, then moxa BL-18 and BL-20 (Liver and Spleen Shu Points)
- Bleed the spine and/or BL-40

*Points Illustrations for treatment of Scoliosis*

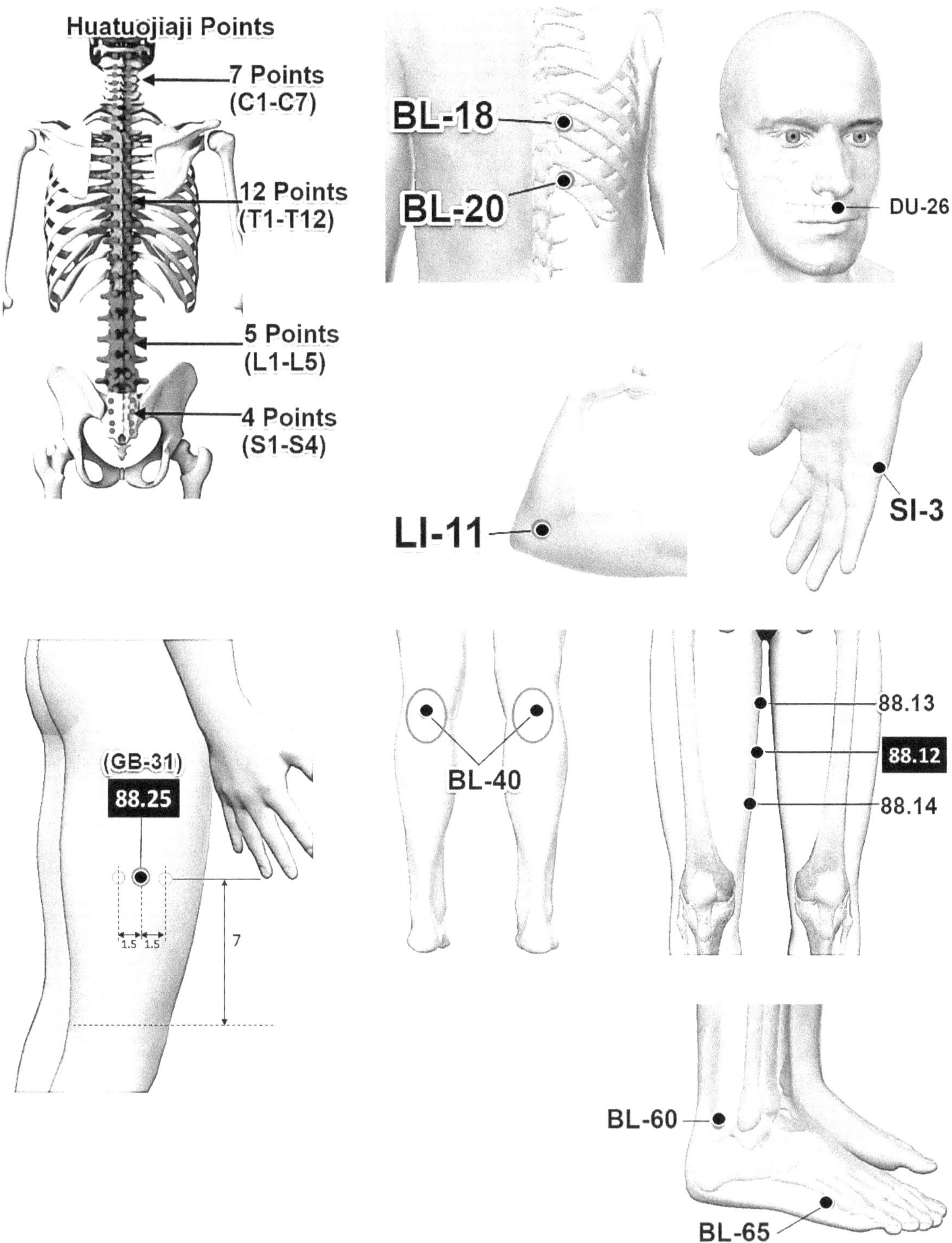

# ARTHRITIS

## Gout

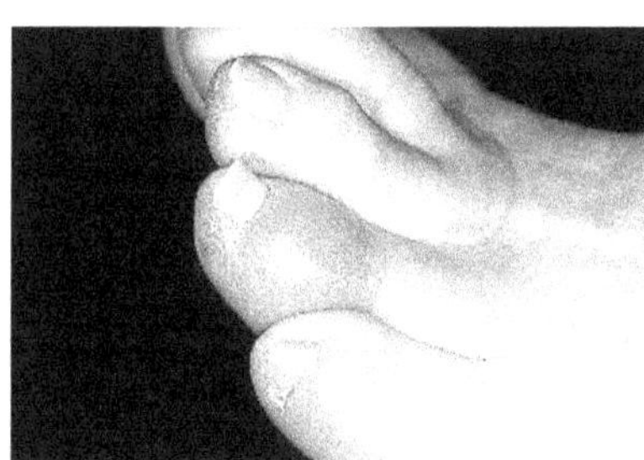

*Gout usually occurs in older men due to high stress and excess consumption of meat and alcohol. The following foods need to be avoided: mushrooms, shrimp, peanuts, internal organs, asparagus, beets, oranges, strawberries, sour fruits, and fructose (especially high fructose corn syrup). Foods that treat gout include: cherry juice, watermelon juice and celery seeds.*

*According to TCM theory, there are several meridians that may be involved in gout. These include:*

***Liver meridian:*** *The liver meridian is responsible for regulating the flow of Qi and blood throughout the body. Imbalances in this meridian may lead to a buildup of toxins and impurities in the blood, which can contribute to the development of gout.*

***Kidney meridian:*** *The kidney meridian is responsible for regulating the flow of Qi and blood through the kidneys, which play a crucial role in filtering toxins and waste products from the body. Imbalances in this meridian may contribute to the buildup of uric acid crystals in the joints.*

***Spleen meridian:*** *The spleen meridian is responsible for regulating the flow of Qi and blood through the digestive system, and plays a key role in the metabolism of nutrients and waste products. Imbalances in this meridian may contribute to the development of gout by affecting the body's ability to eliminate uric acid.*

***Urinary Bladder meridian:*** *The urinary bladder meridian is responsible for regulating the flow of Qi and fluids through the urinary system. Imbalances in this meridian may contribute to the buildup of uric acid crystals in the joints.*

### Treatment

- Needle opposite side 11.27 Wu Hu #3, #4, #5
- Followed by deep needle 77.08 Si Hua Shang (ST-36) on the same side – reduces uric acid. Needle up to 60mm, lifting the needle 50% every 10 minutes to disperse heat.
- Mu Guan and Gu Guan
- Gua sha around BL-18, BL-20, BL-22 and BL-23 (improve metabolism)
- Add 66.11 Huo Ju contralateral to relieve pain.
- LIV-2 (66.03), LIV-3 (66.04), LIV-4, LIV-6, ST-44 – local treatment
- 22.04 Da Bai+22.05 Ling Gu, 22.08 Wan Shun Yi+22.09 Wan Shun Er - for pain relief
- 33.08 Shou Wu Jin and 33.09 Shou Qian Jin - regulate substances in the blood vessels such as cholesterol, uric acid and inflammation markers

### Alternate treatment:

- Needle opposite-side 88.25 Zhong Jiu Li (GB-31);
- 77.18 Shen Guan (Kidney Gate) reduces uric acid.
- If chronic - add SP-4, SP-6

---

### Blood-letting for Gout
- Local wet-cupping as close to the center of the pain as possible.
- Bleed related Jing Well Point

---

*Points Illustrations for treatment of Gout*

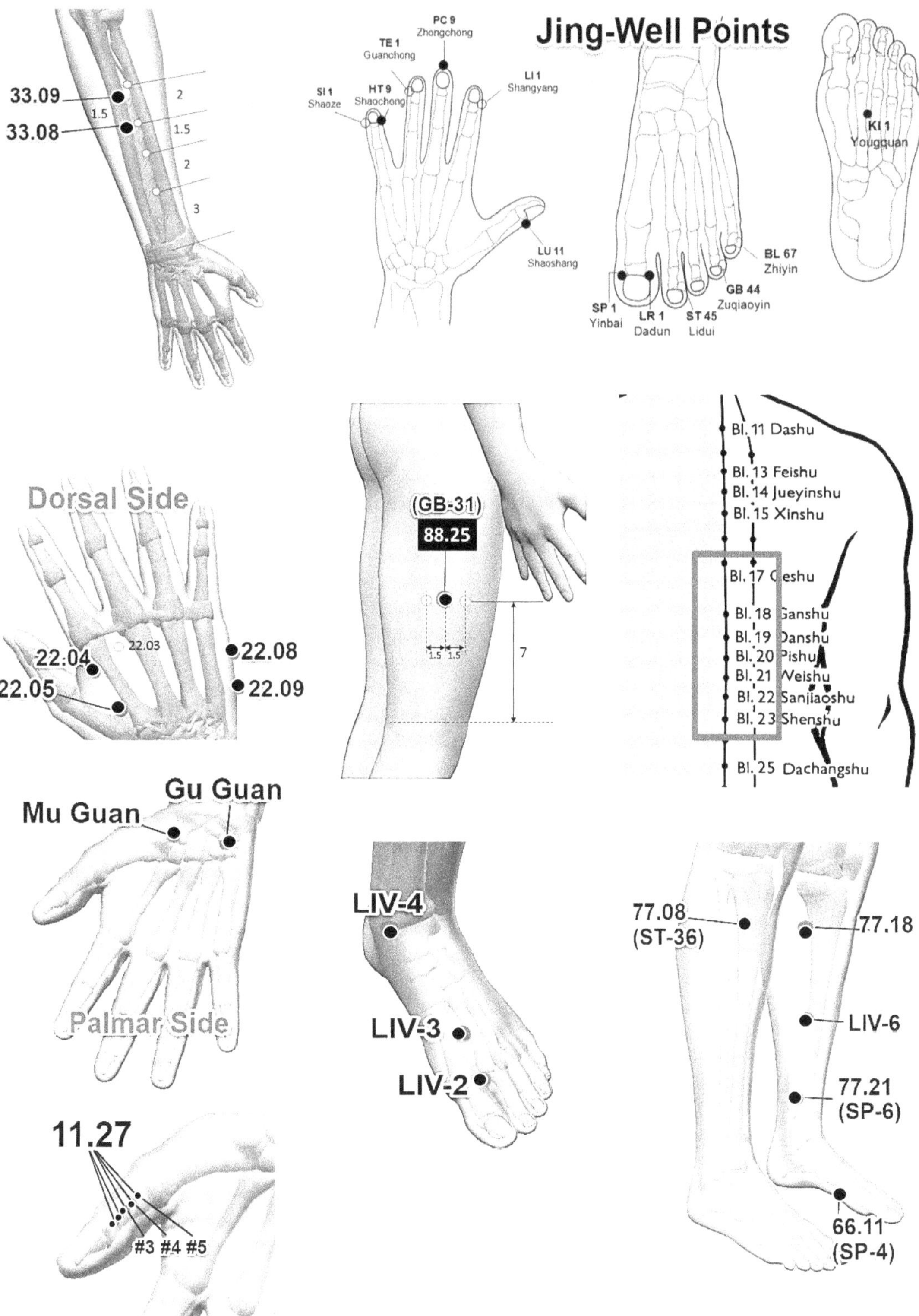

# Rheumatoid arthritis (RA)

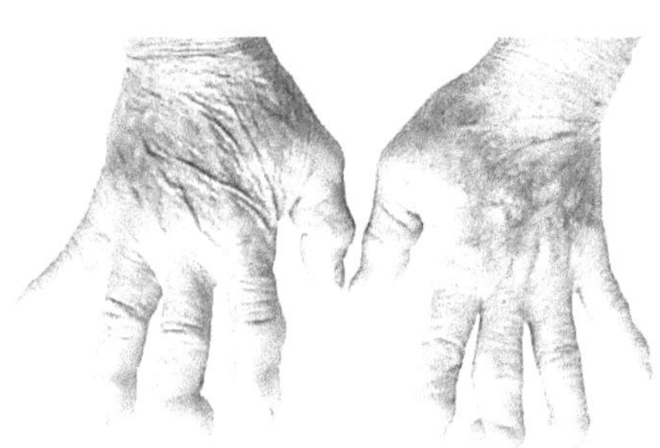

*Rheumatoid arthritis (RA) is a chronic autoimmune disorder that affects the joints, causing pain, inflammation, and stiffness.*

*Affected meridians are:*
*Imbalances in the **Lung meridian** may contribute to RA symptoms in the hands, wrists, and fingers. Imbalances in the **Large Intestine meridian** may contribute to the accumulation of toxins in the body, leading to inflammation and joint damage in RA. Imbalances in the **Spleen meridian** may contribute to the accumulation of dampness and phlegm in the body, leading to joint swelling and stiffness in RA. Imbalances in the **Liver meridian** contribute to the development of RA by causing blood stagnation and inflammation in the joints.*

*Treatment seeks to eliminate the pathogenic influences of cold, damp, and wind and enhances the body's resistance. Because primarily a deficiency is involved, the treatment is based on activation of the Qi by means of moxibustion at tonification points. Needling and moxibustion of general and specific tonification points are carried out daily.*

## Treatment

When a patient has one or two painful joints in the extremities, treat the affected joints. However, if multiple joints are affected, treat for stagnation of qi and blood due to a deficiency or buildup of phlegm.

- 88.01 Tong Guan+88.02 Tong Shan+88.03 Tong Tian (between the Stomach and Spleen meridians). These are the primary points used to treat rheumatoid arthritis. The points' reaction area is the heart, hence have an effect of improving blood circulation.
- Bilateral 33.12 Xin Men (Heart reaction area)
- 11.27 Wu Hu #1, #3, #5 - osteoarthritis, systemic pain and bone swelling.
- 33.08 Shou Wu Jin+33.09 Shou Qian, 66.08 Liu Wan+66.09 Shui Qu - moves blood
- 77.18 Shen Guan+77.19 Di Huang+77.21 Ren Huang
- 88.25 Zhong Jiu Li (GB-31)
- Difficulty opening and closing the hands, sedate or bleed 33.16 Qu Ling (LU-5) on the same side, and then needle 22.01 Chong Zi+22.02 Chong Xian on the opposite side.
- For joint pain in the fingers, and wrist - needle SJ-5.
- Needle Baxie to treat interphalangeal disorders (Rheumatoid Arthritis)

## Moxibustion

- Direct moxibustion is an effective treatment for joint nodules, but proceed with caution. Some patients may have inflammatory rheumatoid arthritis that could aggravate with moxibustion.
- Moxibustion of tonification points: REN-6, REN-8, REN-12, BL-20, BL-22, BL-23, DU-4, DU-13, DU-14, ST-36, KID-7, SP-6.

---

### Blood-letting Treatment

- Cupping of DT.01 Fen Zhi Shang+DT.02 Fen Zhi Xia Toxin Areas.
- Bleeding 11.16 Huo Xi is very effective for rheumatoid arthritis (phlegm) with deformed joints, especially in the hands.
- Bleed 77.14 (ST-40) to reduce phlegm
- BL-43 - arthritic pain
- 99.08 Er San (Ear Apex)
- Taiyang [Ex.2.]. or Ex-HN-5
- Bleed cup BL-40 or surrounding visible veins.
- Wet cup ashi points around the problem joints

*Points Illustrations for treatment of Rheumatoid Arthritis*

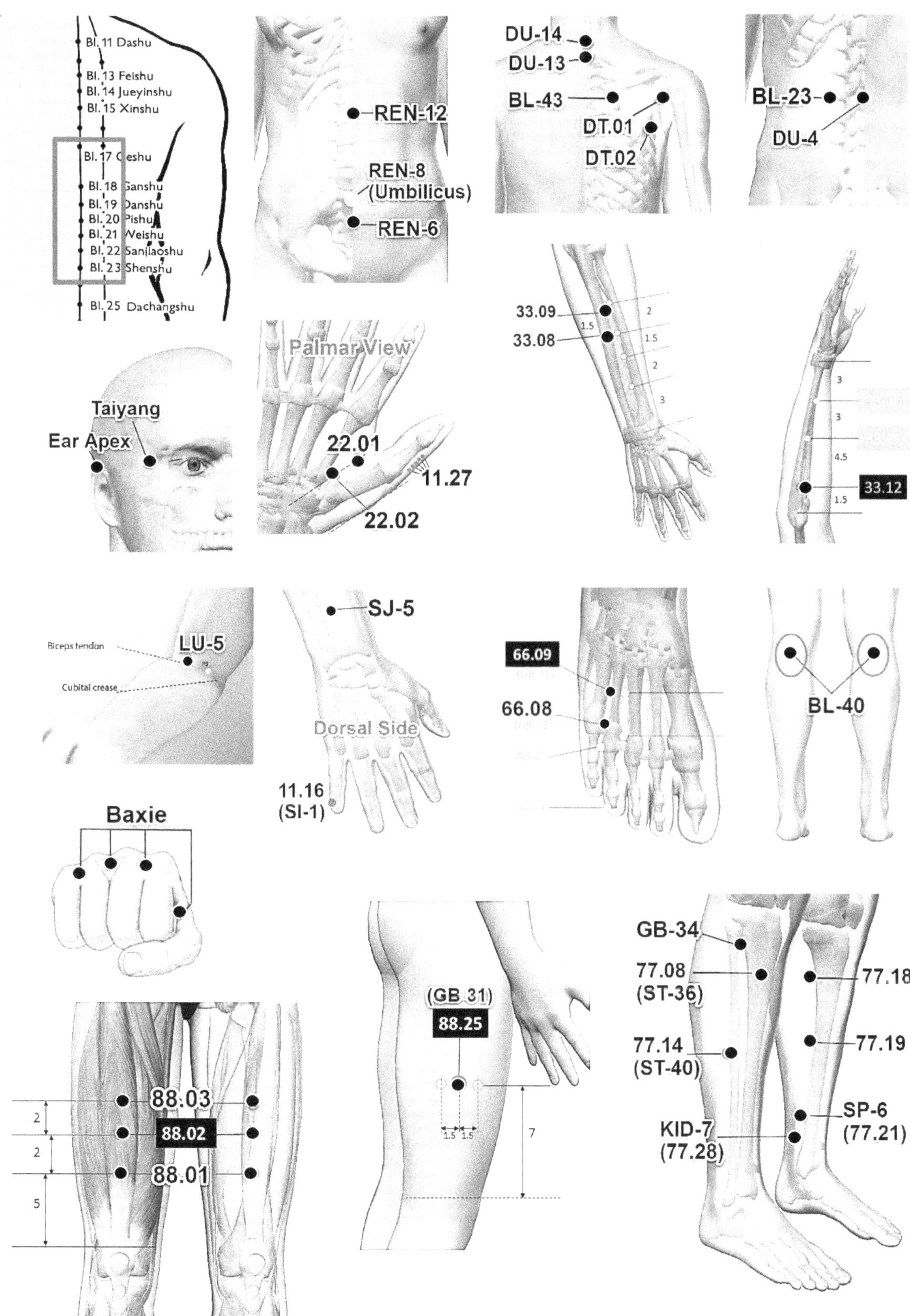

# Bone Spurs and Bone Inflammation

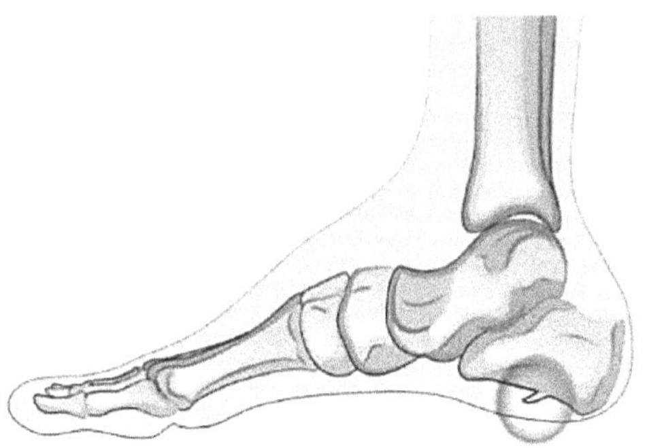

*Bone spurs are bony projections that develop along bone edges.*

*According to TCM theory, bone spurs are caused by the accumulation of Qi stagnation and blood stasis in the affected area. This can result in the formation of calcified deposits or "spurs" on the bone, which can cause pain, inflammation, and reduced range of motion.*

*Bone spurs are also caused by the accumulation of "pathogenic dampness" in the affected area, which leads to the formation of excess bone tissue. This accumulation of dampness can be caused by a variety of factors, including poor diet, overuse or injury of the affected area, and chronic stress.*

*The meridian most commonly associated with bone spurs in TCM is the **Kidney meridian.***

**Bone spur protocol**

- Bilateral SI-3, 22.08, 22.09 – general spurs
- 88.25 (GB-31) + 88.26 + 88.27 – general spurs
- BL-65 – lumbar spurs
- DU-26, REN-24 - if spurs are cervical
- 77.05 Yi Zhong+77.06 Er Zhong+77.07 San Zhong
- 88.12 Ming Huang+88.13 Tian Huang+88.14 Qi Huang – lumbar spurs
- 11.27, Mu Guan and Gu Guan – heel spurs
- Add 77.08 Si Hua Shang+77.09 Si Hua Zhong, 77.11 Si Hua Xia combined with 77.12 Fu Chang These are points on the Stomach Meridians (Earth) which are effective to control Kidney (Water).

All of the points described above must be needled close to the bone to activate the "bone-treating-bone" correspondence. However, when bleeding, never touch the bone with the tip of a bleeding needle; instead bleed the veins nearby. A course of ten treatments might be required to notice a reduction in symptoms.

---

### Blood-letting Treatment

- Bleed locally.
- Bleeding BL-40 is essential in the treatment of bone spurs. BL-40 reduces blood stagnation.
- Bleed DT.05 Shuang Feng
- Bleed visible veins on lateral leg especially around 77.10

*Points Illustrations for treatment of Bone Spurs
and Bone Inflammation*

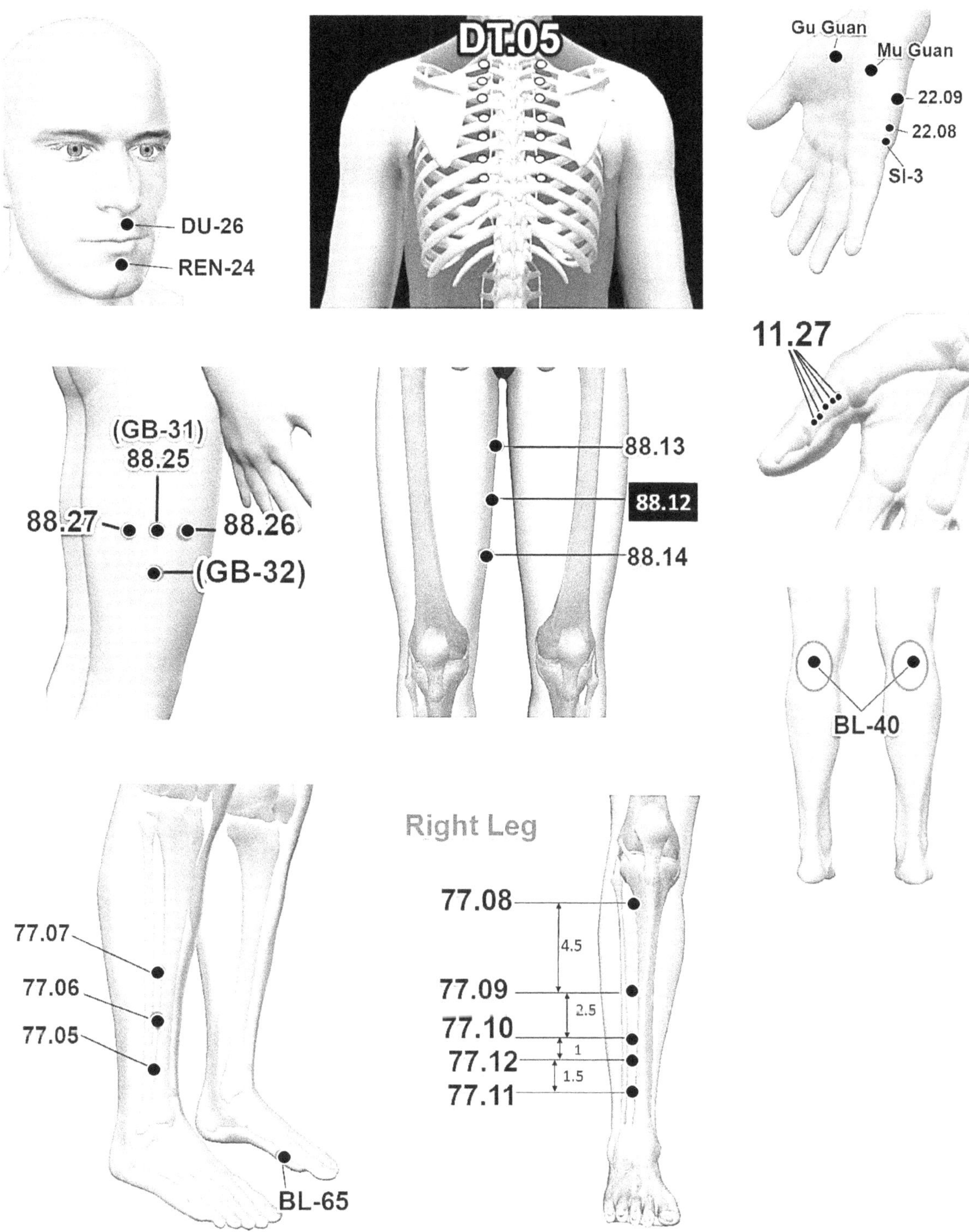

# CHEST AND ABDOMEN

## Chest Pain

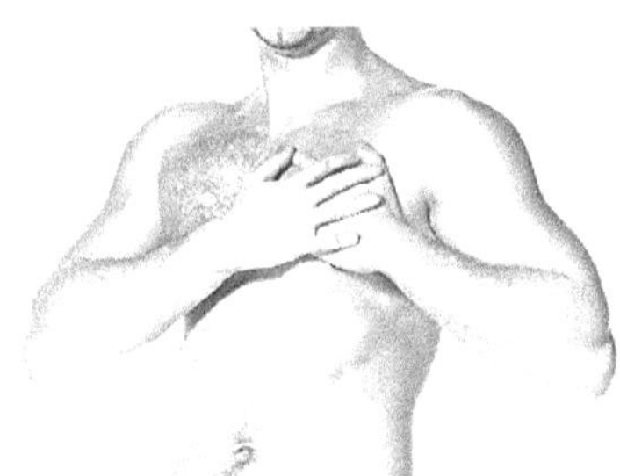

*Chest pain is often related to the lungs and heart. The etiologies of chest pain are qi stagnated in the chest, phlegm obstructed in the lung or blood stasis in collaterals of the heart.*

**Affected (sick) meridians: Pericardium, Lung**

**Chest Pain/Contusion**

- 88.17 Si Ma Zhong+88.18 Si Ma Shang+88.19 Si Ma Xia for pain on the side.  Needle healthy side. Reaction area of the Lung
- 88.01 Tong Guan+88.02 Tong Shan+88.03 Tong Tian for pain in the middle of the chest, possibly heart related. Stomach treats Pericardium (System 2). Reaction area of the Heart.
- P-6 for pain abdomen to chest. Luo-connecting of Pericardium Meridian.
- 22.01 Chong Zi and 22.02 Chong Xian for lung related chest pain
- 33.04 Huo Chuan + 33.05 Huo Ling + 33.06 Huo Shan
- If acute, add 88.28 Jie (ST-34), the Xi-Cleft Point that regulates qi and blood.
- LU-10 (bilateral) - Treats its own (lung) pathway. Chest pain due to lung disorders.
- P-6, St-36 (77.08), SP-4 (66.11), REN-12 -disorders of the chest, heart and stomach
- Corresponding Huatuojiaji Points – back treats the front
- BL-15 – back treats front.

**Chest pain involving the back**

Needle bilaterally or on the opposite side

- 88.17 Si Ma Zhong+88.18 Si Ma Shang+88.19 Si Ma Xia
- 77.18 Shen Guan
- 22.03 Shang Bai
- 22.01 Chong Zi-22.02 Chong Xian
- 22.06 Zhong Bai (treats pain around the back of the heart).

---

### Blood-letting for pain in the chest area

- Bleed 77.09 Si Hua Zhong+77.14 Si Hua Wai - ST treats Pericardium channel (System 2)
- Apex of the ear
- Visible veins in the leg, especially lateral leg
- Visible veins in the BL-40   region
- Visible veins anywhere else on the leg and thigh
- Bleed ST-45, GB-44 followed by needling SJ-6, P-6

*Points Illustrations for treatment of Chest Pain*

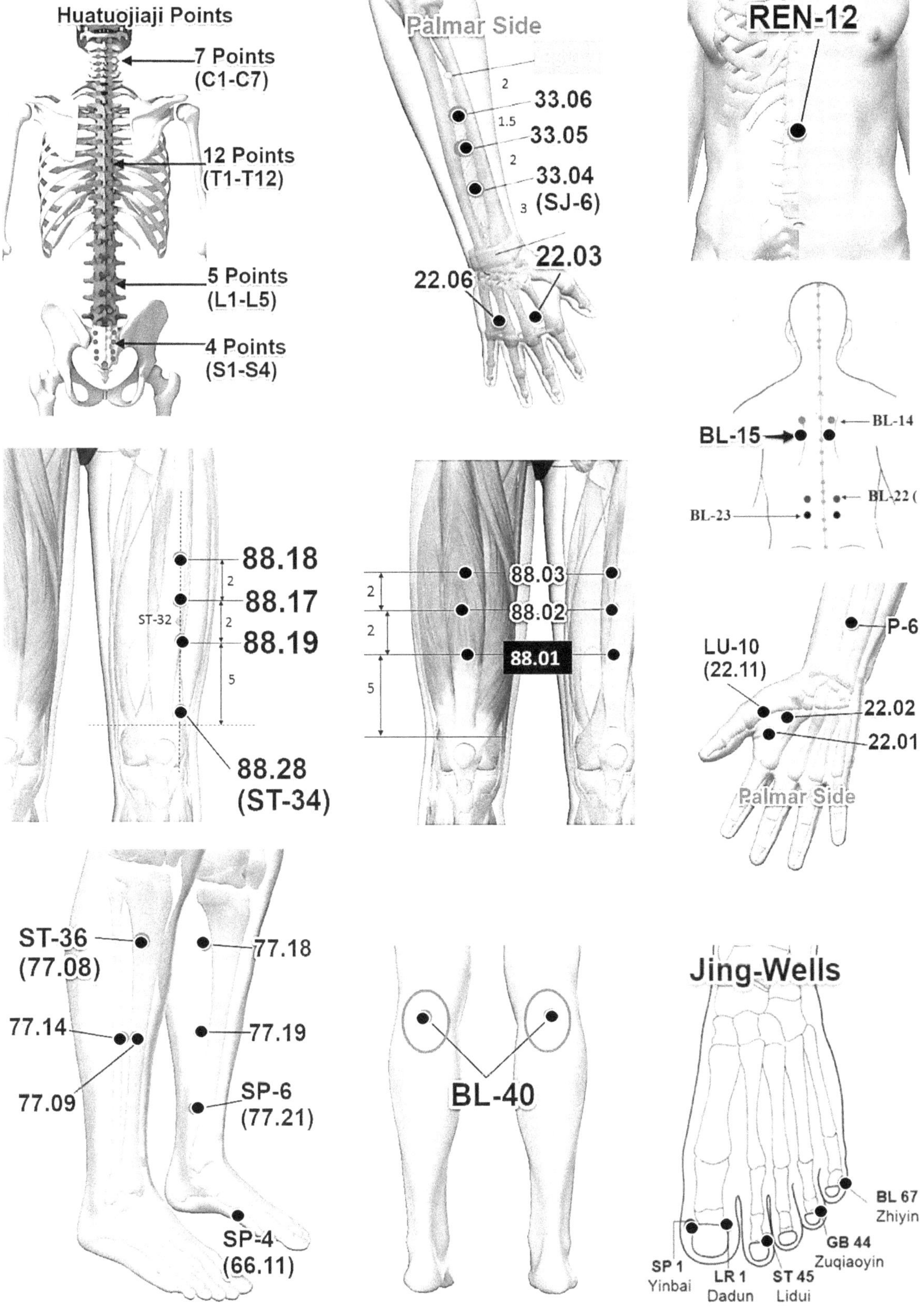

# Lower Abdominal Pain

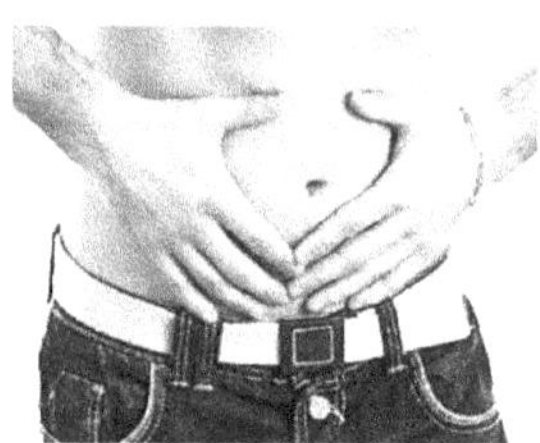

*Abdominal pain syndrome involves multiple organs and is a complicated syndrome. The pain can appear standing alone. It can also be caused by the organic or functional pathological changes of the abdominal organs and can be implicated in a variety of zangfu organs disorders. The pain can be caused by pathological changes stemming from organs external to the abdomen or systemic infection, endocrine and metabolic disorders, allergies, blood disorders and other systemic disorders.*

**Points for abdominal distension, gas and bloating, diarrhea, irritable bowel, and Crohn's disease:**
- 66.05 Men Jin (ST-43), 22.05 with SP-4 (66.11 Huo Ju)
- P-6, deep needling towards SJ-5
- ST-41, ST-44, ST-45 + SP-6+ ST-36

| AFFECTED (SICK) MERIDIANS | TREATMENT POINTS |
|---|---|
| **PERICARDIUM**<br>Hand Jue yin | • P-6 (towards SJ-5)- Luo-connecting point of Pericardium Meridian. Treats its own meridian and pathway which transverses the lower abdomen.<br>• SJ-5 - SJ treats Pericardium (System 3) |
| **STOMACH**<br>Foot Yangming | • ST-34 - Xi-Cleft point. Treats own meridian.<br>• 66.05 Men Jin - Shu-stream point on own stomach meridian.<br>• SP-4 (66.11 Huo Ju) - Spleen treats stomach (System 3) |
| **LARGE INTESTINE**<br>Hand Yang Ming | • Bleed/Moxa around 77.08 Si Hua Shang, 77.09 Si Hua Zhong and 77.14 Si Hua Wai - Stomach treats large intestine (System 1) |
| **SPLEEN**<br>Foot Tai Yin | • SP-6 (77.21). Meeting Point of the Spleen, Liver and Kidney Channels. Moxibustion applicable. |
| **LIVER**<br>Foot Jue Yin | • SP-6 (77.21 Ren Huang. Meeting Point of the Spleen Channel with the Liver and Kidney Channels |
| **KIDNEY**<br>Foot Shao Yin | • SP-6 (77.21 Ren Huang).<br>• KI-10 - He-sea point. Treats own meridian. |
| **REN** | • REN-12 - Alarm point [Mu-Front] of the Stomach that connects with Back Shu. Meeting point of SI, Sanjiao, Stomach and REN. Empirical point.<br>• Moxa around REN-4 and REN-8 over salt and ginger |
| **GALL BLADDER**<br>Foot Shao Yang | • Dannangxue (Ex.35.) or Ex-LE-6 Distal Alarm point of the GB Channel. |

## Blood-letting Treatment
- Bleed 77.08 Si Hua Shang+77.09 Si Hua Zhong + 77.10 Si Hua Fu and 77.14 Si Hua Wai
- Bleed 33.16 Qu Ling or LU-5 - severe case.
- Bleed P-3, BL-40 for acute abdominal pain

*Points Illustrations for treatment of Lower Abdominal Pain*

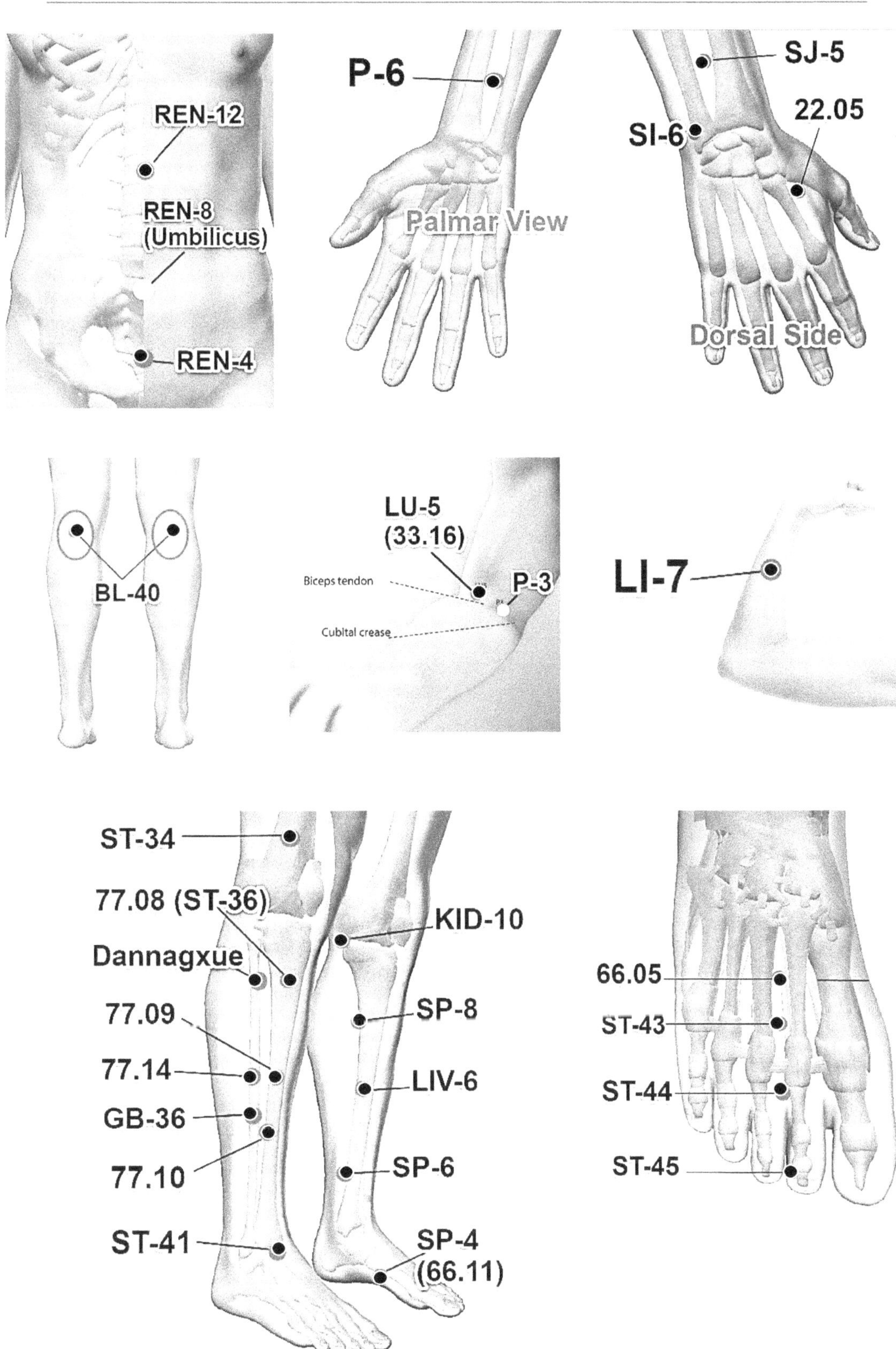

# Hypochondriac Pain

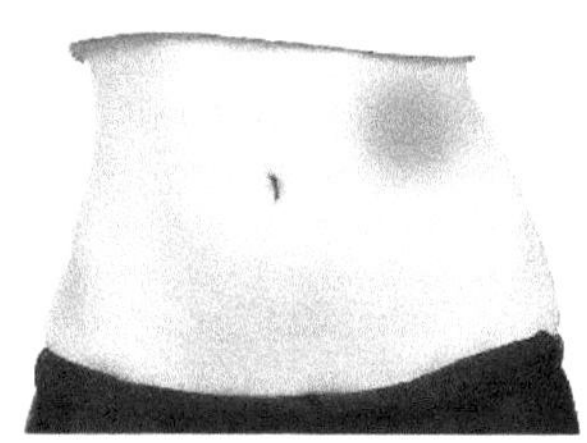

*Hypochondriac (rib) pain is a disorder characterized by pain over the unilateral or bilateral sides of the hypochondriac region. This pain is the result of disorders of the hypochondriac region and chest wall. The etiologies are contusion, strain or injury of the ribs or sift tissues and intercostal neuritis. Also there could be problems with the liver and gallbladder; acute and chronic hepatitis, cholecystitis, cholelithiasis, pleurisy and their after-effects.*

**Commonly used combination:**

- SJ-6, P-6, A.04 San Cha San, LU-10
- LIV-2, GB-34, GB-40, KID-6
- 11.27 Wu Hu contralateral, 77.27 Wai San Guan - rib fracture and ribs pain
- Huatuojiaji points of the affected region

| AFFECTED (SICK) MERIDIANS | TREATMENT POINTS |
|---|---|
| **GALLBLADDER** <br> Foot Shao Yang | • GB-34 (affected side) - Treats own meridian. (Add SJ-6, opposite side, SJ treats GB) <br> • GB-40 (needle towards KID-6) - Yuan source point. Treats own meridian. <br> • SJ-5 - SJ treats GB, System 1 <br> • A.04 San Cha San - SJ treats GB, System 1 |
| **LIVER** <br> Foot Jue Yin | • GB-34 - GB treats Liver (System 3) <br> • P-6 (towards SJ-5) - PC treats liver (System 1) <br> • LIV-2 - Treats own pathway. |
| **KIDNEY** <br> Foot Shao Yin | • KI-6 - Treats kidney pathway |
| **SPLEEN** <br> Foot Tai Yin | • LU-10 (22.11) - Lung treats Spleen (System 1) |

**Blood-letting Treatment**

- Bleed 77.09 Si Hua Zhong+77.14 Si Hua Wai
- Bleed  BL-18
- Gua sha BL-18, BL-19, BL-20

*Points Illustrations for treatment of Hypochondriac pain*

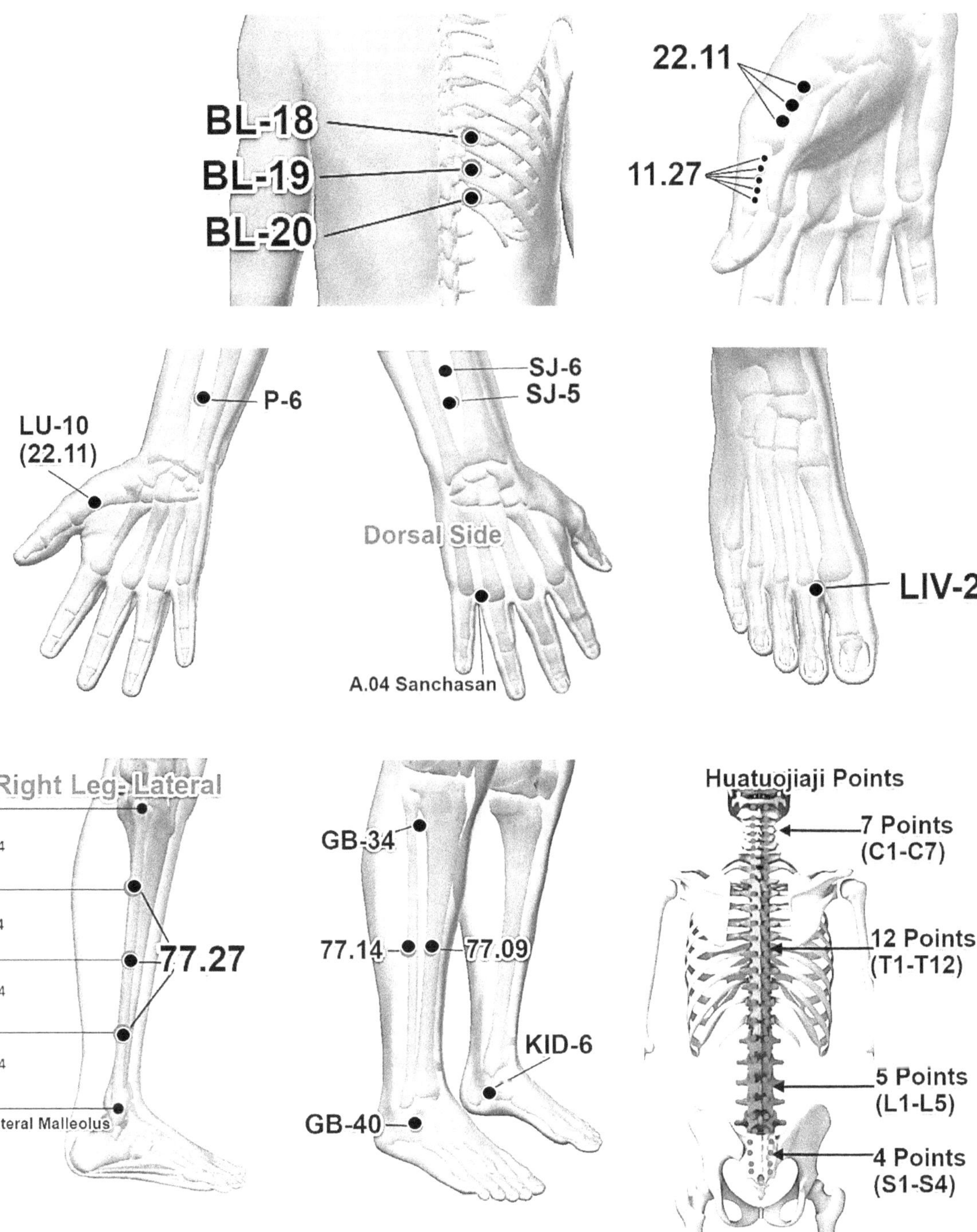

# CARDIOVASCULAR AND STROKE

## Varicose Veins

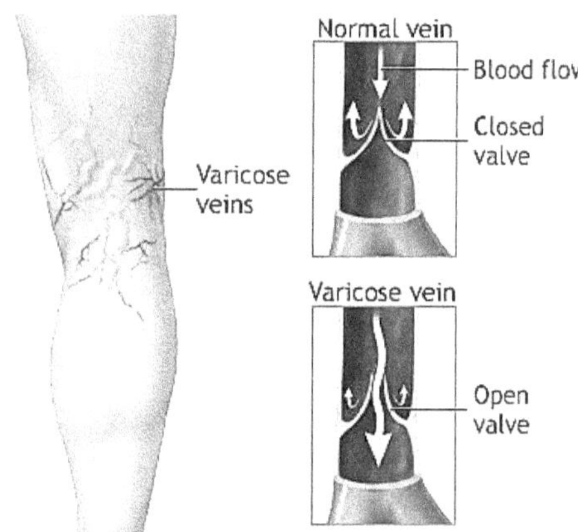


*Varicose veins are superficial veins that have become enlarged and twisted. Typically, they occur just under the skin in the legs. Usually, they result in few symptoms but some may experience fullness or pain in the area.*

*In TCM, varicose veins are believed to be related to an imbalance in the flow of Qi and blood through the meridians or energy channels in the body. The following meridians or channels may be involved in the development of varicose veins:*

***Liver meridian*** *- Any imbalances in the liver meridian can result in the accumulation of Qi and blood in the lower extremities, which can contribute to the development of varicose veins.*

***Spleen meridian*** *- The spleen meridian is also believed to play a role in the development of varicose veins. Any imbalances in this meridian can lead to the accumulation of blood and Qi in the lower extremities.*

***Kidney meridian*** *- The kidney meridian is associated with the regulation of water metabolism in the body, and any imbalances in this meridian can lead to the accumulation of water and the development of edema in the lower extremities.*

***Bladder meridian*** *- Any imbalances in this meridian can result in the accumulation of Qi and blood in the legs, which can contribute to the development of varicose veins.*

***Stomach meridian*** *- The stomach meridian is associated with the digestion of food and the absorption of nutrients, and any imbalances in this meridian can lead to the accumulation of dampness in the body. Dampness can contribute to the development of edema and varicose veins in the lower extremities.*

**Needling Treatment**
- 88.01 Tong Guan+88.02 Tong Shan+88.03 Tong Tian (bilateral)
- SP-6 (Sanyinjiao). This point is said to improve circulation in the lower body and relieve pain.
- BL17 (Geshu) This point is said to regulate blood circulation and strengthen the veins.
- BL18 This point is said to promote the circulation of Qi (vital energy) and blood.
- BL20 (Pishu) This point is said to regulate the spleen and stomach, which are important organs for blood production.
- LI-4 (Hegu): This point is said to stimulate the flow of Qi and blood throughout the body.
- KID-3 (Taixi): This point is said to strengthen the kidneys, which are important organs for blood circulation.
- LIV-3 (66.04), LI-11, ST-36, SP-10

---

### Blood-letting Treatment
- Bleed cup the area or prick fine veins above and below (upstream and downstream) of the varicose veins. Do NOT bleed the bulging varicose veins.

*Point Illustration for treatment of Varicose Veins*

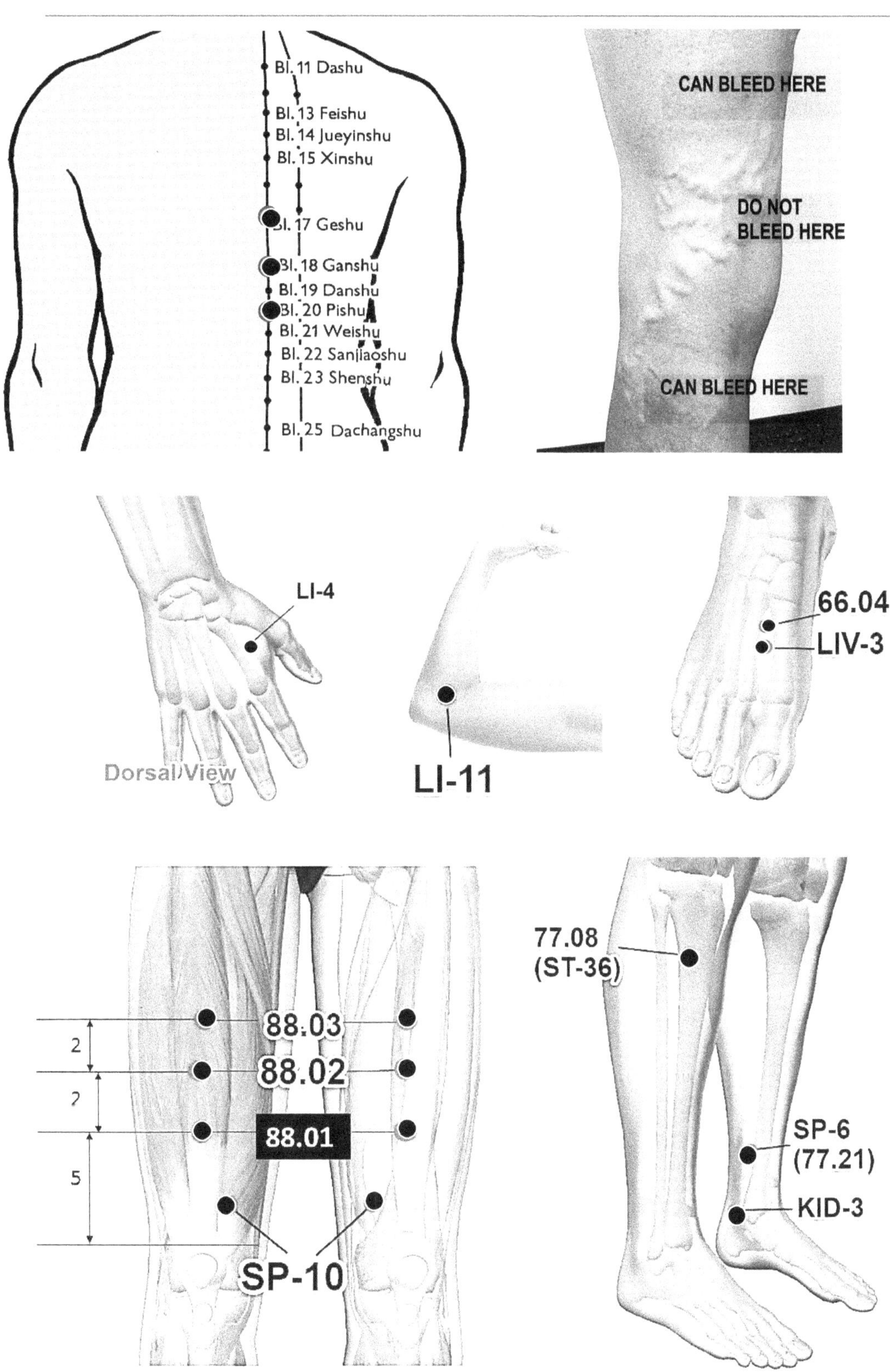

# Heart pain, angina

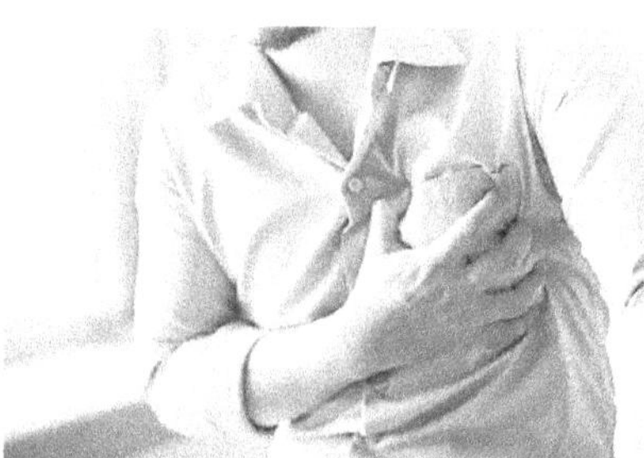

*In Traditional Chinese Medicine (TCM), angina is generally considered to be a type of chest pain caused by Qi and blood stagnation in the chest area. The meridians involved in angina may vary depending on the specific underlying cause, but some of the most commonly implicated meridians include **the Heart meridian, the Pericardium meridian, and the Liver meridian.***

*The **Heart meridian** is responsible for regulating the blood and Qi flow in the chest area, and is often involved in cases of angina caused by emotional factors such as stress or anxiety. The **Pericardium meridian** is closely related to the Heart and is also involved in regulating blood and Qi flow in the chest area. In TCM theory, the Pericardium meridian is considered to be responsible for protecting the Heart and is often targeted in cases of angina caused by physical factors such as overexertion.*

*The **Liver meridian** is also commonly involved in cases of angina in TCM. The Liver is responsible for regulating the smooth flow of Qi throughout the body, and when the Liver meridian becomes blocked or imbalanced, this can lead to stagnation of Qi and blood in the chest area.*

## TREATMENT

### Emergency point for chest pain

- Bleed or finger-nail acupressure 55.01 Huo Bao and/or 11.05 or HT-9
- Deeply needle 77.08 Si Hua Shang+77.09 Si Hua Zhong to release pressure from the chest.
- Acupressure and press needle on DU-9 and/or BL-15 until pain subside.

### Heart (Chest) pain of infarct

- 66.03 Huo Ying+66.04 Huo Zhu
- 88.01 Tong Guan+88.02 Tong Shan+88.03 Tong Tian
- P-4, P-6, HT-7, ST-36
- 33.05 Huo Ling+33.06 Huo Shan
- 44.10 Tian Zong, 44.08 Ren Zong, 44.09 Di Zong
- Moxibustion P-6, REN-17, BL-15

### Palpitation

- 11.05 – stabilize heart rate
- 33.12 Xin Men
- 11.19 Xin Chang

---

### Blood-letting for Cardiac conditions

- Bleed 55.01 Huo Bao and/or 11.05 for acute condition. If dark blood exits, treatment is effective.
- Bleed ear apex
- Bleed visible veins in the left cubital fossa (around LU-5 and P-3)
- DT.11 Hou Xin, particularly to the left of the spine. Palpate and wet-cup where tender
- Visible veins on the lateral left leg
- 77.09 Si Hua Zhong, 77.14 Si Hua Wai
- For enlarged heart and heart disease, bleed DT.07 San Jin (Shu Points close to HT, PC, SI and LU).

*Points Illustrations for treatment of Heart Pain/Angina*

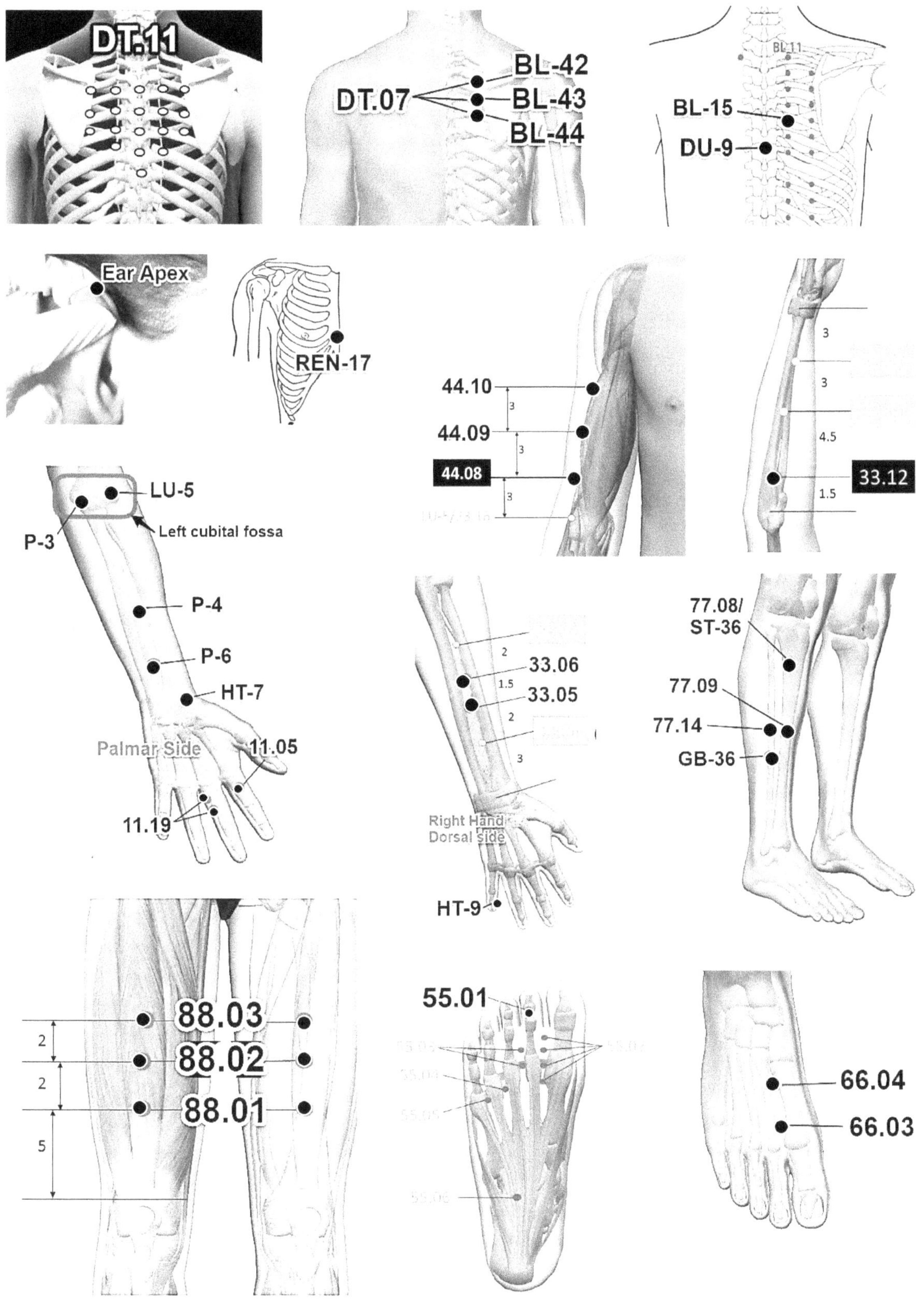

# Hypertension and High Cholesterol

*In Traditional Chinese Medicine (TCM), hypertension and high cholesterol are often viewed as imbalances in the body's energy systems, particularly those related to the **liver, spleen, and kidneys**. Hypertension, or high blood pressure, is typically seen as a result of excess "liver heat" or "liver fire". This can be caused by factors such as stress, anger, and an unhealthy diet. High cholesterol is often seen as a result of excess "dampness" or "phlegm" in the body, which can be caused by factors such as poor diet, lack of exercise, and genetic predisposition.*

### Hypertension and hypercholesterolemia

- 77.14 Si Hua Wai (ST-40) and 66.11 Huo Ju (SP-4) are used together to disperse phlegm and open the blood vessels.
- 77.14 Si Hua Wai (ST-40) lowers cholesterol because it is the Stomach Luo point for phlegm; TCM considers cholesterol as a type of phlegm. Stiff neck and high cholesterol are often related. Best if bled.

### Hypertension (affected meridians/organs: heart, liver and kidney)

- Bilaterally needle 66.03 Huo Ying or 66.04 Huo Zhu (LIV-2/LIV-3) – Reaction: Heart/Liver
- 66.10+66.11 Huo Ju+66.12 Huo San – Reaction: Heart and Kidney
- P-6 and ST-36 (77.08)
- 77.17 (SP-9), 77.18 Shen Guan+77.19 Di Huang+77.21 Ren Huang (SP-6) – Reaction: Kidney
- LI-11, LI-4
- KID-3
- Bilaterally needle BL-65
- GB-34
- Jian Gu (a wood point between LI-3 and LI- 4)
- 22.06 Zhong Bai (SJ-3), SJ-5
- 44.04 (Reaction: Heart/Liver) and 44.05 (Reaction: Heart)

---

### Blood-letting to radically lower blood pressure

- DT.04 Wu Ling
- Visible vein at 99.07 Er Bei and/or 99.08 ear apex
- Bleed fingertips (effective when in emergency)
- Veins found in the vicinity of 77.09 Si Hua Zhong and 77.14 Si Hua Wai (ST-40)
- Visible veins in the legs, especially lower medial and lateral legs near the ankles.
- Bleed from BL-12 to BL-15 and from BL-42 to BL-44
- Bleed around BL-40

*Points Illustrations for treatment of Hypertension and Hypercholesterolemia*

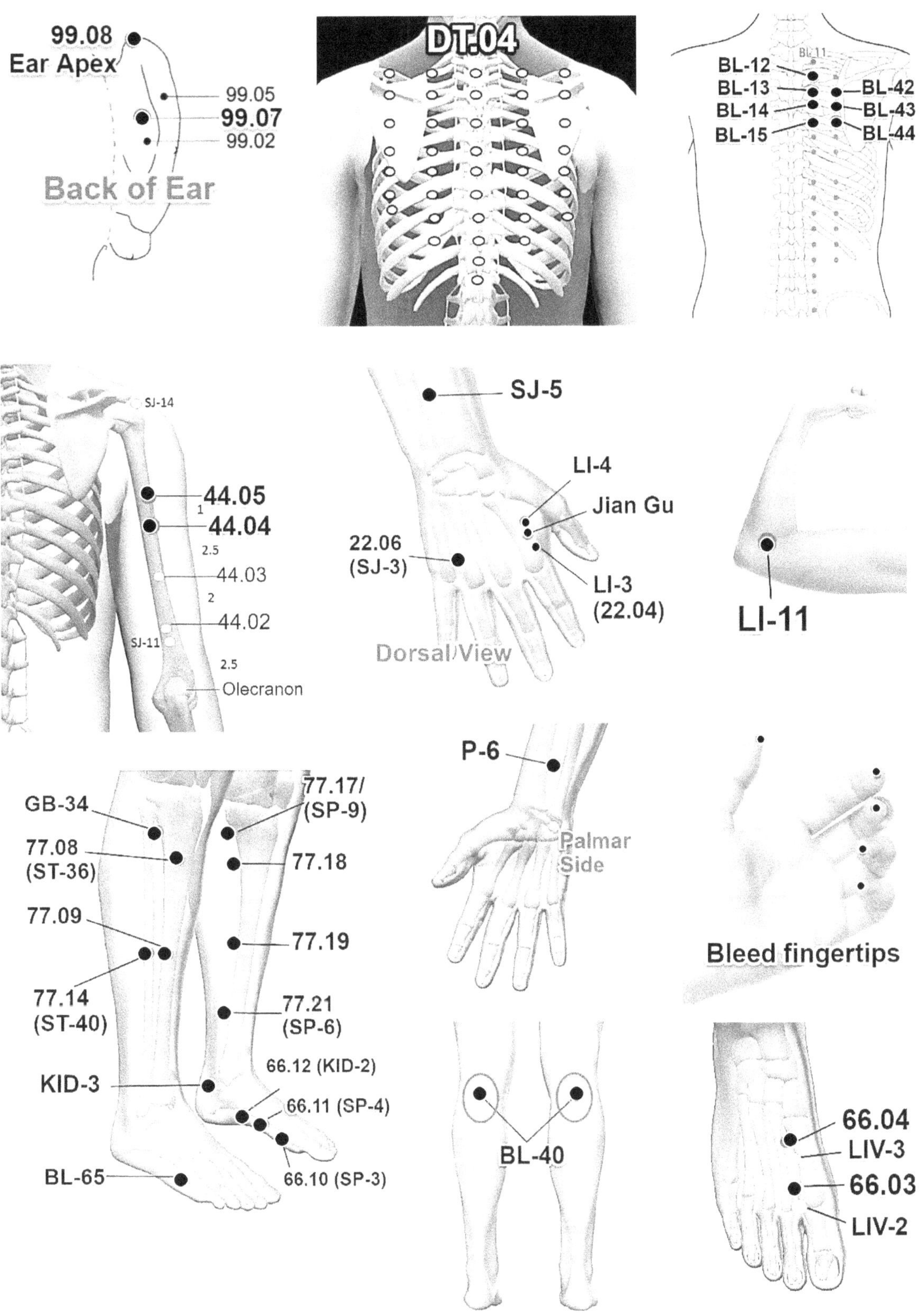

# Hemiplegia from Stroke

*In Traditional Chinese Medicine (TCM), hemiplegia due to stroke is generally considered to be caused by a blockage or obstruction of Qi and blood flow in the brain, resulting in damage to the brain and nervous system. The meridians involved in hemiplegia due to stroke may vary depending on the specific location and severity of the blockage, but some of the most commonly implicated meridians include **the Du meridian, the Ren meridian, the Gallbladder meridian, and the Urinary Bladder meridian.***

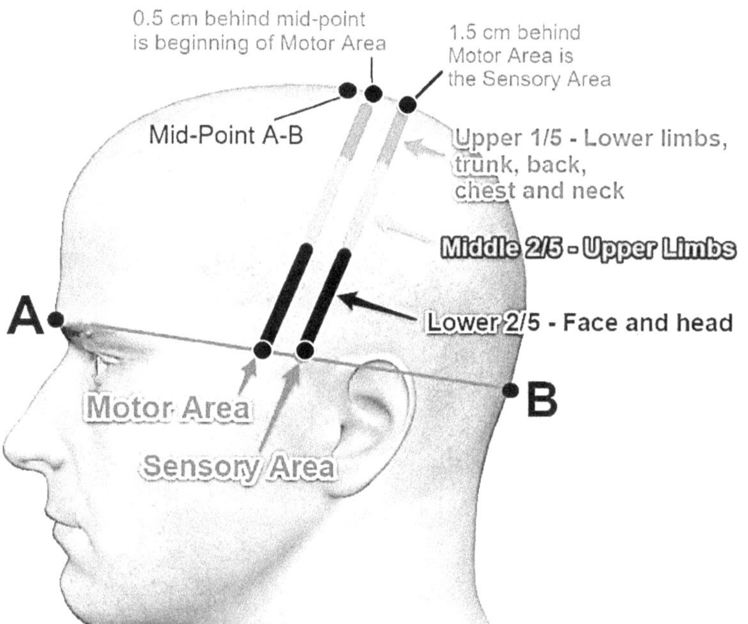


## Preparatory Note

Treating a stroke patient is a lengthy process due to their slow and laborious movements and the various components involved in treatment. You need to be prepared to provide more attention and resources when managing stroke. Before beginning treatment, it is crucial to ensure the patient is adequately hydrated and has stable blood sugar levels.

## Scalp Acupuncture Option 1
### (by Dr.Jiao)

- Thread needles down the **Motor Area** and **Sensory Area Locations** (opposite from the hemiplegia).

- Cross and connect the Motor and Sensory Lines at the targeted levels of the head, shoulder, arm, hand, thumb and fingers (Upper 1/5, Middle 2/5 or Lower 2/5)

- The patient should retain these scalp needles for the duration of the treatment. *Stimulate them regularly while moving the affected arm and leg (Active Qi Moving)*

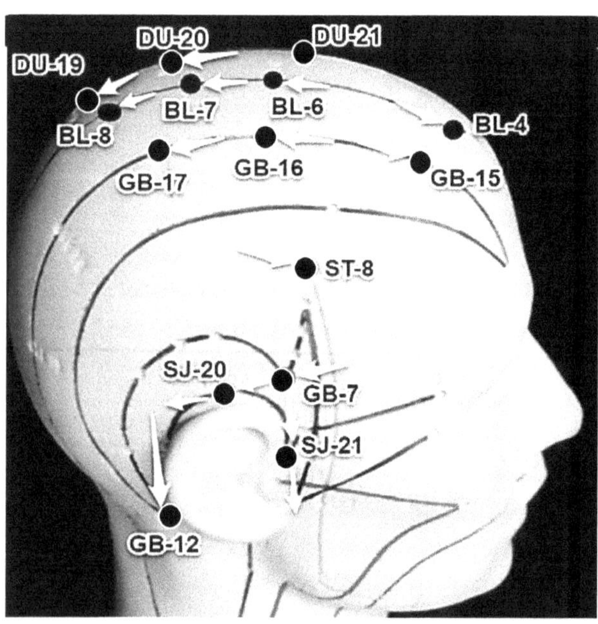


## Scalp Acupuncture Option 2
### (by Dr. Lee Kua Chang)

Dr. Lee Kua Chang uses points on the DU, BL, GB and SJ Meridians on the scalp as per figure. While stimulating the needles, another therapist will tap the spinal cord and another will perform exercises on the affected limbs.

- DU-19, 20, 21
- BL-4, 6, 7,8
- GB-7, 12, 15, 16, 17
- SJ-20, 21
- ST-8

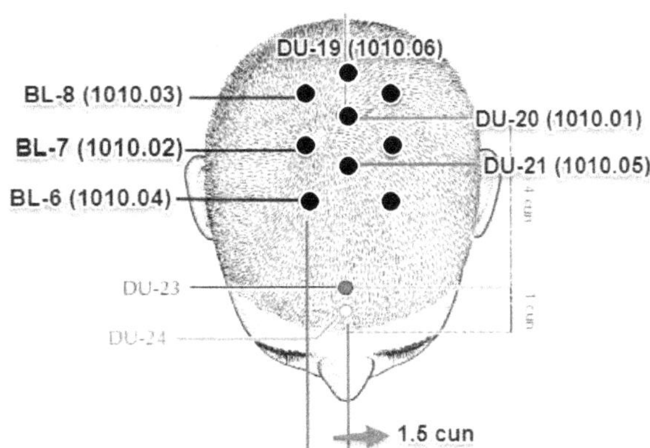


## Scalp Acupuncture Option 3 (Dr. Young)

1010.01 Zheng Hui, 1010.02 Zhou Yuan, 1010.03 Zhou Kun, 1010.04 Zhou Lun, 1010.05 Qian Hui, 1010.06 Hou Hui all have a strong sedative function, as well as the function to activate the circulation and meridians. They are commonly chosen to treat hemiplegia and other wind syndromes". These needles will awaken the brain and stimulate the lower part of the body and urinary bladder.

**Needle 11.10 Mu Huo with Caution**

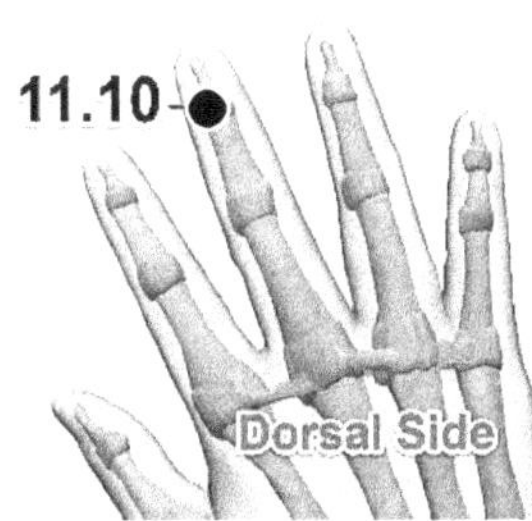


In stroke treatment, an effective point is 11.10 Mu Huo, which can be needled bilaterally. However, it's important to follow the needling protocol precisely since 11.10 (Wood Fire) can also raise blood pressure.

During the first five times of needling 11.10 Mu Huo bilaterally, retain the needles for only five minutes. For the next five times, the retention time should be reduced to three minutes, and after the tenth treatment, the retention time should be one minute only. This gradual reduction in retention time will help the patient adjust to the treatment and prevent any undesired effects. It's safe to needle this point every other day or even once daily, but not more than once each day.

**General treatment for hemiplegia**
- 22.04 Da Bai+22.05 Ling Gu – opposite side
- 88.25 Zhong Jiu Li (GB-31), 88.26 Shang Jiu Li+88.27 Xia Jiu Li
- Bilateral 22.01 Chong Zi+22.02 Chong Xian (effective)
- 77.18 Shen Guan
- 1010.01 Zheng Hui+1010.05 Qian Hui+1010.06 Hou Hui
- 77.05+77.06+77.07 – send blood to the brain
- Needle DU-20 to GB-7 and GB-20
- 44.06 – muscle treats muscle
- See page 196 for discussion on coma.

**Treating Hemiplegia of lower limbs**
- 22.04 Da Bai+22.05 Ling Gu on opposite side with strong qi. Can alternate with LI-4, LI-11, ST-36 with strong stimulation. Can add SP-6.
- Simultaneously stimulate the scalp points and execute qi moving technique. Rest and repeat several times or every 10 minutes.
- Points on Stomach meridian: ST-31, ST-32, ST-36, ST-37, ST-38, ST-39, ST-41, ST-44
- Points on Gall bladder meridian: GB-30, GB-34, GB-37, GB-40
- Point on Liver meridian: LIV-3
- Points on Bladder meridian: BL-30, BL-40, BL-57, BL-60, Huatuojiaji
- Bafeng (Ex. 36.). or Ex-LE-10 - for paralysis of the toes and contraction of foot
- For foot-drop and dysfunction of ankle joints:
  - Electro-acupuncture ST-38 (near 77.09) + LIV-3 (66.04)
  - Needle GB-40 through to KI-6

**Treating Hemiplegia of upper limbs**

- 22.04+22.05 or 22.01+22.02 on healthy side
- Needle opposite-side 88.25 Zhong Jiu Li (GB-31) with A.01 Qi Li (GB-32), strong stimulation.
- Simultaneously stimulate the scalp points and execute qi moving technique.
  Rest and repeat several times or every 10 minutes.
- If found more convenient, use 77.22 Ce San Li+77.23 Ce Xia San Li or GB-34 alternately.
- Points on Large Intestine meridian: LI-4, LI-6, LI-10, LI-11, LI-13, LI-15
- Points on Sanjiao meridian: SJ-3, SJ-5, SJ-14
- Baxie (Ex. 28.) or Ex-UE-9 - for paralysis of the fingers
- Spasticity of the fingers with an inability to stretch – Baxie, P-7, LI-3, LI-4 and SI-3
- Wrist drop – SJ-9, SJ-5

## Gua Sha and Blood-letting Therapy for Stroke

- Bleed-cup all the way down the Large Intestine channel on the arm and the Gallbladder channel on the leg. This treatment is especially helpful in a chronic case. With any kind of bleeding treatment, advisable for patient to be in a reasonably robust state physically (hydrated, rested and not hungry). Can perform gentle gua sha instead.
- Bleed all Jing Well Point, especially during the acute phase and in case of coma.
- DT.04 Wu Ling, alternate week (select different sections, each treatment)
- 99.08 Ear apex
- Bleed LI-11 for severe hemiplegia of arm

*Points Illustrations for treatment of Hemiplegia*

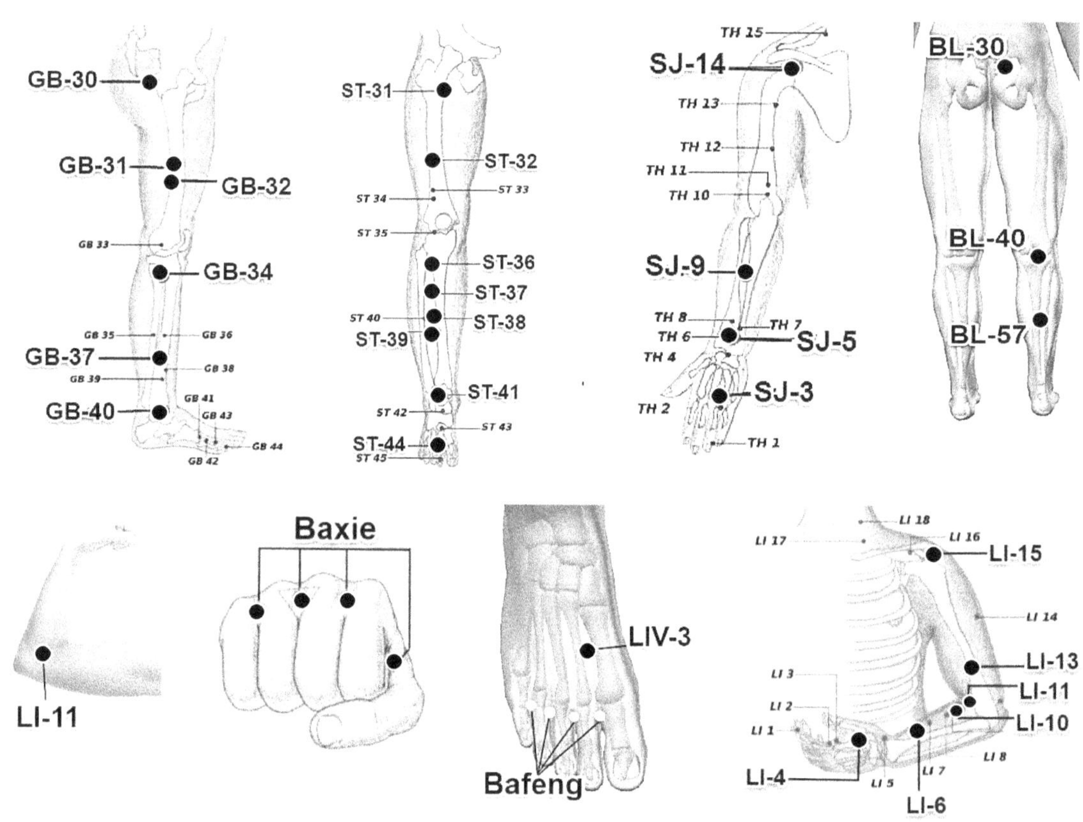

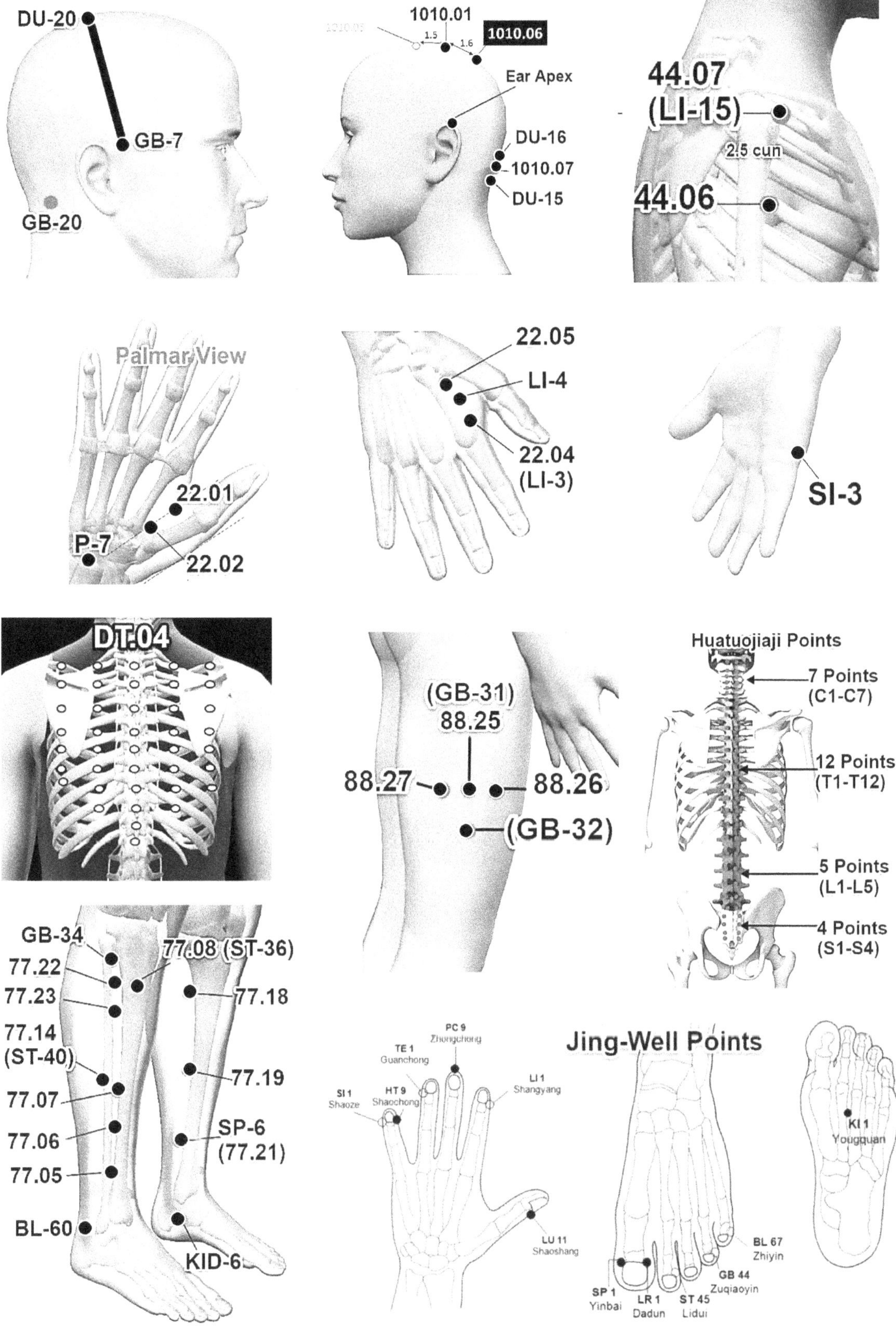
DU-20
GB-7
GB-20
1010.01
1010.06
1.5
1.6
Ear Apex
DU-16
1010.07
DU-15
44.07
(LI-15)
2.5 cun
44.06
Palmar View
22.05
LI-4
22.04
(LI-3)
SI-3
22.01
P-7
22.02
DT.04
(GB-31)
88.25
88.27
88.26
(GB-32)
Huatuojiaji Points
7 Points
(C1-C7)
12 Points
(T1-T12)
5 Points
(L1-L5)
4 Points
(S1-S4)
GB-34
77.08 (ST-36)
77.22
77.23
77.18
77.14
(ST-40)
77.19
77.07
77.06
SP-6
(77.21)
77.05
BL-60
KID-6
PC 9
Zhongchong
TE 1
Guanchong
LI 1
Shangyang
SI 1
Shaoze
HT 9
Shaochong
LU 11
Shaoshang
Jing-Well Points
KI 1
Yougquan
BL 67
Zhiyin
SP 1
Yinbai
LR 1
Dadun
ST 45
Lidui
GB 44
Zuqiaoyin

# Post-Stroke Conditions

**Increase blood circulation to the brain**
- Bleed 99.08 Er San Ear Apex on the side opposite the hemiplegia (bleeding the same side where the stroke occurred within the brain).
- Needle/bleed 77.05 Yi Zhong+77.06 Er Zhong+77.07 San Zhong (GB Channel traverses the head) to increase circulation to the brain. Can treat bilaterally.

**Reduce blood pressure**
- Bleed the Jing Well Point (alternatively can bleed the fingertips
- Bleed 33.16 Qu Ling (LU-5) and BL-40; or bleed DT.04 Wu Ling.
- Bleeding veins found on the Stomach or Gallbladder channels reduce blood pressure.

**Reduce phlegm accumulation**
- Bleed 77.14 Si Hua Wai (ST-40 /phlegm gathering point) to clear phlegm.

**Acute stroke treatment**
- In addition to bleeding Jing Well Point and/or ear apex needle 22.01 Chong Zi+22.02 Chong Xian (because they are opposite 22.04 Da Bai+22.05 Ling Gu) on the side opposite the brain bleed; needle or bleed 33.16 Qu Ling (LU-5) on the same side, to sedate.

**Late-stage stroke treatment**
- In addition to using the standard protocol, also bilaterally needle 77.18 Shen Guan+77.19 Di Huang+77.21 Ren Huang to tonify the Kidneys. Bleeding techniques are effective in cases of long-term blood stagnation.

**Speech Difficulties**
- Needle 44.06 Jian Zhong
- Prick 1010.07 Zong Shu/DT.03 Qi Xing
- 1010.19 Shui Tong+1010.20 Shui Jin

**Swallowing Difficulties**
- Bleed- 1010.01 Zheng Hui+1010.06 Hou Hui, DU-15, DU-16
- Prick 1010.07 Zong Shu/DT.03 Qi Xing

**Hand Contraction**
- 22.01 Chong Zi, 22.02 Chong Xian on the opposite side
- Bloodletting at 33.16 Qu Ling or LU-5

**Clenched jaws**
- Needle/moxa ST-6 (bilateral), ST-7, LI-4, DU-26, DU-20, REN-24, REN-23

**Deviated mouth**
- ST-4 and ST-6

*Points Illustrations for treatment of Post-Stroke Conditions*

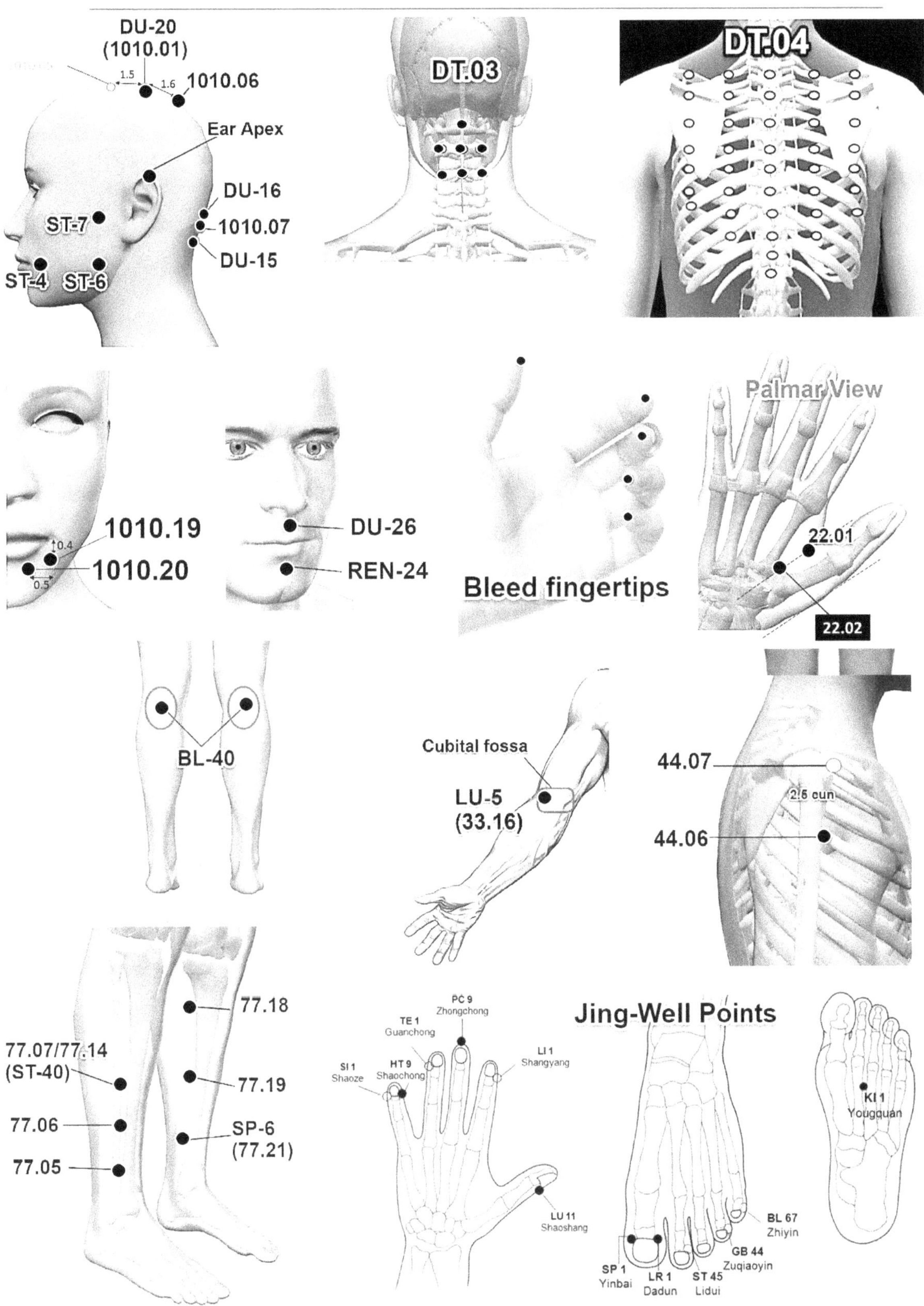

# LIVER AND GALLBLADDER

## Biliary Colic

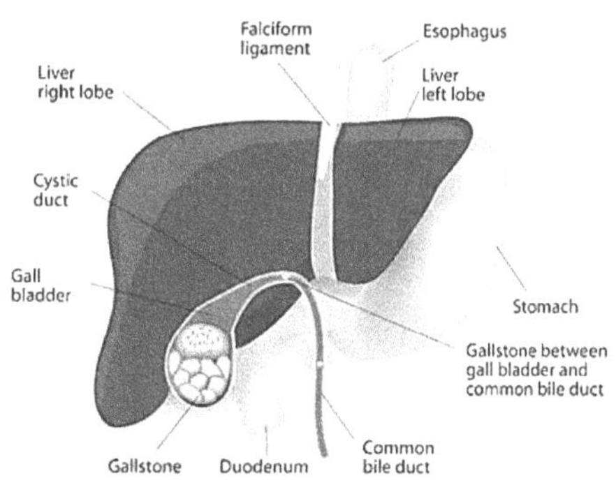


*Biliary colic is a dull pain in the middle to upper right area of the abdomen. It occurs when a gallstone blocks the bile duct, the tube that normally drains bile from the gallbladder to the small intestine. The pain goes away if the stone passes into the small intestine and unblocks the duct.*

**Needling treatment**

| AFFECTED (SICK) MERIDIANS | TREATMENT POINTS |
|---|---|
| **GALL BLADDER** <br> Foot Shao Yang | • Dannang (Ex.35.) or Ex-LE-6. Distal Alarm point of the GB Meridian <br> • 88.14 Qi Huang+88.15 Huo Zhi+88.16 Huo Quan - Liver treats Gallbladder meridian (System 3) <br> • Add 1010.18 Mu Zhi (ST-7) - Meeting point of ST and GB Meridians <br> • 22.06 Zhong Bai + 22.07 Xia Bai - SJ treats GB (System 1) <br> • 88.25, 88.26, 88.27, GB-32 - Treats own meridian. <br> • LIV-3 (66.04 Huo Zhu) - Liver treats GB (System 3) |
| **STOMACH** <br> Foot Yangming | • 1010.18 Mu Zhi - Meeting point of ST and GB Meridians |
| **LIVER** <br> Foot Jue Yin | • 88.14 Qi Huang+88.15 Huo Zhi+88.16- Treats own meridian. <br> • LIV-3 (66.04 Huo Zhu) - Shu-stream point of Liver Meridian. Yuan source point. Treats own meridian. |

### Blood-letting treatment
- Bleed BL-19 - Back Shu of the Gall Bladder
- Visible veins on the lateral right leg
- Palpate the right back area from L2 to L5 and wet-cup tender spots
- Bleed around 77.09 + 77.14
- Moxibustion REN-8 (umbilicus)

*Points Illustrations for treatment of Biliary Colic*

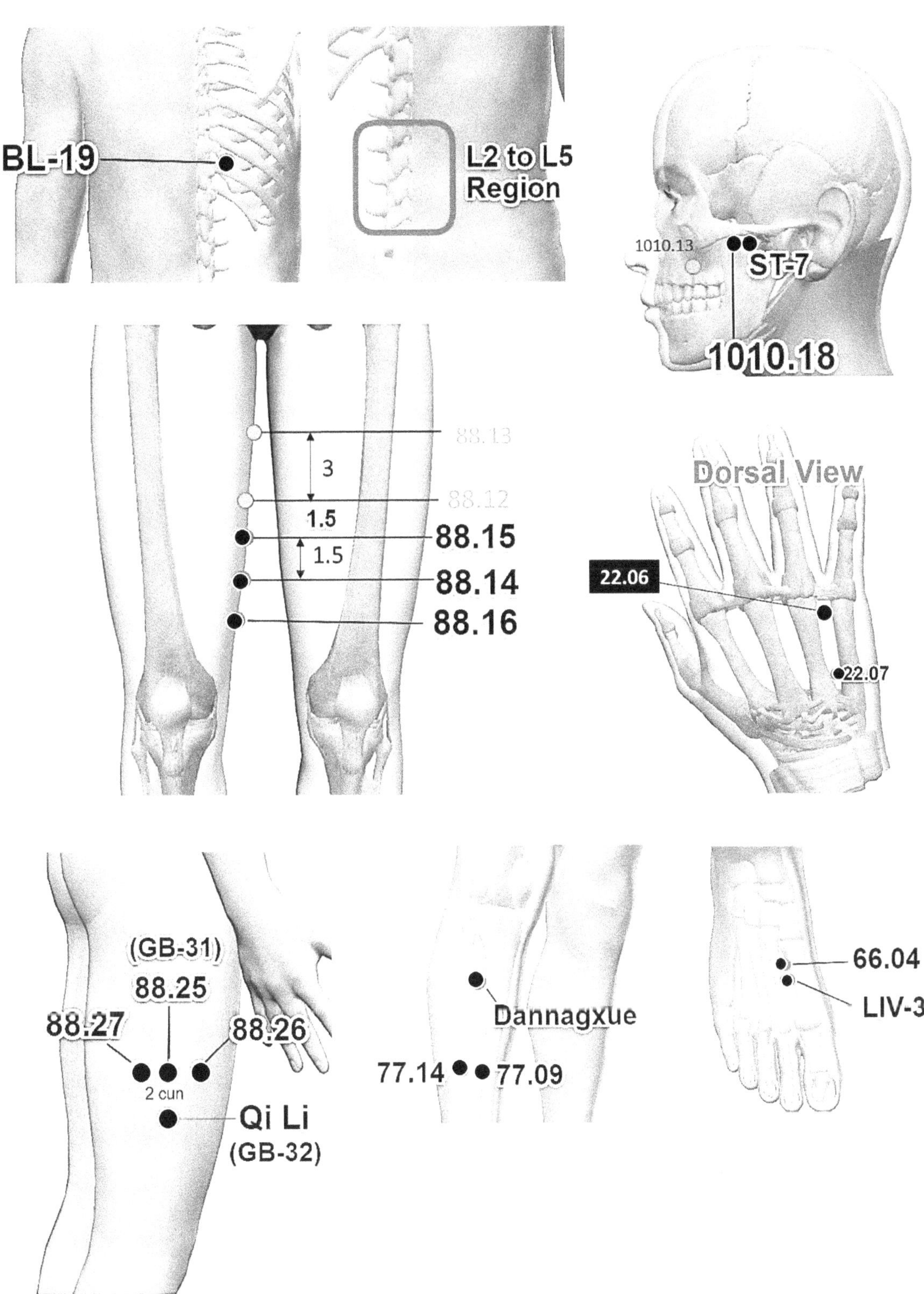

# Gallbladder Inflammation

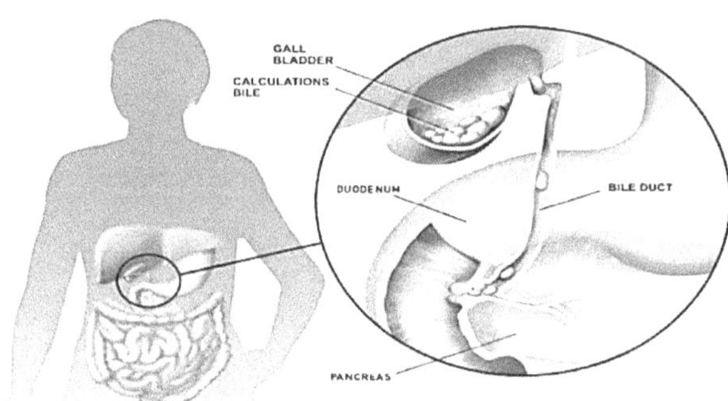


*According to TCM theory, the Gallbladder is a Yang organ and is closely linked to the Liver system. The Liver is responsible for ensuring the smooth flow of Qi (vital energy) throughout the body, and if this flow is disrupted or blocked, it can lead to stagnation and inflammation in the gallbladder.*

*Common TCM patterns associated with gallbladder inflammation include Liver Qi Stagnation, Damp Heat, Blood Stasis, and Yin Deficiency.*

**Treatment for Gallbladder disease, inflammation, sludge or stones**
- 88.14 Qi Huang+88.15 Huo Zhi+88.16 Huo Quan (known as Gallbladder Points)
- 001 Hand Golden Gate +1010.18 Mu Zhi (ST-7)
- 66.03 Huo Ying+ 66.04 Huo Zhu+66.05+001 Hand Golden Gate +1010.18 Mu Zhi (ST-7)
- 001 Hand Golden Gate, needled with 22.07 Xia Bai and Dannang (Ex.35.) or Ex-LE-6
- Bilaterally needle 88.25 Zhong Jiu Li (GB-31)+ A.01 Qi Li (GB-32)+88.26+88.27, 1010.18 Mu Zhi (ST-7)

---

### Blood-letting for Liver/Gall bladder conditions
- Visible veins on the lower leg, especially the GB-34 region
- Palpate the right back area from BL-17 to BL-23 and wet-cup any very tender points
- 55.01 Huo Bao

### Blood-letting for Pain from gallstones
- Palpate the right bladder channel from approximately L2 to L5, and wet-cup any very tender points
- Visible veins in the lateral right leg

---

### <u>Dietary advice for both gallbladder and liver issues</u>

Recommended to avoid consuming greasy, fatty, and spicy foods, and instead opt for cooling foods such as leafy greens, cucumber, celery, and mung bean sprouts to counteract excess heat. Including bitter foods like bitter gourd, dandelion greens, and bitter melon in your diet can aid in clearing heat and toxins from the body. Consuming foods that support the liver system, like beets, carrots, and bitter herbs such as dandelion root and milk thistle, can also be helpful. It is important to avoid alcohol and caffeine, as they can overstimulate the liver and exacerbate inflammation. Eating smaller, more frequent meals throughout the day can help support healthy digestion and prevent stagnation in the gallbladder.

*Points Illustrations for treatment of Gallbladder Inflammation*

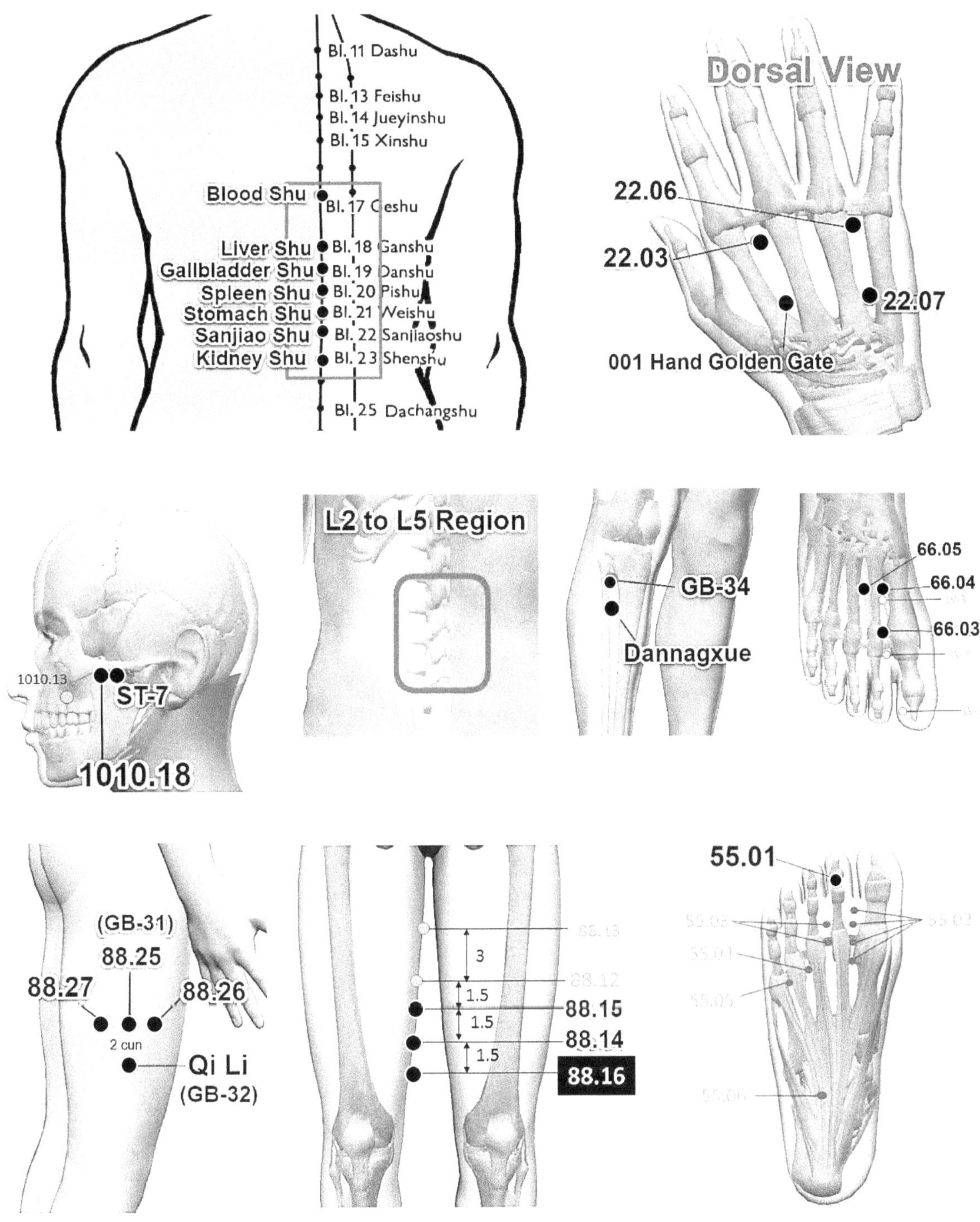

# Liver disease

*In Traditional Chinese Medicine (TCM), liver cirrhosis is viewed as a severe manifestation of chronic liver disease, which can lead to irreversible damage and scarring of the liver tissue. It is generally considered a late-stage condition that is difficult to treat, and TCM treatment focuses on managing symptoms, slowing disease progression, and supporting the body's energy and organ systems.*

*From a TCM perspective, liver cirrhosis is often associated with patterns of Liver Qi stagnation, Liver Yin deficiency, and Blood Stasis. Symptoms may include fatigue, abdominal distension, loss of appetite, nausea, jaundice, and swelling of the legs and abdomen.*

**Affected meridians**: **Liver and Spleen**

### Serious liver disease including liver cirrhosis

For the treatment of severe liver disease, it is recommended to combine the use of 11.20 Mu Yan with 88.12 Ming Huang, 88.13 Tian Huang, and 88.14 Qi Huang. The primary focus should be on the use of 88.12 Ming Huang, 88.13 Tian Huang, and 88.14 Qi Huang, while 11.20 Mu Yan can help manage pain. These points can useful with liver cancer, which can be one of the most painful types of cancer.

### Additional points for Cirrhosis of liver

- After blood-letting, needle 33.11 Gan Men, 88.12 Ming Huang+88.13 Tian Huang+88.14 Qi Huang
- 77.05+77.06+77.07

### Hepatitis

- 33.10 Chang Men, 33.11 Gan Men
- 88.12 Ming Huang+88.13 Tian Huang+88.14 Qi Huang
- SI-4

### Enlarged Liver

- 77.05 Yi Zhong+77.06 Er Zhong+77.07 San Zhong
- 66.06 Mu Liu+66.07 Mu Dou

---

### Blood-letting for Liver Cirrhosis/Gall bladder conditions

- Bleed 44.16 Shang Qu
- Bleed 77.09 Si Hua Zhong, 77.14 Si Hua Wai
- Visible veins on the lower leg, especially the GB-34 region
- Palpate the right back area from BL-17 to BL-23 and wet-cup any very tender points
- 55.01 Huo Bao

### Blood-letting for Hepatitis

- Visible veins on the lower leg, especially the GB-34 region
- Visible veins in the cubital fossa
- Palpate the right back area from BL-17 to BL-23 and wet-cup any tender points

---

*Points Illustrations for treatment of Liver Disease*

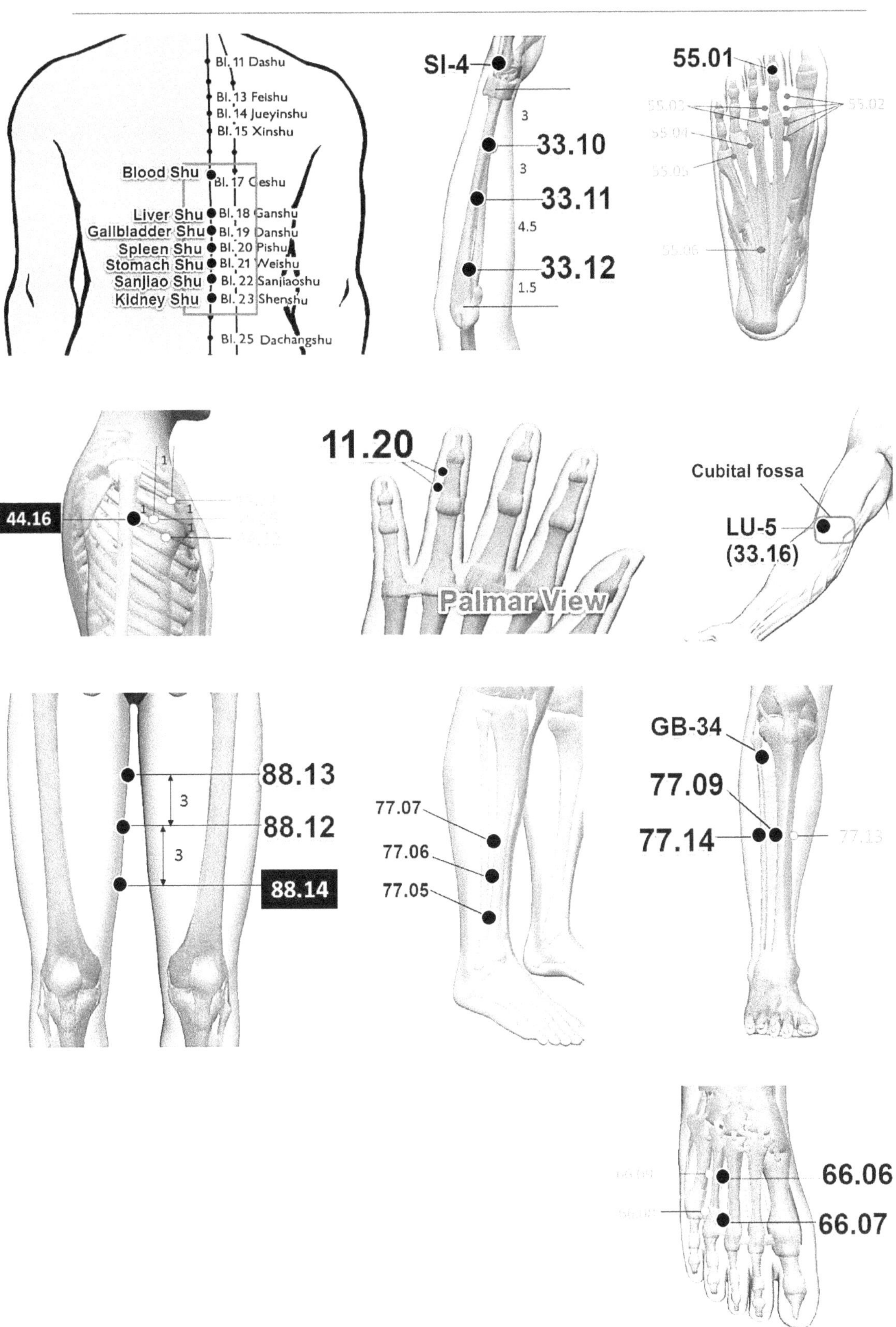

# RESPIRATORY

## Asthma

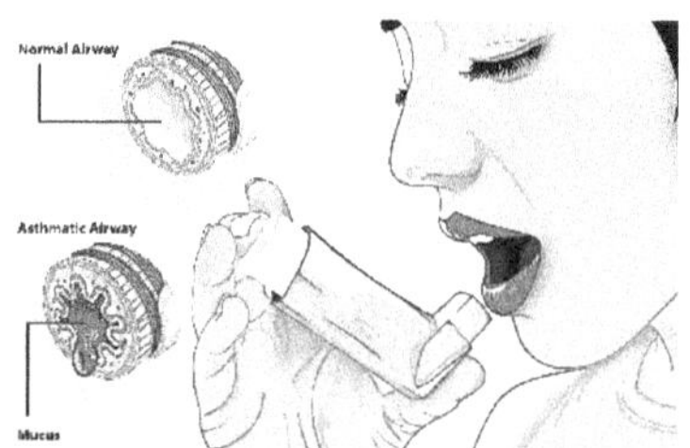

*According to TCM theory, asthma is caused by a combination of external and internal factors that disrupt the balance of Qi in the Lung system and lead to inflammation, constriction, and difficulty breathing.*

*Some common TCM patterns associated with asthma include: Lung Qi Deficiency, Lung Heat and Phlegm-Heat.*

**Needling Treatment**

- 33.13 Ren Shi+33.14 Di Shi+33.15 Tian Shi – due to heart/lung issues.
- Bilateral 1010.19 Shui Tong+1010.20 Shui Jin – due to kidney issues.
- Bilateral 88.17 Si Ma Zhong+88.18 Si Ma Shang+88.19 Si Ma Xia – due to allergic issues
- 22.04 Da Bai+22.05 Ling Gu
- 22.01+22.02 (bilateral) – can be bled in acute situation
- 22.11 Tu Shui (LU-10), insert towards centre of palm– for acute attack.  Can needle bilaterally.
- REN-17
- Bilateral Dingchuan (Ex. 17.) or  Ex-B-1 with electrical stimulation
- Deeply needle 77.08 Si Hua Shang (ST-36)
- Moxa SP-10
- 

---

### Blood-letting Treatment for Asthma/difficulty breathing

- LU-10 (22.11 Tu Shui) can stop wheezing immediately, especially when dark veins are bled.
- 33.16 Qu Ling (LU-5) or around cubital fossa.
- Bleed cup REN-17.  Catgut embedding therapy on REN-17 is beneficial.
- Visible veins in the leg, especially lateral leg or around 77.13 Si Hua Li; 77.14 Si Hua Wai.
- Cup and/or bleed BL-42, BL-43, BL-13 (Lung area), DU-14 every week, needle 2-3 times a week
- Lung area of the back as shown below (palpate for tender) points and wet-cup there.
- 

---

### Dietary advice for asthma in TCM may include

Avoiding dairy products, which can increase phlegm production and exacerbate symptoms.

Eating more pungent foods, such as ginger, garlic, and onions, which can help clear Lung Heat and improve respiratory function.

Eating more cooling foods, such as pears, watermelon, and cucumber, to counteract internal heat and reduce inflammation.

Eating foods that support Lung Qi, such as white radish, honey, and almonds.

Avoiding foods that are difficult to digest or that can cause phlegm, such as greasy or fried foods, sugar, and processed foods.

*Points Illustrations for treatment of Asthma*

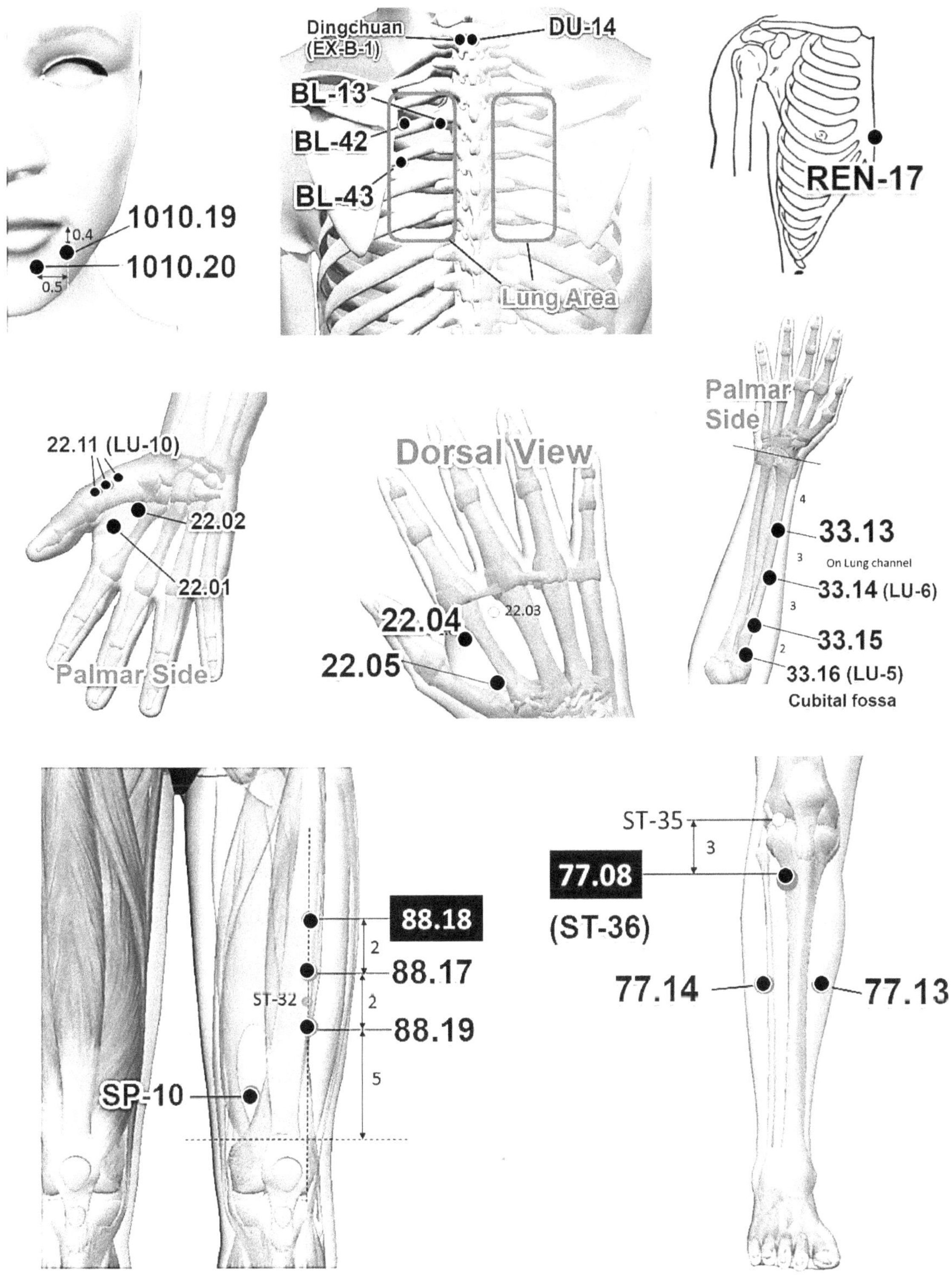

# Sore Throat

*In Traditional Chinese Medicine (TCM), sore throat is considered a symptom of external invasion by a pathogenic factor, such as Wind, Cold, or Heat. It is often associated with patterns of Lung and Stomach imbalances and can be caused by a variety of factors, including viral or bacterial infections, allergies, and environmental irritants.*

*Some common TCM patterns associated with sore throat include: Wind-Heat, Wind-Cold and Stomach Fire:*

**For pain relief**
- 22.04 Da Bai+22.05 Ling Gu,66.03 Huo Ying+66.04 Huo Zhu, 66.05 Men Jin
- LI-5, LI-11, ST-41

## Main Treatment

| AFFECTED (SICK) CHANNELS | TREATMENT POINTS |
|---|---|
| **LUNG** <br> Hand Taiyin | • Bleed LU-11. Jing-well point. Treats own meridian. <br> • LU-10 Ying-spring point. Treats own meridian. Combine with SJ-2. <br> • Or 22.11 (needle or bleed) on one side and A.04 San Cha San on other side. |
| **LARGE INTESTINE** <br> Hand Yangming | • Bleed LI-1. Jing-well point. Treats own meridian. |
| **LIVER** <br> Foot Jueyin | • LIV-3 (66.04 Huo Zhu) - Shu-stream point of Liver Meridian. Yuan source point. <br> • Treats own meridian. Combine with KID-6 and DU-20. |
| **SAN JIAO** <br> Hand Shaoyang | • SJ-2 Ying-spring point. Treats own meridian. <br> • Needle/bleed SJ-1 - Treats own meridian. |
| **KIDNEY** <br> Foot Shaoyin | • KID-3 - Shu Stream Point on the Kidney Channel. Yuan Source on the Kidney Channel. Treats own meridian. Can bleed. <br> • KID-6 - Treats own meridian. Combine with LU-7 |
| **REN** | • REN-23 - Treats own meridian. |

### Blood-letting for Tonsillitis, pharyngitis
- Apex of the ear
- LU-11, LI-1
- Visible veins in the cubital fossa
- Visible veins on the leg, especially ST 36/GB 34/77.24/77.25/77.07 region and BL-40 region
- VT.01 Hou'e Jiu (Throat Moth)

*Points Illustrations for treatment of Sore Throat*

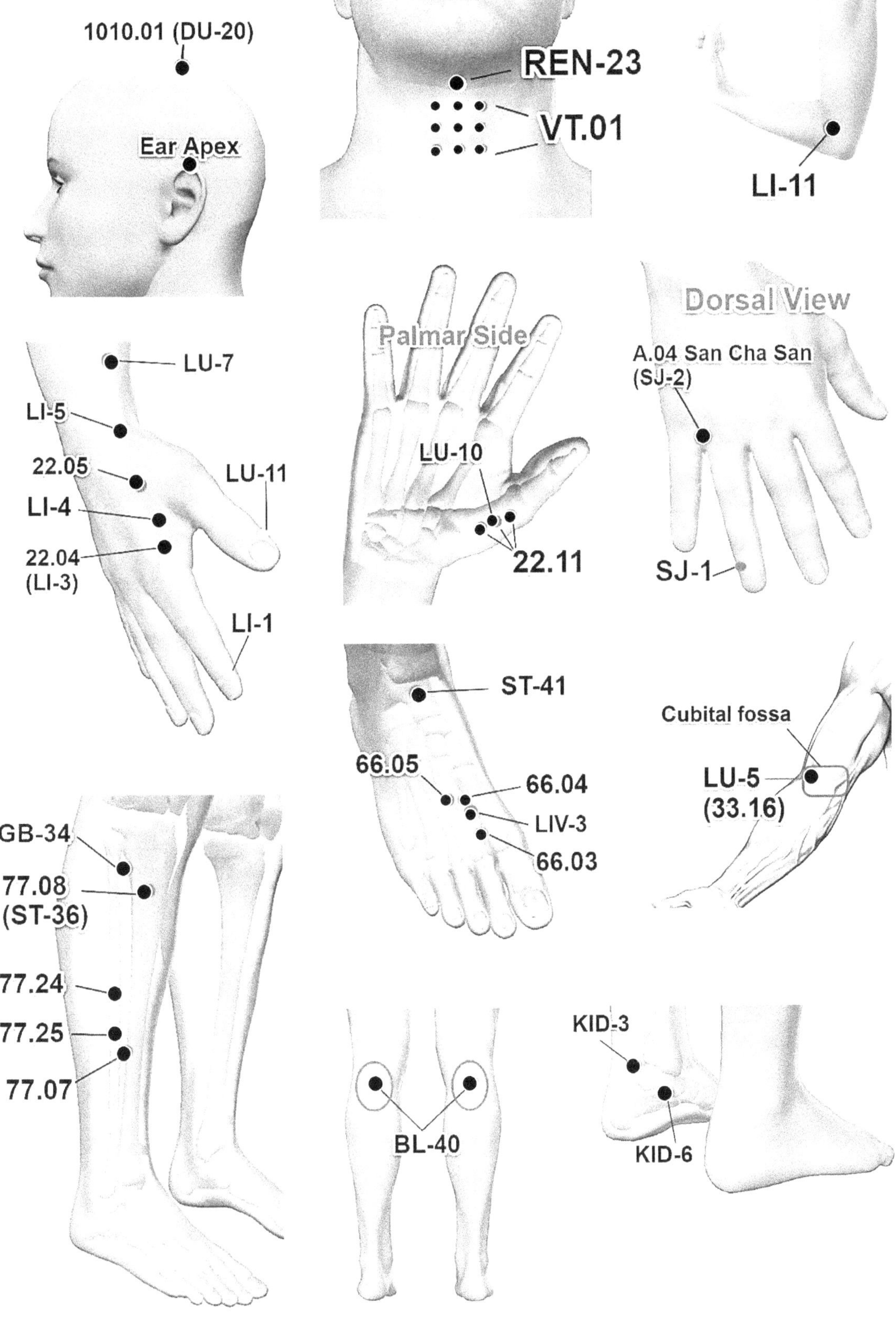

# Common Cold

*According to Traditional Chinese medicine (TCM), the common cold affects the lung meridian, which is responsible for respiratory function and immune system function. When the **lung meridian** is weak or blocked, the body is more susceptible to the invasion of external pathogens, leading to the development of a cold.*

*In addition to the lung meridian, the **spleen and stomach meridians** may be affected.*

**Prevention**

Taking a very hot shower with water focused on the upper back and neck within a few hours of feeling chilled may prevent illness. Sweating profusely during the shower may alleviate the chills. *(Susan Johnson)*

| Accompanying symptoms | Treatment |
|---|---|
| Common cold, allergies | • A.04 San Cha San+ 22.04 Da Bai+22.05 Ling Gu<br>• Bilaterally 88.17 Si Ma Zhong+88.18 Si Ma Shang+88.19 Si Ma Xia<br>• Bilaterally needle ST-36, SP-6, LI-11, LI- 4, LU-7 |
| With running nose and nasal congestion | • Add 77.22 Ce San Li+77.23 Ce Xia San Li,<br>• Add Unilaterally needle 66.05 Men Jin (ST-43).<br>• Add Bilaterally needle proximal point 11.17 Mu (Anger).<br>• Add Bleed EX-HN-6 ERJIAN ear Apex and/or Yintang [Ex. 1.] or Ex-HN-3<br>• Add 1010.15 Fu Kuai (LI-20) as Guiding Points |
| With sore throat | • Add 77.24 Qian Jin+77.25 Zu Wu Jin<br>• Add 88.17 Si Ma Zhong+88.18 Si Ma Shang+88.19 Si Ma Xia, 77.07<br>• Bleed tender spots on VT.01 Hou'e Jiu (Throat Moth), LU-11 and LI-1 |
| With asthma | • Add 22.11 Tu Shui |
| With coughing | • Add 33.13 Ren Shi+33.14 Di Shi+33.15 Tian Shi<br>• Add 22.01+22.02, 11.01+11.05+11.02 (with yellow phlegm) |
| Nausea/stomach pain | • Add 22.11 Tu Shui, 22.10 Shou Jie |
| With headache | • Add GB-20, LI-4.  22.04 Da Bai and A.04 San Cha San |
| To alleviate fever | • Blood-let DT.04, ear apex<br>• Add DU-14, LI-11, LI-4 |

---

### Blood Letting Treatment

- Bleed-cup  DU-14  and  BL-13 especially with headache and alleviate fever
- Bleed  LU-10 or  LU-11 - for sore throat
- Bloodlet: BL-41 to BL-44, BL-11 to BL-15 - severe common cold
- Bleed 99.08 Er San (Ear Apex), bleed LU-11 to accelerate recovery

*Points Illustrations for treatment of Common Cold*

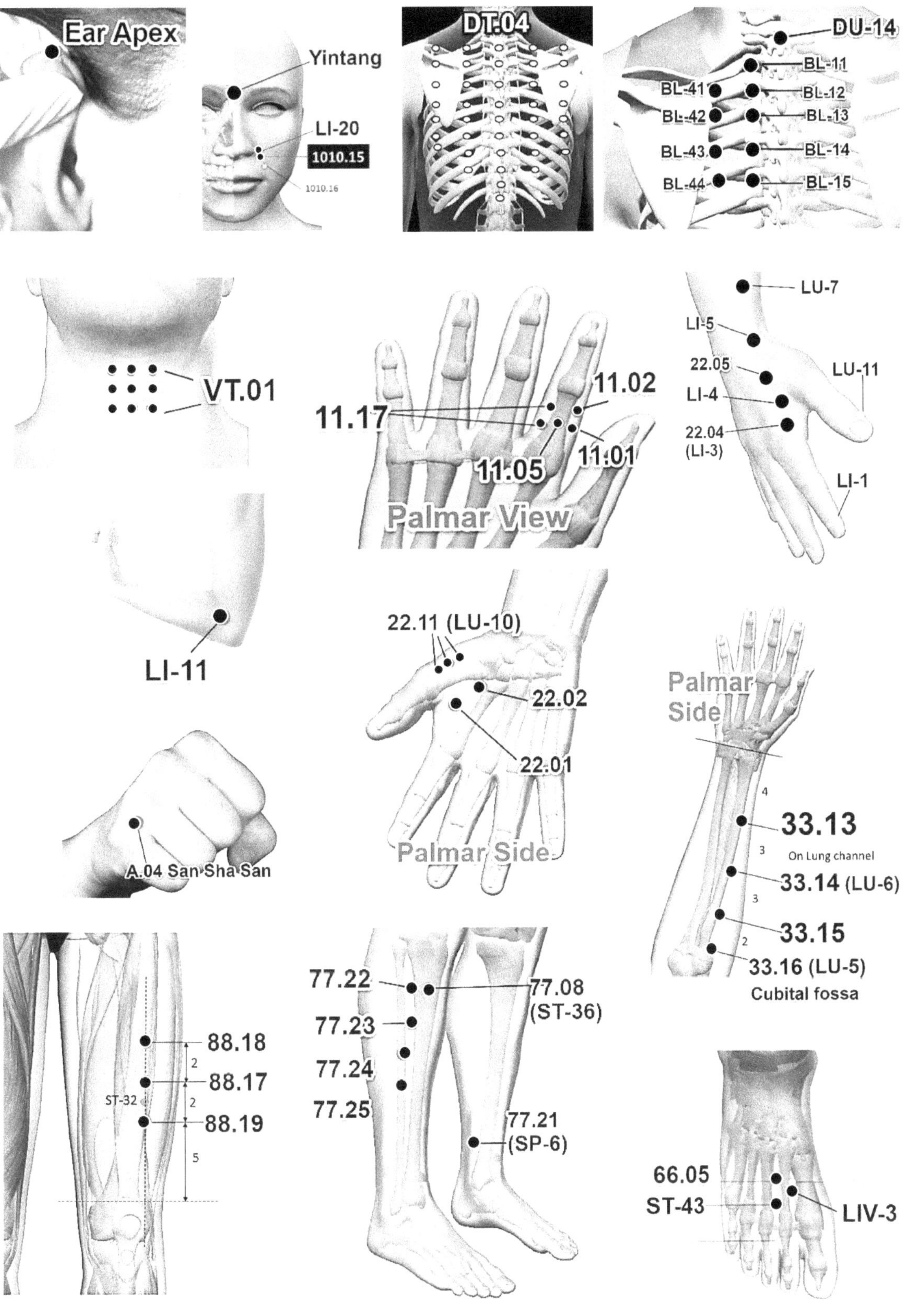

# Nasal Issues

*The meridians (energy pathways) that are commonly involved in nasal issues include:*

***Lung meridian:*** *The Lung meridian governs the respiratory system, and is closely related to the nose and sinuses. When there is an imbalance in the Lung meridian, it can result in symptoms such as coughing, wheezing, and nasal congestion.*

***Large Intestine meridian:*** *The Large Intestine meridian is connected to the nose and sinuses, and an imbalance in this meridian can lead to symptoms such as nasal discharge and congestion.*

***Stomach meridian:*** *The Stomach meridian runs through the face and nose, and an imbalance in this meridian can result in symptoms such as nasal inflammation and swelling.*

***Triple Warmer meridian:*** *The Triple Warmer meridian governs the body's overall energy flow and is closely related to the immune system. When there is an imbalance in this meridian, it can result in symptoms such as nasal congestion, runny nose, and sinusitis.*

**Effective points for nasal issues are:**
- 88.17 Si Ma Zhong+88.18 Si Ma Shang+88.19 Si Ma Xia.
- LI-20 (1010.15) -Guide point
- 11.17
- 4 Gates (LI-4 and LIV-3)

**Treatment for Nasal obstruction**
- 44.06 Jian Zhong
- LI-20, 11.17 Mu
- 88.17 Si Ma Zhong+88.18 Si Ma Shang+88.19 Si Ma Xia
- 66.03 Huo Ying+66.04 Huo Zhu + 66.05 Men Jin +ST-44
- 77.22 + 77.23
- Point 33.07 Huo Fu Hai (LI-10) is effective.

**Treatment for Sinusitis, allergic rhinitis**
- 88.17 Si Ma Zhong+88.18 Si Ma Shang+88.19 Si Ma Xia
- 88.01 Tong Guan+88.02 Tong Shan+88.03 Tong Tian
- 11.17 Mu, LI-20
- SP-3 and 66.04 Huo Zhu

**Nose bleeding**
- 44.06
- 66.04 (LIV-3), LI-4 (4 Gates), 66.08

---

### Blood-letting Treatment for nose obstruction and allergy
- 99.08 Er San (Ear Apex), BL-4
- 22.11 Tu Shui
- Blue veins around 77.14 Si Hua Wai - *chronic rhinitis*
- Yintang [Ex. 1.] or Ex-HN-3
- 1010.12 Zheng Ben
- Around DT.07 San Jin
- BL-2

*Points Illustrations for treatment of Nasal Issues*

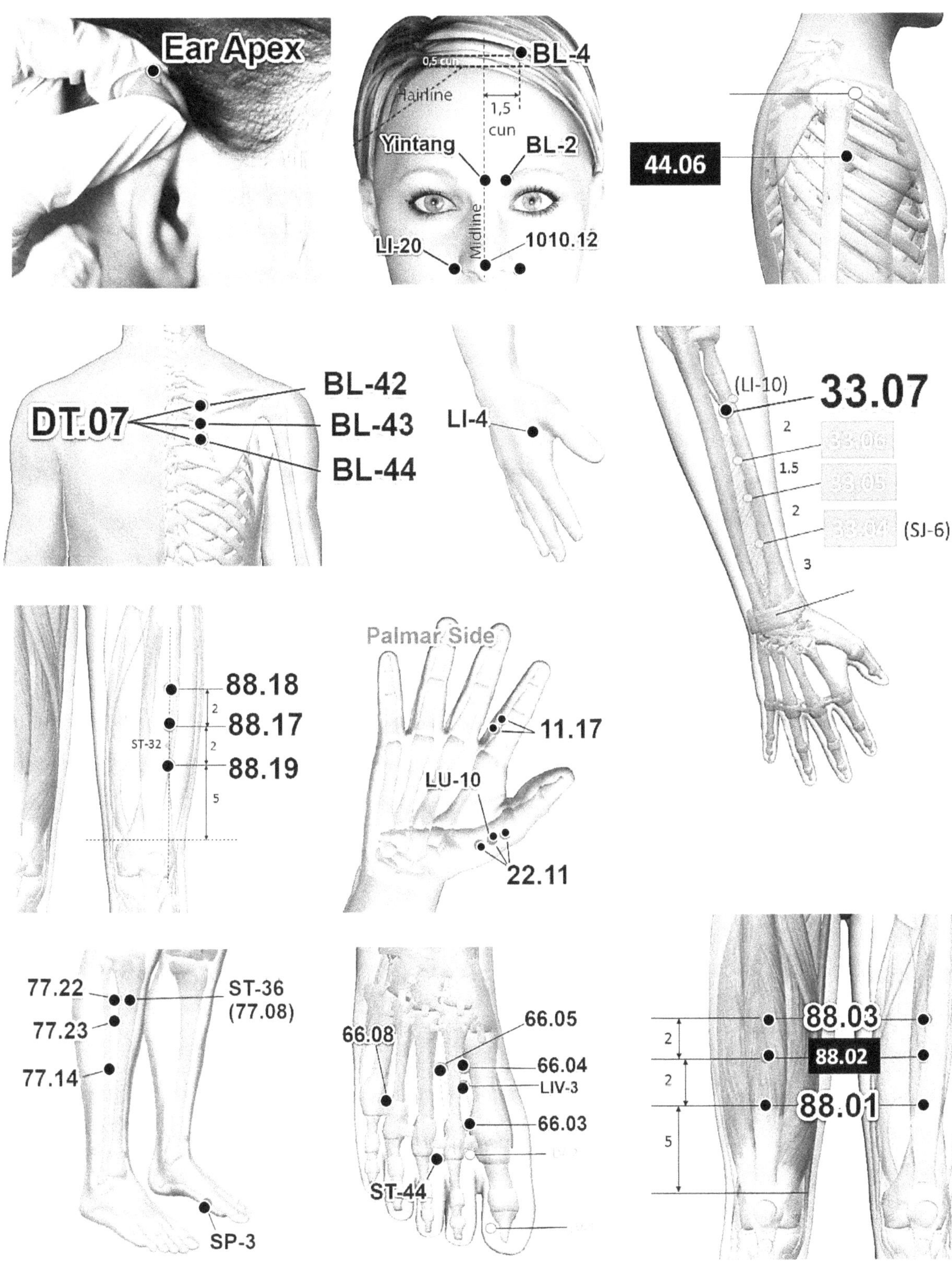

# Cough, Bronchitis

*The **Lung channel(meridian)** is considered to be the primary channel affected by cough, as it is responsible for the flow of Qi and oxygen to the respiratory system.  The **Large Intestine channel** is also thought to be affected by cough, as it is closely related to the Lung channel in TCM theory.*

*Other channels that may be affected by cough include the **Stomach channel** and the **Spleen channel.***

**Needling Treatment**

- 1010.20 Shui Jin with 22.11 Tu Shui (LU-10) - For cough in the morning (Dr. Young)
- 1010.20 Shui Jin and 33.16 Qu Ling (LU-5) - For cough in the afternoon (Dr. Young)
- 1010.19 Shui Tong+1010.20 Shui Jin with 88.17 Si Ma Zhong+88.18 Si Ma Shang+88.19 Si Ma Xia or A.04 San Cha San - effective combination for severe common cold, bronchitis, cough, pleurisy, or emphysema.
- 33.13 Ren Shi+33.14 Di Shi+33.15 Tian Shi, 1010.19 Shui Tong+1010.20 Shui Jin - chronic cough
- 33.13 Ren Shi+33.14 Di Shi+33.15 Tian Shi, 22.01 Chong Zi+22.02 Chong Xian- cough with upper back and/or chest pain)
- BL-11 +BL-12+BL-13
- REN-17, REN-22

**Cupping Neck/ Upper Back**

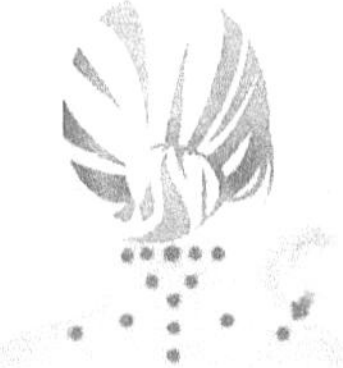

**Cupping and Blood-letting for Cough/Bronchitis**

- Cup the entire neck and upper back (with the patient sitting upright)
- Lung area of the back as shown on opposite page. Wet-cup tender points.
- Cubital fossa, around 33.16 Qu Ling (LU-5)
- Visible veins in the leg, especially lateral leg

*Points Illustrations for treatment of Cough, Bronchitis*

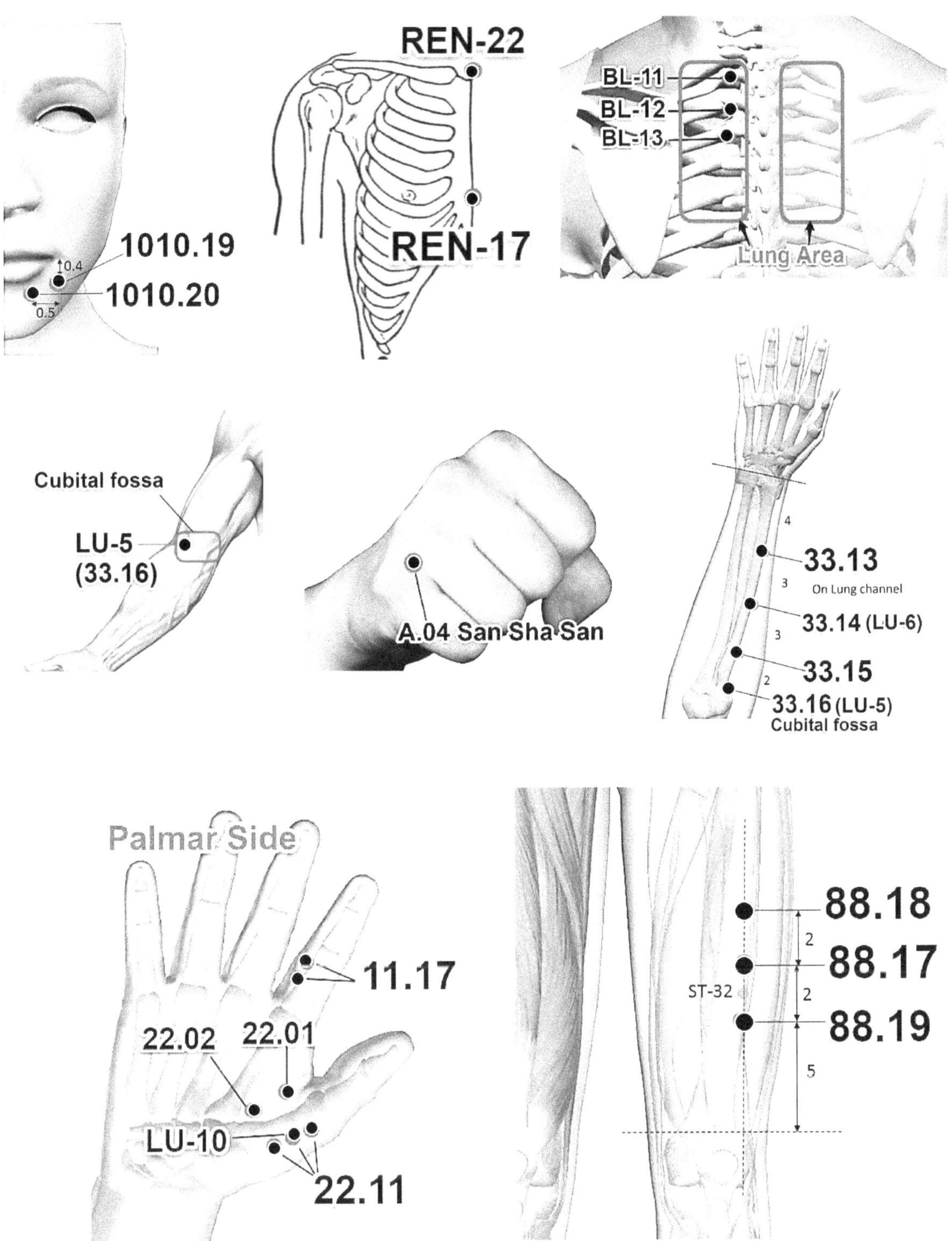

# GASTRO-INTESTINAL

## Nausea and Vomiting

*The **Stomach channel** is closely related to the digestive system and is often used to treat nausea and vomiting caused by improper diet or digestive disorders. The **Pericardium channel** is associated with the heart and emotional health and is often used to treat nausea and vomiting caused by emotional stress or anxiety.*

*Other channels that may be involved in the treatment of nausea and vomiting include the **Liver channel** and the **Gallbladder channel.***

**Treatment for Nausea and vomiting**

- Needle 1010.19 Shui Tong+1010.20 Shui Jin
- Needle P-5, P-6, P-7, P-8
- REN-12
- LIV-13
- ST-36

---

### Blood-letting Treatment
- Bleed DT.03 Qi Xing or 1010.07 Zong Shu or bleed DU-16. Pinch the skin when pricking. Gua sha the area can be helpful.
- Bleed 77.09 Si Hua Zhong, then needle 1010.19 Shui Tong+1010.20 Shui Jin

*Points Illustrations for treatment of Nausea and Vomiting*

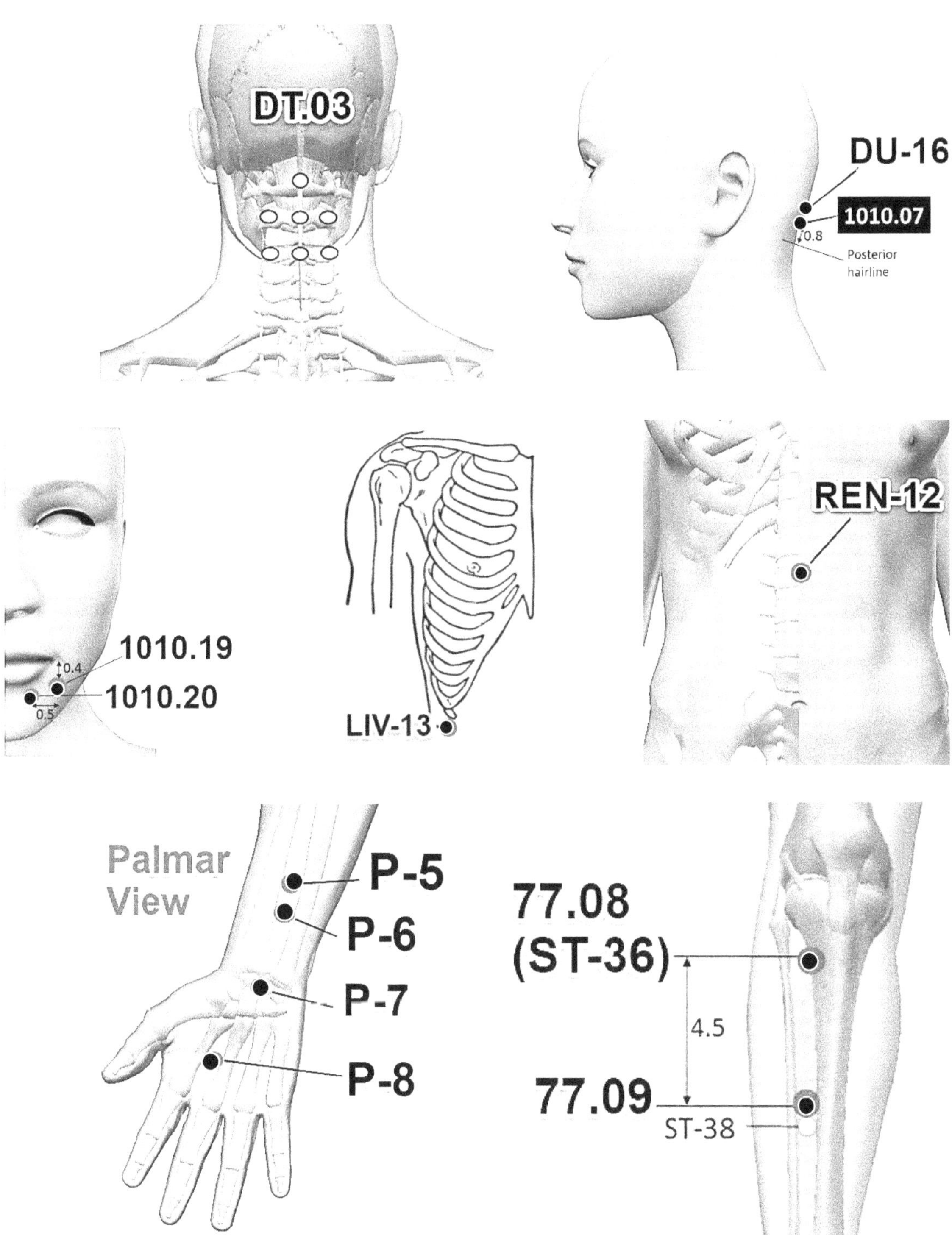

# Rectal (Anus) Pain/Hemorrhoids

*Swollen veins in the lower part of rectum and anus that causes bleeding and discomfort. Sharp pain in the anus is mostly caused by anal fissure or external hemorrhoids while burning pain of the anus is often caused by anal fissure or abscess at the anus. Hemorrhoids are essentially varicose veins of the anus and lower rectum and, like varicose veins, they respond exceptionally well to bloodletting.*

*The **Large Intestine channel** is closely related to the digestive system and is often used to treat hemorrhoids and other digestive disorders. The **Liver channel** is associated with the smooth flow of Qi and blood in the body and is often used to treat stagnation in the lower part of the body.*

*Other channels that may be involved in the treatment of rectal pain and hemorrhoids include the **Spleen channel and the Kidney channel.***

**Treatment for Hemorrhoids and constipation**

- Extra point EX-UE-2 ERBAI (located four cun proximal to P-7 on both sides of the tendon)
- Combine with 33.04 Huo Chuan (SJ-6)
- 33.01 Qi Men+33.02 Qi Jiao+ 33.03 Qi Zheng
- 1010.01 Zheng Hui (DU-20) – Top treats bottom
- 77.04 Bo Qiu and BL-57 (specific for hemorrhoids)
- 66.05 Men Jin ( ST-44) - anal prolapse
- Needle around the umbilucus (holographic umbilucus to anus). Moxibustion applicable.
- BL-25, BL-32, BL-54 (moxibustion applicable)

---

### Blood-letting Treatment - Highly effective

- Bleeding in the popliteal crease, BL-40 area (esp. if dark veins present) is highly effective in treating hemorrhoids.
- Bleed all bleed-able veins around BL-40 to BL-57 and around 77.04, weekly.
- Bleed BL-25, BL-32
- Bleed veins around SP-7, SP-8, SP-9 and back of calf
- Bleed DU-28 if there are blisters- Meeting point of REN, DU and ST (Foot Yang Ming) meridians
- Bleed 77.09 and 77.14 for bleeding before and after bowel movement. Followed by needling 88.04+88.05+88.06
- Prick 11.26 to assist wound healing

*Points Illustrations for treatment of Hemorrhoids*

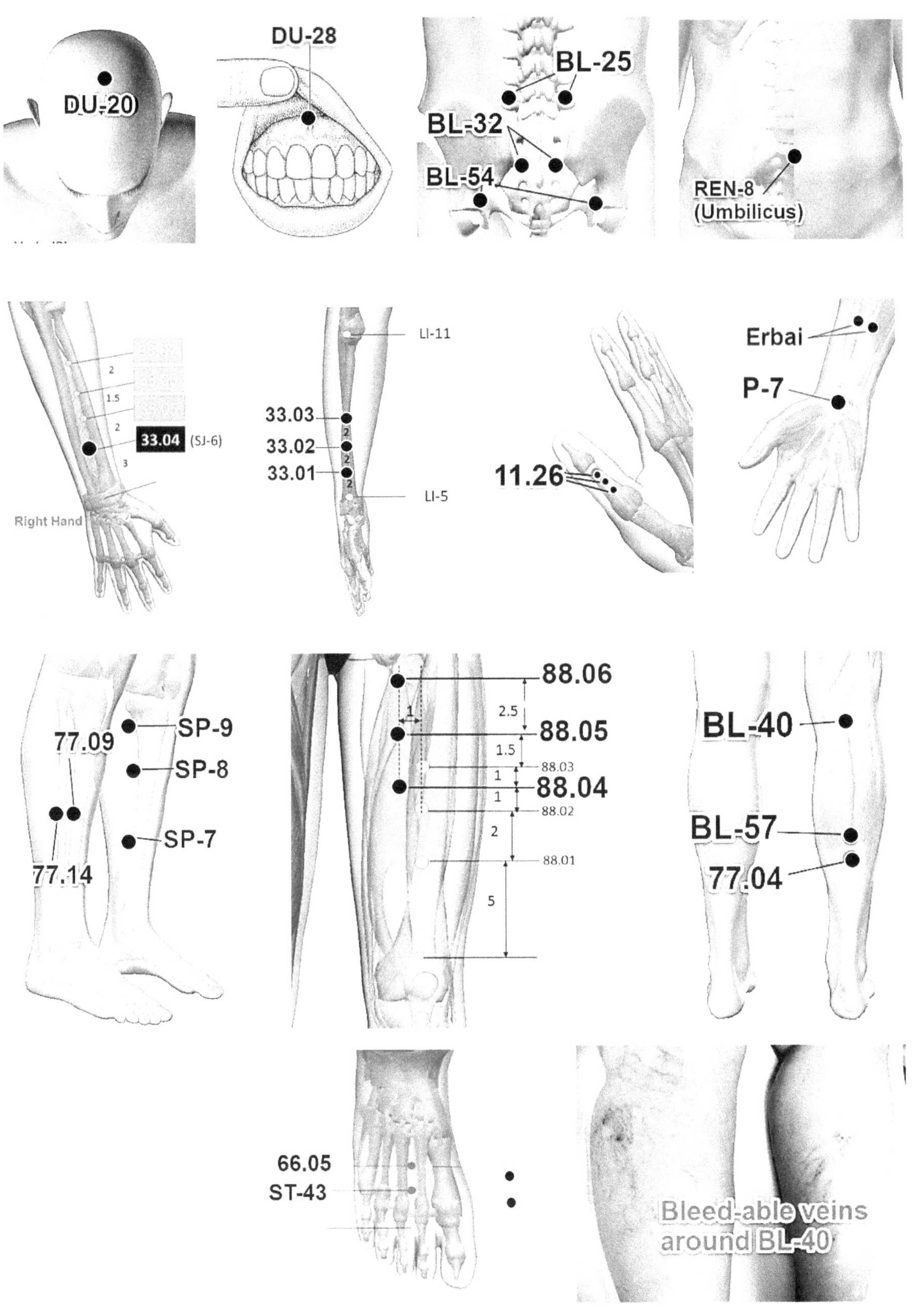

# Constipation

*The **Stomach channel** is closely related to the digestive system and is often used to promote digestion and regulate bowel movements. The **Large Intestine channel** is associated with the elimination of waste from the body and is often used to stimulate peristalsis and promote regular bowel movements.*

*Other channels that may be involved in the treatment of constipation include the **Spleen channel and the Kidney channel.***

*Dietary changes can be an effective way to address this imbalance and promote regular bowel movements. Here are some dietary recommendations for constipation according to TCM:*

*Eat warm, cooked foods: In TCM, warm and cooked foods are believed to be easier to digest and promote Qi flow in the digestive system. Raw and cold foods are thought to weaken the digestive system and contribute to Qi stagnation*

*Increase fiber intake: Fiber is important for maintaining regular bowel movements and preventing constipation. However, do not over-consume as they can be hard to digest.*

*Stay hydrated: Drinking plenty of fluids, especially warm water, can help to promote bowel movements and prevent constipation. Avoid drinking too many cold or iced beverages, as they can weaken the digestive system and contribute to Qi stagnation.*

*Eat on a regular schedule.*

*Avoid greasy or fatty foods.*

**Treatment**

- 33.04 Huo Chuan (SJ-6) and 33.05 is primarily used for constipation because it regulates qi and controls fire.
- 33.01 Qi Men.jpg+33.02 Qi Jiao+ 33.03 Qi Zheng.jpg -stubborn constipation
- REN-12, ST-25, ST-36 – abdominal pain and constipation
- 22.05 Ling Gu + 66.05 Men Jin
- 66.13 Shui Jing (KI-6) can be added; together they regulate qi and tonify fluids.
- SJ-5+ST-25+KID-6
- Acupressure ST-25 or SP-15 bilateral, first thing in the morning in a comfortable lying down position with a below underneath the knees

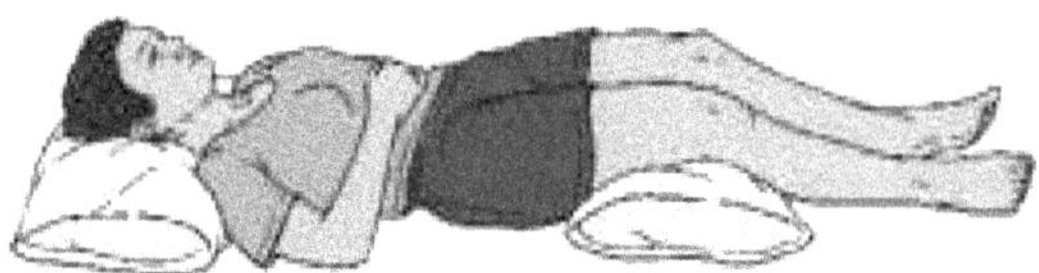

**Blood-letting Treatment**

1. Bleed over sacrum - chronic constipation
2. Bleed DT.13 Shui Zhong, DT.14 Shui Fu
3. LI-1
4. Moxibustion RN-8

*Points Illustrations for treatment of Constipation*

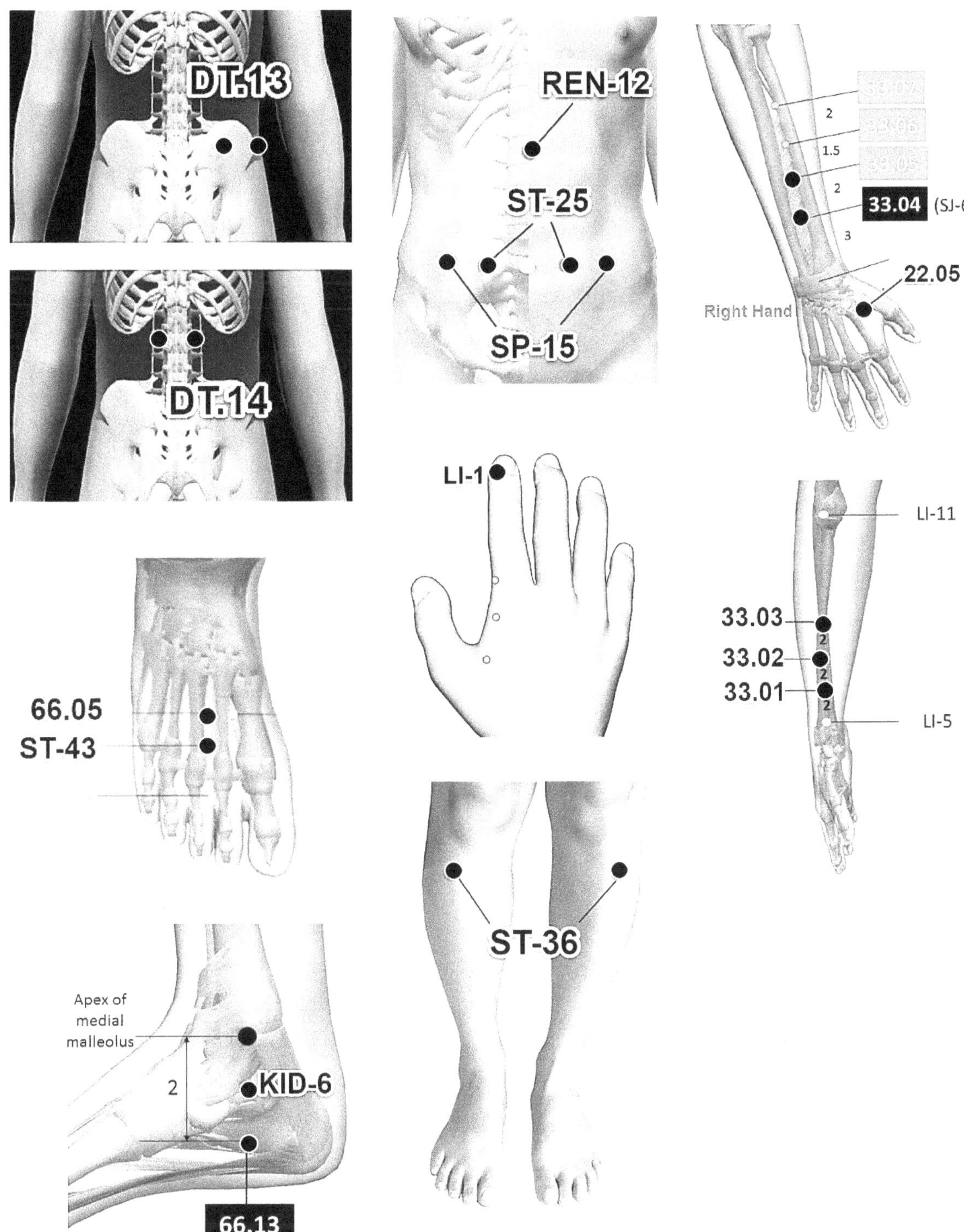

# Diarrhea

*The **Spleen channel** is closely related to the digestive system and is often used to regulate the flow of Qi and promote healthy digestion. The **Stomach channel** is also closely related to digestion and is often used to regulate the stomach and intestines and promote the elimination of waste.*

*Other channels that may be involved in the treatment of diarrhea include **the Large Intestine channel and the Kidney channel.***

### Acute diarrhea (non-pathogenic cold-type)

- Bilateral (ST-36) 77.08, 77.09, 77.11 Si Hua Xia+77.12 Fu Chang
- ST-25+ST-36+SP-4
- Moxa between REN-4–REN-12
- Diarrhea Experience Point (Draw a straight line from the center of exterior malleolus to planta, the place at which it meets the border of red and white line of sole is Diarrhea Experience Point). Needling and Moxibustion applicable.

### Severe diarrhea

- 66.05 Men Jin (ST-43), 22.11 Tu Shui
- 33.10 Chang Men+33.11 Gan Men
- LI-11
- 77.11 Si Hua Xia+77.12 Fu Chang
- Add P-6 if there is vomiting
- Gua sha/Moxa from BL-20 to BL-25 area.

---

**Blood-letting Treatment**
1. Bleed 77.09 Si Hua Zhong and 77.14 Si Hua Wai for severe acute case.
2. 22.11 Tu Shui (Bleed blue vein)

*Points Illustrations for treatment of Diarrhea*

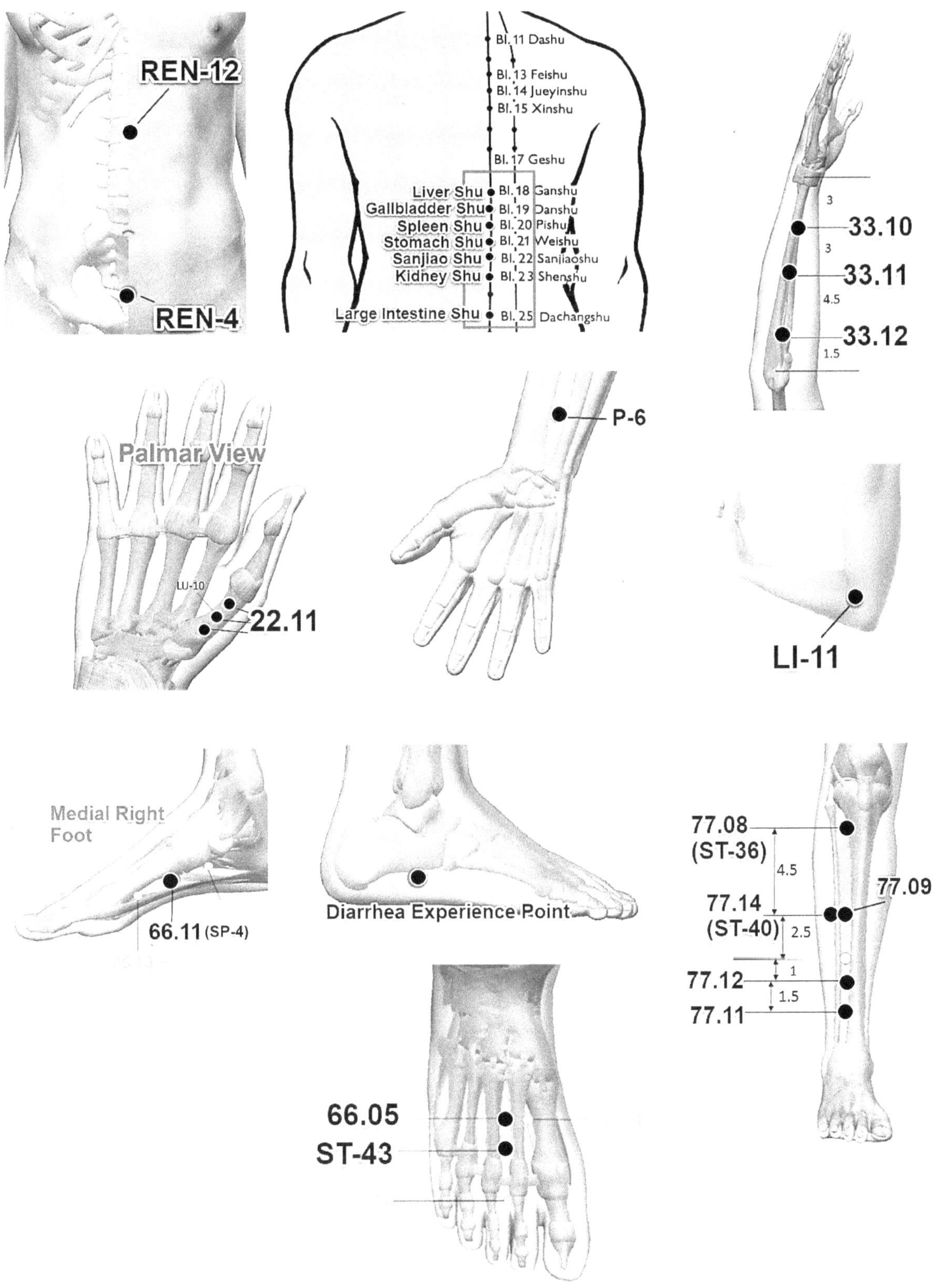

# Gastritis and Stomach-ache

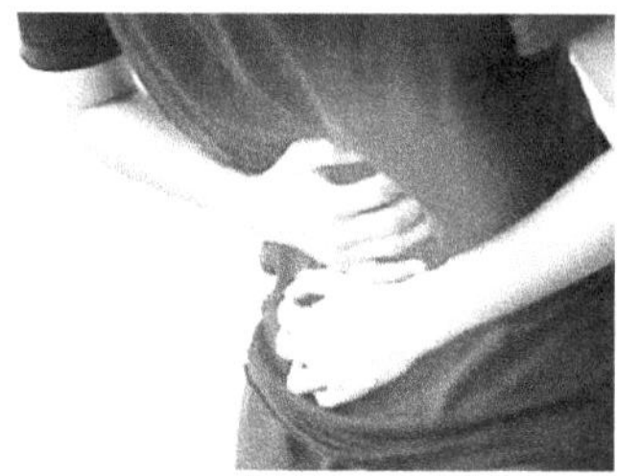

*Related channels include:*

***Stomach Meridian:*** *As the name suggests, this meridian is closely related to the digestive system and is often targeted in the treatment of gastritis.*

***Spleen Meridian****: The spleen meridian is another important channel for the digestive system, as it is responsible for transforming food into Qi and blood.*

***Pericardium Meridian:*** *This meridian is often used in the treatment of emotional imbalances that may contribute to gastritis, as it is closely associated with the heart and emotions*

***Gallbladder Meridian:*** *The gallbladder meridian is often targeted in cases where there is excess heat or inflammation in the digestive system.*

***Liver Meridian:*** *The liver meridian is also closely related to the digestive system, as it is responsible for storing and regulating the flow of blood.*

**Common TCM Treatment Points**
- Needle REN-12, ST-25, LI-11, ST-34, ST-36, P-6, SP-6, GB-34, LIV-3
- Moxibustion REN-12, LIV-13, ST-36, BL-17, BL-20, BL-21. Gua sha is applicable.

| AFFECTED (SICK) MERIDIANS | TREATMENT POINTS |
|---|---|
| **STOMACH**<br>Foot Yangming | • ST-44, 66.05 (ST-43)<br>• ST-34 - Xi-Cleft point. Treats own meridian. For acute pain, ulcers.<br>• ST-36 - He-sea point. Treats own meridian. Even better if bleed around ST-36.<br>• REN-12 - Treats the stomach. Alarm point [Mu-Front] of the Stomach.<br>• 77.01 Zheng Jin - Treating tendons reduces spasm pain.<br>• Bleed around 77.08, 77.09 and 77.14 Si Hua Wai - Treats own meridian. |
| **LUNG**<br>Hand Tai Yin.<br>Pathway connects to the stomach | • Yintang [Ex. 1.] or Ex-HN-3 associated with lung disorders<br>• 22.11 Tu Shui (LU-10) - Treats the Lung pathway |

### Blood-letting for Gastric and digestive conditions and pain
- Visible veins on the lower leg, especially ST-36 region, also BL-40 region.
- Bleed any visible veins around 22.11 (LU-10)
- Bleed around 77.08 Si Hua Shang, 77.09 Si Hua Zhong and 77.14 Si Hua Wai - Treats own meridian.
- DT.15 San Jiang. Palpate and wet-cup where tender.
- Bleed 11.26 if there are ulcers.

*Points Illustrations for treatment of Gastritis and Stomach-ache*

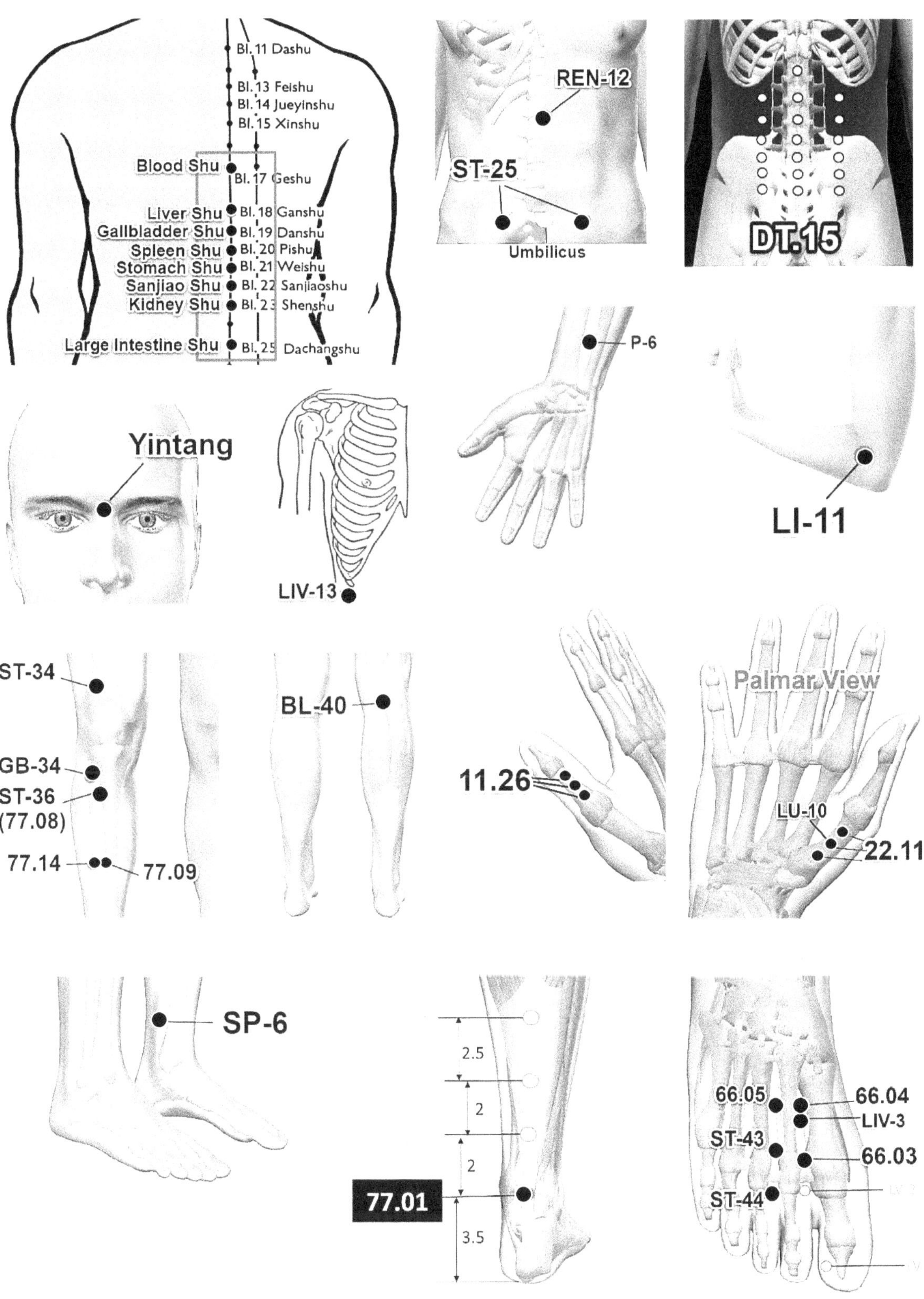

# <u>SKIN</u>

## Psoriasis

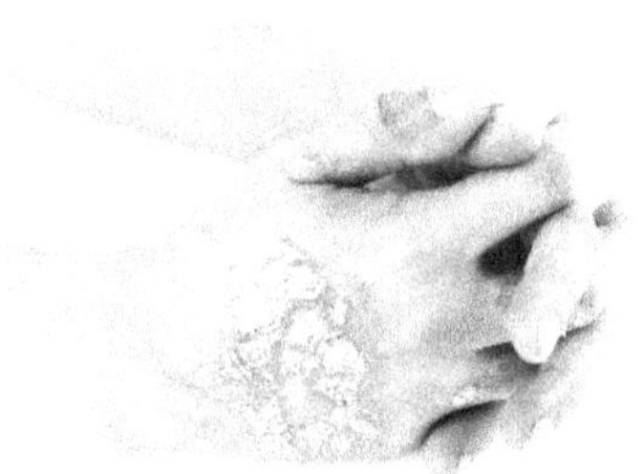

*Psoriasis is an autoimmune condition that causes inflammation in your skin. Symptoms of psoriasis include thick areas of discolored skin covered with scales. These thick, scaly areas are called plaques.*

*In Traditional Chinese Medicine (TCM), psoriasis is often considered as a manifestation of "Blood Heat" syndrome. This syndrome is believed to arise from a combination of internal heat, stagnation of blood and wind, and may involve the **Lung, Stomach, and Liver channels.***

*The **Lung channel** is responsible for regulating the skin and hair, and its function is often compromised in psoriasis. The **Stomach channel** is responsible for digestion and absorption of nutrients, and its dysfunction can result in a buildup of internal heat, leading to psoriasis. The **Liver channel** is responsible for the free flow of Qi (vital energy) and blood, and its stagnation can contribute to the development of psoriasis.*

**Treatment for psoriasis**

- 33.13, 33.14 (LU-6), 33.15, 33.16 (LU-5) – On Lung Meridian. LU-6 is Xi-Cleft point.
- Bilateral 88.17 Si Ma Zhong+88.18 Si Ma Shang+88.19 Si Ma Xia – Lung Reaction Area
- Bilaterally needle A.04 San Cha San
- LI-11, SP-6
- SP-10 (specific point for allergy)
- ST-36
- 77.21 Ren Huang (SP-6)
- LIV-3 (66.04), 11.17 Mu - psoriasis on hands
- "Surround the dragon" needling of affected area.
- Moxa affected area over garlic paste

---

### Cupping/Blood-letting for Psoriasis

- Bleed 99.07 Er Bei and/or Ear Apex
- Bleed-cup BL-13, BL-14
- Bleed LU-5 area
- Bleed BL-40 area
- Bleed cup affected area
- Cup DT.01 Fen Zhi Shang+DT.02 Fen Zhi Xia if free of psoriasis.
- To promote healing in areas with larger lesions, use a technique known as "seven-star hammer" on the healthy skin just outside of the affected area ("surrounding the dragon"). Avoid lesions that are injured or bleeding.

*Points Illustrations for treatment of Psoriasis*

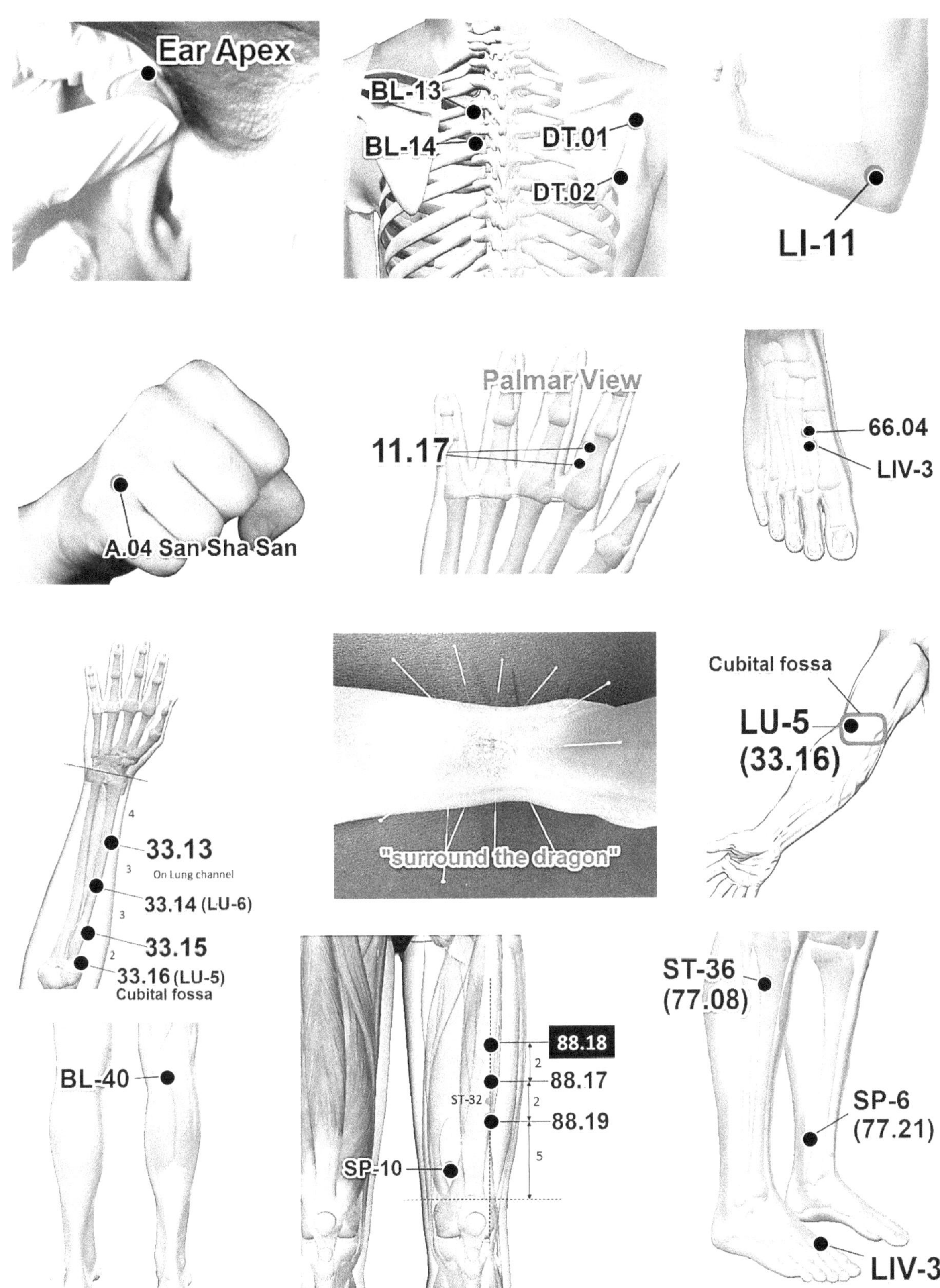

# Skin Diseases

*Acne: In TCM, acne is often considered as a manifestation of "Damp-Heat" syndrome, which involves **the Stomach, Spleen, and Lung channels.***

*Eczema: Eczema is a chronic skin condition characterized by dry, itchy, and inflamed skin. In TCM, eczema is often related to "Blood Heat" syndrome, which involves the **Liver and Gallbladder channels***

**Acne**
- LI-11, ST-36, SP-10, SP-6
- 88.17 Si Ma Zhong+88.18 Si Ma Shang+88.19 Si Ma Xia
- A.04 San Cha San
- 1010.15 Fu Kuai (LI-20) - Guide Point and treat 1-3 times weekly.
- Local points applicable.
- Gua sha BL-13, BL-20, BL-21, BL-25 zones

**Itching and rashes (eczema)/urticaria (hives)**
- 88.17 Si Ma Zhong+88.18 Si Ma Shang+88.19 Si Ma Xia - bilateral
- SP-6 strengthens the Spleen and eliminates dampness.
- SP-10 cools the blood and removes dampness to stop itching.
- A.04 San Cha San
- 88.25 (GB-31) – wind point
- LI-11 Qu Chi clears heat, cools the blood, expels wind and alleviates itching.
- HT-8 is very good for itching because itching and pain belong to the Heart.
- 44.06 Jian Zhong
- 11.17 (needle disease side)
- LI-20 – itching on face
- Cup the navel
- Gua sha BL-13, BL-20, BL-21, BL-25 zones

---

### Blood-letting for itching and skin conditions
- Bleed 99.07 Er Bei, 99.08 Er San Ear Apex once a week.
- For severe itching, seven-star hammer or plum blossom affected, light tapping on perimeter of the eczema and moxibustion is applicable.
- Plum blossom both sides of the spinal column, affected area
- Bleed cup DT.01 Fen Zhi Shang+DT.02 Fen Zhi Xia
- Bleed DU-14, BL-13, BL-14, BL-40
- Visible veins on the legs
- Bleed 11.26, 77.14 for shingles
- Plum blossom or wet-cup shingles affected area after scabs have fallen off.

*Points Illustrations for treatment of Skin Diseases*

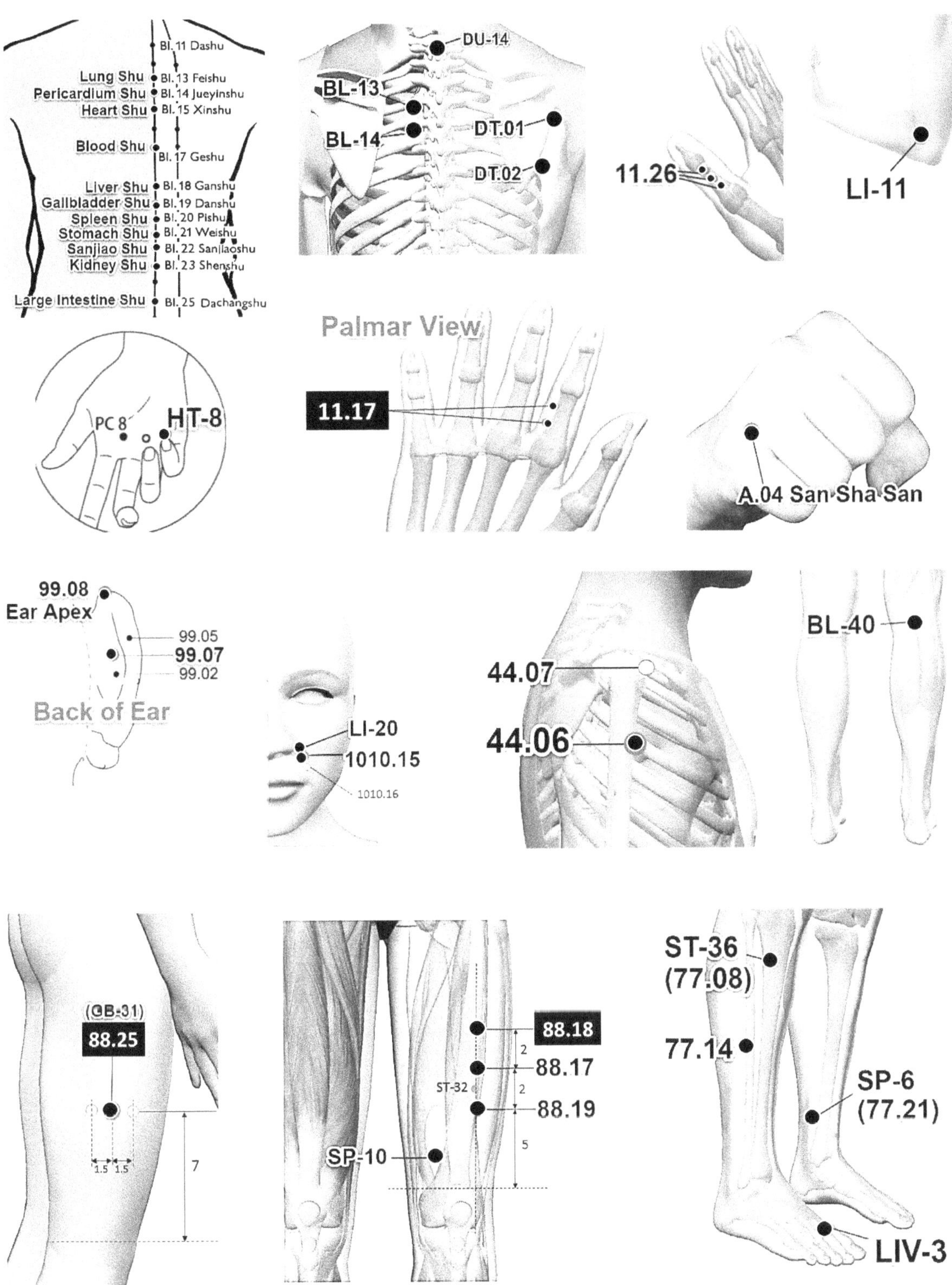

# KIDNEY AND URINARY

## Renal Colic

*Renal colic is usually related to the presence of kidney stones, which cause sudden and severe pain in the back and abdomen. According to TCM theory, the **Urinary Bladder and Kidney channels** are closely related and form a functional unit that regulates the body's water metabolism. Therefore, the treatment of renal colic in TCM aims to clear the obstruction and restore the normal flow of Qi and blood in the Urinary Bladder and Kidney channels. This is believed to help eliminate the dampness and heat accumulation, reduce inflammation, and alleviate pain.*

**Pain relief for Kidney stone with back pain**

- 88.09+88.10+88.11
- 1010.13 Ma Jin Shui +1010.14 Ma Kuai Shu
- BL-23 – specific point for acute renal colic
- KID-5 – Xi-Cleft point
- EX-UE-7 Yaotongdian- same side as pain
- Moxa REN-3, REN-4, REN-10

| AFFECTED (SICK) MERIDIANS | TREATMENT POINTS |
|---|---|
| **URINARY BLADDER** <br> Foot Taiyang | <ul><li>BL-57 - Treats own meridian</li><li>BL-23 - Back Shu of the Kidney. Treats own meridian</li><li>1010.13 Ma Jin Shui +1010.14 Ma Kuai Shui- SI channel treats Bladder</li></ul> |
| **KIDNEY** <br> Foot Shao Yin | <ul><li>22.06 Zhong Bai + 22.07 Xia Bai - SJ treats Kidney (System 2)</li><li>SJ-3 - SJ treats Kidney (System 2)</li><li>KID-3 - Shu Stream Point on the Kidney Channel. Yuan Source on the Kidney Channel. Treats own meridian.</li><li>KID-5 – Xi Cleft point fort pain relief</li><li>SJ-5 - Luo-connecting point. SJ treats Kidney (System 2)</li><li>BL-57 - BL treats Kidney (System 3)</li><li>BL-23 - BL treats Kidney (System 3)</li><li>BL-25, BL-28, BL-32, BL-54</li></ul> |
| **LIVER** <br> Foot Jue Yin | <ul><li>LIV-3 (66.04 Huo Zhu) - Shu-stream point of Liver Meridian. Yuan source point. For ureter stones, biliary colic and renal colic.</li><li>Treats own meridian.</li></ul> |
| **STOMACH** <br> Foot Yang Ming | <ul><li>ST-36 - He-sea point. Treats abdominal issues.</li></ul> |

---

**Blood-letting for Pain from kidney stones**

- Palpate VT.05 Fu Chao'er Shi San (Bowel Nest 23) area and bleed-cup tender points
- 44.17 Shui Yu (same as SI-10)
- Visible veins on the leg, especially the lateral leg
- Veins to between the medial malleolus and SP-6.
- Bleed BL-40

*Points Illustrations for treatment of Renal Colic*

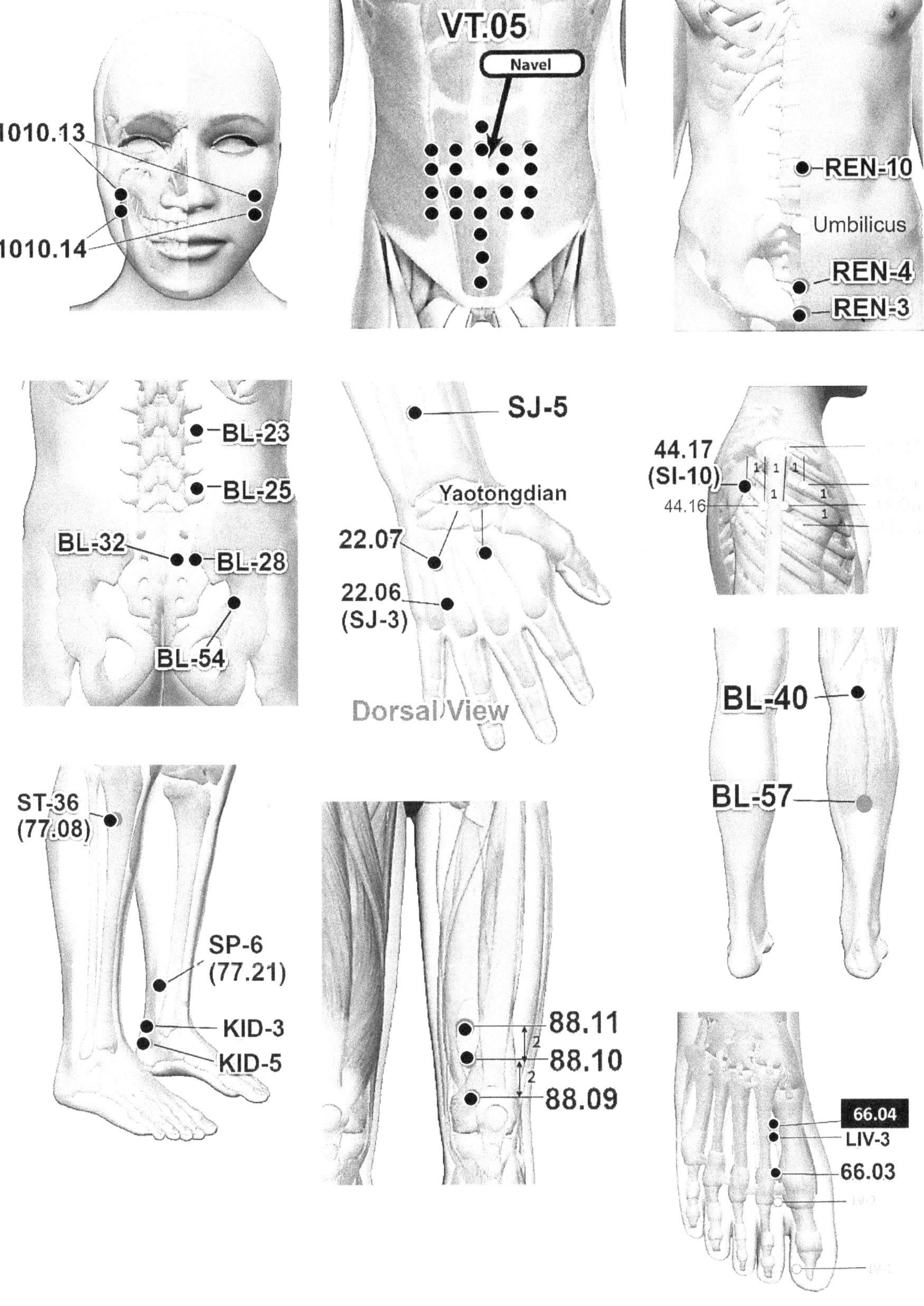

# Kidney Failure

*In TCM, the **Kidney channel** is closely related to the Kidney organ and is responsible for regulating the flow of Qi and blood to the Kidney and other related organs. It is connected with the **Bladder channel**, which also plays an important role in regulating water metabolism and eliminating waste products from the body.*

*Other related channels that may be involved in kidney failure in TCM include: **Ren Mai (Conception Vessel), Du Mai (Governing Vessel) and Chong Mai (Penetrating Vessel.***

**Treatment for cysts in kidney and liver**
- Cup DT.01 Fen Zhi Shang+DT.02 Fen Zhi Xia Toxin Areas because with the liver and kidneys compromised, toxins may increase in the body.
- Cupping over the ribs on top of the liver, and gently cup the lower back over the kidneys.
- Combine 11.20 Mu Yan and 88.12 Ming Huang+88.13 Tian Huang+88.14 Qi Huang with 77.18 Shen Guan+77.19 Di Huang+77.21 Ren Huang

**Kidney failure**
- Needle 88.09+88.10+88.11 or 77.18+77.19+77.21 (Kidney reaction areas)
- 66.14 Shui Xiang (KI-3)
- 77.17 Tian Huang (SP-9)
- Burn moxa on the navel (over salt and covered with a slice of ginger that is pierced with holes)
- ST-36 (77.08), SP-9 (77.17), REN-9, KI-7 (77.28) – TCM treatment combination

**Nephritis (inflammation of the kidneys)**
- Bilaterally needle 88.09 Tong Shen+88.10 Tong Wei+88.11 Tong Bei
- Or 77.18 Shen Guan or 77.18 Shen Guan+77.19 Di Huang+77.21 Ren Huang
- If chronic with no edema: Bilaterally needle 22.06 Zhong Bai+22.07 Xia Bai, add SI-3 (22.08)
- Acute nephritis: Bleed 44.17 Shui Yu (effective if yellow discharge appears) or bleed BL-40.

**Kidney failure causing edema**
- Moxa REN-9 (effective TCM point for edema)
- Bilateral 88.09 Tong Shen+88.10 Tong Wei+88.11 Tong Bei
- 77.17 Tian Huang or 77.18 Shen Guan+77.19 Di Huang+77.21 Ren Huang
- 77.28 Guang Ming
- 88.03 Tong Tian and 22.06 Zhong Bai+22.07 Xia Bai to treat edematous limbs.
- 77.08 Si Hua Shang (ST-36) and moxibustion REN-8 – assist urination
- Bleed 44.17 Shui Yu to strengthen the kidneys, for edema, nephritis and proteinuria

---

### Blood-letting for Kidney conditions/nephritis
- 44.17 Shui Yu (same as SI-10)
- Palpate VT.05 Fu Chao'er Shi San (Bowel Nest 23) palpate for very tender point and bleed-cup.
- Visible veins on the leg, especially the lateral leg and between the medial malleolus and SP-6.
- Palpate the bladder channel from approximately L2 to S4 and bleed any tender points
- Gua sha BL-23 Shen Shu, BL-52 Zhi Shi and DU-4 Ming Men

*Points Illustrations for treatment of Kidney Failure*

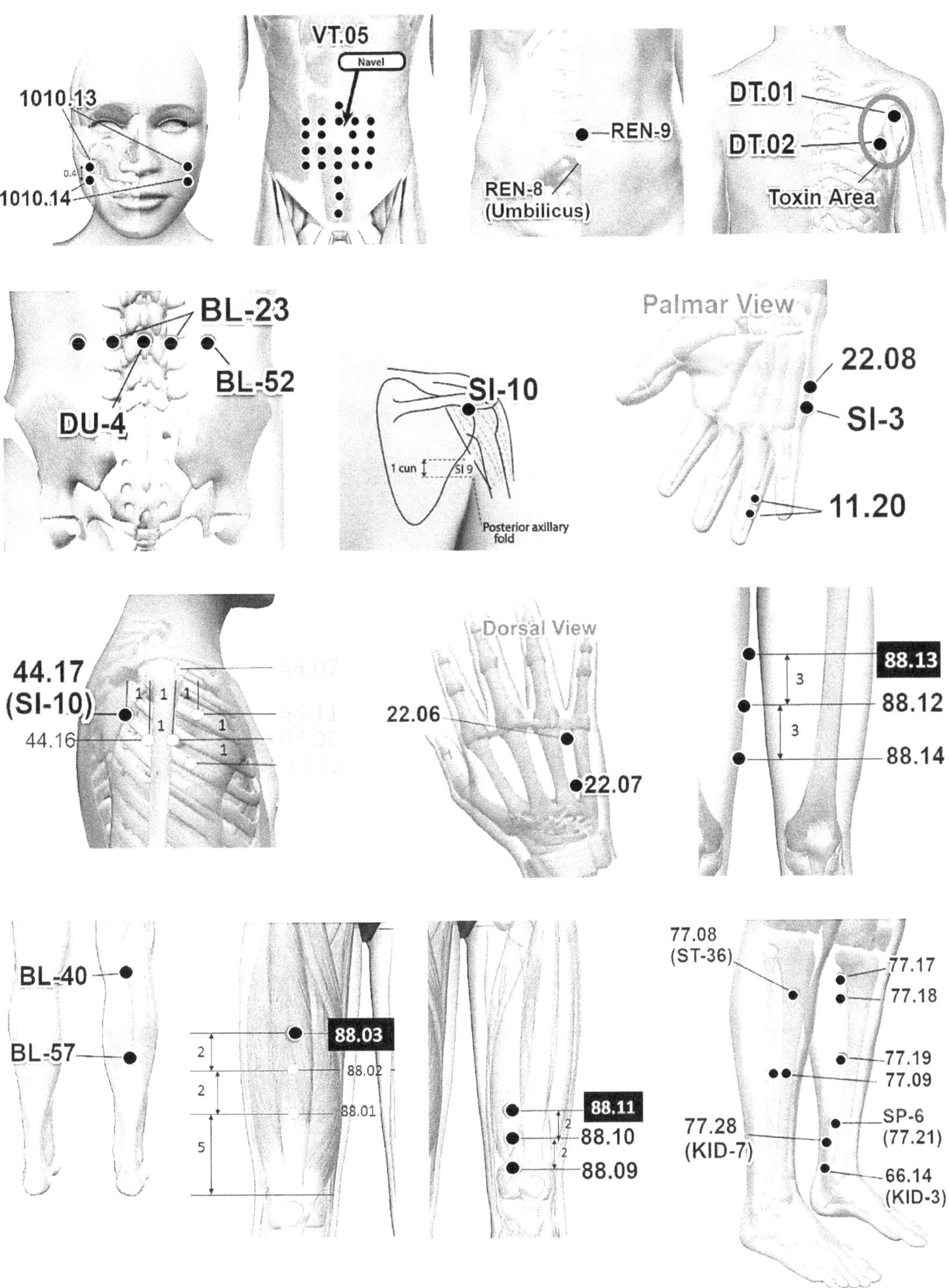

# Urinary Issues

## General Urinary Disorders

- 1010.13 Ma Jin Shui+1010.14 Ma Kuai Shui and/or 77.18 +77.19 +77.21 - for any urinary disorders.
- Add 66.03 +66.04 - for urinary stones, infection or inflammation (including prostatitis)

## Bladder prolapse

- Moxa 1010.01 Zheng Hui (DU-20), DU-4, BL-23 - for bladder prolapse

## Urinary stones

- 001 Hand Golden Gate with 22.07 Xia Bai relieves the pain of kidney stones or gallbladder stones.
- Add 1010.13 Ma Jin Shui+1010.14 Ma Kuai Shui (bladder stone), and 1010.16 Liu Kuai for stones
- Add 11.17 Mu (Anger) for burning urine due to anger.
- REN-3 or REN-4

## Urinary tract infection (UTI)

- 11.17 Mu (Anger) and LI- 4 /LIV-3 or LI-3 /LIV-2 (Anxiety Four Gates) - if there is irritability
- 66.02 Mu Fu, 66.03, 66.04
- 77.18 Shen Guan+77.19 Di Huang+77.21 Ren Huang
- 1010.13 Ma Jin Shui+1010.14 Ma Kuai Shui
- REN-3 or REN-4

## Frequent Urination

- 22.04 Da Bai+22.05 Ling Gu, 77.18 Shen Guan+77.19 Di Huang+77.21 Ren Huang

## Urinary incontinence

- 1010.13 Ma Jin Shui+1010.14 Ma Kuai Shui
- 77.18 Shen Guan+77.19 Di Huang+77.21 Ren Huang for the elderly (weak kidneys)

## Urethralgia (Pain of the urethra)

- 66.03 Huo Ying+66.04 Huo Zhu and 22.04 Da Bai+22.05 Ling Gu – 4 Gates
- 11.01 Da Jian with 11.04 Wai Jian
- 44.11 Yun Bai, 44.12 Li Bai

---

**Blood Letting Treatment**

**Interstitial cystitis** (A chronic, painful bladder condition with increased urinary urgency and frequency)
- Visible veins in the legs, especially the ST-36/GB-34 area and between the medial malleolus and SP-6.
- Visible veins in the BL-40 region

**Kidney conditions/nephritis**
- VT.05 Fu Chao'er Shi San (Bowel Nest 23) palpate for very tender point and wet-cup there, most likely the point above and to the left or right of the navel, depending on which side the pain is.
- 44.17 Shui Yu (same as SI-10)
- Visible veins on the leg, especially the lateral leg and between the medial malleolus and SP-6.
- Palpate the bladder channel from approximately L2 to S4 and bleed any tender spots

**Pain from kidney stones**
- VT.05 Fu Chao'er Shi San (Bowel Nest 23) palpate for a very tender point and wet-cup there
- 44.17 Shui Yu (same as SI-10)
- Visible veins on the leg, especially the lateral leg and between the medial malleolus and SP-6.

*Points Illustrations for Urinary Issues*

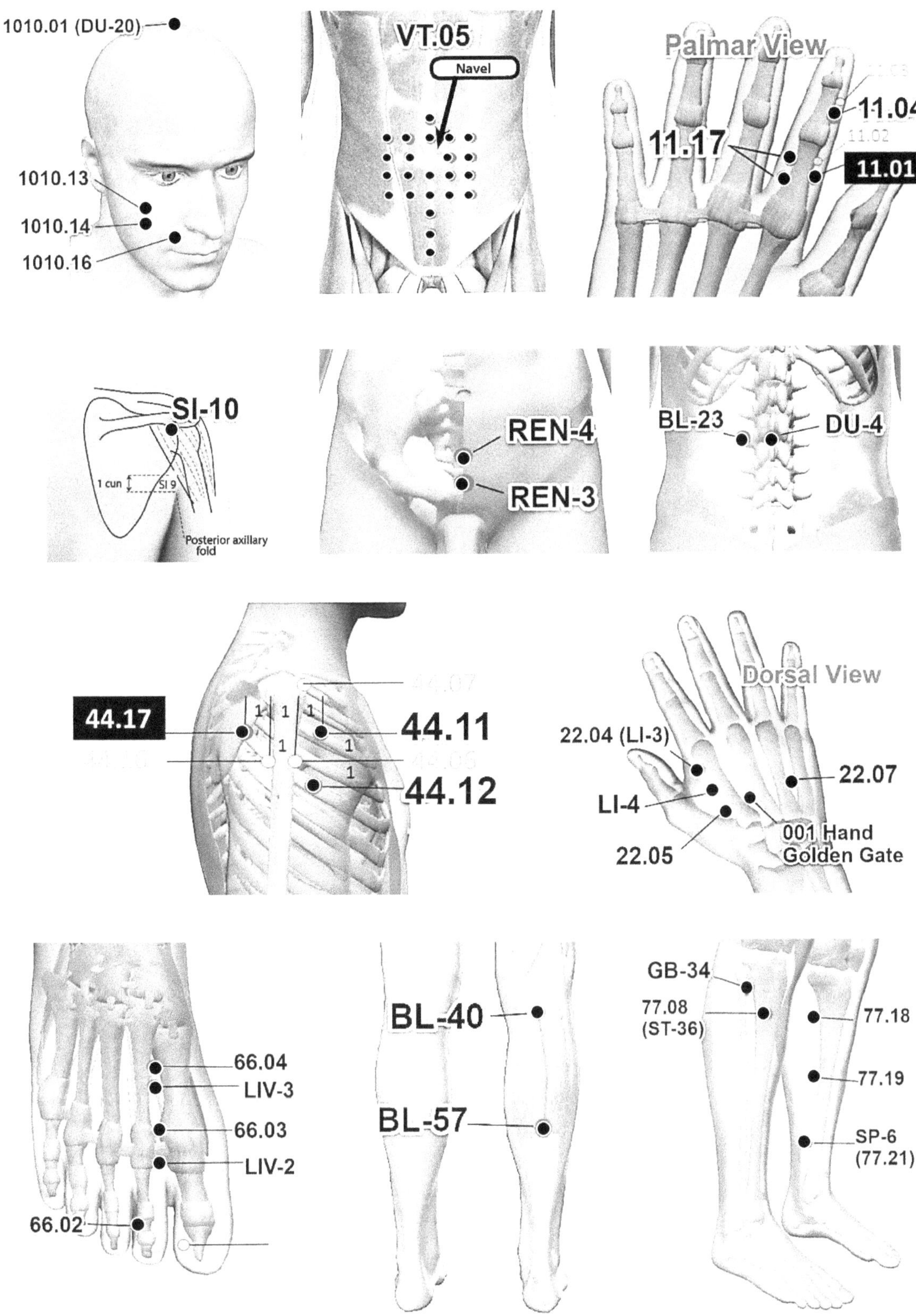

# <u>GYNECOLOGICAL</u>

## Female Infertility

*The Kidney, Liver, Spleen, and Heart channels* are responsible for regulating the body's reproductive functions.

*Kidney Channel:* The Kidney channel is considered the foundation of reproductive energy and is responsible for regulating the menstrual cycle, supporting ovulation, and promoting fertility.

*Liver Channel:* The Liver channel is responsible for regulating the smooth flow of Qi and blood throughout the body, including the reproductive organs. It also plays an important role in regulating the menstrual cycle and promoting the release of the egg.

*Spleen Channel:* The Spleen channel is responsible for transforming and transporting nutrients and fluids throughout the body, including the reproductive organs.

*Heart Channel:* The Heart channel is responsible for regulating the blood circulation and nourishing the uterus and other reproductive organs. It also plays an important role in regulating the emotional state and reducing stress, which can affect fertility.

*Ren Mai (Conception Vessel)* - located on the midline of the body, running from the pubic bone to the lower lip. It is used to tonify the reproductive energy and regulate the menstrual cycle.

**Points to strengthen and regulate Spleen, Liver and Kidney**

- 11.06 Huan Chao + 11.24 Fu Ke - Gynecological Points, one on each side (alternate sides daily for two months; stop after conception).
- 88.04 Jie Mei Yi+88.05 Jie Mei Er+88.06 Jie Mei San
- Three Plum Blossom
- 88.09 Tong Shen+88.10 Tong Wei+88.11 Tong Bei
- 77.18 Shen Guan+77.19 Di Huan+77.21 Ren Huang
- SP-6, KID-3, LIV-3
- 66.13 Shui Jing+66.14 Shui Xiang+66.15 Shui Xian (uterus, kidney, brain issues)
- Dry cupping on REN-4, BL-18 and BL-23 can be helpful

**Moxibustion**

Indirect moxibustion with ginger is used on Guanyuan (REN-4). The ginger should be about 2 cm in diameter and 2-3 mm in thickness. Prick holes in the ginger, before placing a big moxa cone on top. Five cones are used per treatment twice daily, morning and evening before sleep. Ten treatments are one course. Usually, one to five courses are needed. No treatments should be done during the woman's menstruation.

---

### Blood-letting for Infertility

- DT.15 San Jiang. Because bleeding the abdomen is not recommended, we bleed the back to treat the front for intestinal disease, amenorrhea or ovarian disease and male or female infertility.
- Visible veins in the leg, especially the BL-40 region and ST-36 region
- Visible veins around the area between the medial malleolus and SP-6

*Points Illustrations for treatment of Female Infertility*

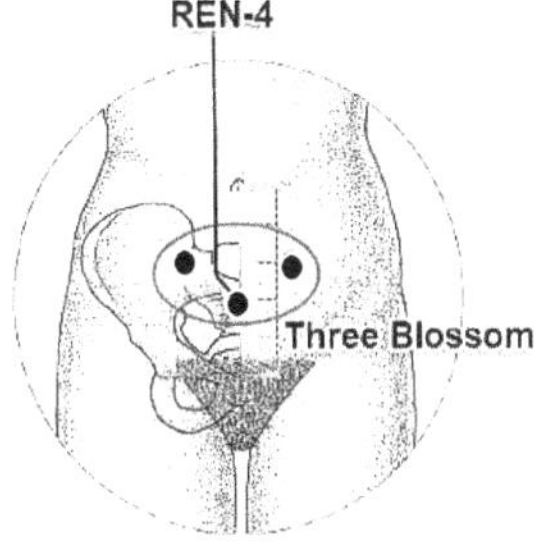


**Three Plum Blossom.** This three-point unit is located on the abdomen. The first point is 3.0 cun inferior to the navel; the other two points are found bilaterally, 2.0 cun inferior to the navel and 2.0 cun lateral to the midline. When treating infertility, Three Plum Blossom clears uterine stagnation and cleans the womb, treating damp heat conditions such as endometriosis and pelvic inflammatory disease (PID). Three Plum Blossom points are not used after ovulation when patients are trying to conceive. *(Credit to Dr. Susan Johnson)*

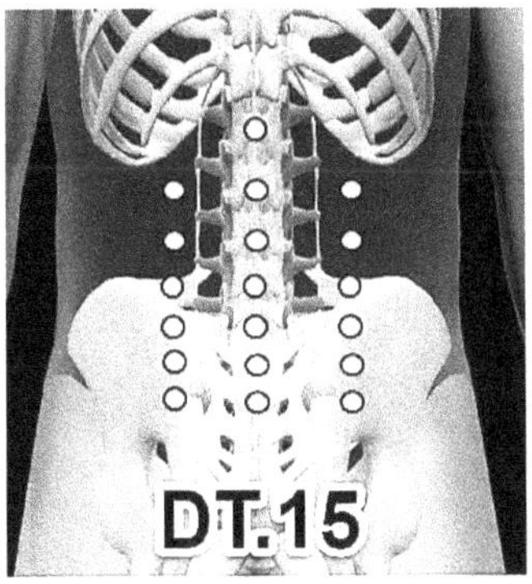

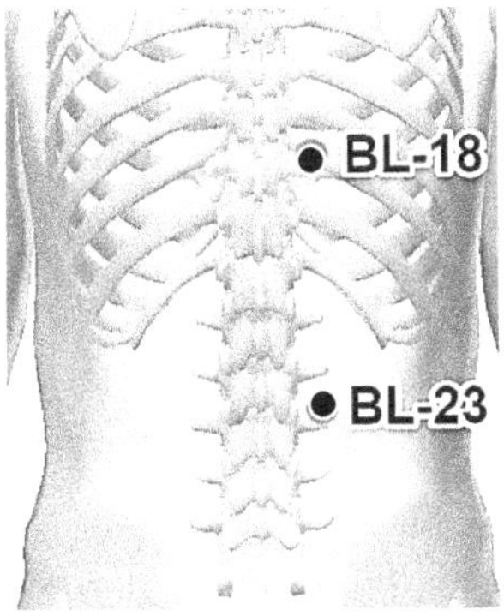

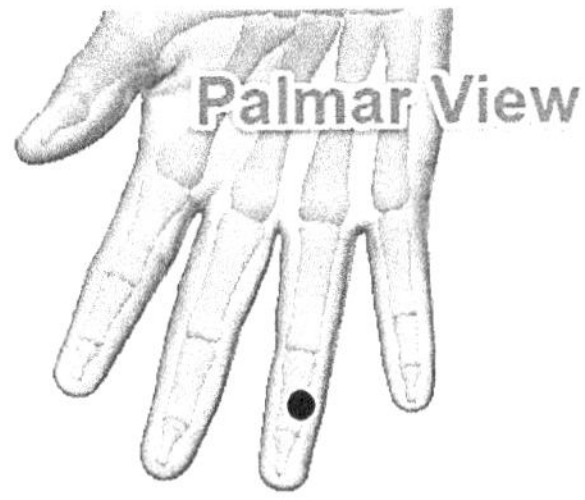

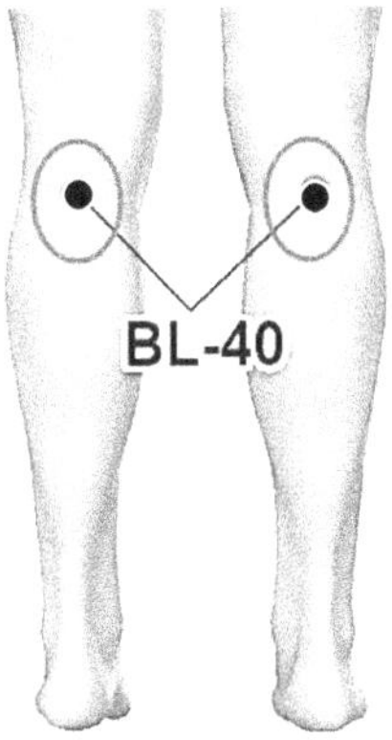

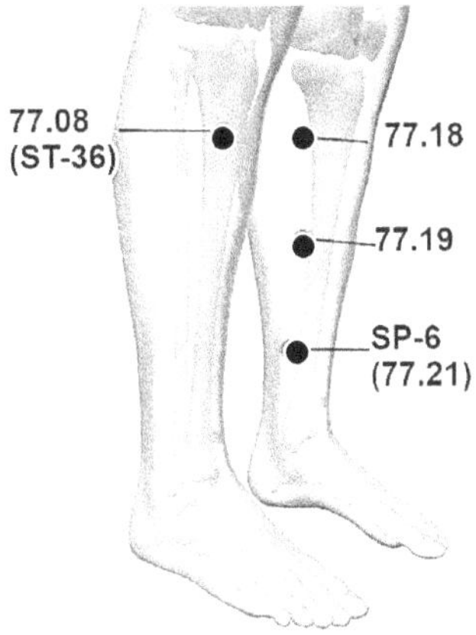

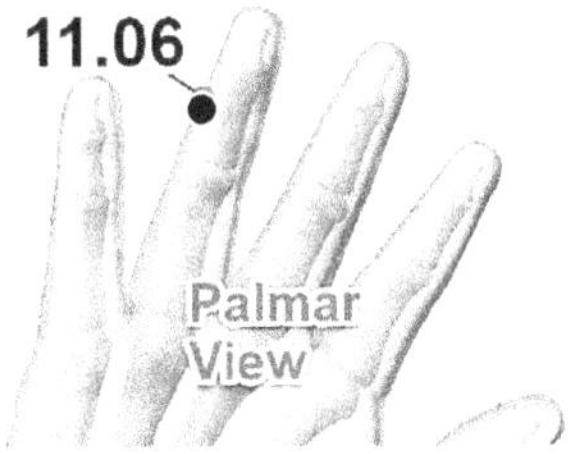

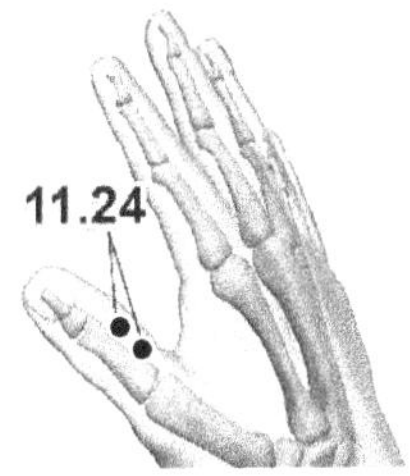

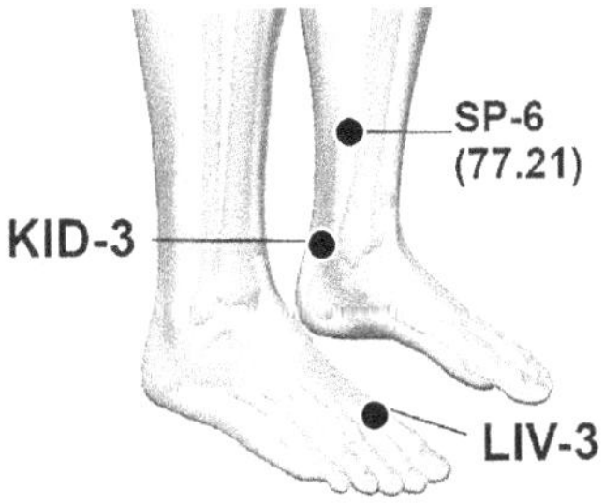

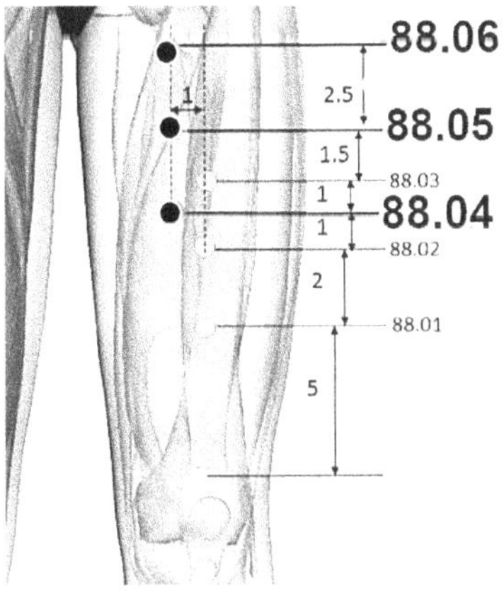

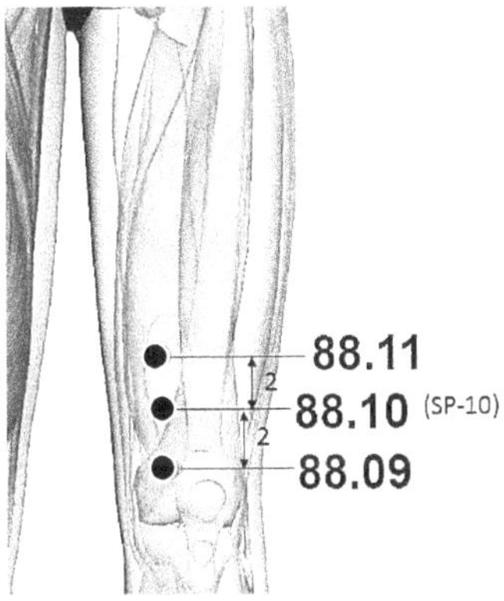

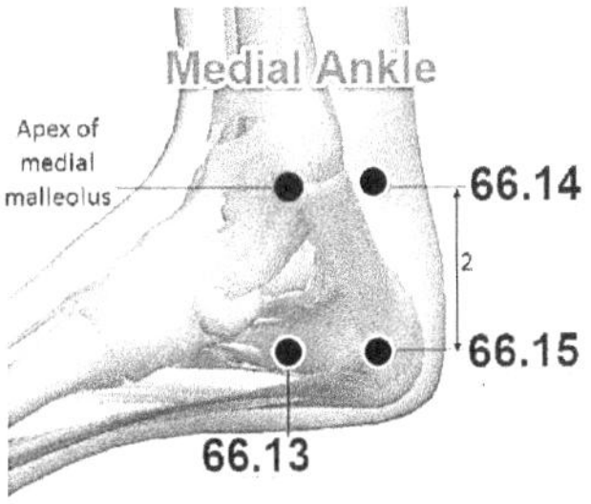

# Dysmenorrhea

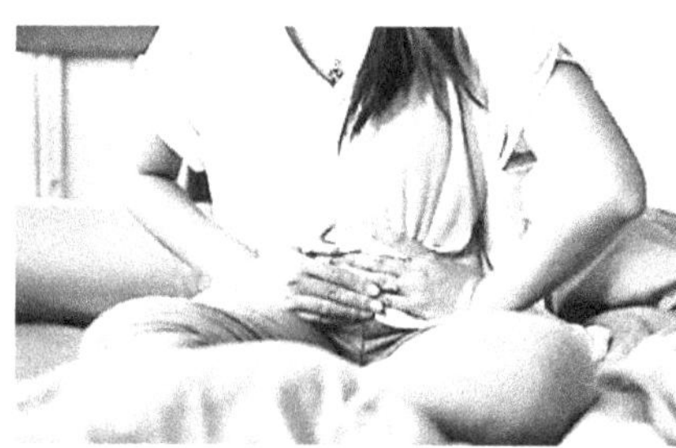

*Dysmenorrhea refers to the lower abdominal pain before, during or after menstruation.*

*Dysmenorrhea, also known as painful menstrual cramps, is a common gynaecological condition that affects many women. In Traditional Chinese Medicine (TCM), dysmenorrhea is believed to be caused by an imbalance or stagnation of Qi and blood in the body, which can lead to menstrual cramps and pain. The main meridians involved in dysmenorrhea are the **Ren, Chong, Liver, and Spleen channels.***

| AFFECTED MERIDIANS | TREATMENT POINTS |
| --- | --- |
| **STOMACH** <br> Foot Yangming | • 66.02 66.05 Men Jin (ST-43, Shu-stream point on ST meridian). <br> • 77.08+77.09+77.11 (on the ST meridian) <br> • ST-44 - Ying-Spring Point. Treats own meridian. <br> • 22.04+22.05 – LI treats ST (System 1) |
| **URINARY BLADDER** <br> Foot Tai Yang | • BL-67 (can moxibustion) - Jing-well point. Bladder relates to the uterus. <br> • BL-57 - Empirical point for cramps. Treats own meridian. <br> • 11.24 Fu Ke - Lung treats Bladder (Sys 2). Treats all diseases of uterus. <br> • BL-32 - Treats lumbago, gynecological and urinary disorders. |
| **KIDNEY** <br> Foot Shao Yin. | • BL-67 (moxibustion is effective)- Jing-well point. Bladder treats Kidney (System 3) |
| **LIVER** <br> Foot Jue Yin | • LIV-2 - Ying-spring point. Treats own meridian pathway. <br> • LIV-3 (66.04 Huo Zhu) - Shu-stream/Yuan source point. Treats own meridian. |
| **SPLEEN** <br> Foot Tai Yin | • SP-6 (77.21 Ren Huang) Meeting Point on the Spleen Channel with the Liver and Kidney Channels. Moxibustion applicable. |
| **REN** | • REN-3, REN-4, REN-6, REN-12. Moxibustion applicable. <br> • EX-B-8 SHIQIZHUI SHIQIZHUIXIA - DU treats REN. Moxa applicable. |

**Blood-letting for Dysmenorrhea** (painful periods, menstrual cramps)
- DT.15 San Jiang (Back treats front)
- Visible veins in the leg, especially the BL-40 region and ST-36 region
- Visible veins between the medial malleolus and SP-6, SP-8, SP-9

*Points Illustrations for treatment of Dysmenorrhea*

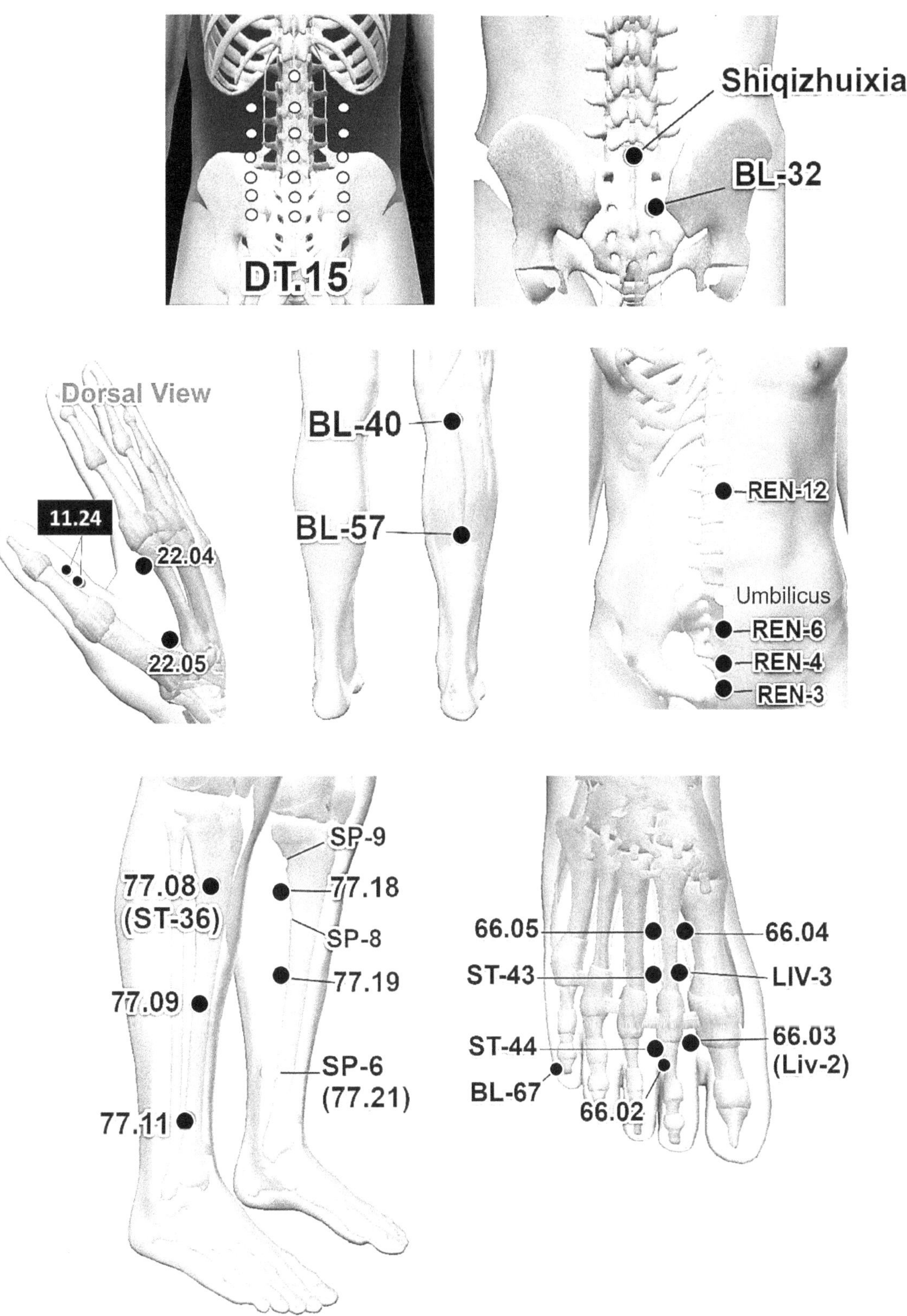

# Amenorrhea

*In Traditional Chinese Medicine (TCM), amenorrhea, which is the absence of menstruation, is often related to the* ***Kidney and Liver meridians.***

*The Kidney meridian is believed to be responsible for the reproductive system, and any imbalances in this meridian can affect the menstrual cycle. The Kidney meridian also controls the body's water metabolism, and its deficiency or excess can lead to conditions like edema or dehydration, respectively.*

*The Liver meridian is responsible for the smooth flow of Qi (energy) and blood throughout the body. When the Liver Qi is stagnant or deficient, it can lead to menstrual irregularities, including amenorrhea.*

*TCM practitioners may also consider the* ***Spleen and Heart meridians****, as they are involved in the production of blood and emotional well-being, respectively.*

**Needling for Amenorrhea**
- 11.06 Huan Chao+11.24 Fu Ke
- Or 88.04 Jie Mei Yi+88.05 Jie Mei Er+88.06 Jie Mei San (on alternate days)
- 66.14 Shui Xiang+66.15 Shui Xian (near KD-5 Shui Quan, the Xi-Cleft point on the Kidney meridian)
- 88.12 Ming Huang+88.13 Tian Huang+88.14 Qi Huang (Reaction: Liver)
- 77.17 Tian Huang, 77.18 Shen Guan+77.19 Di Huang+77.21 Ren Huang (Reaction: Kidney)
- ST-25 (the Mu Point for the Large Intestine, and it regulates qi and blood)
- REN-24 is effective because the Stomach and Large Intestine meridians (Yang Ming) have more qi and more blood, and both travel around the mouth.
- SP-6 (Sanyinjiao), REN-4 (Guanyuan), REN-6 (Qihai), LIV-3 (Taichong), GB-41 (Zulinqi), LI-4 (Hegu) – commonly used TCM combination.
- BL-23 and BL-32
- Moxibustion/gua sha around REN-4, REN-3, ST-29 and SP-6

---

### Blood-letting for Amenorrhea
- DT.15 San Jiang (over sacrum)– Bleeding the back is therapeutic for the front.

*Points Illustrations for treatment of Amenorrhea*

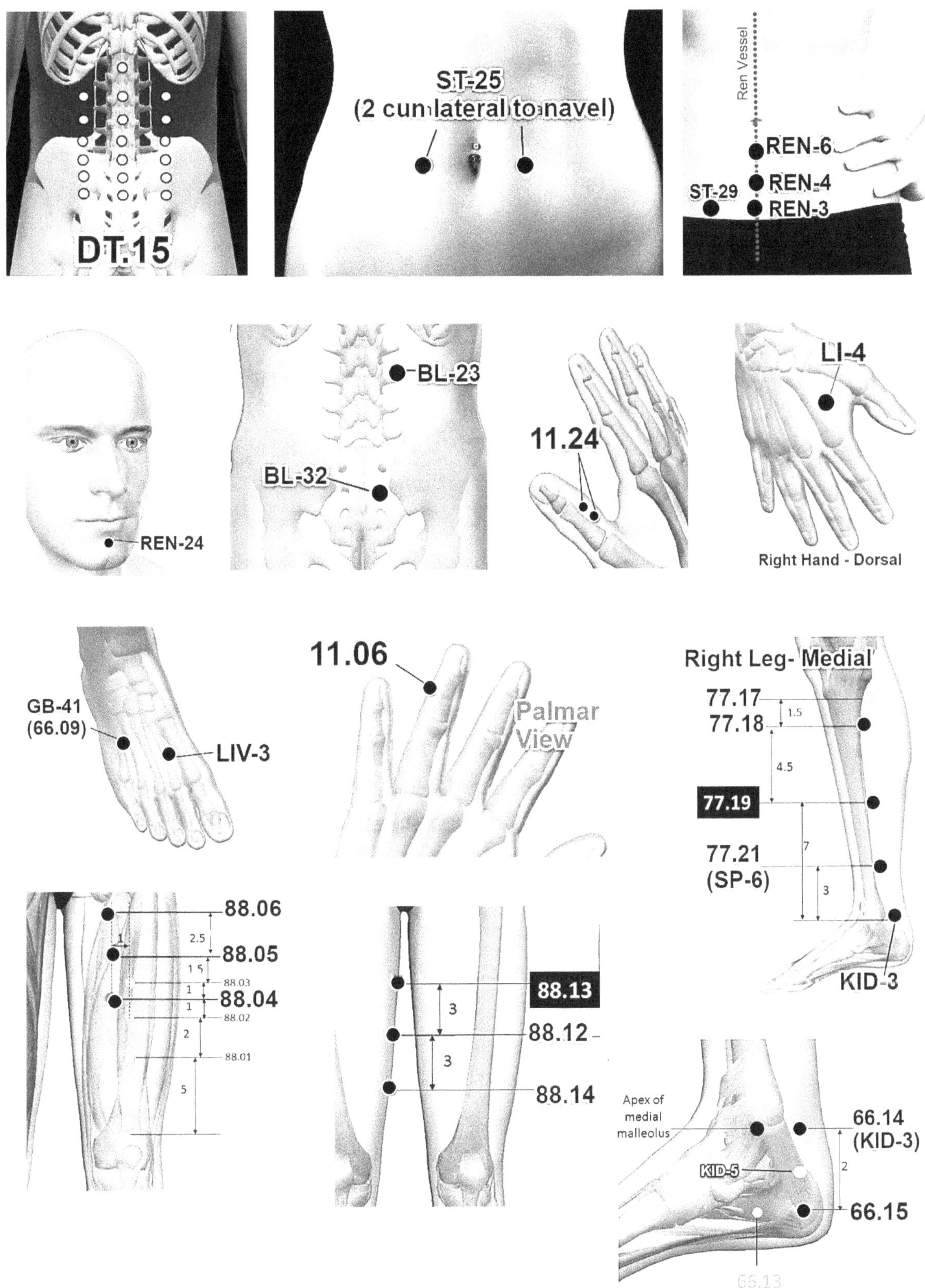

# Uterine cysts, fibroid

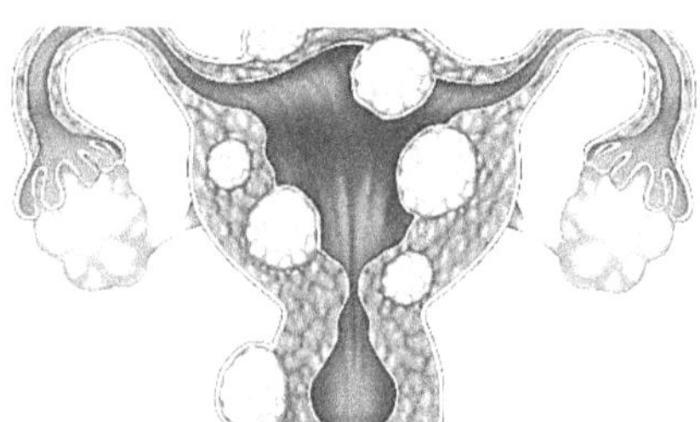

*In Traditional Chinese Medicine (TCM), uterine cysts are believed to be caused by various factors, including Qi and blood stagnation, dampness and phlegm accumulation, and Kidney and Spleen Qi deficiency. The meridians or channels involved in uterine cysts are primarily **the Liver channel and the Spleen channel**.*

*When the Liver Qi becomes stagnant, it can lead to the formation of cysts in the uterus. Therefore, regulating the Liver Qi is an important aspect of treating uterine cysts in TCM.*

*The Spleen channel is also involved in the formation of uterine cysts, as the Spleen is responsible for transforming and transporting food and fluids in the body. When the Spleen Qi becomes deficient, it can lead to the accumulation of dampness and phlegm, which can contribute to the formation of cysts in the uterus.*

**Treatment**

- 88.04 Jie Mei Yi+88.05 Jie Mei Er+88.06 Jie Mei San
- 11.06 Huan Chao+ 11.24 Fu Ke
- 66.03 Huo Ying+66.04 Huo Zhu (LIV-3)
- ST-44, ST-43, 66.05
- 77.27
- 66.13 Shui Jing+66.14 Shui Xiang+66.15 Shui Xian (uterus, kidney, brain issues)
- SP-6, REN-3, REN-6, SP-9, GB-39, ST-36
- Moxibustion: around BL-40, REN-3, REN-4, KID-8

---

### Blood-letting Treatment

- Visible veins in the leg, esp. around BL-40, ST-36 and between medial malleolus and SP-6
- Prick area between 22.01 Chong Zi+22.02 Chong Xian
- 77.09 Si Hua Zhong+77.14 Si Hua Wai or ST-40- in severe cases
- Blood-let over the lower abdomen and the sacrum
- 66.13 Shui Jing

*Points Illustrations for treatment of Uterine Cysts/fibroid*

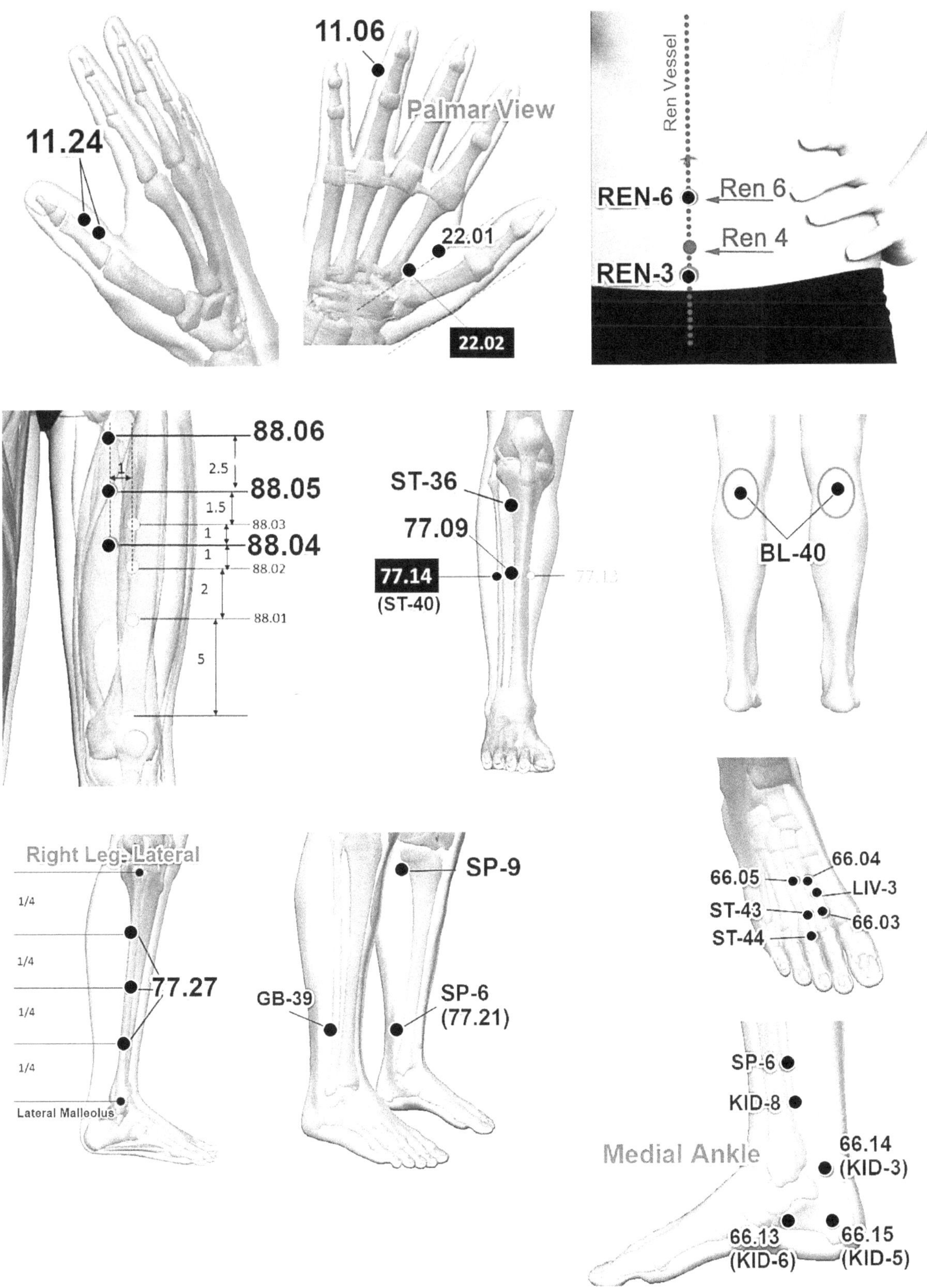

# MALE ISSUES
## Genital Pain

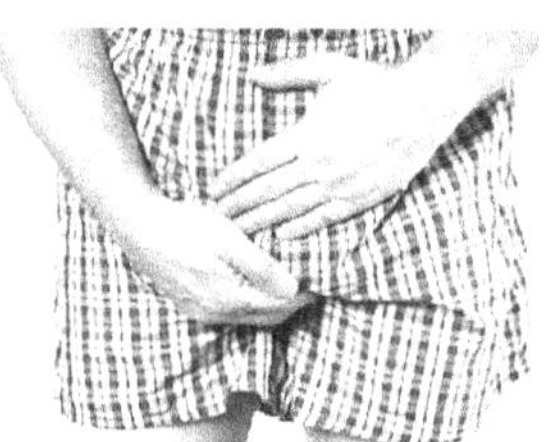

*Genital pain can be caused by inflammation such as urinary tract infection, orchitis, epididymitis and prostatitis. It can also be caused by traumatic injuries and pruritus disorders such as genital abscesses. The following meridians may be involved in cases of genital pain:*

***Kidney Meridian:*** *Imbalances in this meridian can lead to a range of issues, including impotence, infertility, and pain in the genitals.* ***Liver Meridian:*** *Imbalances in this meridian can lead to painful menstrual periods, impotence, and other issues related to the reproductive organs.* ***Spleen Meridian:*** *Imbalances in this meridian can lead to a range of issues, including digestive problems, infertility, and other reproductive disorders.* ***Bladder Meridian:*** *Imbalances in this meridian can lead to pain and inflammation in the genitals, as well as urinary tract infections and other related issues.*

| AFFECTED (SICK) MERIDIANS | TREATMENT POINTS |
|---|---|
| **LIVER**<br>Foot Jue Yin | • LIV-2 - Ying-spring point. Treats own meridian pathway.<br>• 11.03 Fu Jian + 11.04 Wai Jian - LI treats Liver (System 2). Treats penis and testicles.<br>• LIV-3 (66.04 Huo Zhu) - Shu-stream and yuan source point.<br>• 22.05 Ling Gu - LI treats Liver (System 2)<br>• GB-41 (66.09) – GB treats Liver.<br>• Bleed/moxibustion LIV-1 – pain at tip of penis, testicular pain |
| **REN** | • REN-3, REN-4, REN-6 - treats urinary tract and reproductive disorders |
| **LUNG**<br>Hand Tai Yin | • LU-7 - Treats REN meridian. Communicates with KID-6. |
| **SPLEEN** | • SP-6<br>• 77.18 Shen Guan+77.19 Di Huang+77.21 Ren Huang (inflammation of the glans penis, testicular pain) |
| **BLADDER** | • BL-23, BL-32 |

### Blood-letting treatment for Herpes and sores of the lips and genitals
• 77.15 Shang Chun+77.16 Xia Chun
• 99.08 Er San (Ear Apex) (lesions on the lips of the mouth)

*Points Illustrations for treatment of Genital Pain*

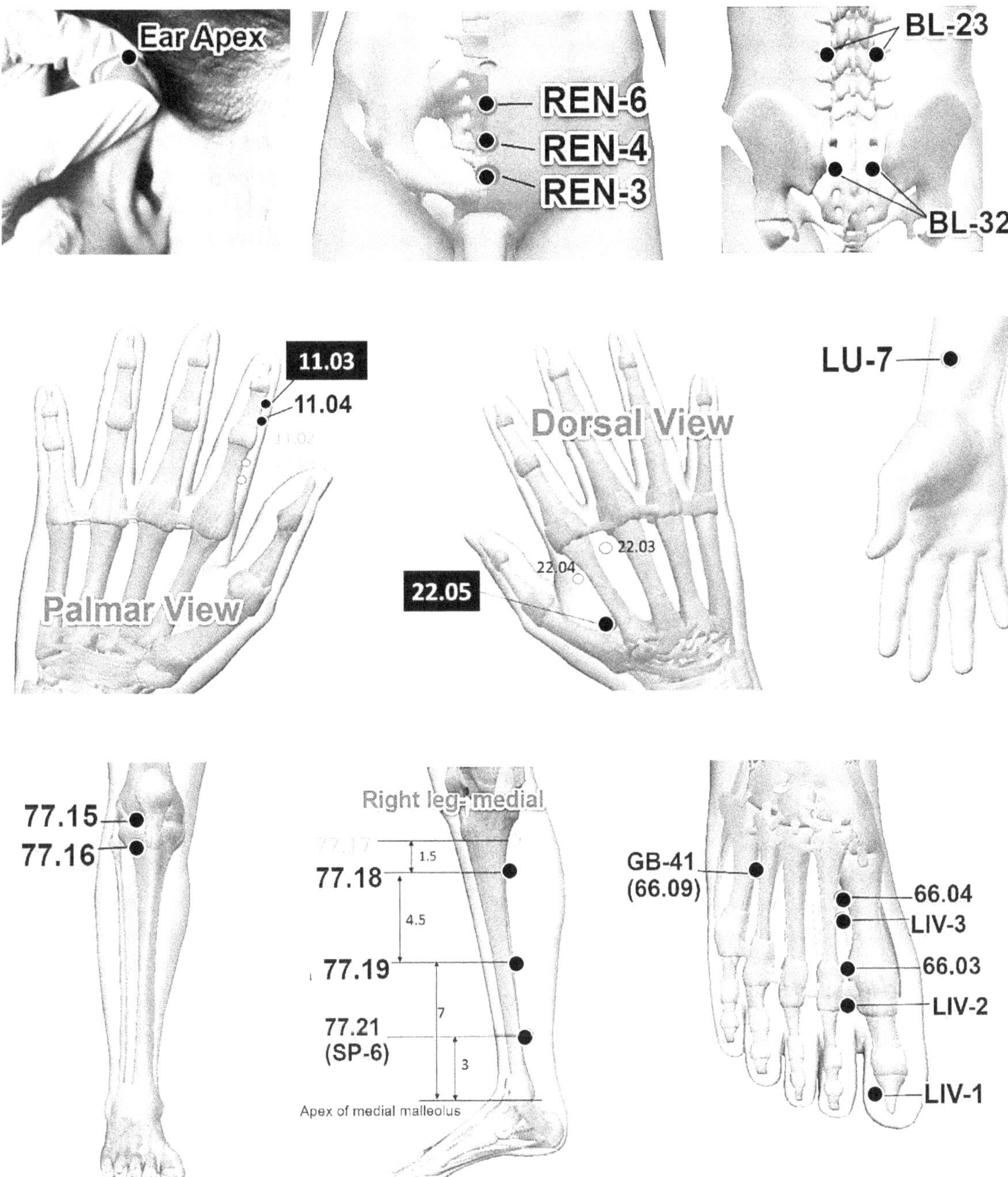

# Impotence and premature ejaculation

*The following meridians may be involved in cases of impotence and premature ejaculation:*

***Kidney Meridian****: Imbalances in this meridian can lead to impotence, premature ejaculation and other sexual dysfunction.*

***Liver Meridian:*** *Imbalances in this meridian can lead to sexual dysfunction, including impotence and premature ejaculation.*

***Spleen Meridian****: Imbalances in this meridian can lead to a range of issues, including digestive problems, which can impact sexual function.*

***Bladder Meridian:*** *Imbalances in this meridian can lead to sexual dysfunction, including impotence and premature ejaculation.*

**Treatment**

- LIV-1 - effective point for impotence. The Liver channel passes through and around the genitals, and being a Jing-Well point it clears congestion and calms the spirit.
- 1010.19 Shui Tong + 1010.20 - tonifies deficient Kidney qi, increasing energy (including sexual energy), and it is used to treat impotence, paralysis, and weakness in the legs.
- 1010.13 Ma Jin Shui+1010.14 Ma Kuai Shui. Kidney reaction area.
- Needle 77.18 Shen Guan+77.19 Di Huang+77.21 Ren Huang – Kidney reaction area.
- Needle and moxibustion REN-3 and REN-4. Catgut embedding therapy applicable.
- SP-6 + DU-4+REN-4 – combination for impotence.  Moxibustion applicable.
- REN-4 + REN-6 +BL-23+ST-36 – for low sexual ability. Moxibustion applicable.
- REN-3+BL-52 + HT-7 + SP-6 – nocturnal emission
- REN-3 + BL-52 + BL-23 – premature ejaculation

*Points Illustrations for Impotence and Premature Ejaculation*

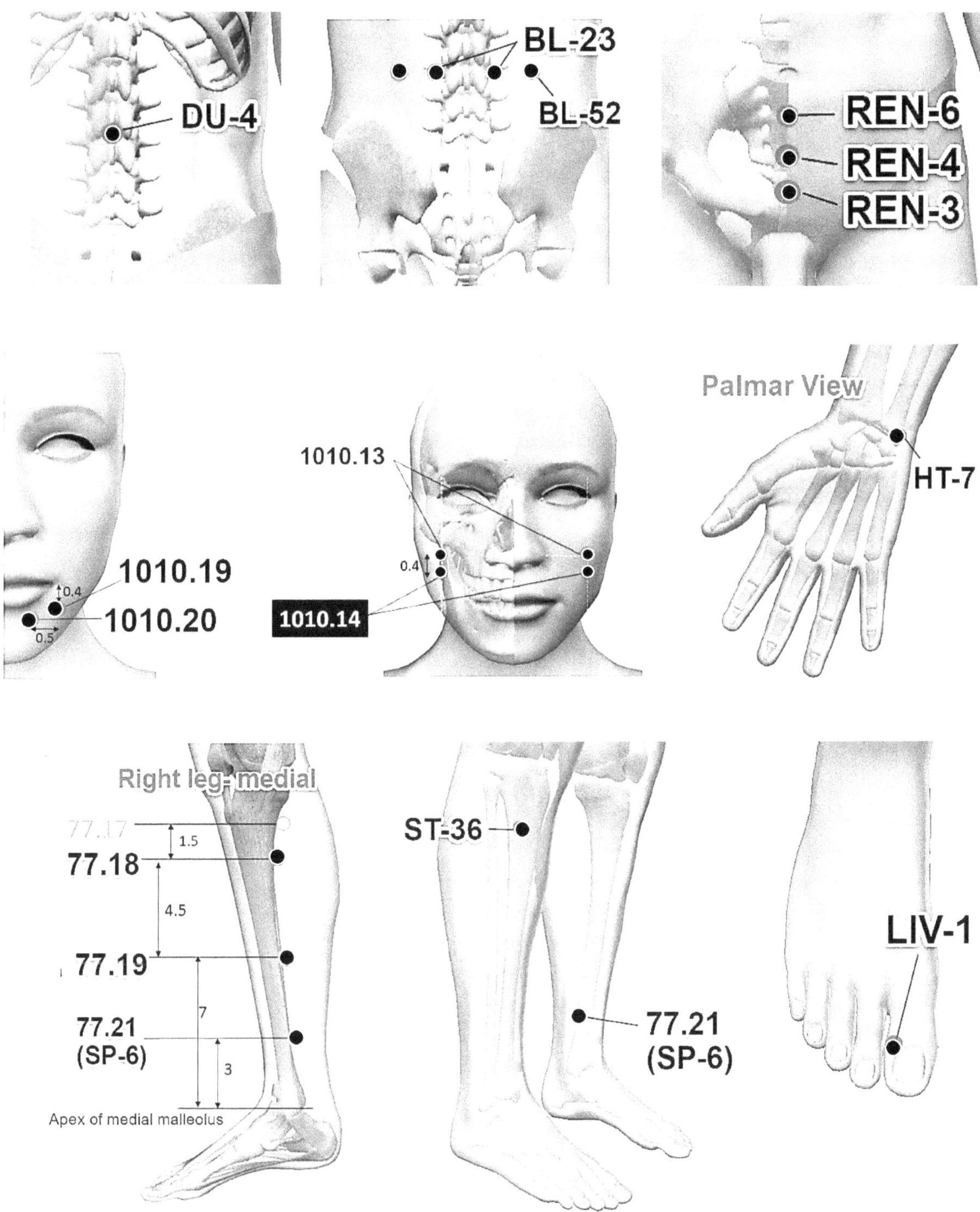

# Prostate Issues

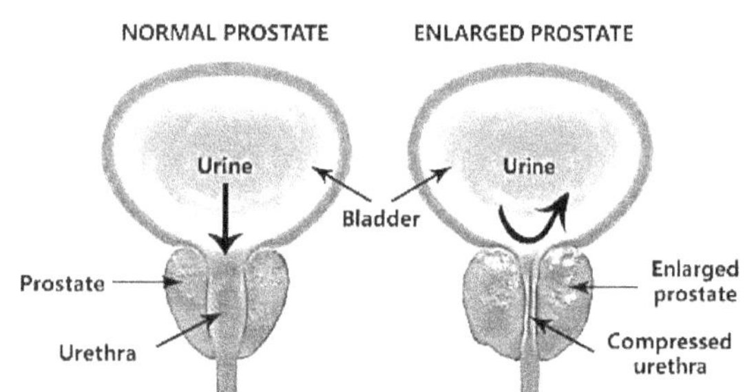



*The following meridians may be involved in cases of prostate issues:*

***Kidney Meridian****: Imbalances in this meridian can lead to inflammation, enlargement, and other prostate issues.*

***Spleen Meridian****: Imbalances in this meridian can lead to dampness and stagnation in the lower body, which can contribute to prostate issues.* ***Liver Meridian****: Imbalances in this meridian can lead to stagnation in the lower body, which can contribute to prostate issues.*

**Prostate enlargement** - A condition in which the flow of urine is blocked due to the enlargement of prostate gland. The symptoms include increased frequency of urination at night and difficulty in urinating.

**Needling combinations for prostate enlargement:**
- Bilaterally needle 1010.13 Ma Jin Shui+1010.14 Ma Kuai Shui
- Or 77.18 Shen Guan+77.19 Di Huang+77.21 Ren Huang
- REN-3, REN-4 or REN-6. BL-28 +BL-23, KID-3 (choose a few)
- Bilaterally needle 66.04 Huo Zhu, 77.17 Tian Huang (SP-9)
- Sedate 77.08 Si Hua Shang (ST-36) to promote immediate urination.
- 11.06, 11.24 and 11.05
- Bilaterally needle 22.05 Ling Gu with 77.18 Shen Guan+77.19 Di Huang+77.21 Ren Huang.
- Bilaterally needle 88.13 Tian Huang, 77.08 Si Hua Shang (ST-36)
- Bilaterally needle 44.06 Jian Zhong, 44.11 Yun Bai
- Bilaterally needle 66.03 Huo Ying-66.04 Huo Zhu
- BL-65 (Shu-stream point on the Urinary Bladder channel).
- LIV-1 can be used as a Guiding Point with any of the above treatments.
- Moxa BL-23, DU-4, REN-4 and/or REN-6

**Prostatitis**: A condition resulting from inflammation or swelling of the prostate gland. This condition is usually caused by damp heat in the Liver and Gallbladder. It is characterized by radiating medial thigh pain, blood in the semen and sometimes tailbone pain. If it is chronic or Kidney qi deficient, there may be a white discharge.

**Needling combinations for prostatitis**
- Bilaterally needle 66.03 Huo Ying-66.04 Huo Zhu Fire Hardness/Fire Master
- Or 77.18 Shen Guan+77.19 Di Huang+77.21 Ren Huang
- Unilaterally needle left-side 11.01 Da Jian+11.02 Xiao Jian
- 11.06, 11.24, LIV-2 (66.03), LIV-3 (66.04)
- Bilaterally needle LIV-1 as a Guiding Point
- Moxibustion: REN-3, REN-4, REN-6, REN-8

---

### Blood-letting Treatment for Prostate Issues
- Bilaterally bleed small veins from the medial malleolus up to SP-6 San Yin Jiao

*Points Illustrations for treatment of Prostate Issues*

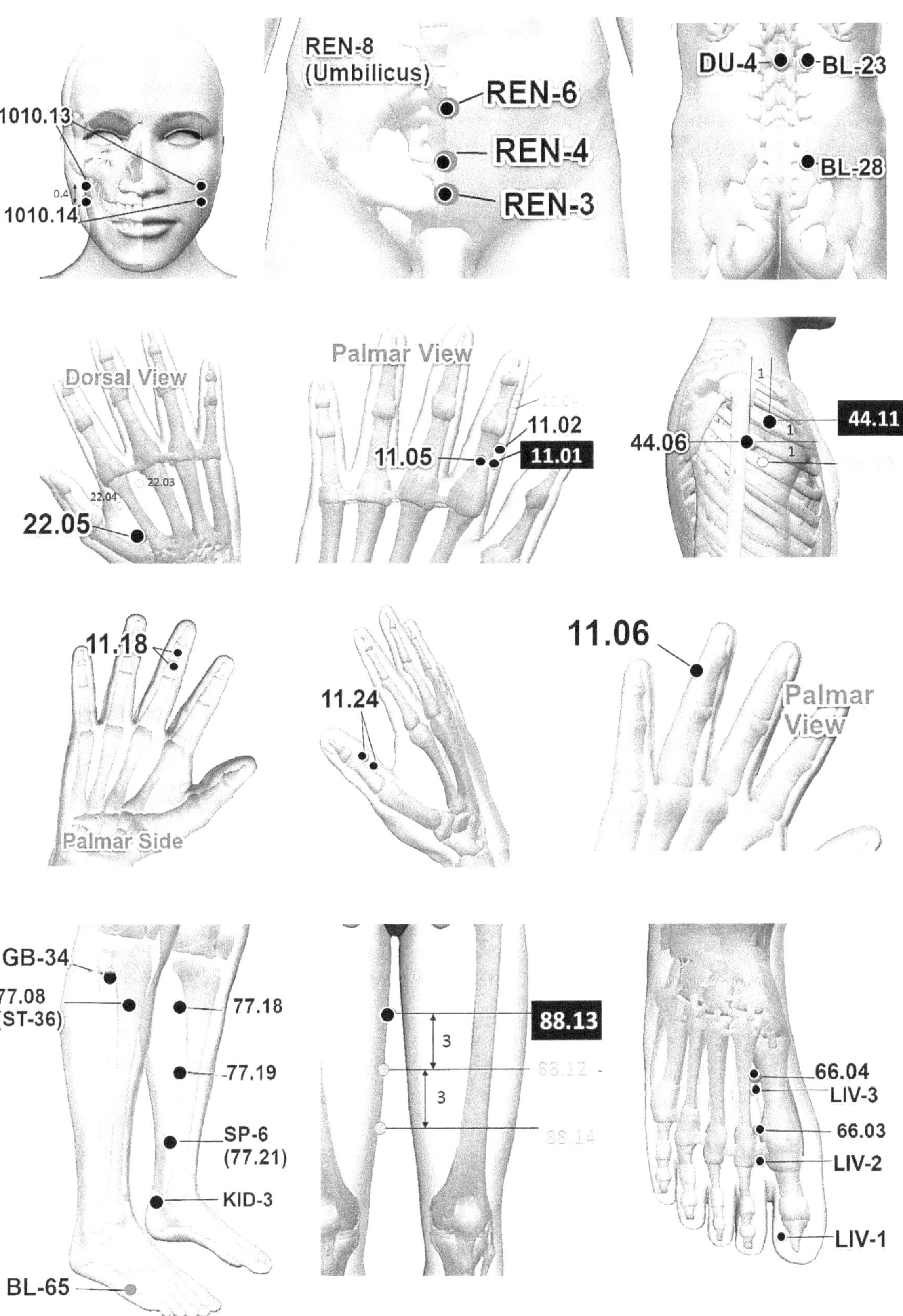

# NEUROLOGICAL

## Insomnia

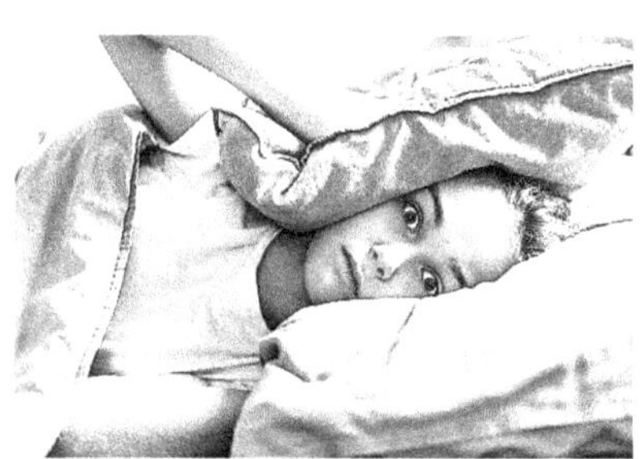

*The following are some of the meridians that may be involved in cases of insomnia:*

***Heart Meridian****: The Heart Meridian governs the spirit and emotions in TCM, and is closely linked to sleep. Imbalances in this meridian can lead to anxiety, overthinking, and difficulty falling asleep.*

***Liver Meridian:*** *The Liver Meridian is responsible for the smooth flow of Qi throughout the body, and is closely linked to the body's stress response. Imbalances in this meridian can lead to stress, tension, and difficulty relaxing.*

***Spleen Meridian:*** *The Spleen Meridian is responsible for the transformation and transportation of nutrients in the body. Imbalances in this meridian can lead to digestive issues and can impact the body's ability to properly nourish itself, which can contribute to insomnia.*

***Lung Meridian:*** *The Lung Meridian is responsible for the regulation of breathing and oxygen exchange in the body. Imbalances in this meridian can lead to shallow breathing or disruptions in the body's circadian rhythms, which can contribute to insomnia.*

**Treatment options for insomnia**

- Needle 1010.08 Zhen Jing (Yintang [Ex. 1.] or Ex-HN-3) with 1010.01 Zheng Hui (DU-20)
- Bilaterally needle Jian Gu (Extra Point), it is located by palpating the second metacarpal bone between 22.04 Da Bai and 22.05 Ling Gu to find the most sensitive point. Can use a press needle.
- 77.18 Shen Guan+77.19 Di Huang+77.21 Ren Huang (symptoms of Kidney yin deficiency)
- 88.25 Zhong Jiu Li, 88.26 Shang Jiu Li, 88.27 Xia Jiu Li
- 55.06
- LI- 4 /LIV-3 - if related to a digestive function
- LI-3 (22.04) with LIV-2 (66.03) - if related to anxiety (Anxiety Four Gates)
- Needle left-side 11.17 Mu.
- HT-7 (both sides) with GB-44 and BL-62
- P-6, SP-6, LU-7, BL-15, Anmian, Yintang
- A press needle at ear Shenmen is helpful with acupuncture
- Moxa at ST-36, KID-1, KID-6

---

### Blood-letting Treatment
- Bleed 99.07 Er Bei, 99.08 (ear apex) weekly.

*Points Illustrations for treatment of Insomnia*

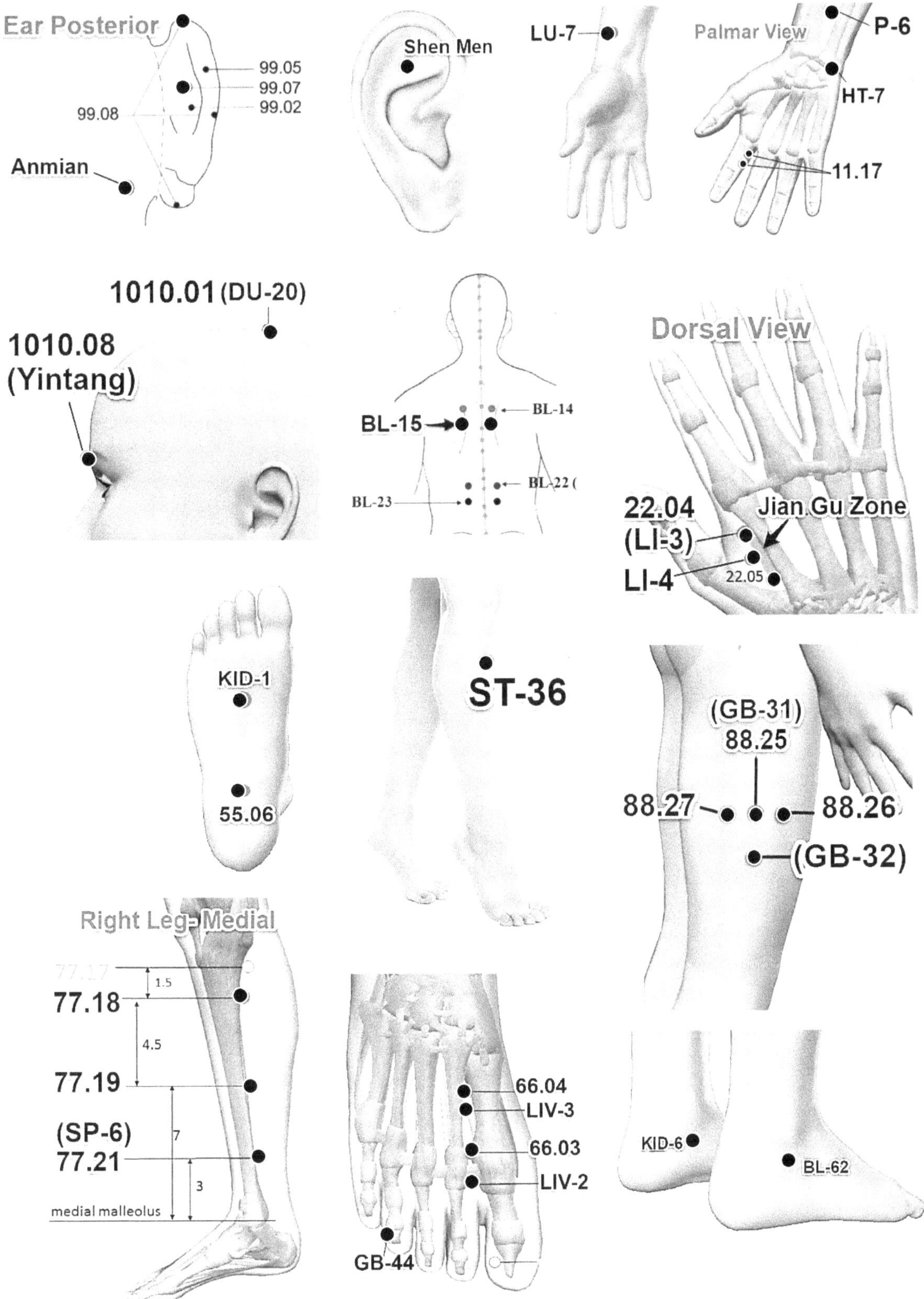

# Anxiety and Anger

*Anxiety is often associated with imbalances in the **Heart and Kidney meridians.** The **Heart meridian** is responsible for regulating emotions and the **Kidney meridian** is responsible for providing a foundation for the body's Qi. When there is an imbalance in these meridians, it can lead to symptoms such as palpitations, insomnia, and nervousness.*

*Anger, on the other hand, is often associated with imbalances in the **Liver meridian**. The **Liver meridian** is responsible for regulating the flow of Qi in the body and is particularly sensitive to emotional stress. When there is an imbalance in the **Liver meridian**, it can lead to symptoms such as irritability, headache, and high blood pressure.*

**Needling treatment**

- 1010.01 Zheng Hui (DU-20) + 1010.05 Qian Hui+1010.06 Hou Hui, 1010.08 Zhen Jing
- HT-7 + Yintang [Ex. 1.] or Ex-HN-3 + SP-6
- P-6, P-4 + DU-26 - neurosis (mental illness)
- LIV-3, 11.17 Mu- reducing anger, irritability, and depression
- KID-6, BL-62
- 88.01 Tong Guan+88.02 Tong Shan+88.03 Tong Tian
- Add 11.05 if there is palpitation
- 88.25 Zhong Jiu Li (GB-31) – stress
- ST-45 - bipolar disorder

---

### Blood-letting Treatment

- 99.08 Er San (Ear Apex)
- P-3, ST-40, GB-34, GB-35 (select dark veins)
- BL-40 (select dark veins)
- 1010.12 Zheng Ben – feeling possessed

*Points Illustrations for treatment of Anxiety and Anger*

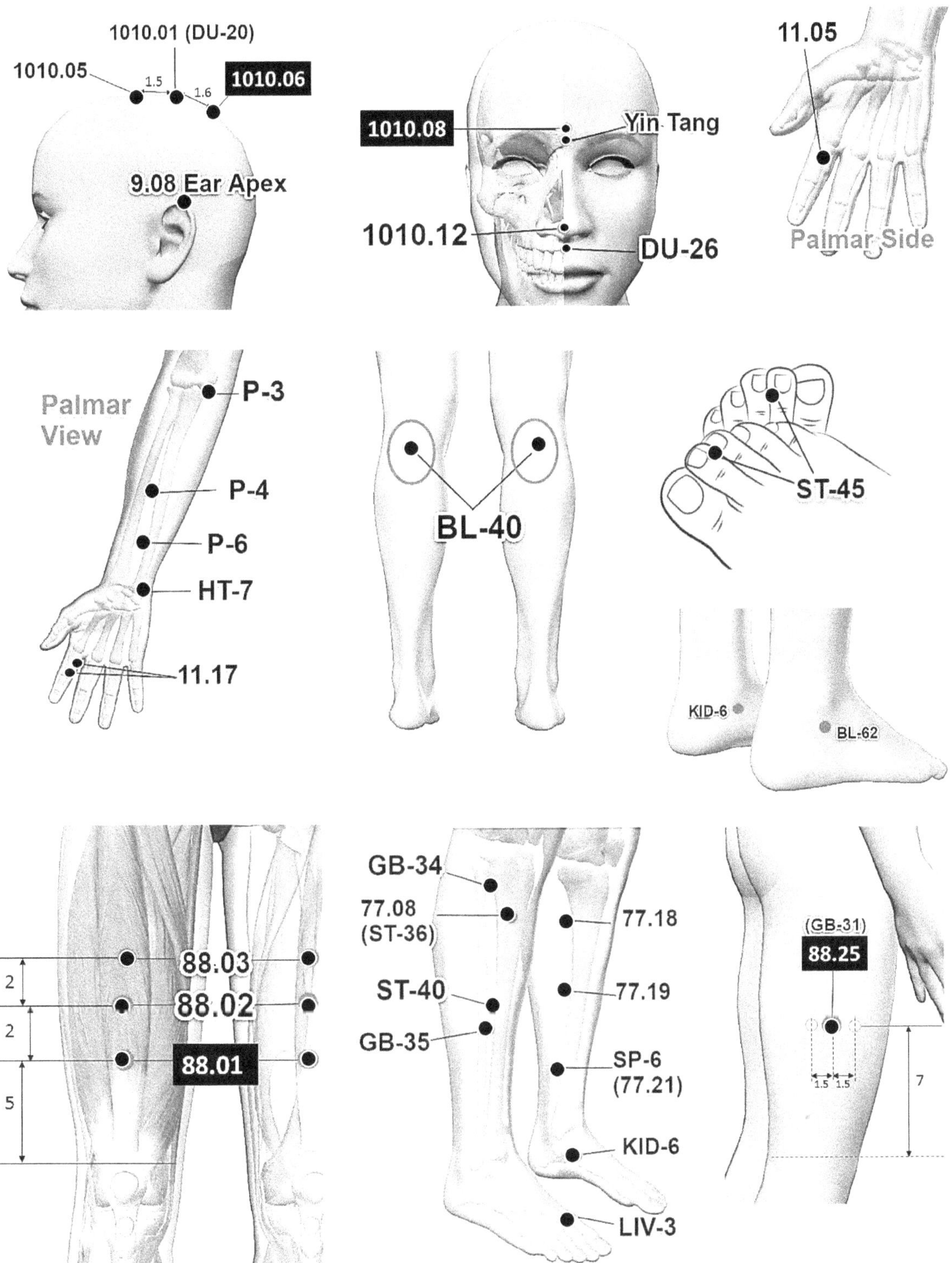

# Parkinson's and Alzheimer's disease

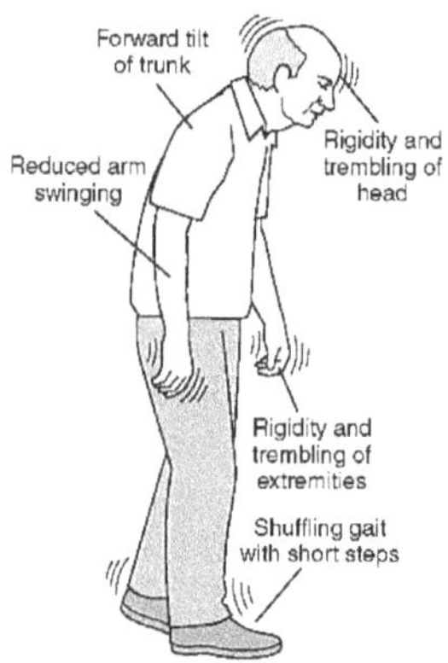


*It is recognized today that neurological disorders such as Alzheimer's disease and Parkinson's disease are caused by brain toxicity. For complete recovery from conditions like Parkinson's and multiple sclerosis, a slow but steady detoxification is absolutely essential. (Dr. Susan Johnson)*

*According to TCM theory, the meridians involved in these conditions are the **Liver meridian, Kidney meridian, and Spleen meridian.***

**Treatment for Temor and Parkinson's**

- 1010.01 Zheng Hui with 88.12 Ming Huang+88.13 Tian Huang+88.14 Qi Huang and/or 88.25 Zhong Jiu Li (GB-31)
- Alternate with 77.18 Shen Guan+77.19 Di Huang+77.21 Ren Huang
- 1010.01 Zheng Hui+1010.05 Qian Hui+1010.06 Hou Hui (DU-20, DU-19, DU-21)
- 11.17 Mu (Anger) to address feelings of frustration and despair.
- LIV-3 and LI-4 (Four Gates) to resolve tremors and calm the nervous system.
- KID-3
- Weakness of the extremities (Parkinson's disease): Thread needles from 1010.02 Zhou Yuan (BL-7) toward BL-5 in the beginning phase of treatment of Parkinson's.
- Unilaterally needle 33.10 Chang Men, 33.11 Gan Men, 1010.01 Zheng Hui+1010.05 Qian Hui+1010.06 Hou Hui (DU-20, DU-19, DU-21) – drain damp heat

**Treatment for Alzheimer's and Memory Loss**

- 1010.12 Zheng Ben (DU-25) – needle or bleed for declining brain power
- 77.17 Tian Huang 77.18 Shen Guan+77.19 Di Huang+77.21 Ren Huang
- 22.04 Da Bai+22.05 Ling Gu
- 1010.01 Zheng Hui+1010.05 Qian Hui+1010.06 Hou Hui
- 77.05 Yi Zhong+77.06 Er Zhong+77.07 San Zhong
- KI-1 (Acupressure or Moxa)
- HT-7, LU-7, P-6, Sishencong [Ex. 6] or Ex-HN-1, DU-20
- Dementia - Sishencong [Ex. 6] or Ex-HN-1, BL-15, BL-20, ST-36, BL-23, KID-6 (Reinforce)

## Cupping/Bleeding Treatment

- Cup DT.01 Fen Zhi Shang+DT.02 Fen Zhi Xia Toxin Areas until the skin no longer colors.
- Bleeding of 99.08 Er San Ear Apex, Taiyang [Ex.2.]. or Ex-HN-5 (temple area, avoiding the artery)
- LU-5
- BL-40

*Points Illustrations for treatment of Parkinson's and Alzheimer's disease*

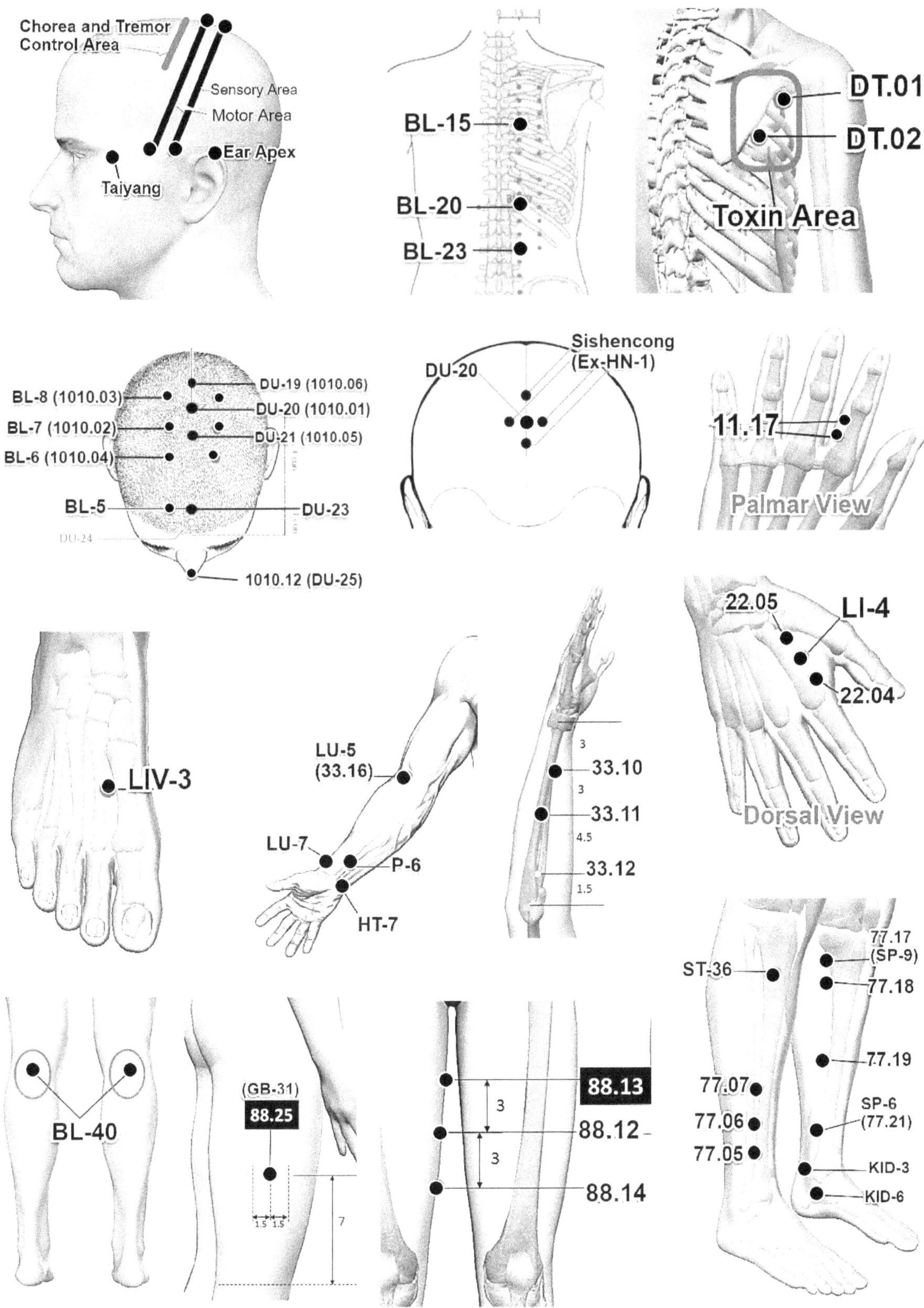

# Dizziness and Vertigo

*Dizziness and vertigo are common symptoms that can be caused by various factors, including inner ear problems, blood pressure changes, medication side effects, and neurological disorders.*

*The **Liver meridian** is responsible for the smooth flow of Qi and blood throughout the body, and any obstruction or stagnation in this flow can result in dizziness or vertigo. The Liver is also considered to be closely related to emotions, particularly anger and stress, which can affect the flow of Qi and blood and lead to these symptoms.*

*The Spleen meridian is responsible for transforming food and fluids into Qi and blood, and any imbalance in this meridian can lead to a deficiency of Qi and blood. There will be symptoms such as fatigue, weakness, and dizziness.*

*A deficiency or imbalance in the **Kidney meridian** can lead to symptoms such as dizziness, vertigo, and tinnitus.*

### Effective points for vertigo
- 22.04+22.05 (improves blood-circulation to the brain)
- LI-11 (LI treats itself and LIV, System 2)+DU-20+LIV-3 (66-04)
- Add P-6 for Meniere's.

### Meniere's Disease Treatment
- 88.12 Ming Huang+88.13 Tian Huang+88.14 Qi Huang – reaction area is Liver.
- Add either LI-11 unilaterally or 22.05 Ling Gu, needled unilaterally.
- P-6 unilaterally - treats nausea and vomiting
- Alternatively, consider 88.17 Si Ma Zhong+88.18 Si Ma Shang+88.19 Si Ma Xia
- 88.25 Zhong Jiu Li (GB-31) for wind diseases and internal ear pathologies

### Dizziness due to Kidney deficiency or weakness of cerebral nerves
*Kidney deficiency is the most commonly seen cause of dizziness in the clinic and it most frequently affects the elderly. Kidney dominates the brain.*
- Bilateral 77.18 Shen Guan+77.19 Di Huang+77.21 Ren Huang – Tung's Master Kidney points.
- 88.12 Ming Huang+88.13 Tian Huang+88.14 Qi Huang
- 22.06 Zhong Bai+22.07 Xia Bai

### Dizziness due to blood diseases
- 88.12 Ming Huang+88.13 Tian Huang+88.14 Qi Huang - best for treating blood diseases
- 77.05 Yi Zhong+77.06 Er Zhong+77.07 San Zhong or 66.06 Mu Liu+66.07 Mu Dou.
- Dr. Miriam Lee's Ten Great Needles Treatment (bilateral ST-36, SP-6, LI-11, LI- 4, LU-7), with or without moxa on ST-36 and SP-6.
- Moxa on the DU-4 Ming Men and REN-4 -REN-8 is also very useful in building blood.

### Vertigo due to cerebral anemia
- 88.01+88.02+88.03

## Bleeding Treatment
- Bleed ear apex
- Bleed BL-10, DU-16
- Bleed 77.07 or around ST-40 (77.14)
- In severe case - 77.05 Yi Zhong+77.06 Er Zhong+77.07 San Zhong bleed if unconsciousness occurs (look for blood vessels in the area
- Bleed 44.07 Bei Mian (LI-15) – Meniere's.
- Bleed LIV-1, needle 22.05 Ling Gu with LI-11 or LIV-3
- In case of hypertensive vertigo, bleed DT.04 Wu Ling then needle LIV-2+LIV-3 (66.04)

*Points Illustrations for treatment of Dizziness and Vertigo*

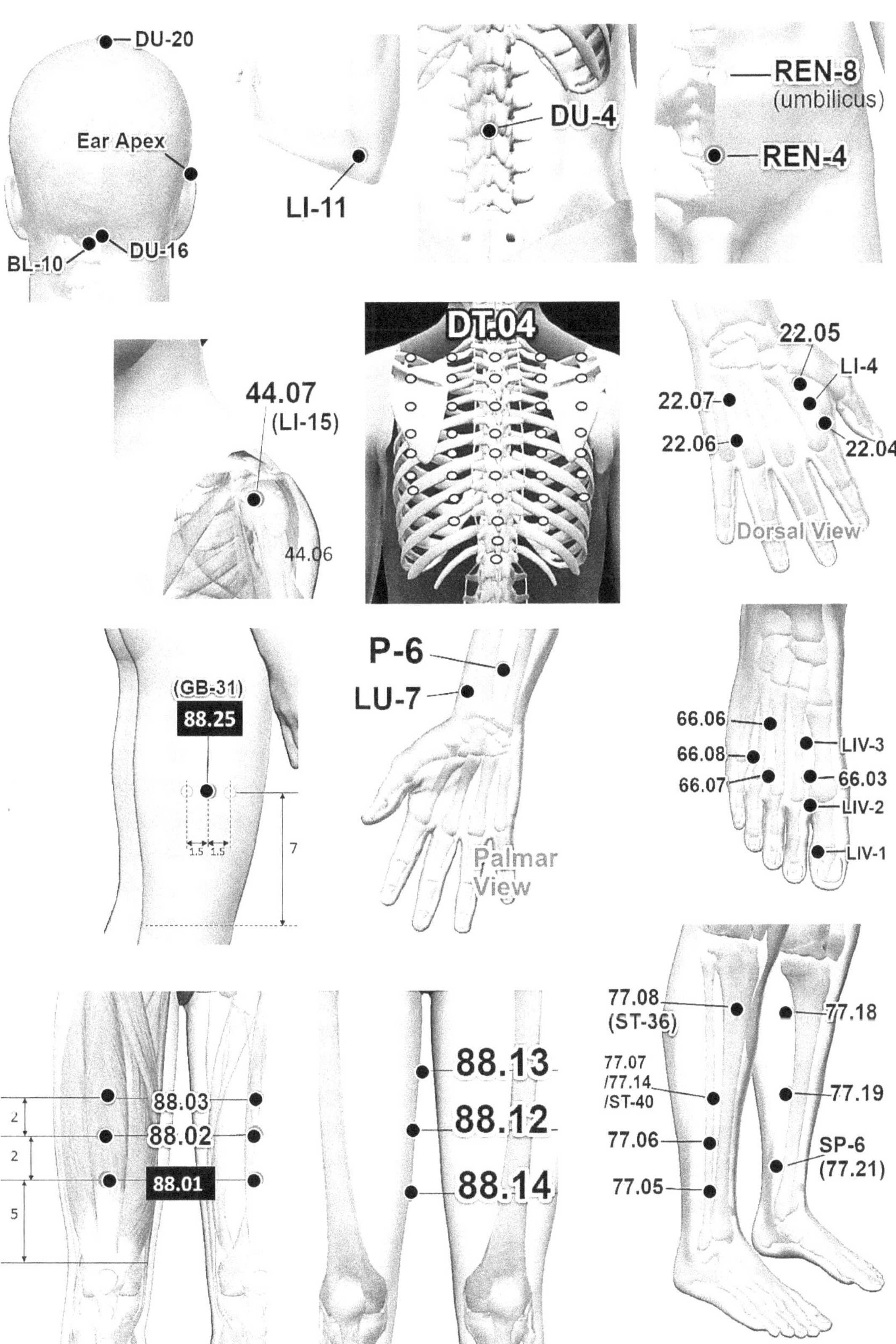

# <u>OTHER DISEASES</u>
## Fibromyalgia, multiple sclerosis, and muscle atrophy

*Fibromyalgia is a disorder characterized by widespread pain, fatigue, and tenderness in the muscles, tendons, and ligaments. Multiple Sclerosis is a disorder of the central nervous system that affects the myelin sheath, which covers and protects nerve fibers. Muscle Atrophy is a condition characterized by a loss of muscle mass and strength.*

*In TCM, Fibromyalgia, Multiple Sclerosis (MS), and Muscle Atrophy are considered to be disorders related to the imbalance of Qi (vital energy) and blood in the body. The meridians involved in these conditions are primarily the **Spleen meridian, Kidney meridian, and Bladder meridian.** Other meridians are involved too.*

**Treatment for fibromyalgia, multiple sclerosis, and muscle atrophy**
- 88.17 Si Ma Zhong+88.18 Si Ma Shang+88.19 Si Ma Xia -Located very near the Stomach meridian, in the large quadriceps muscles. "Muscles treat muscles".
- A.04 San Cha San

**Fibromyalgia**
Liver stagnation causes fibromyalgia, which is especially exacerbated by stress. Treatment is directed toward soothing the Liver and clearing stagnation.
- LI- 4 /LIV-3
- GB-41 (66.09) + 66.08
- A.04 San Cha San if whole-body pain
- 66.06 Mu Liu can be added to regulate the Liver
- 88.17 Si Ma Zhong+88.18 Si Ma Shang+88.19 Si Ma Xia
- 77.05+77.06+77.07
- SP-6, LIV-3, DU-20
- Cup along GB and BL meridians. Gua sha is applicable.

**Multiple sclerosis**
The basic principle is to tonify the Spleen and Kidneys, detoxify the liver and brain, and strengthen nerves, tendons and muscles.
- 77.18 Shen Guan+77.19 Di Huang+77.21 Ren Huang
- 88.17 Si Ma Zhong+88.18 Si Ma Shang+88.19 Si Ma Xia
- A.04 San Cha San
- If it is difficult for the patient to extend their muscles, add 22.05 Ling Gu and 66.04 (LIV-3).
- If there is numbness, add 77.05 Yi Zhong+77.06 Er Zhong+77.07 San Zhong with 66.06 Mu Liu+66.07 Mu Dou to wake up the brain and circulate the blood.
- KID-3, BL-23, LI-4, GB-34 (Moxibustion applicable)

**Muscle atrophy**
- 22.04 Da Bai+22.05 Ling Gu
- 44.06 Jian Zhong
- Supporting Points: 44.11 Yun Bai, 44.12 Li Bai, 44.15 Xia Qu, 44.16 Shang Qu
- 88.17 Si Ma Zhong+88.18 Si Ma Shang+88.19 Si Ma Xia
- ST-36, LI-11, BL-52 (Moxibustion applicable)
- Cup along GB and BL meridians. Gua sha is applicable.

*Points Illustrations for treatment of Fibromyalgia,
multiple sclerosis, and muscle atrophy*

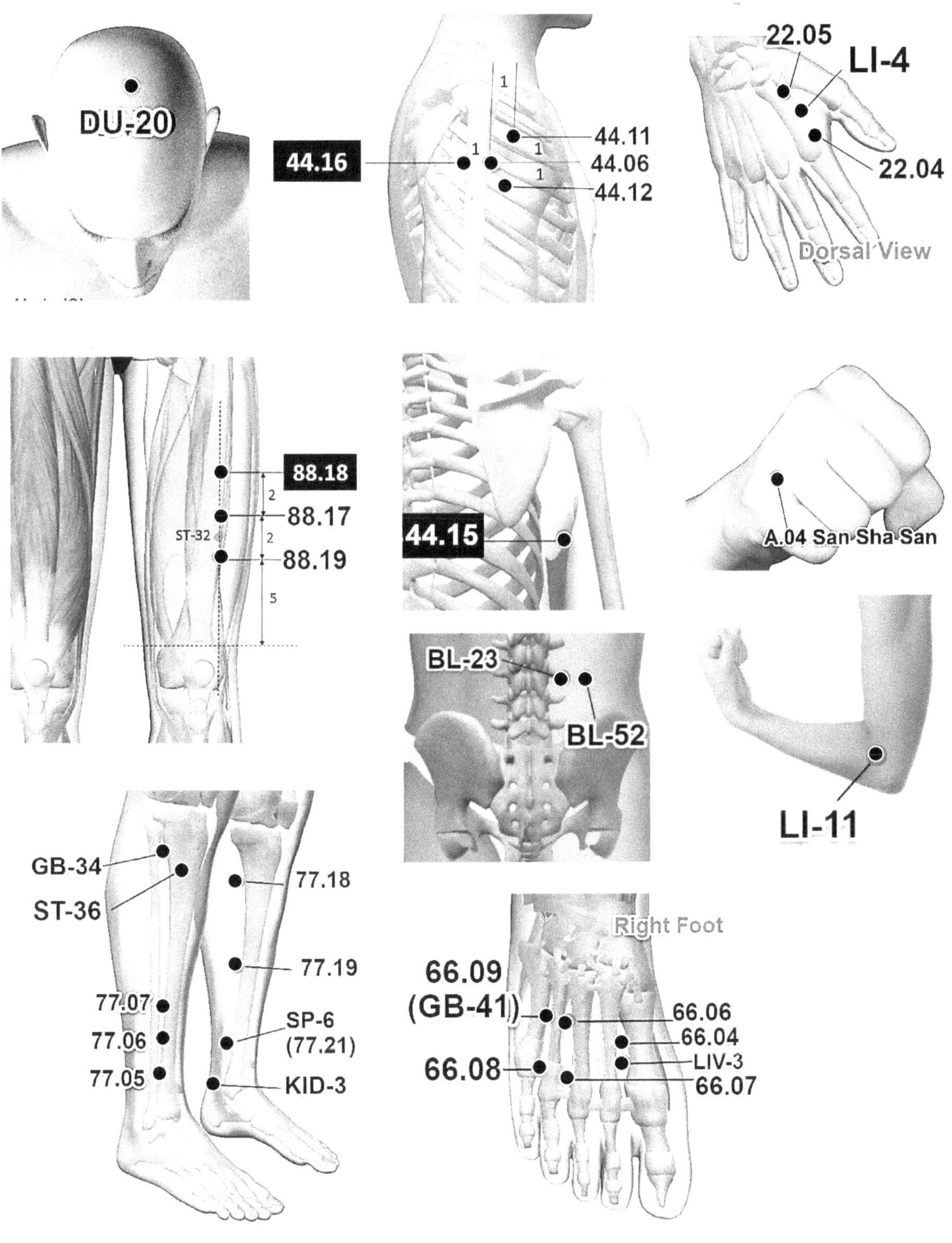

# Edema

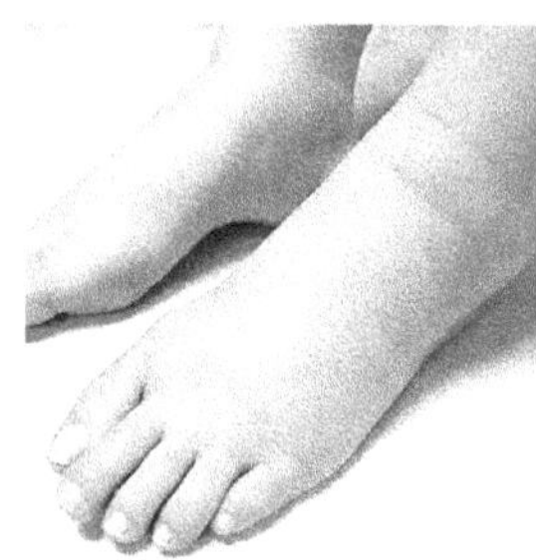

*Swelling caused due to excess fluid accumulation in the body tissues. Edema can occur in any parts of the body.*

*When edema is heart related, it may show up on only one leg, or on both legs. Fluid may leak from acupuncture needle sites when the situation is severe. Chronic leg edema may be due to Kidney weakness in addition to the Heart; for that reason, we choose from both **Heart and Kidney** points listed below.*

**Effective combination for edema and ascites**
- REN-5, REN-9, SP-9, BL-20.  Apply cupping at REN-5 and REN-9 for 10 minutes after needling. Moxibustion applicable.

**Heart-related edema in the legs and feet**
- 88.01 Tong Guan+88.02 Tong Shan+88.03 Tong Tian
- 77.18 Shen Guan+77.19 Di Huang+77.21 Ren Huang (SP-6)
- 77.08 Si Hua Shang (ST-36)
- 33.12

**Kidney-related edema**
- Moxa REN-9 (effective TCM point for edema)
- Bilateral 88.09 Tong Shen+88.10 Tong Wei+88.11 Tong Bei - swelling of body and limbs
- 77.17 Tian Huang or 77.18 Shen Guan+77.19 Di Huang+77.21 Ren Huang -peripheral edema
- 77.28 Guang Ming
- 88.03 Tong Tian and 22.06 Zhong Bai+22.07 Xia Bai to treat swollen, edematous limbs.
- 77.08 Si Hua Shang (ST-36) can be used to induce urination
- Bleed 44.17 Shui Yu to strengthen the kidneys, for edema, nephritis and proteinuria
- KID-3, BL-20, BL-23
- Moxa KID-7, KID-1, KID-3

**Liver -related ascites or abdominal edema**
- 88.12 Ming Huang+88.13 Tian Huang+88.14 Qi Huang
- 11.20 Mu Yan Wood Inflammation

**Facial edema**
- Add DU-26 and DU-21
- Bleed ST-43

**Foot edema**
- Add GB-41 (66.09), SP-5, SP-6 (77.21)

*Points Illustrations for treatment of Edema*

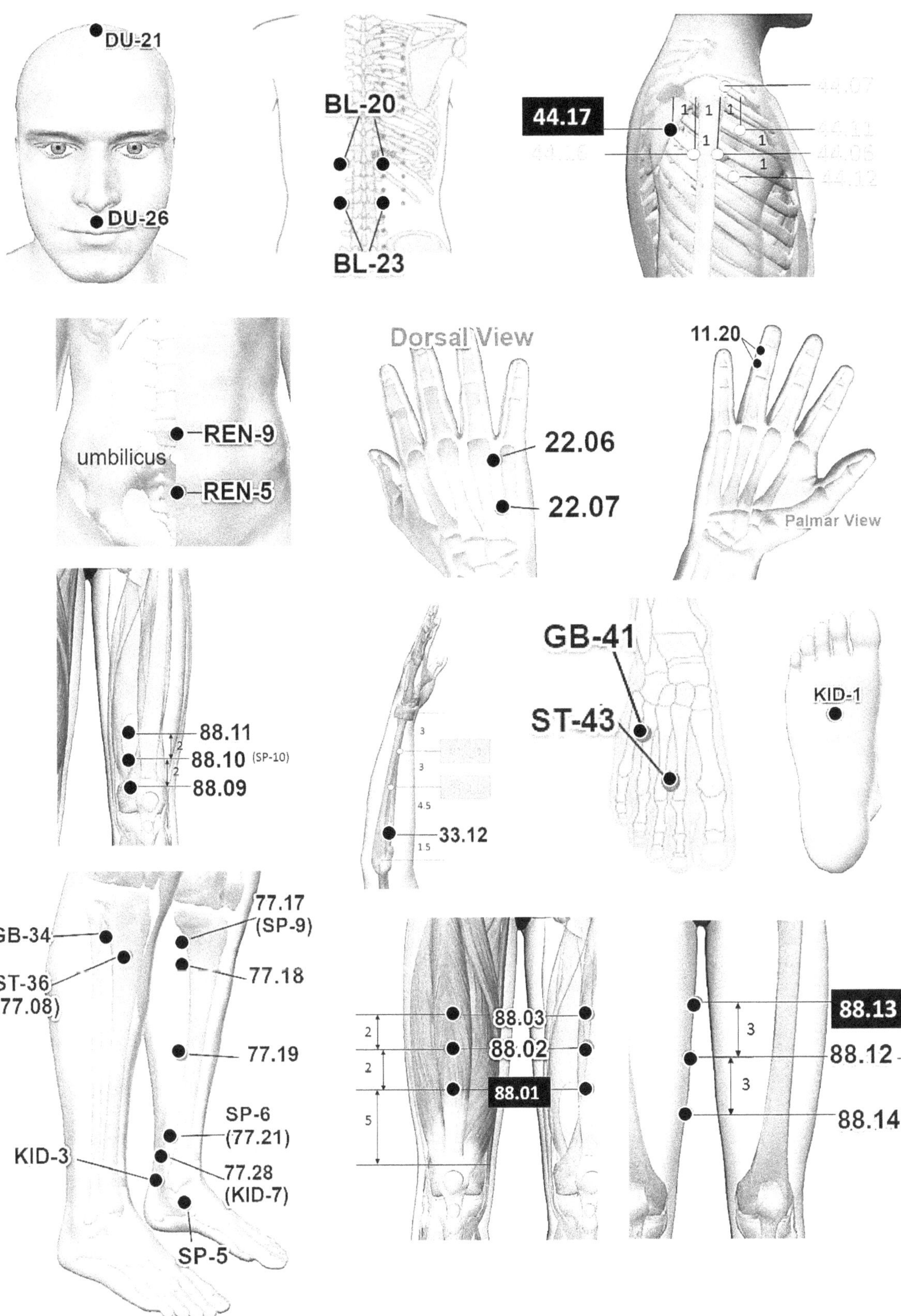

# Diabetes

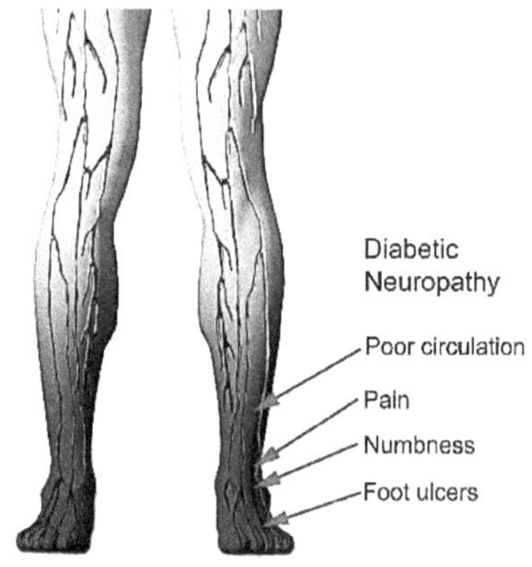


*In Traditional Chinese Medicine (TCM), diabetes is considered to be a condition caused by imbalances in the **Spleen and Kidney meridians,** which are responsible for the body's energy production and fluid metabolism.*

*The Spleen is responsible for transforming food into energy, or Qi, and transporting it throughout the body. In TCM, the Spleen is also responsible for the production and transportation of fluids in the body. Weak Spleen Qi can lead to imbalances in blood sugar levels, causing diabetes.*

*The Kidneys are responsible for storing and releasing the body's vital energy, or Jing, which is necessary for healthy metabolism. The Kidneys are also responsible for regulating the body's water metabolism, which affects the production and excretion of urine. Weak Kidney Qi can cause imbalances in blood sugar levels, leading to diabetes.*

**Diabetes**

- Combine:
  88.09 Tong Shen+88.10 Tong Wei+88.11 Tong Bei (Kidney reaction area)
  77.18 Shen Guan+77.19 Di Huang+77.21 Ren Huang (SP-6) – Kidney reaction area
  88.12 Ming Huang+88.13 Tian Huang+88.14 Qi Huang – Liver reaction area
- 66.14 Shui Xiang
- SJ-4, REN-24 to regulate the qi.
- KID-3, ST-36
- BL-17, BL-18, BL-20, BL-21, BL-23. Moxibustion and gua sha applicable.
- 11.18 Pi Zhong -treats spleen, good for diabetes
- Bleed 1010.07 and/or DT.14

**Diabetic neuropathy (nerve damage)**

- Gentle massage affected area with finger and oil
- Bilateral 77.18 Shen Guan+77.19 Di Huang+77.21 Ren Huang (SP-6)
- Bleed Jing Well Point (avoid lower extremities)
- LI-10, LI-11, LI-4, SJ-5 (needle then moxa) - Neuropathy in the upper limbs
- GB-34, SP-9, GB-39, KI-3, GB-30 (needle then moxa) - Neuropathy in the lower limbs
- Bleed 11.26 Zhi Wu - diabetic wounds

**Homeostatis combination**

- Baihui (DU-20.), Jianjrng (GB-21.), Quchi (LI-11.), Taichong (LIV-3 .), Sanyinjiao SP-6), Zusanli (ST-36.), Dazhui (DU-14), Zhangmen (LIV-13.)

*Points Illustrations for treatment of Diabetes*

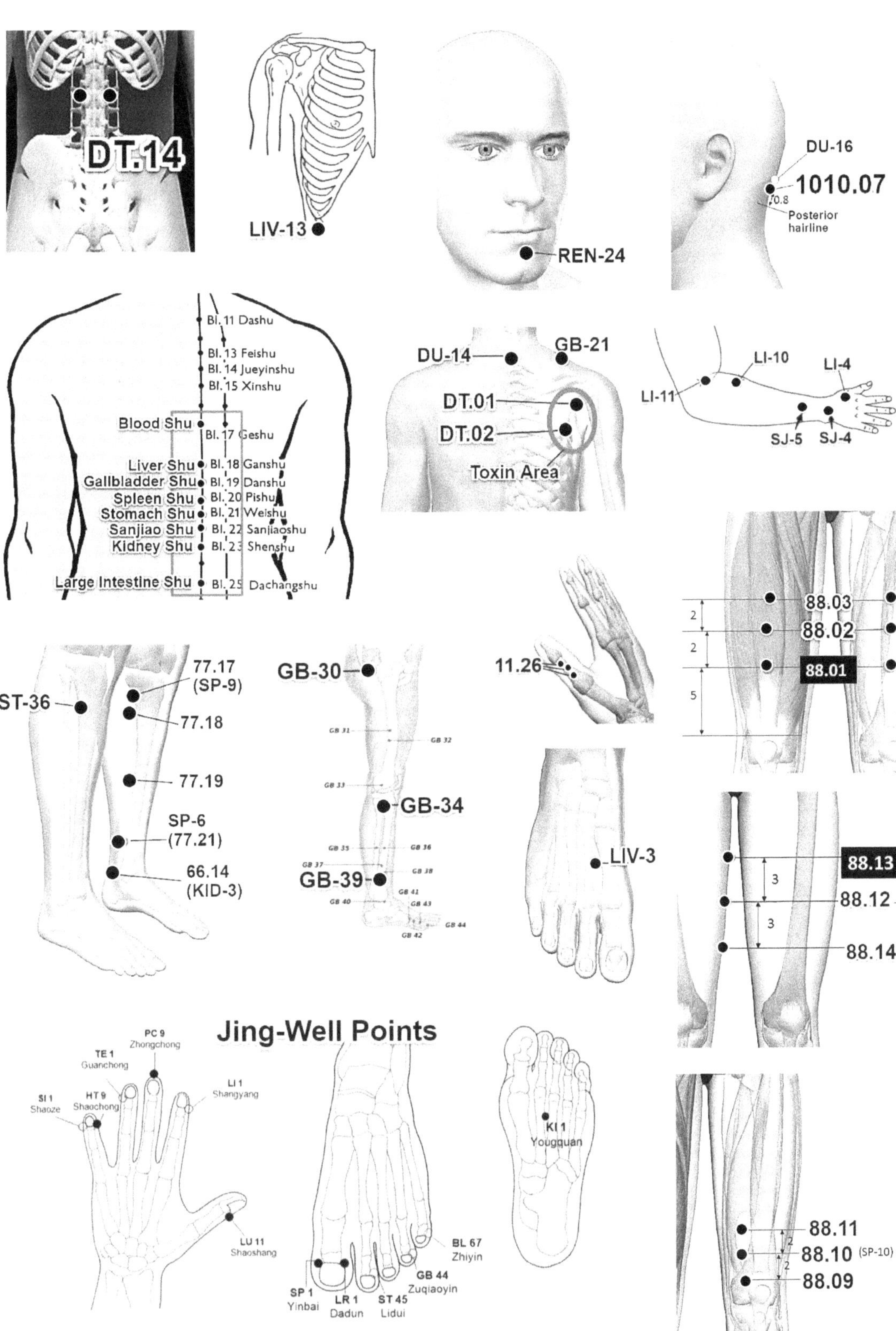

# Cancer

**To address malignancy**
- Bilateral needling of 77.27 Wai San Guan is recommended daily, does not interfere with chemotherapy or radiation treatment. Usually needled after needling of specific tumor treatment.
- Press needle or bleed 11.26 for cancer malignancies.
- Use press needles on affected organ base on Reaction areas (usually finger points)
- 66.09 Shui Qu (GB-41) + 88.25 Zhong Jiu Li (GB-31) - early cancer pain
- Bilateral 77.05 Yi Zhong+77.06 Er Zhong+77.07 San Zhong for lumps or masses malignancies

**Detoxification following chemotherapy and/or radiation**
- For detoxification following rounds of cancer treatment, P-6 can be needled, and DT.01 Fen Zhi Shang+DT.02 Fen Zhi Xia Toxin Areas can be cupped during breaks in treatment.

**Can treat side effects of chemotherapy and radiation**
- Bleed 1010.07 Zong Shu - if there is nausea and vomiting during the treatment
- Bleed either LU-5 or the Stomach channel to clear heat - if there are mouth ulcers
- Bilateral needling of 77.18+77.19 +77.21 - peripheral neuropathy
- Needle LU-5, LU-10 and ST-34 - for acute stomach pain

## <u>For tumors, use points specific to the malignant organ</u>

**Malignant brain tumor**
- Bilateral 55.06 Shang Liu with 77.05 Yi Zhong+77.06 Er Zhong+77.07 San Zhong
- Or bilateral 55.06 Shang Liu+77.27 Wai San Guan
- Unilaterally needle: 66.10 Huo Lian+66.11 Huo Ju+66.12 Huo San (SP-3, SP-4, KI-2)

**Malignancy in the bladder-** 1010.13 +1010.14 and then 77.27 Wai San Guan.

**Stomach Cancer -** 66.05 Men Jin (ST-43) and 77.27 Wai San Guan

**Female reproductive cancers.** Cancers can occur in any part of the female reproductive system—the vulva, vagina, cervix, uterus, fallopian tubes, or ovaries.
- Begin with 11.06 Huan Chao+11.24 Fu Ke, and followed by
- 77.27 Wai San Guan

**Liver cancer**
- Begin with 11.20 Mu Yan.
- 88.12 Ming Huang+88.13 Tian Huang+88.14 Qi Huang. Followed by 77.27 Wai San Guan

**Breast cancer**
- 6.06 Mu Liu+66.07 Mu Dou
- Bilateral 77.05 Yi Zhong+77.06 Er Zhong+77.07 San Zhong
- Bleed 88.17 Si Ma Zhong+88.18 Si Ma Shang+88.19 Si Ma Xia (preferably when there are bleed-able vessels)

**Lung tumor/cancer**
- Bleed 77.09 Si Hua Zhong;
- Needle 22.04 Da Bai+22.05 Ling Gu.
- Pain from lung cancer: 22.01 Chong Zi+22.02 Chong Xian

*Points Illustrations for treatment of Cancer*

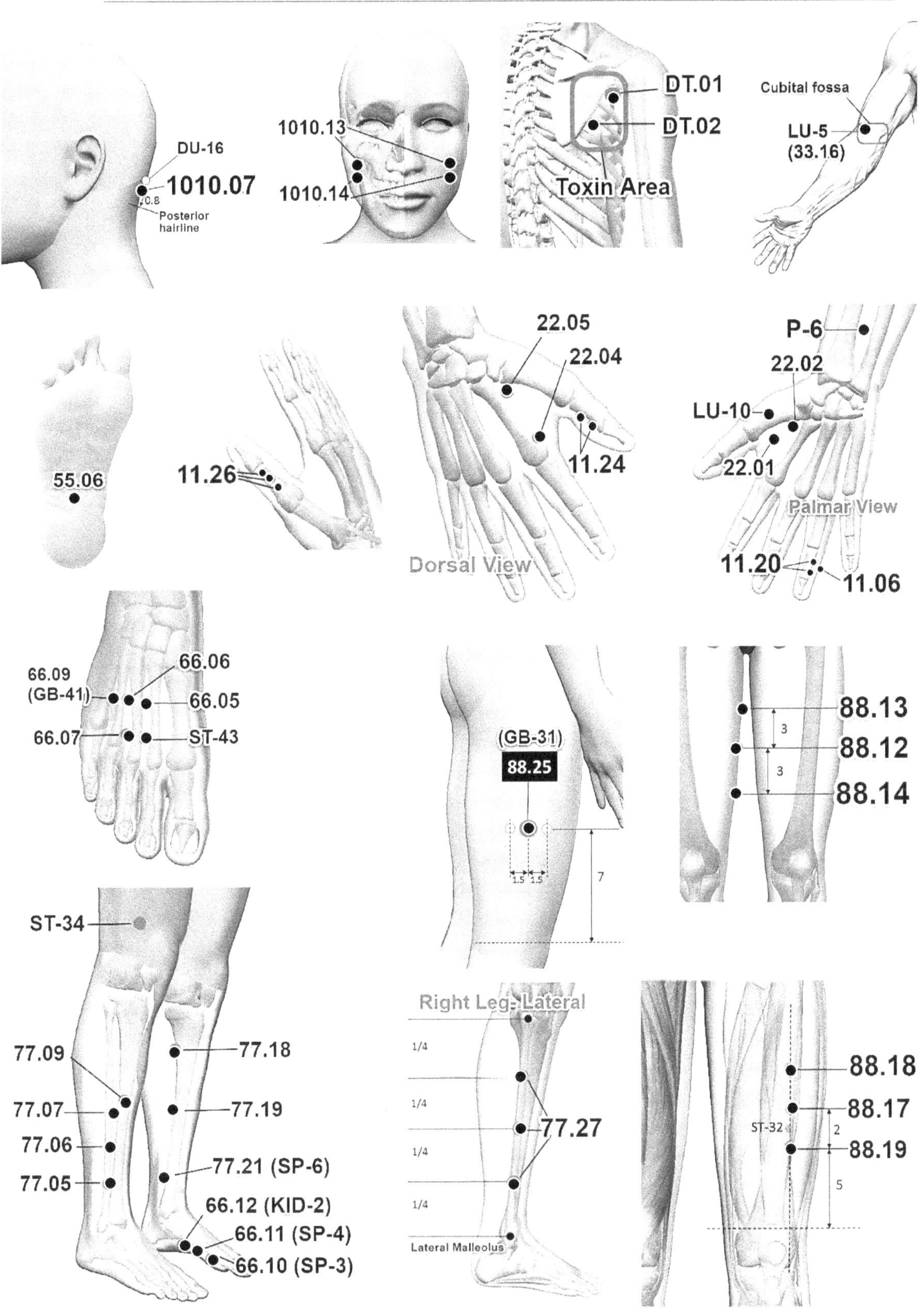

# Coma

*A state of prolonged unconsciousness where the patient cannot respond to external stimuli.*

*Objective in coma treatment - to move the blood and disperse wind and phlegm.*

*In Traditional Chinese Medicine (TCM), a coma is considered a severe and potentially life-threatening condition that indicates a disruption in the flow of vital energy or Qi throughout the body. Coma can be caused by a variety of factors, including trauma, stroke, or other underlying medical conditions.*

**Option 1**

Stimulate Liver and Pericardium meridians. Bilateral needling of P-6 is recommended, followed by needling LIV-3 (or 66.04) and/either 66.03 in the direction towards KI-1. KI-1 is a specific point for coma treatment, as it opens sensory orifices, calms the spirit, and revives collapsed yang, helping to wake up the brain. Additionally, the Liver channel runs through the brain and connects to DU-20. Can add 55.06.

**Option 2**

DU-26 is needled first, followed by 1010.01 (DU-20), 1010.06 Hou Hui (DU-19) and 1010.05 Qian Hui (DU-21).  Needling the DU meridian regulates qi and blood.

**Option 3: Restoring consciousness and inducing resuscitation.**
- Main points: P-6 (bilateral), DU-26, SP-6 – with moderate to strong stimulation
- HT-1, LU-5, LI-4, BL-40 – secondary points

**Option 4**
- Moxa ST-36, REN-4, KI-1, SP-6

---

### Blood-letting Treatment
- Bleed the twelve Jing Well Point (start with P-6 and then LU-11). LU-11, on the thumb is holographically related to the brain.
- Bleed DT.04 Wu Ling

*Points Illustrations for treatment of Coma*

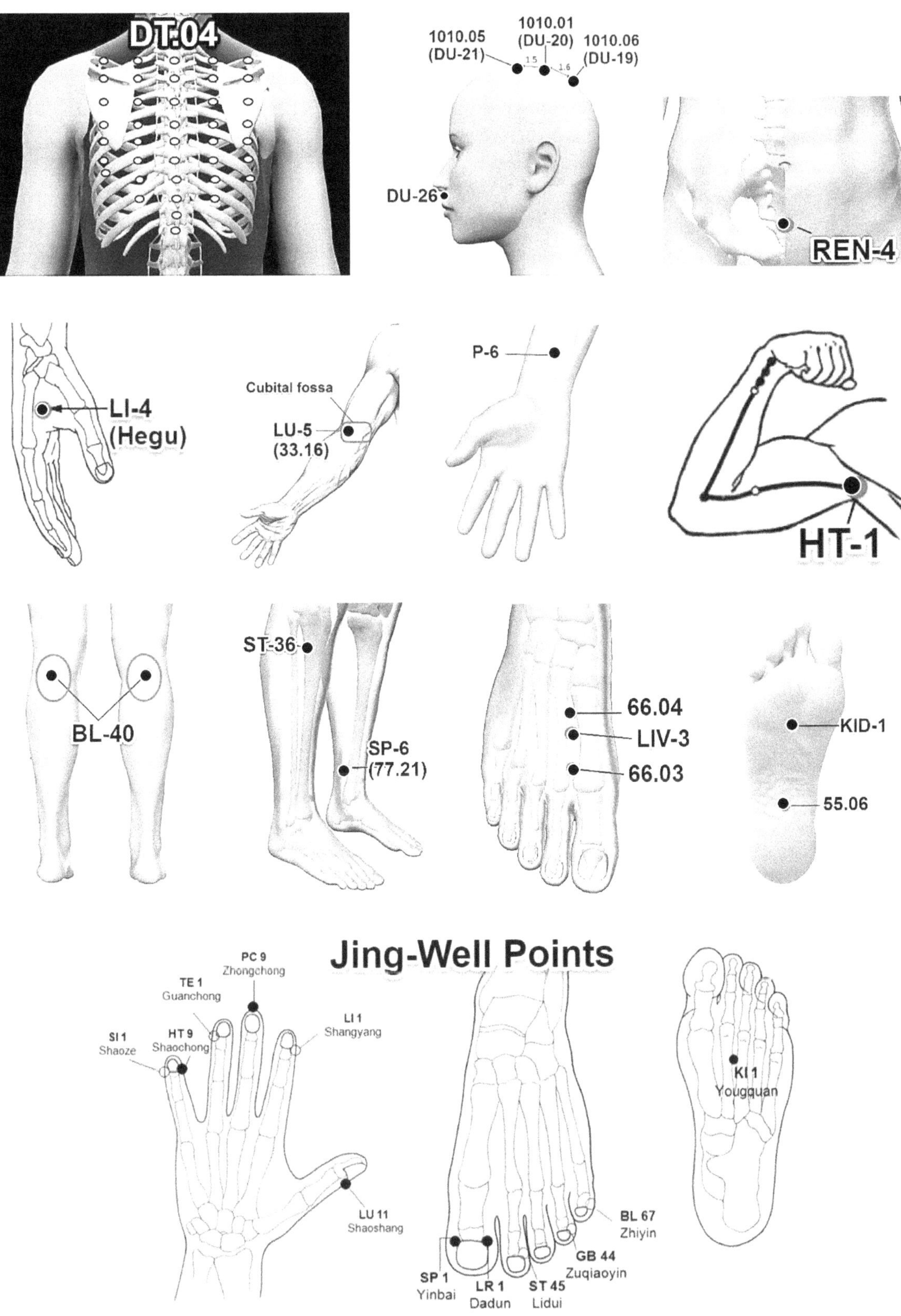

## INDEX FOR DISEASES

# <u>Bibliography</u>


Beijing College of Traditional Chinese Medicine (1980). *Essentials of Chinese Acupuncture.* Foreign Languages Press, Beijing.

Bleecker, Deborah (2018). *Tung Acupuncture Points.* Draycott Publishing, LLC.

Carson, P. (1988). *Tung's Orthodox Acupuncture.* Taiwan: Lien Ho Press Company.

Deadman, P., Baker, K. & Al-Khafaji, M (2007). *A Manual of Acupuncture.* JOCM, Hove.

Ellis, Andrew & Others (1991). *Fundamentals of Chinese Acupuncture.* Paradigm Publications.

Focks, C (2008). *Atlas of Acupuncture.* Churchill Livingstone, Edinburgh.

Jarmey, Chris and Bouratinos, Haira (2023). *The Definitive Guide to Acupuncture Points.* Healing Arts Press.

Jayasuriya, Anton (2001). *Clinical Acupuncture.* B. Jain Publishers (P) Ltd.

Johns, Robert (2005). *The Art of Acupuncture Techniques.* North Atlantic Books.

Johnson, Susan (2019). *Master Tung's Magic Points, A definitive clinical guide.* Magic Points Press.

Lee, M. (1992). *Insights of a Senior Acupuncturist: One Combination of Points Can Treat Many Diseases.* Boulder, CO: Blue Poppy Press.

Lee, M. (1992). *Master Tong's Acupuncture: An Ancient Alternative Style in Modern Clinical Practice.* Boulder, CO: Blue Poppy Press.

Maher, J.H. (2005). *Advanced Tung Style Acupuncture: The Dao Ma Needling Technique of Master Tung Ching Chang:* RBC.

McCann, H., & Ross, H. (2018). *Practical Atlas of Tung's Acupuncture.* Bonn, Germany: Verlag Muller & Steinicke.

Mouscher, Dean (2018). *The Complete Guide to Chinese Medicine Bloodletting.* Crandon Publishing.

Wang, C. M., & Vasilakis, S. (2013) *Introduction to Tung's Acupuncture.* Lombard, IL: Chinese Tung Acupuncture Institute.

Shudo Denmei (2003). Finding Effective Acupuncture Points. Eastland Press, Inc.

Stux, Gabriel (2003). *Basics of Acupuncture.* Springer- Verlag Berlin Heidelberg

Whisnant, Brad (2021). *Top Tung Acupuncture Points.* SN Books Publishing.

Yang Zhenguo (2004). *English-Chinese Layer Anatomical Atlas of Acupoints of the Human Body.* Shanghai University of Traditional Chinese Medicine Press

Young, W.C. (2006). *Illustrated Tung's Acupuncture Points.* Rowland Heights, CA: American Chinese Medical Culture Center.

Young, W.C. (2008). *Lectures on Tung's Acupuncture: Points Study.* Rowland Heights, CA: American Chinese Medical Culture Center.

Young, W.C. (2008). *Lectures on Tung's Acupuncture: Therapeutic System.* Rowland Heights, CA: American Chinese Medical Culture Center.

Yu-Lin Lian & Others (2005). *The Pictorial Atlas of Acupuncture, An illustrated manual of acupuncture points.* Tandem Verlag GmbH.